Different **types of images:**
- Realistic and detailed anatomical illustrations for in-depth views
- Schematic illustrations to see functional relationships
- Photos of surface anatomy
- Orientation sketches
- Photographs of imaging processes

The figures

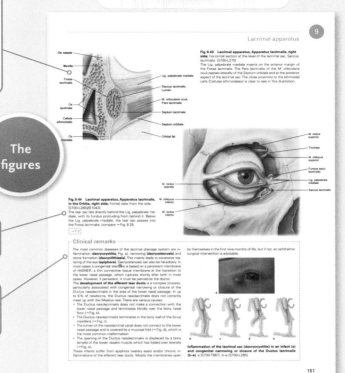

Detailed figure captions clarify the most important structures and topographical relationships.

The **illustrated Clinical remarks** feature shows a picture of the affected body area, which helps you to remember what you have learnt.

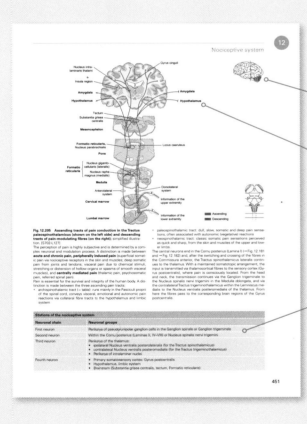

Orientation sketches give you the anatomical section depicted at a glance.

Learning tip: important structures are shown in **bold**.

Tables help to identify the relevant relationships.

Sample questions from the exam

Sample questions from an **oral anatomy exam** are given at the end of each chapter to test your knowledge.

Sample exam questions

To check that you are completely familiar with the content of this chapter, sample questions from an oral anatomy exam are listed here.

Explain the structure of a bone:
- How do you distinguish bones according to their form and structure?
- How can you classify a long tubular bone?
- What happens in fracture-healing?
- What types of bone joints do you know?
- How can bone adapt functionally to increased stress?

Describe the structure of a joint:
- What specific joint types do you know?
- What is the structure of the joint capsule?
- What is meant by the neutral-zero-method?
- What is an amphiarthrosis?
- What auxiliary structures do you know in joints?
- How is a bursa structured?

Explain the structure of a skeletal muscle:
- What types of muscle do you know and how can you classify muscles?
- How is a tendon sheath structured?
- What is meant by muscle activity?
- What is a lever arm?
- What is meant by dynamic muscle activity?

Explain different circulatory systems:

What is meant by portal vein circulation?
- What pathway does the lymph take from the periphery of the body?
- Can you describe the general structure of a lymph node?

Explain the lymphatic drainage pathways in the neck:
- How many lymph nodes are there in the neck area?
- What lymph node groups exist in the neck area?
- Why is the throat area divided into lymphatic drainage regions (compartments)?
- What structures drain their lymph into the cervical lymph nodes?

Explain the structure of the nervous system:
- How is the nervous system divided up?
- What is a dermatome?
- What is meant by the autonomic nervous system?
- What is the enteric nervous system?

Explain imaging methods:
- Name some imaging methods used in routine clinical practice.
- How does computer tomography differ from magnetic resonance imaging?
- What is contrast agent imaging?
- What advantages does ultrasound imaging offer compared to conventional X-ray imaging?

Explain the skin and its derivatives:

You will find these topics in the 17ᵗʰ edition

General Anatomy and Musculoskeletal System — Volume 1

General Anatomy

Anatomical planes and positions → Surface anatomy → Development → Musculoskeletal system → Neurovascular pathways → Imaging methods → Skin and its derivatives

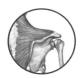

Trunk

Surface → Development → Skeleton → Imaging methods → Musculature → Neurovascular pathways → Topography, dorsal trunk wall → Female breast → Topography, ventral trunk wall

Upper Limb

Surface → Development → Skeleton → Musculature → Neurovascular pathways → Topography → Cross-sectional images

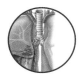

Lower Limb

Surface → Skeleton → Musculature → Neurovascular pathways → Topography → Cross-sectional images

Inner Organs — Volume 2

Organs of the thoracic cavity

Topography → Heart → Lung → Oesophagus → Cross-sectional images

Organs of the abdominal cavity

Development → Topography → Stomach → Intestines → Liver and gallbladder → Pancreas → Neurovascular pathways → Cross-sectional images

Retroperitoneal space and pelvic cavity

Topography → Kidney and adrenal gland → Efferent urinary tracts → Rectum and anal canal → Male genitalia → Female genitalia → Cross-sectional images

Head, Neck and Neuroanatomy — Volume 3

Head

Overview → Skeleton and joints → Adipose tissue and scalp → Musculture → Topography → Neurovascular pathways → Nose → Mouth and oral cavity → Salivary glands

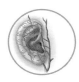

Eye

Development → Skeleton → Eyelids → Lacrimal gland and lacrimal apparatus → Muscles of the eye → Topography → Eyeball → Visual pathway

Ear

Overview → Outer ear → Middle ear → Auditory tube → Inner ear → Hearing and equilibrium

Neck

Overview → Musculature → Pharynx → Larynx → Thyroid gland → Topography

Learning Tables

Brain and spinal cord

Development → General principles → Brain → Meninges and blood supply → Cerebral areas → Cranial nerves → Spinal cord → Sections

Learning Tables for Muscles, Joints and Nerves

Head → Neck → Trunk → Upper limb → Lower limb → Cranial nerves

F. Paulsen, J. Waschke

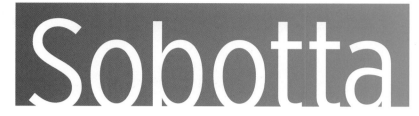

Atlas of Anatomy

Translated by
T. Klonisch and S. Hombach-Klonisch

Friedrich Paulsen, Jens Waschke (eds.)

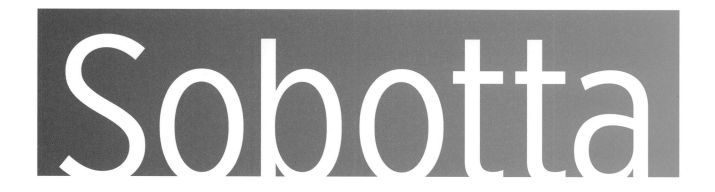

Atlas of Anatomy

General Anatomy and Musculoskeletal System

17th Edition

English version with Latin nomenclature

Translated by
T. Klonisch and S. Hombach-Klonisch,
Winnipeg, Canada

ELSEVIER

Original Publication
Sobotta Atlas der Anatomie, 25. Auflage
© Elsevier GmbH, 2022.
All rights reserved.
ISBN 978-3-437-44130-1

This translation of Sobotta Atlas der Anatomie, 25th edition by Friedrich Paulsen and Jens Waschke was undertaken by Elsevier GmbH.

Elsevier GmbH, Bernhard-Wicki-Str. 5, 80636 Munich, Germany
We are grateful for any feedback and suggestions sent to:
kundendienst@elsevier.com

ISBN 978-0-7020-6765-5

Notice
Practitioners and researchers must always rely on their own experience and knowledge in evaluating and using any information, methods, compounds or experiments described herein. Because of rapid advances in the medical sciences, in particular, independent verification of diagnoses and drug dosages should be made. To the fullest extent of the law, no responsibility is assumed by Elsevier, authors, editors or contributors for any injury and/or damage to persons or property as a matter of products liability, negligence or otherwise, or from any use or operation of any methods, products, instructions, or ideas contained in the material herein.

Bibliographical information published by the Deutsche Nationalbibliothek
The Deutsche Nationalbibliothek lists this publication in the Deutsche Nationalbibliografie: detailed bibliographic data are available on the internet at https://www.dnb.de

23 24 25 26   5 4 3 2

Content strategist: Sonja Frankl
Project management: Dr. Andrea Beilmann, Sibylle Hartl
Editing and translating: Marieke O'Connor, Oxford, U.K.
Media rights management: Sophia Höver, Munich, Germany
Production management: Dr. Andrea Beilmann, Sibylle Hartl
Design: Nicola Kerber, Olching, Germany
Typesetting: abavo GmbH, Buchloe, Germany
Printing and binding: Drukarnia Dimograf Sp. z o. o., Bielsko-Biała, Poland
Cover design: Stefan Hilden, hilden_design, Munich; SpieszDesign, Neu-Ulm, Germany

Updated information is available on the internet at **www.elsevier.de**

This atlas was founded by Johannes Sobotta †, former Professor of Anatomy and Director of the Anatomical Institute of the University in Bonn, Germany.

German editions:
1st Edition: 1904–1907 J. F. Lehmanns Verlag, Munich, Germany
2nd–11th Edition: 1913–1944 J. F. Lehmanns Verlag, Munich, Germany
12th Edition: 1948 and following editions Urban & Schwarzenberg, Munich, Germany
13th Edition: 1953, ed. H. Becher
14th Edition: 1956, ed. H. Becher
15th Edition: 1957, ed. H. Becher
16th Edition: 1967, ed. H. Becher
17th Edition: 1972, eds. H. Ferner and J. Staubesand
18th Edition: 1982, eds. H. Ferner and J. Staubesand
19th Edition: 1988, ed. J. Staubesand
20th Edition: 1993, eds. R. Putz and R. Pabst, Urban & Schwarzenberg, Munich, Germany
21st Edition: 2000, eds. R. Putz and R. Pabst, Urban & Fischer, Munich, Germany
22nd Edition: 2006, eds. R. Putz and R. Pabst, Urban & Fischer, Munich, Germany
23rd Edition: 2010, eds. F. Paulsen and J. Waschke, Urban & Fischer, Elsevier, Munich, Germany
24th Edition: 2017, eds. F. Paulsen and J. Waschke, Elsevier, Munich, Germany
25th Edition: 2022, eds. F. Paulsen and J. Waschke, Elsevier, Munich, Germany

Foreign Editions:
Arabic
Chinese
Croatian
Czech
English (nomenclature in English or Latin)
French
Greek
Hungarian
Indonesian
Italian
Japanese
Korean
Polish
Portuguese
Russian
Spanish
Turkish
Ukrainian

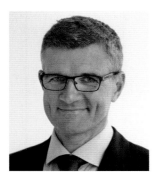

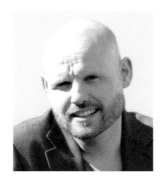

Prof. Dr. Friedrich Paulsen
Dissecting courses for students

In his teaching, Friedrich Paulsen puts great emphasis on students actually being able to dissect the cadavers of body donors. *'The hands-on experience in dissection is extremely important not only for the three-dimensional understanding of anatomy and as the basis for virtually every medical profession, but for many students also clearly addresses the issue of death and dying for the first time. The members of the dissection team not only study anatomy but also learn to deal with a particular situation. Medical students will never again come into such close contact with their classmates and teachers.'*

Friedrich Paulsen was born in Kiel in 1965. After completing his school education in Brunswick he first trained as a nurse. He then studied human medicine at the Christian-Albrecht University of Kiel (CAU). After acting as an AiP (Doctor in Practice) at the university clinic for Oral and Maxillofacial Surgery, and after acting as a doctor's assistant at the University ENT Clinic, he took on the position of assistant at the Anatomical Institute of the CAU in 1998, during an *'Ärzteschwemme'*, obtaining a qualification in the subject of anatomy under Prof Dr Bernhard Tillmann, MD. In 2003 he was appointed to the posts of C3-Professor for Anatomy at the Ludwig-Maximilians-University in Munich and the Martin Luther University, Halle-Wittenberg. In Halle he founded a further Education Centre for Clinical Anatomy. Further posts followed at the ordinariat at the Universities of Saarland, Tübingen and Vienna, as well as at the Friedrich Alexander University (FAU), Erlangen-Nuremberg, where he has been the Professor for Anatomy and the Institute Director since 2010. From 2016 to 2018 he was Vice President for Education and from 2018 until 2022 Vice President for the People, and thereby a part of the FAU university leadership. Since 2006 he has been the publisher of the magazine 'Annals of Anatomy' and since 2014 he has belonged to the Commission of Experts of the IMPP (Institute for medical and pharmaceutical examination issues). Friedrich Paulsen is honorary member of the Anatomical Society (Great Britain and Ireland) as well as of the Societatea Anatomistilor (Rumania). Since 2006 he has been the secretary of the Anatomical Society, from 2009 to 2019 he was the Secretary-General of the International Federation of Associations of Anatomy (IFAA), the international governing body of the anatomists and since 2021 he has been the president of the European Federation of Experimental Morphology (EFEM), the governing body of European anatomists. In addition, he is the Visiting Professor at the Department of Topographic Anatomy and Operative Surgery of the Sechenov University (Moscow/Russia) and was Visiting Professor at the Wroclaw Medical University (Wroclaw/Poland) and the Khon-Kaen University (Khon-Kaen/Thailand). He has received numerous scientific awards, including the Dr. Gerhard Mann SICCA research award from the professional organisation of ophthalmologists in Germany (Berufsverband der Augenärzte Deutschland), the Golden Lion from the German Ophthalmosurgeons, the Commemorative Medal from the Comenius University Bratislava as well as numerous awards for outstanding teaching.

His areas of focus in research concerns the surface of the eye, the protein and peptides in tears and the lacrimal system, as well as the causes of dry eyes.

Prof. Dr. med. Friedrich Paulsen

Prof. Dr. Jens Waschke
More clinical relevance in teaching

For Jens Waschke, one of the most important challenges of modern anatomy is to target the actual demands of clinical training and practice. *'The clinical aspects in the atlas direct the students within the first semester towards anatomy and show them how important the subject is for clinical practice in the future. The biggest challenge for modern anatomy is to focus on the relevant educational objectives. In our books we want to consolidate the important anatomical details, leaving out the unnecessary clinical knowledge aimed at specialists. At the start of their training, students are unable to differentiate between basic and specialist knowledge, and we need to avoid our young colleagues being overloaded instead of concentrating on the basics.'*

Jens Waschke (born 1974 in Bayreuth) studied medicine at the University of Würzburg and graduated in 2000 in Anatomy. After his AiP in Anatomy and Internal Medicine, he became qualified in 2007 in Anatomy and Cell Biology. Between 2003 and 2004 he completed a nine-month research placement in Physiology at the University of California in Davis, USA. From 2008 he held the newly founded Chair III at the University of Würzburg, before being appointed to the Ludwig-Maximilians-University in Munich, where he has been the head of Chair I at the Institute of Anatomy. He has turned down further appointments to Vienna (MUW) and Hanover (MHH).

Since 2012 he has been the head of the software company quo WADIS-Anatomie with Dr. Andreas Dietz. In 2018, Jens Waschke was chosen to be the president of the Anatomical Society and is a member of its board until 2022. In addition, he is a honorary founding member of the Anatomical Society of Ethiopia and member of the Commission of Experts of the IMPP.

In 2019, Jens Waschke published the book *Humans – Simply Genius!*, to make anatomy more easily understandable to the wider public. In 2021 he published his first anatomical crime novel *One Leg*. In his research as a cell biologist, Jens Waschke examines the mechanisms controlling the adherence between cells and the binding function of the outer and inner barriers of the human body. His main focus of interest is the mechanisms leading to the malfunctioning of cell adherence which variously cause the blister-forming skin disease pemphigus, arrhythmogenic cardiomyopathy or CROHN's disease. His goal is to understand cell adherence better and to discover new forms of treatment.

Prof. Dr. med. Jens Waschke

Translators

Prof. Dr. Thomas Klonisch

Professor Thomas Klonisch studied human medicine at the Ruhr-University Bochum and the Justus-Liebig-University (JLU) Giessen. He completed his doctoral thesis at the Institute of Biochemistry at the Faculty of Medicine of the JLU Giessen before joining the Institute of Medical Microbiology, University of Mainz (1989–1991). As an Alexander von Humboldt Fellow he joined the University of Guelph, Ontario, Canada, from 1991–1992 and, in 1993–1994, continued his research at the Ontario Veterinary College, Guelph, Ontario. From 1994–1996, he joined the immunoprotein engineering group at the Department of Immunology, University College London, UK, as a senior research fellow. From 1996–2004 he was a scientific associate at the Department of Anatomy and Cell Biology, Martin Luther University of Halle-Wittenberg, where he received his accreditation as anatomist (1999), completed his habilitation (2000), and held continuous national research funding. In 2004, he was appointed Full Professor and Head at the Department of Human Anatomy and Cell Science (HACS) at the College of Medicine, Faculty of Health Science, University of Manitoba, Winnipeg, Canada, where he was the Department Head until 2019. He remains a Professor at HACS and is currently the director of the Histology Services and Ultrastructural Imaging Platform.

His research areas include mechanisms employed by cancer stem/progenitor cells to enhance tissue invasiveness and survival strategies in response to anticancer treatments. A particular focus is the role of endocrine factors, such as the relaxin-like ligand-receptor system, in promoting carcinogenesis.

Prof. Dr. Sabine Hombach-Klonisch

Teaching clinically relevant anatomy and clinical case-based anatomy learning are the main teaching focuses of Sabine Hombach-Klonisch at the Rady Faculty of Health Sciences of the University of Manitoba. Since her appointment in 2004, Professor Hombach has been nominated annually for teaching awards by the Manitoba Medical Student Association (MMSA) and received the MMSA award for teaching in the small group setting in 2020 and 2021.

Sabine Hombach graduated from Medical School at the Justus-Liebig-University Giessen in 1991 and successfully completed her doctoral thesis in 1994. Following a career break to attend to her two children she re-engaged as a sessional lecturer at the Department of Anatomy and Cell Biology of the Martin-Luther-University Halle-Wittenberg in 1997 and received a post-doctoral fellowship from the province of Saxony-Anhalt 1998–2000. Thereafter, she joined the Department of Anatomy and Cell Biology as a scientific associate. Professor Hombach received her accreditation as anatomist in 2003 from the German Society of Anatomists and from the Medical Association of Saxony-Anhalt, and completed her habilitation at the Medical Faculty of the Martin-Luther-University Halle-Wittenberg in 2004. In 2004, Professor Hombach was appointed to the Department of Human Anatomy and Cell Science, Faculty of Medicine of the University of Manitoba. Appointed as department head in January 2020, she strongly promotes postgraduate clinical anatomy training for residents.

Her main research interests are in the field of breast and brain cancer. Her focus is to identify the molecular mechanisms that regulate metastasis and cell survival under treatment stress. She employs unique cell and animal models and human primary cells to study the influence of the tumour microenvironment on brain metastatic growth.

Preface of the 25ᵗʰ German edition

In the foreword to the first edition of his atlas, Johannes Sobotta wrote in May 1904: 'Many years of experience in anatomical dissection prompted the author to create a pictorial representation of the peripheral nervous system and blood vessels in the way that the student has got used to seeing the relevant parts on a dissection, i.e. showing vessels and nerves in the same area in conjunction to each other. In addition, the atlas alternately contains text and tables. The images form the core of the atlas, with additional ancillary and schematic illustrations, and the figure legends give a short and succinct clarification for quick orientation when using the book in the dissection lab.'

As with fashion, students' reading and study habits change regularly. The multimedia presence and availability of information as well as stimuli are surely the main reasons for these habits to be changing more quickly than ever before. These developments and thereby also the changing requirements students demand from the atlases and textbooks they wish to use, as well as the digital availability of the contents, need to be taken into consideration by the authors, editors and publishers. Interviews and systematic surveys with students are useful in gauging their expectations. Until now, the textbook market has also been an indicator for change: detailed textbooks claiming complete integrity are brushed aside for textbooks and lecture notes targeted at the didactic needs of the students at particular universities as well as the study content of human medicine, dentistry and biomedical sciences and the corresponding examinations involved. Equally, the illustrations in atlases such as the Sobotta, which have fascinated many generations of doctors and health professionals from all over the world with their exact and naturalistic depictions of real anatomical specimens, are sometimes regarded by students as too complicated and detailed. This realisation requires some consideration as to how to adapt the strengths of the atlas – which has developed over 25 editions into a reference work of accuracy and quality – to modern didactic concepts without comprimising its unique characteristics and originality.

Looking at it didactically, we have retained the concept of the three volumes, as used by Sobotta in his first edition: General Anatomy and Musculoskeletal System (1), Internal Organs (2) and Head, Neck and Neuroanatomy (3). We have also adopted although slightly modified the approach mentioned in the preface of the first edition of combining the figures in the atlas with explanatory text, a trend which has regained popularity. Hereby each image is accompanied by a short explanation which gives an introduction to the image and explains why the particular dissection and area were chosen. The individual chapters were systematically divided according to current study habits and various images were supplemented or replaced. Most of these new images are conceptualised in such a way that the studying of the relevant pathways supplying blood and innervation is made easier pedagogically. In addition, we have reviewed many existing figures, shortened the descriptions and have highlighted the important terms, to make the anatomical content more accessible. Numerous clinical cases are referred to, most now including illustrations, and turn the sometimes lifeless subject of anatomy into a clinical and lively one. This helps the beginner to visualize a possible future career and gives them a taste of what's to come. Introductions to the individual chapters gives a succinct overview of the contents and the most important themes, as well as presenting a relevant case in everyday clinical practice. Each chapter ends with a number of typical questions as they may be given in an oral or written anatomy exam. As with the 24ᵗʰ edition, every chapter contains a short introduction to the embryology of the relevant theme. Included for the first time are the lifesize poster of the skeleton and musculature of a woman and a man, as well as the instructional poster.

Two points should be taken into account:
1. The atlas in the 25ᵗʰ edition does not replace any accompanying textbook.
2. No matter how good the didactical concept, it cannot replace the study process, but it can at least try to make it more vivid. To study anatomy is not difficult but it is very time-consuming. Time well worth spending, as both the doctor and the patient will eventually benefit. The goal of the 25ᵗʰ edition of the Sobotta Atlas is not only to ease the study process but also to make it an exciting and interesting time, so that one turns to it eagerly when studying, as well as in the course of one's professional career.

Erlangen and Munich in the summer of 2022,
exactly 118 years after publication of the first German edition.

Friedrich Paulsen and Jens Waschke

Any errors?

https://else4.de/978-0-7020-6765-5

We demand a lot from our contents. Despite every precaution it is still possible that an error can slip through or that the factual contents needs updating. For all relevant errors, a correction will be provided. With this QR code, quick access is possible.

We are grateful for each and every suggestion which could help us to improve this publication. Please send your proposals, praise and criticism to the following email address: kundendienst@elsevier.com

Acknowledgements of the 25th German edition

It has again been very exciting to work on the 25th edition of the Sobotta Atlas, with which we feel increasingly closely connected.

Now more than ever, a comprehensive atlas such as the Sobotta demands a dedicated team run by a well-organised publishing company. The entire process for this 25th edition has been coordinated by the content strategist Sonja Frankl, to whom we are very grateful. Additionally, not much would have been possible without the longstanding and all-encompassing experience of Dr Andrea Beilmann, who was entrusted with many of the previous editions and who forms the foundation of the Sobotta team. We thank her warmly for all her help and support. We fondly remember the monthly telephone conferences in which Dr Beilman and Sonja Frankl were on hand to lend support with the design, bringing together their distinct and diverse working styles in a quite remarkable fashion. Along with Dr Beilmann, Sibylle Hartl coordinated the project and was responsible for the production as a whole. We thank her wholeheartedly. Without the determination and vigilance of Kathrin Nühse, this edition would not have been possible in its present form. We are further enormously grateful to Martin Kortenhaus (editing), the team at the abavo GmbH (formal image processing and setting), and Nicola Kerber (layout development), who were involved with the editorial side and in making the outcome a success.

In particular, we are grateful to our illustrators, Dr Katja Dalkowski, Anne-Kathrin Hermanns, Martin Hoffmann, Sonja Klebe and Jörg Mair, who helped us to revise many existing images as well as creating numerous new ones.

For their help in creating the clinical images, we sincerely thank: PD Dr Frank Berger, MD, Institute for Clinical Radiology at the Ludwig-Maximilians-University, Munich; Prof Dr Christopher Bohr, MD, Clinic and Polyclinic for Ear, Nose and Throat, University Hospital, Regensburg – previously UK-Erlangen/FAU; Dr Eva Louise Brahmann, MD, Clinic for Ophthalmology at the Heinrich Heine University, Düsseldorf; Prof Dr Andreas Dietz, MD, Director of the Clinic and Polyclinic for Ear, Nose and Throat, University of Leipzig; Prof Dr Arndt Dörfler, MD, Institute for Radiology, Neuroradiology, Friedrich Alexander University, Erlangen-Nuremberg; Prof Dr Gerd Geerling, MD, Clinic for Ophthalmology at the Heinrich-Heine University of Düsseldorf; Dr Berit Jordan, MD, University Clinic and Polyclinic for Neurology, Martin Luther University of Halle-Wittenberg; Prof Dr Marco Kesting, MD, Dentistry, Oral Maxillofacial Clinic, Friedrich Alexander University, Erlangen-Nuremberg; PD Dr Axel Kleespies, MD; Surgical Clinic, Ludwig-Maximilians-University, Munich; Prof Dr Norbert Kleinsasser, MD, University Clinic for Ear, Nose and Throat, Julius Maximilian University, Würzburg; PD Dr Hannes Kutta, MD, ENT Practice, Hamburg-Altona/Ottensen; Dr Christian Markus, MD, Clinic for Anaesthesiology, Julius Maximilian University, Würzburg; MTA Hong Nguyen and PD Doctor of Science Martin Schicht, Institute for Functional and Clinical Anatomy, Friedrich Alexander University at Erlangen-Nuremberg; Jörg Pekarsky, Institute for Anatomy, Functional and Clinical Anatomy, Friedrich Alexander University, Erlangen-Nuremberg; Dr Dietrich Stövesand, MD, Clinic for Diagnostic Radiology, Martin Luther University of Halle-Wittenberg; Prof Dr Jens Werner, MD, Surgical Clinic, Ludwig-Maximilians-University, Munich; Dr Tobias Wicklein, MD Dentristry, Erlangen, and Prof Dr Stephan Zierz, MD, Director of University Clinic and Polyclinic for Neurology, Martin Luther University of Halle-Wittenberg.

Finally we thank our families, who have had to share us with the Sobotta Atlas in the context of the 25th edition, as well as being on hand with advice when needed and strong support.

Erlangen and Munich, summer of 2022

Friedrich Paulsen and Jens Waschke

Adresses of the editors in chief

Prof. Dr. Friedrich Paulsen
Institute of Anatomy, Department of Functional and Clinical Anatomy
Friedrich Alexander University Erlangen-Nuremberg
Universitätsstraße 19
91054 Erlangen
Germany

Prof. Dr. Jens Waschke
Institute of Anatomy and Cell Biology, Department I
Ludwig-Maximilians-University (LMU) Munich
Pettenkoferstraße 11
80336 Munich
Germany

Adresses of the translators

Prof. Dr. Thomas Klonisch
Dept. of Human Anatomy and Cell Science
Max Rady College of Medicine, Rady Faculty of Health Sciences
University of Manitoba
130–745 Bannatyne Avenue
Winnipeg, Manitoba, R3E 0J9, Canada

Prof. Dr. Sabine Hombach-Klonisch
Dept. of Human Anatomy and Cell Science
Max Rady College of Medicine, Rady Faculty of Health Sciences
University of Manitoba
130–745 Bannatyne Avenue
Winnipeg, Manitoba, R3E 0J9, Canada

True-to-life representation is the top priority

Sabine Hildebrandt*, Friedrich Paulsen, Jens Waschke

'To practise as a doctor without profound anatomical knowledge is unthinkable. For the diagnosing, treatment and prognosis of illnesses, a detailed knowledge of the structure, positional relationships and the neurovascular pathways which supply the regions and organs of the body is central.'

Anatomical knowledge is gained through cognitive, tactile and especially visual learning processes, and can only be fully acquired when working with the human body itself. Images, graphics and three-dimensional programmes depicting the essential elements help to develop a three-dimensional perception of the relationships in the human body, and help the student to memorise and name structures.

The visual principle of learning did not always apply in anatomical teaching. The writings of the great anatomists of antiquity, such as the school of **Hippocrates of Kos** (460–370 BC) and **Galen of Pergamon** (131–200), did not include any illustrations of human anatomy, because a life-like representation of the human form in books was technically impossible; nor did these authors perform dissections on humans.[1,2,3,4] Even the reformer of anatomy, **Mondino di Luzzi** (1270–1326), had to do without illustrations. He introduced the dissection of human bodies for anatomical education in Bologna and wrote the first modern anatomy 'book' in 1316. This 77-page collection of folios became the standard reference for medical training for the next few centuries.[1,4] Images from another contemporary medical compendium were included for visual instruction; however, their lack of detail and overt inaccuracies did not add much of practical value to the volume.

The Renaissance brought an increased awareness of nature and the relevance of trueness to life in art, and in this it was **Leonardo da Vinci** (1452–1519) who emphasised the visual representation of anatomy. His depictions of human anatomy were based on his own dissections.[5] Unfortunately, he never completed his planned anatomical volume, but did leave behind his anatomical sketches. It was thus in 1543 that **Andreas Vesalius'** (1514–1564) '*De humani corporis fabrica libri septem*' became the first book to depict human anatomy entirely based on the dissection of bodies. The numerous illustrations were high-quality woodcut prints but were not coloured.[6,7] Image quality evolved over the next few centuries and reached another peak with the work of anatomist **Jean Marc Bourgery** (1797–1849) and his draftsman **Nicolas Henri Jakob** (1782–1871). Bougery and Jakob jointly created an eight-volume anatomy atlas over a period of more than 20 years. However, this work as well as the one created by Vesalius, were published in folio format and thus so expensive and unwieldy that they were – and still are – highly valued by wealthy doctors and art connoisseurs, but unsuitable for students and their foundational anatomy education. In the English-speaking world this changed in 1858, when **Henry Gray** (1827–1861) published the textbook 'Anatomy, Descriptive and Surgical'. It contained non-coloured illustrations based on dissections of the human body, and was quickly established as an affordable and popular alternative for students.[8]

Around 1900, **August Rauber** (1841–1917), along with **Friedrich Wilhelm Kopsch** (1868–1955), **Carl Heitzmann** (1836–1896), as well as **Carl Toldt** (1840–1920), **Werner Spalteholz** (1861–1940) and several other authors, created volumes on anatomy for various publishers. These atlases, sometimes in combination with a textbook, claimed to present human anatomy in full. The anatomist **Johannes Sobotta** (1869–1945), who worked in Würzburg, complained that the books were too detailed and therefore unsuitable for foundational medical education. In addition, he believed the prices for these volumes were unjustifiably high for the quality of the images. Sobotta therefore endeavored to '*produce an atlas with lifelike images and suitable for use by medical students in the dissecting room*'.[9] The publishers and editors of the Sobotta Atlas have followed this basic principle ever since.

The first edition of the Sobotta Atlas was published in 1904 by J.F. Lehmanns under the title 'Atlas of the descriptive anatomy of humans in 3 volumes' and contained 904 mostly coloured illustrations. The majority of these were created by the illustrator **Karl Hajek** (1878 –1935), who thus had a large share in the quality and success of the Sobotta Atlas. The atlas seems to have had a ground-breaking effect after its publication in that it brought the further development of anatomical textbooks a big step forward.

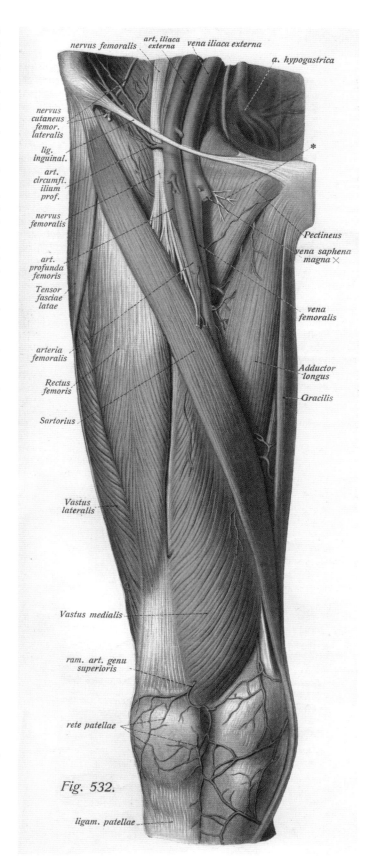

Fig. 1 Illustration of the ventral femoral musculature based on a dissection (1st edition of the Sobotta Atlas). [S700]

At the time of the first edition of the Sobotta Atlas, there were other atlases featuring muscles that were coloured, and neurovascular bundles highlighted in colour. However, it was only the Sobotta atlas which gave a complete and true-to-life colouring of the images of a situs or extremity, and this was only possible through a high-quality printing technique. This is illustrated by → Fig. 1 from the first edition with the example of the dissection of an anterior thigh. Even more than 100 years later, these images still look fresh and life-like and are therefore timeless. Many illustrations were added over the following editions, and the existing illustrations were continuously revised and adapted to match contemporary learning habits and aesthetic perceptions.

Unfortunately, we cannot mention all the illustrators over the course of 25 editions who have made the Sobotta Atlas what it is today; there are simply too many. Individual artists will therefore be singled out as being representative for all. From 1925, **Erich Lepier** (1898–1974) worked as illustrator for Urban & Schwarzenberg; first for various clinicians and then for the anatomist Eduard Pernkopf. After the Second World War, when Urban & Schwarzenberg had taken over publication of the Sobotta Atlas from J.F. Lehmanns, Lepier produced numerous illustrations for this atlas. Late in life he was awarded the title of professor because of his outstanding work.

From the 20th edition in 1993, **Sonja Klebe** contributed to the atlas and her outstanding creations need to be highlighted. The editors still work with her in a productive collaborative team, as can be seen in → Fig. 2, with an image of the topography of the head.

For later editions, images from other works by the Elsevier publishing company have also been included in the Sobotta Atlas. Since the turn of the millennium, most anatomical images from many of the publishing houses have been created digitally. Technical advances make it possible to create anatomical images in an inverse way to before. Previously, as in the Sobotta Atlas, new images were drawn exclusively using real human specimens. Schematic representations for simplification were derived by deduction.

Today, simple line drawings and schematics are first drawn up by computer programmes, to then incorporate the textures of various tissues by induction. Ultimately this produces the impression of a real representation of an anatomical specimen. The results are remarkably vivid despite being artificial. It is an attractive option for organisational as well as economic reasons. Today – in contrast to the times leading up to the postwar period – hardly any anatomical institute still employs its own illustrators, who, along with the anatomists and the dissected specimen, would create images of the quality required for the Sobotta Atlas. In addition, there are hardly any anatomists whose work time can be dedicated to producing anatomical specimens of the highest quality. Anatomists today are not only university professors and textbook

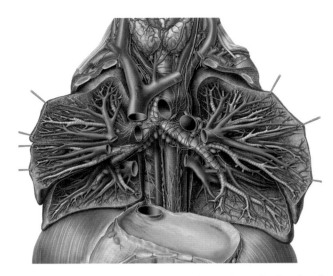

Fig. 3 Illustration of a dissection of the lungs from the Pernkopf Atlas (25th edition of the Sobotta Atlas, → Fig. 5.113). [S700-L238]/ [Q300]

authors, but scientists who conduct research and depend on performance-oriented financial resources. Due to these developments, it is next to impossible for today's anatomists to collaborate with illustrators over several months in the creation of a single optimal illustration. As a result, this manner of image creation has been almost entirely abandoned, and there are practically no representations that exceed or even compete with the images in older atlases. This is also the reason for the Sobotta Atlas to continue including images from atlases such as the Pernkopf Atlas as a model for new editions. The quality of some of the Pernkopf images is still unsurpassed, as → Fig. 3 shows, with a dissection of the lungs as an example – the editors know of no other comparable illustration of the lung structure and its associated neurovasculature that represents all vascular details, including the lymphatics, correctly.

This decision to reproduce an illustration from the Pernkopf Atlas can only be justified on the basis of a conscious examination[10] of the egregious ethical transgressions of anatomy during National Socialism (Nazi Germany), in memory of the victims of the Nazi regime whose bodies are depicted here. Since this applies to all anatomical representations in atlases that already existed and were further developed during this period, we discuss this historical background in more detail here.[11]

Anatomical work in teaching and research, as well as in the production of new teaching materials, including atlases, was and is dependent on an adequate supply of dead human bodies. Traditional legal anatomical body procurement in Germany and worldwide was based on the bodies of so-called 'unclaimed' people, i.e. those who died in public institutions and whose relatives did not claim them for a burial. It was only in the second half of the 20th century that this changed fundamentally – in Germany as in other countries – with the advent of effective body donation programmes.[12,13] Before that, the sources of anatomical body procurement primarily included psychiatric institutions, prisons, people who committed suicide and – historically the first legally regulated source – bodies of the executed. Anatomy laws were repeatedly adapted by the respective governments, including Nazi Germany.[14,15] With rare exceptions, a constant theme in the history of anatomy has been the lack of bodies for teaching and research. This changed significantly under National Socialism. In the first years after 1933 there were still the usual missives by anatomists to the authorities, complaining about the scant body supply. Very soon, however, their inquiries became specific, and they asked for access to execution sites and the bodies of the executed, or asked for the bodies of prisoners of war to be delivered to their institutes. Thus, anatomists were not only passive recipients of the bodies of Nazi victims, but actively requested them for teaching, and above all for research.[16]

In the 'Third Reich', the bodies from psychiatric hospitals included those of people murdered as part of the 'euthanasia' killing programme, as documented for various anatomical institutes.[17,18] From 1933 on there

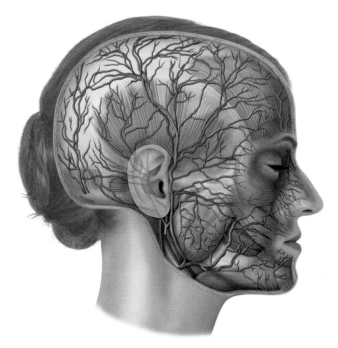

Fig. 2 Illustration by Sonja Klebe of the vascular pathways of the head (25th edition of the Sobotta Atlas, → Fig. 8.83). [S700-L238]

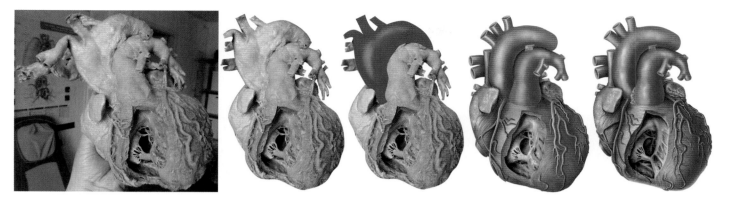

Fig. 4 Step-by-step development of one of Sonja Klebe's drawings of the topography of the heart, based on a plastinate and photos. [L238]

was also an increase in persecuted Jewish citizens among the suicides.[19] Due to the changes in Nazi legislation and the persecution of the so-called 'enemies of the German people', the number of political prisoners increased, not only in the normal penal system and in the Gestapo prisons, but above all in the constantly expanding network of concentration camps and decentralised camps for prisoners of war and forced labourers. The escalating violence and inhumane living conditions in these facilities resulted in high death rates, and the dead were delivered to many of the anatomical institutes. The number of executions after civilian and military trials also rose exponentially under the National Socialists, especially during the war years.[20] All anatomical institutes received the bodies of the executed, without exception, and regardless of the political convictions of the individual anatomists who worked with these bodies.

More than 80% of the anatomists who remained in Nazi Germany had joined the NSDAP, the Nazi party, but not all of them were such avid National Socialist ideologues as **Eduard Pernkopf** (1888–1955), the Viennese Dean of the Medical Faculty and Director of the Institute of Anatomy. He used the unrestricted access to the bodies of executed Nazi victims not primarily for scientific studies, as many of his colleagues did, but instead created the subsequent volumes of his 'Topographical Anatomy of Humans'. Together with his assistants and a group of medical illustrators, he had begun this work in the early 1930s. It is highly likely that the majority of the pictures in the atlas created during the war years show victims of the Nazi regime, because Pernkopf's institute received the bodies of more than 1,377 executed people from the Vienna prison system between 1938 and 1945, more than half of them convicted of treason.[21] Erich Lepier and his illustrator colleagues Karl Endtresser (1903–1978) and Franz Batke (1903–1983) left clear signs of their political sympathies with the Nazi regime in their signatures on images that were created during the war. Lepier often integrated a swastika in his signature, and Endtresser and Batke SS runes. These peculiarities of the atlas initially remained without comment, and the work enjoyed great popularity with anatomists, surgeons and medical illustrators alike, due to the true-to-nature details, a colour palette intensified by a new printing process, and Pernkopf's so-called 'stratigraphic' method of representation, in which a body region is presented in dissection steps from the surface to the deep layers in a sequence of dissections. After the war, Lepier copied a number of Pernkopf originals for the Sobotta Atlas to replace illustrations by Karl Hajek. Interestingly, very detailed illustrations of the body cavities and their organs which also depicted the neurovascular system were not copied. Leaving out these drawings across many editions of the Sobotta Atlas can be explained by the fact that, for many years, the relevance of neurovascular structures to the diagnostics and treatment of malignant tumours were not fully explored. As this very important function of the lymph vessels is now well-known, the current publishers regard further appropriation of the high-quality Pernkopf images as well-justified.

Soon after the publication of the first American edition of the Pernkopf Atlas in 1963/64, questions arose about the political background of the work. The rumours were only followed up on in the 1980s with investigations by American authors, before a public debate on the ethics of the use of the Pernkopf Atlas ensued in the mid-1990s.[22] Recommendations ranged from complete removal of the atlas from libraries to its historically informed use.[23] Urban and Schwarzenberg ended the publication of the work, but this did not stop its use, especially by surgeons.[24,25] When results of the systematic study of anatomy in Nazi Germany became known to a wider audience, a new inquiry emerged about the ethical use of the Pernkopf images in special surgical situations in 2016.[26] This question found an answer, based on Jewish medical ethics, in the *Responsum Vienna Protocol* by Rabbi Joseph Polak.[27,28,29] A responsum is a traditional scholarly and legal answer to a question put to a rabbi. Rabbi Polak concludes that most authorities would certainly allow the use of the Pernkopf images if they help save human life (according to the principle of *piku'ach nefesh*). However, this use is tied to the absolute condition that it is made known to one and all what these images are. Only in this way will the dead be granted at least some of the dignity to which they are entitled.

Following the argument of the *Vienna Protocol* and the condition that the victims of National Socialism whose bodies are shown in the images of the Pernkopf Atlas are remembered explicitly, the editors see it as justifiable to include new re-drawn copies of Pernkopf images in this new edition of the Sobotta Atlas: **to save future patients through the best possible anatomical visual instruction, in memory of the victims.**

In the 25th edition, the number of images has now grown to 2,500. It remains the highest priority to continue creating images with the various illustrators and graphic artists that are in no aspect inferior to dissected specimens. → Fig. 4 shows the example of a plastinated heart from a body donor, which the illustrator Sonja Klebe used, together with photographs from different perspectives, to create a new image. The spatial depth allows for three-dimensional understanding of the anatomy. It is the result of the artist's exploration process, in which she was able to observe, 'grasp' and understand the specimen.

The editors would like to thank all the illustrators and artists involved, as well as the Elsevier publishing team, without whom the atlas would not have been possible in this form.

Boston, Erlangen and Munich, 2022

Sabine Hildebrandt*, Friedrich Paulsen and Jens Waschke

Literature

1   Persaud TVN. Early history of human anatomy. Springfield: Charles C Thomas, 1984.

2   Persaud TVN. A history of human anatomy: the post-Vesalian era. Springfield: Charles C Thomas, 1997: 298, 309.

3   Rauber A, Kopsch F. Anatomie des Menschen. 7. Aufl. Leipzig: Thieme, 1906.

4   Roberts KB, Tomlinson JDW. The fabric of the body. Oxford: Oxford University Press, 1992.

5   Clayton M, Philo R. Leonardo da Vinci Anatomist. London: Royal Collection Trust, 2017.

6   Garrison DH, Hast MH. The fabric of the human body (kommentierte Übersetzung des Werks von Andreas Vesalius). Basel: Karger, 2014.

7   Vollmuth R. Das anatomische Zeitalter. München: Verlag Neuer Merkur, 2004.

8   Hayes B. The Anatomist: A True story of Gray's Anatomy. Ballantine, 2007. ISBN 978-0-345-45689-2

9   Sobotta, J. Atlas der Anatomie des Menschen. 1. Aufl. München: J. F. Lehmanns-Verlag, 1904–1907.

10 Arbeitskreis »Menschliche Präparate in Sammlungen« (2003): Empfehlungen zum Umgang mit Präparaten aus menschlichem Gewebe in Sammlungen, Museen und öffentlichen Räumen, in: Deutsches Ärzteblatt 2003; 100: A1960–A1965. As well as other points, it explains: 'If it is shown that the deceased has died because of their genealogy, ideology or political persuasion due to state-controlled and-managed acts of violence or due to the well-founded probability of this having been the case, this is seen as a grave injury to their personal dignity. If such a context of wrongdoing is established, the specimens from the collections in question will be removed and interred in a dignified manner or will cease to be used, in a comparably dignified manner.' Distinct priority is especially given to specimens from the Nazi era, 'dealing with these specimens in a specialised way – after extensive research of the source – indiscriminately removing all dissections from collections between 1933 and 1945.' For specimens with an uncertain source and date of origin, the following is recommended: 'If after a first assessment, the specimen is of unknown origin and appears to be from the 20th century, it should then be separated and be subjected to a thorough examination. If no unambiguous allocation can be made, these specimens need to be categorically interred, unless there are certain cases in which contradictory overall aspects can be presented, documented and established.'

11 A full presentation of the history of anatomy in Nazi Germany is here: Hildebrandt S. The Anatomy of Murder: Ethical Transgressions and Anatomical Science in the Third Reich. New York: Berghahn Books, 2016.

12 Garment A, Lederer S, Rogers N, et al. Let the Dead Teach the Living: The Rise of Body Bequeathal in 20th-century America. Academic Medicine 2007; 82, 1000–1005.

13 Habicht JL, Kiessling C, Winkelmann A. Bodies for anatomy education in medical schools: An overview of the sources of cadavers worldwide. Acad Med 2018; 93: 1293–1300.

14 Stukenbrock K. Der zerstückte Coerper: Zur Sozialgeschichte der anatomischen Sektionen in der frühen Neuzeit (1650–1800). Stuttgart: Franz Steiner Verlag, 2001.

15 Hildebrandt S. Capital Punishment and Anatomy: History and Ethics of an Ongoing Association. Clinical Anatomy 2008; 21: 5–14.

16 Noack T, Heyll U. Der Streit der Fakultäten. Die medizinische Verwertung der Leichen Hingerichteter im Nationalsozialismus. In: Vögele J, Fangerau H, Noack T (Hrsg.). Geschichte der Medizin – Geschichte in der Medizin. Hamburg: Literatur Verlag, 2006: 133–142.

17 Overview in: Hildebrandt S. The Anatomy of Murder: Ethical Transgressions and Anatomical Science in the Third Reich. New York: Berghahn Books, 2016.

18 Czech H, Brenner E. Nazi victims on the dissection table – the anatomical institute in Innsbruck. Ann Anat 2019; 226: 84–95.

19 Goeschel C. Suicide in Nazi Germany. Oxford: Oxford University Press, 2009.

20 Numbers in Hildebrandt 2016 , see footnote 17.

21 Angetter DC. Anatomical Science at University of Vienna 1938–45. The Lancet 2000; 355: 1445–57.

22 Weissmann G. Springtime for Pernkopf. Reprinted 1987. In: Weissmann G (ed.). They All Laughed at Christopher Columbus. New York: Times Books; Williams, 1988: 48–69.

23 Hildebrandt S. How the Pernkopf Controversy Facilitated a Historical and Ethical Analysis of the Anatomical Sciences in Austria and Germany: A Recommendation for the Continued Use of the Pernkopf Atlas. Clinical Anatomy 2006; 19: 91–100.

24 Yee A, Coombs DM, Hildebrandt S, et al. Nerve surgeons' assessment of the role of Eduard Pernkopf 's Atlas of Topographic and Applied Human Anatomy in surgical practice. Neurosurgery 2019; 84: 491–498.

25 Yee A, Li J, Lilly J, et al. Oral and maxillofacial surgeons' assessment of the role of Pernkopf's atlas in surgical practice. Ann Anat 2021; 234: 1–10.

26 Complete documentation pertaining to this enquiry and the history of the perception of the Pernkopf Atlas, as well as the 'Vienna Protocol' in: Vol. 45 No. 1 (2021): Journal of Biocommunication Special Issue on Legacies of Medicine in the Holocaust and the Pernkopf Atlas, https://journals.uic.edu/ojs/index.php/jbc/article/view/10829 (last assessed: 27. November 2021).

27 Polak J. A. Vienna Protocol for when Jewish or possibly-Jewish human remains were discovered. Wiener Klinische Wochenschrift 2018; 130: S239–S243.

28 Vienna Protocol 2017. How to deal with Holocaust era human remains: recommendations arising from a special symposium. 'Vienna Protocol' for when Jewish or Possibly-Jewish Human Remains are Discovered. Im Internet: https://journals.uic.edu/ojs/index.php/jbc/article/view/10829/9795 (last assessed: 21. October 2021).

29 Hildebrandt S, Polak J, Grodin MA, et al. The history of the Vienna Protocol. In: Hildebrandt S, Offer M, Grodin MA (eds.). Recognizing the past in the present: medicine before, during and after the Holocaust. New York: Berghahn Books, 2021: 354–372.

*   Sabine Hildebrandt, MD;
    Associate Scientific Researcher, Assistant Professor of Pediatrics, Harvard Medical School; Boston, U.S.A.

1. List of abbreviations

Singular:			Plural:					
A.	=	Arteria	Aa.	=	Arteriae	♀	=	female
Lig.	=	Ligamentum	Ligg.	=	Ligamenta	♂	=	male
M.	=	Musculus	Mm.	=	Musculi			
N.	=	Nervus	Nn.	=	Nervi			
Proc.	=	Processus	Procc.	=	Processus			
R.	=	Ramus	Rr.	=	Rami			
V.	=	Vena	Vv.	=	Venae			
Var.	=	Variation						

Percentages:

In the light of the large variation in individual body measurements, the percentages indicating size should only be taken as approximate values.

2. General terms of direction and position

The following terms indicate the position of organs and parts of the body in relation to each other, irrespective of the position of the body (e.g. supine or upright) or direction and position of the limbs. These terms are relevant not only for human anatomy but also for clinical medicine and comparative anatomy.

General terms

anterior – posterior = in front – behind (e.g. Arteriae tibiales anterior et posterior)
ventralis – dorsalis = towards the belly – towards the back
superior – inferior = above – below (e.g. Conchae nasales superior et inferior)
cranialis – caudalis = towards the head – towards the tail
dexter – sinister = right – left (e.g. Arteriae iliacae communes dextra et sinistra)
internus – externus = internal – external
superficialis – profundus = superficial – deep (e.g. Musculi flexores digitorum superficialis et profundus)
medius, intermedius = located between two other structures (e.g. the Concha nasalis media is located between the Conchae nasales superior and inferior)
medianus = located in the midline (Fissura mediana anterior of the spinal cord). The median plane is a sagittal plane which divides the body into right and left halves.
medialis – lateralis = located near to the midline – located away from the midline of the body (e.g. Fossae inguinales medialis et lateralis)
frontalis = located in a frontal plane, but also towards the front (e.g. Processus frontalis of the maxilla)

longitudinalis = parallel to the longitudinal axis (e.g. Musculus longitudinalis superior of the tongue)
sagittalis = located in a sagittal plane
transversalis = located in a transverse plane
transversus = transverse direction (e.g. Processus transversus of a thoracic vertebra)

Terms of direction and position for the limbs

proximalis – distalis = located towards or away from the attached end of a limb or the origin of a structure (e.g. Articulationes radioulnares proximalis et distalis)

for the upper limb:
radialis – ulnaris = on the radial side – on the ulnar side (e.g. Arteriae radialis et ulnaris)

for the hand:
palmaris – dorsalis = towards the palm of the hand – towards the back of the hand (e.g. Aponeurosis palmaris, Musculus interosseus dorsalis)

for the lower limb:
tibialis – fibularis = on the tibial side – on the fibular side (e.g. Arteria tibialis anterior)

for the foot:
plantaris – dorsalis = towards the sole of the foot – towards the back of the foot (e.g. Arteriae plantares lateralis et medialis, Arteria dorsalis pedis)

3. Use of brackets

[ ]: Latin terms in square brackets refer to alternative terms as given in the Terminologia Anatomica (1998), e.g. Ren [Nephros]. To keep the legends short, only those alternative terms have been added that differ in the root of the word and are necessary to understand clinical terms, e.g. nephrology. They are primarily used in figures in which the particular organ or structure plays a central role.

( ): Round brackets are used in different ways:
– for terms also listed in round brackets in the Terminologia Anatomica, e.g. (M. psoas minor)
– for terms not included in the official nomenclature but which the editors consider important and clinically relevant, e.g. (Crista zygomaticoalveolaris)
– to indicate the origin of a given structure, e.g. R. spinalis (A. vertebralis).

4. Colour chart

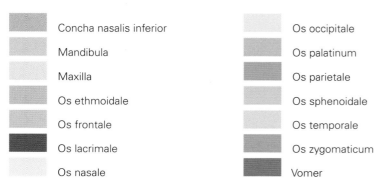

Concha nasalis inferior

Mandibula

Maxilla

Os ethmoidale

Os frontale

Os lacrimale

Os nasale

Os occipitale

Os palatinum

Os parietale

Os sphenoidale

Os temporale

Os zygomaticum

Vomer

In the newborn the following cranial bones are indicated by only one colour:

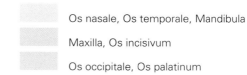

Os nasale, Os temporale, Mandibula

Maxilla, Os incisivum

Os occipitale, Os palatinum

Picture credits

The reference for all image sources in this work appears at the end of each figure legend in square brackets.
Explanation of the special characters:
[…]/[…] = after submission of
[…/…] = collaboration between author and illustrator
[…~…] = modified by author and/or illustrator
[…-…] = work combined with illustrator

All unlabelled graphics and illustrations © Elsevier GmbH, Munich. We are very grateful to all clinical colleagues named below who have made available ultrasound, computed tomographic and magnetic resonance images as well as endoscopic images and colour photos of operation sites and patients.

B500	Benninghoff-Archiv: Benninghoff A, Drenckhahn D. Anatomie, div. Bd. und Aufl. Elsevier/Urban & Fischer
B501	Benninghoff. Drenckhahn D, Waschke J. Taschenbuch Anatomie, div. Aufl. Elsevier/Urban & Fischer
C155	Földi M, Kubik S. Lehrbuch der Lymphologie. 3. A. Gustav Fischer, 1993
C185	Voss H, Herrlinger R. Taschenbuch der Anatomie. Gustav Fischer, 1963
E102-005	Silbernagl S. Taschenatlas der Physiologie. 3. A. Thieme, 2009
E107	Blechschmidt E. Die vorgeburtlichen Entwicklungsstadien des Menschen. S. Karger AG, 1961
E262-1	Rauber A, Kopsch F. Anatomie des Menschen. Band I. Thieme, 1987
E282	Kanski, J. Clinical Ophthalmology: A Systematic Approach. 5th ed. Butterworth-Heinemann, 2003
E288	Forbes C, Jackson W. Color Atlas and Text of Clinical Medicine. 3rd A. Elsevier/Mosby, 2003
E329	Pretorius ES, Solomon JA. Radiology Secrets Plus. 3rd ed. Elsevier/Mosby, 2011
E336	LaFleur Brooks, M.: Exploring Medical Language. 7th ed. Elsevier/Mosby, 2008
E339-001	Asensio JA, Trunkey DD. Current Therapy of Trauma and Surgical Critical Care. 1st ed. Elsevier/Mosby, 2008
E347-09	Moore KL, Persaud TVN, Torchia MG. The Developing Human. 9th ed. Elsevier/Saunders, 2013
E347-11	Moore KL, Persaud TVN, Torchia MG. The Developing Human. 11th ed. Elsevier/Saunders, 2020
E377	Eisenberg RL, Johnson N. Comprehensive Radiographic Pathology, Skeletal System. Elsevier/Mosby, 2012
E380	Eiff MP, Hatch RL. Fracture Management for Primary Care. 3rd ed. Elsevier/Saunders, 2012
E393	Adam A, Dixon AK. Grainger & Allison's Diagnostic Radiology. 5th ed. Elsevier/Churchill Livingstone, 2008
E402	Drake R, Vogl AW, Mitchell A. Gray's Anatomy for Students. 1st ed. Elsevier, 2005
E402-004	Drake R, Vogl AW, Mitchell A. Gray's Anatomy for Students. 4th ed. Elsevier, 2020
E404	Herring JA. Tachdijan's Pediatric Orthopaedics. 4th ed. Elsevier/Saunders, 2008.
E458	Kelley LL, Petersen C. Sectional Anatomy for Imaging Professionals. 2nd ed. Elsevier, 2007
E460	Drake R, et al. Gray's_Atlas of Anatomy. 1st ed. Elsevier, 2008
E475	Baren JM, et al. Pediatric Emergency Medicine. 1st ed. Elsevier/Saunders, 2008
E513-002	Herring W. Learning Radiology- Recognizing the Basics. 2nd ed. Elsevier/Saunders, 2012
E530	Long B, Rollins J, Smith B. Merrill's Atlas of Radiographic Positioning and Procedures. 11th ed. Elsevier/Mosby, 2007
E563	Evans R. Illustrated Orthopedic Physical Assessment. 3rd ed. Elsevier/Mosby, 2008
E602	Adams JG, et al. Emergency Medicine. Expert Consult. Elsevier/Saunders, 2008
E625	Myers E, Snyderman C. Operative Otolaryngology: Head and Neck Surgery. 3rd ed. Elsevier/Saunders, 2008
E633-002	Tillmann BN. Atlas der Anatomie. 2. A. Springer, 2010
E633-003	Tillmann BN. Atlas der Anatomie. 3. A. Springer, 2017
E684	Herrick AL, et al. Orthopaedics and Rheumatology in Focus. 1st ed. Elsevier/Churchill Livingstone, 2006
E708	Marx J, Hockberger RS, Walls RM. Rosen's Emergency Medicine 7th revised ed. Elsevier/Mosby, 2009
E748	Seidel H, et al. Mosby's Guide to Physical Examination. 7th ed. Elsevier/Mosby, 2011
E761	Fuller G, Manford MR. Neurology. An Illustrated Colour Text. 3rd ed. Elsevier/Churchill Livingstone, 2010
E813	Green M, Swiontkowski M. Skeletal Trauma in Children. 4th ed. Elsevier/Saunders, 2009
E821	Pauwels F. Gesammelte Abhandlungen zur funktionellen Anatomie des Bewegungsapparates. Springer, 1965
E838	Mitchell B, Sharma R. Embryology. An Illustrated Colour Text. 1st ed. Elsevier/Churchill Livingstone, 2005
E867	Winn HR. Youmans Neurological Surgery. 6th ed. Elsevier/Saunders, 2011
E908-003	Corne J, Pointon K. Chest X-ray Made Easy. 3rd ed. Elsevier/Churchill Livingstone, 2010
E943	Kanski J. Clinical Ophthalmology. A Systemic Approach. 6th ed. Butterworth-Heinemann, 2007
E984	Klinke R, Silbernagl S. Lehrbuch Physiologie. 5. A. Thieme; 2005
E993	Auerbach P, Cushing T, Harris NS. Auerbach's Wilderness Medicine. 7th ed. Elsevier, 2016
E1043	Radlanski RJ, Wesker KH. Das Gesicht. Bildatlas klinische Anatomie. 2. A. KVM, 2012
F201-035	Abdul-Khaliq H, Berger F. Angeborene Herzfehler: Die Diagnose wird häufig zu spät gestellt. Dtsch Arztebl 2011;108:31-2
F264-004	Hwang S. Imaging of Lymphoma of the Musculoskeletal System. Radiologic Clinics of North America 2008;46/2:75-93
F276-005	Frost A, Robinson C. The painful shoulder. Surgery 2006;24/11:363-7
F276-006	Marsh H. Brain tumors. Surgery. 2007; 25/12:526-9
F276-007	Hobbs C, Watkinson J. Thyroidectomy. Surgery 2007;25/11:474-8
F698-002	Meltzer CC, et al. Serotonin in Aging, Late-Life Depression, and Alzheimer's Disease: The Emerging Role of Functional Imaging. Neuropsychopharmacology 1998;18:407-30
F702-006	Stelzner F, Lierse W. Der angiomuskuläre Dehnverschluss der terminalen Speiseröhre. Langenbecks Arch. klin. Chir. 1968;321:35–64
F885	Senger M, Stoffels HJ, Angelov DN. Topography, syntopy and morphology of the human otic ganglion: A cadaver study. Ann Anat 2014;196: 327-35
F1062-001	Bajada S, Mofidi A, Holt M, Davies AP. Functional relevance of patellofemoral thickness before and after unicompartmental patellofemoral replacement. The Knee. 2012;19/3:155-228
F1067-001	Lee MW, McPhee RW, Stringer MD. An evidence-based approach to human dermatomes. Clin Anat 2008;21(5):363-73
F1082-001	Weed LH. Forces concerned in the absorption of cerebrospinal fluid. Am J Physiol 1935;114/1:40-5
G056	Hochberg MC, et al. Rheumatology. 5th ed. Elsevier/Mosby, 2011
G123	DeLee JC, Drez D, Miller MD. DeLee & Drez's Orthopaedic Sports Medicine. 2nd ed. Elsevier/Saunders, 2003
G159	Forbes A. et al. Atlas of Clinical Gastroenterology. 3rd ed. Elsevier/Mosby, 2004
G198	Mettler F. Essentials of Radiology. 2nd ed. Elsevier/Saunders, 2005
G210	Standring S. Gray's Anatomy. 42nd ed. Elsevier, 2020

G211 Ellenbogen R, Abdulrauf S, Sekhar L. Principles of Neuro-logical Surgery. 3rd ed. Elsevier/Saunders, 2012

G217 Waldman S. Physical Diagnosis of Pain. 2nd ed. Elsevier/Saunders, 2009

G305 Hardy M, et al.: Musculoskeletal Trauma. A guide to assessment and diagnosis. 1st ed. Elsevier/Churchill Livingstone, 2011

G322 Larsen WJ. Human embryology. 1st ed. Elsevier/Churchill Livingstone, 1993

G343 Netter FH. Atlas of Human Anatomy. 5th ed. Elsevier/Saunders, 2010

G435 Perkin GD, et al. Atlas of Clinical Neurology. 3rd ed. Elsevier/Saunders, 2011

G463 DeLee JC, Drez D, Miller MD. DeLee & Drez's Orthopaedic Sports Medicine. Principles and Practices. 3rd ed. Elsevier/Saunders, 2010

G465 Tang JB, et al. Tendon Surgery of the Hand. 1st ed. Elsevier/Saunders, 2012

G548 Swartz MH. Textbook of Physical Diagnosis. 7th ed. Elsevier, 2014

G558 Applegate E. J. The Sectional Anatomy Learning System-Concepts. 3rd ed. Elsevier/Saunders, 2009

G570 Wein AJ, et al. Campbell-Walsh Urology. 10th ed. Elsevier/Saunders, 2012

G617 Folkerth RD, Lidov H. Neuropathology. Elsevier, 2012

G645 Douglas G, Nicol F, Robertson C. Macleod's Clinical Examination. 13th ed. Elsevier/Churchill Livingstone, 2013

G704 Hagen-Ansert SL. Textbook of Diagnostic Sonography. 7th ed. Elsevier/Mosby, 2012

G716 Pagorek S, et al. Physical Rehabilitation of the Injured Athlete. 4th ed. Elsevier/Saunders, 2011

G717 Milla S, Bixby S. The Teaching Files- Pediatrics. 1st ed. Elsevier/Saunders, 2010

G718 Soto J, Lucey B. Emergency Radiology- The Requisites. 1st ed. Elsevier/Mosby, 2009

G719 Thompson SR, Zlotolow A.: Handbook of Splinting and Casting (Mobile Medicine). 1st ed. Elsevier/Mosby, 2012

G720 Slutsky DJ. Principles and Practice of Wrist Surgery. 1st ed. Elsevier/Saunders, 2010

G721 Canale ST, Beaty J. Campbell's Operative Orthopaedics (Vol.1). 11th ed. Elsevier/Mosby, 2008

G723 Rosenfeld JV. Practical Management of Head and Neck Injury. 1st ed. Elsevier/Churchill Livingstone, 2012

G724 Broder J. Diagnostic Imaging for the Emergency Physician. 1st ed. Elsevier/Saunders, 2011

G725 Waldmann S, Campbell R. Imaging of Pain. 1st ed. Elsevier/Saunders, 2011

G728 Sahrmann S. Movement System Impairment Syndromes of the Extremities, Cervical and Thoracic Spines. 1st ed. Elsevier/Mosby, 2010

G729 Browner BD, Fuller RP. Musculoskeletal Emergencies. 1st ed. Elsevier/Saunders, 2013

G744 Weir J, et al. Imaging Atlas of Human Anatomy. 4th ed. Elsevier/Mosby, 2011

G749 Le Roux P, Winn H, Newell D. Management of cerebral aneurysms. Elsevier/Saunders, 2004

G1C60-001 Schünke M, Schulte E, Schumacher U. Prometheus. All-gemeine Anatomie und Bewegungsapparat. Band 1. 5. A. Thieme, 2018

G1060-002 Schünke M, Schulte E, Schumacher U. Prometheus. Innere Organe. Band 2. 5. A. Thieme, 2018

G1060-003 Schünke M, Schulte E, Schumacher U. Prometheus. Kopf, Hals, Neuroanatomie. Band 3. 5. A. Thieme, 2018

G1061 Debrunner HU. Orthopädisches Diagnostikum. 4. A. Thieme, 1982

G1062 Liniger H, Molineus G. Der Unfallmann. J.A. Barth, 1974

G1063 Vossschulte KF, et al. Lehrbuch der Chirurgie. Thieme, 1982

G1064 Schmidt H-M, Lanz U. Chirurgische Anatomie der Hand. Hippokrates, 1992

G1065 Tubiana R. The Hand, Vol. 1. Saunders, 1981

G1066 Gegenbaur C, Göpfert E. Lehrbuch der Anatomie des Menschen, Band III/1: Das Blutgefäßsystem. W. Engel-mann, 1913

G1067 Baumgartl E. Das Kniegelenk. Springer, 1964

G1068 Tandler J. Lehrbuch der systematischen Anatomie, 3. Band. Das Gefäßsystem. F.C.W. Vogel, 1926

G1069 Loeweneck H, Feifel G. Bauch. In: Praktische Anatomie (begründet von von Lanz T, Wachsmuth W). Springer, 2004

G1070 Debrunner HU, Jacob AC. Biomechanik des Fußes. 2. A. Ferdinand Enke, 1998

G1071 Carpenter MB. Core Text of Neuroanatomy. 2nd ed. Williams & Wilkins, 1978

G1072 Schultze O, Lubosch W. Atlas und kurzgefasstes Lehrbuch der topographischen und angewandten Anatomie. 4. A. Lehmanns, 1935

G1073 Kubik S. Visceral lymphatic system. In: Viamonte Jr M, Rüttmann A (eds.). Atlas of Lymphography. Thieme, 1980

G1076 Schiebler TH, Korf H-W. Anatomie. 10. A. Steinkopff bei Springer, 2007

G1077 Zilles K, Rehkämper G. Funktionelle Neuroanatomie. 3. A. Springer, 1998

G1078 Stelzner F. Die anorectalen Fisteln. 3. A. Springer, 1981

G1079 Bourgery JM, Jacob NH. Atlas of Human Anatomy and Surgery. TASCHEN, 2007

G1080 Tillmann B. Farbatlas der Anatomie: Zahnmedizin – Humanmedizin. Thieme, 1997

G1081 Purves D, et al. NeuroScience. 3rd ed. Sinauer Associates Inc, 2004

G1082 von Hagens G, Whalley A, Maschke R, Kriz W. Schnitt-anatomie des menschlichen Gehirns. Steinkopff, 1990

G1083 Braus H, Elze C. Anatomie des Menschen, Band 3. Periphere Leitungsbahnen II, Centrales Nervensystem, Sinnesorgane. Springer, 1960

G1084 Martini FH, Timmons MJ, Tallitsch RB. Anatomie. 1. A. Pearson, 2017

G1085 Brodmann K. Vergleichende Lokalisationslehre der Groß-hirnrinde in ihren Prinzipien, dargestellt aufgrund des Zellenbaues. J.A. Barth, 1909

G1086 Rohen JW. Anatomie für Zahnmediziner. Schattauer, 1994

G1087 Spoendlin H. Strukturelle Organisation des Innenohres. In: Oto-Rhino-Laryngologie in Klinik und Praxis. Band 1. (Hrsg. Helms J, Herberhold C, Kastenbauer E). Thieme, 1994: 32-74

G1088 Nieuwenhuys R, Voogd J, van Huijzen C. Das Zentral-nervensystem des Menschen. Ein Atlas mit Begleittext. 2. A. Springer, 1991

G1089 Berkovitz KB, et al. Oral Anatomy, Histology and Embryology. 5th ed. Elsevier/Mosby, 2017

G1091 Kandel ER, Koester JD, Mack SH, Siegelbaum SA. Principles of Neuroscience. 6th ed. McGraw Hill, 2021

G1192 O'Dowd G, Bell S, Wright S. Wheater's Pathology: A Text, Atlas and Review of Histopathology. 6th ed. Elsevier, 2019

H043-001 Mutoh K, Hidaka Y, Hirose Y, Kimura M. Possible induction of systemic lupus erythematosus by zonisamide. Pediatr Neurol 2001; 25(4):340-3

H061-001 Dodds SD, et al. Radiofrequency probe treatment for subfailure ligament injury: a biomechanical study of rabbit ACL. Clin Biomech 2004; 19(2):175-83

H062-001 Sener RN. Diffusion MRI: apparent diffusion coefficient (ADC) values in the normal brain and a classification of brain disorders based on ADC values. Comput Med Imaging Graph 2001; 25(4):299-326

H063-001 Heller AC, Kuether T, Barnwell SL, Nesbit G, Wayson KA. Spontaneous brachial plexus hemorrhage-case report. Surg Neurol 2000; 53(4):356-9

H064-001 Philipson M, Wallwork N. Traumatic dislocation of the sternoclavicular joint. Orthopaedics and Trauma 2012; 26(6):380-4

H081 Yang B, et al. A Case of Recurrent In-Stent Restenosis with Abundant Proteoglycan Component. Korean Circulation 2003; 33(9):827-31

H084-001 Custodio C, et al. Neuromuscular Complications of Cancer and Cancer Treatments. Physical Med Rehabilitation Clin North America 2008; 19(1):27-45

H102-002 Armour JA, et al. Gross and microscopic anatomy of the human intrinsic cardiac nervous system. Anat Rec 1997; 247:289–98

H230-001 Boyden EA. The anatomy of the choledochoduodenal junction in man. Surg Gynec Obstet 1957; 104:641–52

H233-001 Perfetti R, Merkel P. Glucagon-like peptide-1: a major regulator of pancreatic b-cell function. Eur J Endocrinol 2000; 143:717–25.

H234-001 Braak H. Architectonics as seen by lipofuscin stains. In: Peters A, Jones EG (eds.): Cerebral Cortex. Cellular Components of the Cerebral Cortex. Cellular Components of the Cerebral Cortex, Vol I. Plenum Press, 1984:59–104

J787 Colourbox.com

J803 Biederbick & Rumpf, Adelsdorf, Germany

K383 Cornelia Krieger, Hamburg, Germany

L106 Henriette Rintelen, Velbert, Germany

L126 Dr. med. Katja Dalkowski, Buckenhof, Germany

L127 Jörg Mair, München, Germany

L131 Stefan Dangl, München, Germany

L132 Michael Christof, Würzburg, Germany

L141 Stefan Elsberger, Planegg, Germany

L157 Susanne Adler, Lübeck, Germany

L190 Gerda Raichle, Ulm, Germany

L231 Stefan Dangl, München, Germany

L238 Sonja Klebe, Löhne, Germany

L240 Horst Ruß, München, Germany

L266 Stephan Winkler, München, Germany

L271 Matthias Korff, München, Germany

L275 Martin Hoffmann, Neu-Ulm, Germany

L280 Johannes Habla, München, Germany

L281 Luitgard Kellner, München, Germany

L284 Marie Davidis, München, Germany

L285 Anne-Katrin Hermanns, „Ankats Art", Maastricht, Netherlands

L303 Dr. med. Andreas Dietz, Konstanz, Germany

L316 Roswitha Vogtmann, Würzburg, Germany

L317 H.-C. Thiele, Gießen, Germany

L318 Tamas Sebesteny, Bern, Suisse

L319 Marita Peter, Hannover, Germany

M282 Prof. Dr.med. Detlev Drenckhahn, Würzburg, Germany

M492 Prof. Dr. med. Peter Kugler, Würzburg, Germany

M580 Prof. Dr. med. W. Kriz, Heidelberg, Germany

M1091 Prof. Dr. Reinhard Pabst, Hannover, Germany

O534 Prof. Dr. Arnd Dörfler, Erlangen, Germany

O548 Prof. Dr. med Andreas Franke, Kardiologie, Klinikum Region Hannover, Germany

O1107 Dr. Helmuth Ferner- Privatklinik Döbling, Wien, Austria

O1108 Prof. Hans-Rainer Duncker, Gießen, Germany

O1109 August Vierling (1872–1938), Heidelberg, Germany

P310 Prof. Dr. med. Friedrich Paulsen, Erlangen, Germany

P498 Prof. Dr. med. Philippe Pereira, SLK-Kliniken, Klinik für Radiologie, Heilbronn, Germany

Q300 Pernkopf-Archiv: Pernkopf E. Atlas der topgraphischen und angewandten Anatomie des Menschen, div. Bd. und Aufl. Elsevier/Urban & Fischer

R110-20 Rüther W, Lohmann C. Orthopädie und Unfallchirurgie. 20. A. Elsevier, 2014

R170-5 Welsch U, Kummer W, Deller T. Histologie – Das Lehrbuch: Zytologie, Histologie und mikroskopische Anatomie. 5. A. Elsevier/Urban & Fischer, 2018

R234 Bruch H-P, Trentz O. Berchtold Chirurgie. 6. A. Elsevier/Urban & Fischer, 2008

R235 Böcker W, Denk H, Heitz P, Moch H. Pathologie. 4. A. Elsevier/Urban & Fischer, 2008

R236 Classen M, Diehl V, Kochsiek K. Innere Medizin. 6. A. Elsevier/Urban & Fischer, 2009

R242 Franzen A. Kurzlehrbuch Hals-Nasen-Ohren-Heilkunde 3. A. Elsevier/Urban & Fischer, 2007

R247 Deller T, Sebesteny T. Fotoatlas Neuroanatomie. 1. A. Elsevier/Urban & Fischer, 2007

R252 Welsch U. Atlas Histologie. 7. A. Elsevier/Urban & Fischer, 2005

R254 Garzorz N. Basics Neuroanatomie. 1. A. Elsevier/Urban & Fischer, 2009

R261 Sitzer M, Steinmetz H. Neurologie. 1. A. Elsevier/Urban & Fischer, 2011

R306 Illing St, Classen M. Klinikleitfaden Pädiatrie.8. A. Elsevier/Urban & Fischer, 2009

R314 Böckers T, Paulsen F, Waschke J. Sobotta Lehrbuch Anatomie. 2. A. Elsevier/Urban & Fischer, 2019

R316-007 Wicke L. Atlas der Röntgenanatomie. 7. A. Elsevier/Urban & Fischer, 2005

R317 Trepel M. Neuroanatomie. 5. A. Elsevier/Urban& Fischer, 2011

R331 Fleckenstein P, Tranum-Jensen J. Röntgenanatomie. 1. A. Elsevier/Urban & Fischer, 2004

R333 Scharf H-P, Rüter A. Orthopädie und Unfallchirurgie. 2. A. Elsevier/Urban & Fischer, 2018

R349 Raschke MJ, Stange R. Alterstraumatologie – Prophylaxe, Therapie und Rehabilitation 1. A. Elsevier/Urban & Fischer, 2009,

R388 Weinschenk S. Handbuch Neuraltherapie. Diagnostik und Therapie mit Lokalanästhetika. 1. A. Elsevier/Urban & Fischer, 2010

R389 Gröne B. Schlucken und Schluckstörungen: Eine Einführung. 1. A. Elsevier/Urban & Fischer, 2009

R419 Menche N. Biologie- Anatomie- Physiologie. 9. A. Elsevier/Urban & Fischer, 2020

R449 Hansen JT. Netter's Clinical Anatomy. 4th ed. Elsevier/Urban & Fischer, 2018

R476 Kienzle-Müller B, Wilke-Kaltenbach G. Babies in Bewegung. 4. A. Elsevier, 2020

S002-5 Lippert H. Lehrbuch Anatomie. 5. A. Elsevier/Urban & Fischer, 2000

S002-7 Lippert H. Lehrbuch Anatomie. 7. A. Elsevier/Urban & Fischer, 2006

S008-4 Kauffmann GW, Sauer R, Weber WA. Radiologie. 4. A. Elsevier/Urban & Fischer, 2008

S100 Classen M, et al. Differentialdiagnose Innere Medizin 1. A. Urban & Schwarzenberg, 1998

S124 Breitner B. Chirurgische Operationslehre, Band III, Chirurgie des Abdomens. 2. A. Urban & Schwarzenberg, 1996

S130-6 Speckmann E-J, Hescheler J, Köhling R. Physiologie. 6. A. Elsevier/Urban & Fischer, 2013

S133 Wheater PR, Burkitt HG, Daniels VG. Funktionelle Histologie. 2. A. Urban & Schwarzenberg, 1987.

S700 Sobotta-Archiv: Sobotta. Atlas der Anatomie des Menschen, div. Aufl. Elsevier/Urban & Fischer

S701 Sobotta-Archiv: Hombach-Klonisch S, Klonisch T, Peeler J. Sobotta. Clinical Atlas of Human Anatomy. 1st ed. Elsevier/Urban & Fischer, 2019

S702 Sobotta-Archiv: Böckers T, Paulsen F, Waschke J. Sobotta. Lehrbuch Anatomie, div. Aufl. Elsevier/Urban & Fischer

T127 Prof. Dr. Dr. Peter Scriba, München, Germany

T419 Jörg Pekarsky, Institut für Anatomie LST II, Universität Erlangen-Nürnberg, Germany

T534 Prof. Dr. med. Matthias Sitzer, Klinik für Neurologie, Klinikum Herford, Germany

T663 Prof. Dr. Kurt Fleischhauer, Hamburg, Germany

T719 Prof. Dr. Norbert Kleinsasser, HNO-Klinik, Universitätsklinikum Würzburg, Germany

T720 PD Dr. med. Hannes Kutta, Universitätsklinikum Hamburg-Eppendorf, Germany

T786 Dr. Stephanie Lescher, Institut für Neuroradiologie, Klinikum der Goethe-Universität, Frankfurt, Prof. Joachim Berkefeld, Institut für Neuroradiologie, Klinikum der Goethe-Universität, Frankfurt, Germany

T832 PD Dr. Frank Berger, Institut für Klinische Radiologie der LMU, München, Germany

T863 C. Markus, Uniklinik Würzburg, Germany

T867 Prof. Dr. Gerd Geerling, Universitätsklinikum Düsseldorf, Germany

T872 Prof. Dr. med. Micheal Uder, Universitätsklinikum Erlangen, Germany

T882 Prof. Dr. med Christopher Bohr, Universitätsklinikum Regensburg, Germany

T884 Tobias Wicklein, Erlangen, Germany

T887 Prof. Dr. med Stephan Zierz, Dr. Jordan, Uniklinik Halle, Germany

Table of content

General anatomy

Anatomical planes and positions 4
Surface anatomy 14
Development 18
Musculoskeletal system 20
Neurovascular pathways 48
Imaging methods 70
Skin and its derivatives 76

Trunk

Surface 84
Development 88
Skeleton 90
Imaging methods 124
Musculature 132
Neurovascular pathways 160
Topography, dorsal trunk wall 170
Female breast 182
Topography, ventral trunk wall 186

Upper limb

Surface 200
Development 202
Skeleton 204
Musculature 236
Neurovascular pathways 276
Topography 308
Cross-sectional images 338

Lower limb

Surface 346
Skeleton 348
Musculature 414
Neurovascular pathways 452
Topography 476
Cross-sectional images 500

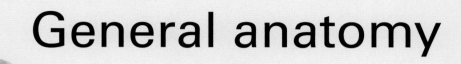

General anatomy

Anatomical planes and positions 4

Surface anatomy 14

Development 18

Musculoskeletal system 20

Neurovascular pathways 48

Imaging methods 70

Skin and its derivatives 76

1

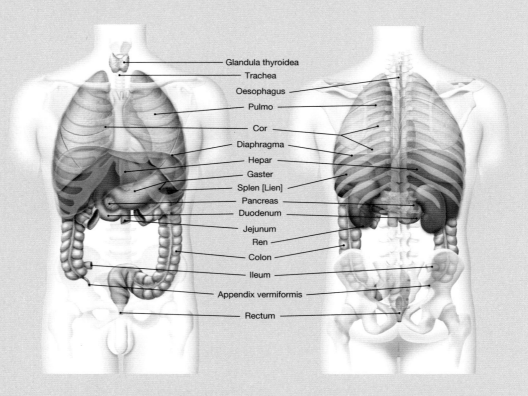

Glandula thyroidea
Trachea
Oesophagus
Pulmo
Cor
Diaphragma
Hepar
Gaster
Splen [Lien]
Pancreas
Duodenum
Jejunum
Ren
Colon
Ileum
Appendix vermiformis
Rectum

Overview

The Greek word 'ανατεμνειν' (anatemnein) means 'cut open' and describes the oldest method in the subject of anatomy, already practised in ancient times. Anatomy is the study of the structure of the healthy body. Without the knowledge of anatomy, one cannot learn about functions, and without the knowledge of structure and function, no pathological changes can be understood. In order to learn a new language, one needs to have a foundation of vocabulary and grammatical knowledge. The same is true of anatomy. One will need to know all the principles and have functional knowledge. Not only do planes, axes and orientation lines on the body, descriptions, as well as possibilities of movement play a role in clinical practice, but also knowledge of the musculoskeletal system, including biomechanical processes, the location of internal organs and their surface projection, the circulatory systems of the body and the structure of the nervous system. They form the basis for any diagnostic (especially imaging techniques, e. g. X-ray, ultrasound, scintigraphy, computed tomography, magnetic resonance imaging) as well as therapeutic measures.

Main topics

After working through this chapter, you should be able to:

- orientate yourself on the human body, divide the body into different sections and describe its plan or 'blueprint', know the main axes and planes, describe directions of movement and know directional terms as well as the location of the parts of the body, and the general anatomical terms;
- divide the surface into regions and describe the surface projection of inner organs;
- explain the basic principles of embryonic development, starting with fertilisation;
- know the basic principles of the musculoskeletal system, such as the classification of bones, structure of a long or tubular bone, names of bones of the skeleton, structure of a joint, joint types, documentation of joint motion and auxiliary structures of joints (intervertebral discs, labra, bursae, ligaments);
- explain basic concepts of general muscle theory, such as the structure of a skeletal muscle, muscle types, tendon attachment sites, auxiliary muscles and tendons, and describe the principles of muscle mechanics;
- describe the various circulatory systems, such as systemic circulation, including the heart and major arteries and veins, pulmonary circulation, organisation of the prenatal cardiovascular system, portal vein circulation and lymphatic vessel system (lymph circulation) with lymph nodes;
- understand the nervous system (structure, somatic and autonomous nervous system) and know the dermatomes on the body surface;
- describe the principles of diagnostic imaging techniques such as conventional X-ray, ultrasound, computed tomography, magnetic resonance imaging, scintigraphy;
- describe the structure of the skin and its derivatives.

Clinical relevance

In order not to lose touch with prospective everyday clinical life with so many anatomical details, the following describes a typical case that shows why the content of this chapter is so important.

A patent (open) Ductus arteriosus (BOTALLI) (PDA)

Case study
A premature infant, born in the 34th week of pregnancy plus two days (34+2 WOP) develops increased shortness of breath and poor feeding shortly after birth (fourth day of life). The infant is very pale, and her hands and feet are relatively cold.

Result of examination
The on-duty paediatrician at the neonatal station notices on palpation of the abdomen an enlargement of the liver and spleen (hepatosplenomegaly), and auscultation of the heart reveals a loud machine-like murmur (systolic crescendo and diastolic decrescendo murmur) in the second intercostal space on the left, which is accompanied by a tactile vibration across the chest. Palpation of the pulse shows a fast pulse with high blood pressure (Pulsus celer et altus). He immediately takes further diagnostic steps.

Diagnostic procedure
The electrocardiogram (ECG) shows left-ventricular stress. The chest X-ray indicates an enlarged pulmonary vessel and a left-sided widening of the heart. The completed echocardiography (colour Doppler test, → Fig. a) shows blood flow between the aorta and pulmonary vessels, enabling a direct image of a shunt.

 A shunt is a short circuit connection between normally separate vessels or cavities.

The diagnosis of a patent Ductus arteriosus (BOTALLI) (PDA) (→ Fig. b) is thus confirmed.

Diagnosis
A patent Ductus arteriosus (BOTALLI).

Treatment
A drug treatment with the prostaglandin synthesis inhibitor ibuprofen is initiated to close the haemodynamically effective PDA.

Further developments
Although the symptoms improve slightly under treatment, a pronounced systolic heart murmur can still be heard and the PDA is detectable in the colour Doppler test. For this reason, an interventional closure by means of cardiac catheterisation is introduced the following day by inserting an umbrella system. Shortly after the procedure, the pulse of the infant is already within the normal range, breathing is calm and no heart murmur is detectable. She remains for some time on the neonatal ward and progresses well, and can therefore be discharged.

Dissection lab
Examine the pressure and flow conditions in the large and small circulation with the heart as the central organ and consider how the blood flows in the baby girl with PDA.

 Consider which other shunts are obliterated after birth.

Back in the clinic
After birth, the increasing oxygen concentration arising from the lungs unfolding and the first breaths normally cause the Ductus arteriosus to contract and close. In premature babies, many organs are not yet fully developed. The cause of the persistence of a PDA is therefore attributed to the fact that the vessel muscles here contract less well, as they are less developed, and a relatively high prostaglandin concentration leaves the Ductus arteriosus open.

 From the 28th week of pregnancy, women should not take prostaglandin synthesis inhibitors (e.g. ibuprofen) for pain medication, so that the Ductus arteriosus does not close too early.

After birth, the prostaglandin levels normally drop quickly and the Ductus arteriosus closes up spontaneously. Therefore, therapeutic measures with prostaglandin synthesis inhibitors are often successful.

 Immediately after birth, initial examination of the newborn is carried out in order to determine whether all vital functions, such as the respiratory and cardiovascular systems, are in order.

In the case of a haemodynamically effective PDA, a left-to-right shunt occurs due to high pressure in the systemic circulation and low pressure in the pulmonary circulation with volume overload on the left side of the heart, so that blood from the aorta flows into the lungs, which causes increased pulmonary blood flow and increased pressure in the pulmonary circulation. Thus a certain amount of blood from the lungs, reaching the left ventricle and from there the aorta, flows back into the lungs via the PDA (machine-like murmur). There is a lack of circulating blood in the systemic circulation (cold hands and feet). As a reaction, the heart rate increases (Pulsus celer et altus) in order to transport enough oxygen to the periphery of the body. If the PDA is not treated, the continual increased pressure leads to damage of the vessels in the lungs. This remodelling (or modification) of the vessel structure further 'fixes' the increased pressure and may make it exceed the pressure of the systemic circulation, resulting in a shunt reverse (right-to-left shunt), whereby blood reaches the systemic circulation directly from the pulmonary circulation, without being pre-saturated with oxygen. The result is cyanosis (bluish discolouration of the skin, lips and mucous membranes) and a rapid decrease in capacity. At some point the heart undergoes decompensation.

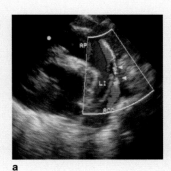 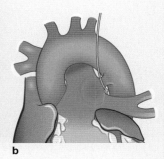

a b

Fig. a A colour Doppler test. [O548]
Fig. b A patent Ductus arteriosus (BOTALLI). [S700-L126]

Anatomical planes and positions

Parts of the body

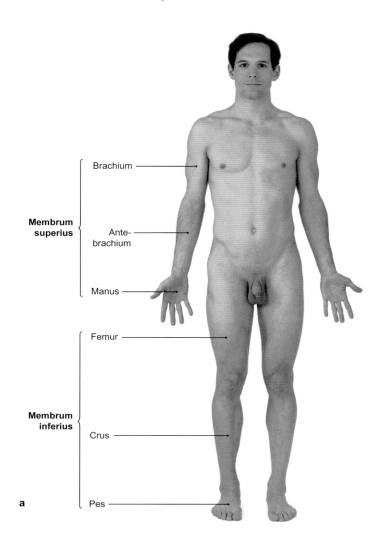

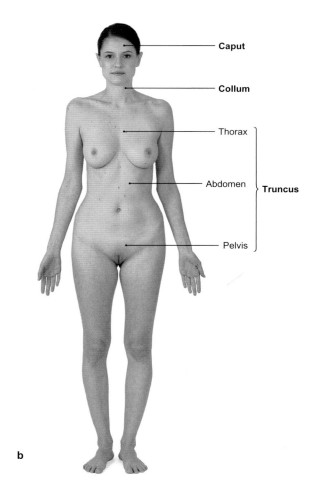

Brachium

Membrum
superius

Ante-
brachium

Manus

Femur

Membrum
inferius

Crus

a   Pes

Caput

Collum

Thorax

Abdomen   Truncus

Pelvis

b

Fig. 1.1a and b   Surface anatomy; ventral view. [S702-J803]
a Male anatomy.
b Female anatomy.
Usually anatomical descriptions relate to an upright position; facing forward, with the arms hanging down, with palms turned towards the body or forwards, the legs parallel and the feet facing forward.
The body is divided up into the head (Caput), neck (Collum), trunk (Truncus) including the chest (thorax), stomach (abdomen), hips (pelvis) and back (Dorsum), and the upper limbs (Membrum superius) and lower limbs (Membrum inferius). The limbs are sub-divided into the upper arm (Brachi-

um), forearm (Antebrachium) and hand (Manus), and the thigh (femur), lower leg (crus) and foot (Pes).
Secondary sexual characteristics: the external appearance of a human being is identified in the different stages of life by physical attributes. These occur in men and women as gender dimorphism (gender differences, especially after sexual maturity). The development of sexual organs is genetically determined. Responsible for their development are the primary sex organs (ovaries and testes), which are referred to as the primary sexual characteristics. Developing in puberty, it is mainly the secondary sexual characteristics (→ table) which are responsible for the outer appearance.

Outer appearance	
Man	**Woman**
Beard growth	Mammary gland (Mamma)
Hair growth on the front thorax and abdomen (varies greatly between individuals) and also on the back and extremities	Distribution of subcutaneous fat (more consistent, smoother outlines)
Pubic hair growth up to the navel	Pubic hair growth up to the height of the mons pubis
Reduced hairline (receding hairline, pattern baldness)	Even hairline
Larger body size	Smaller body size and muscle mass
Narrower pelvis	Horizontally oval pelvis

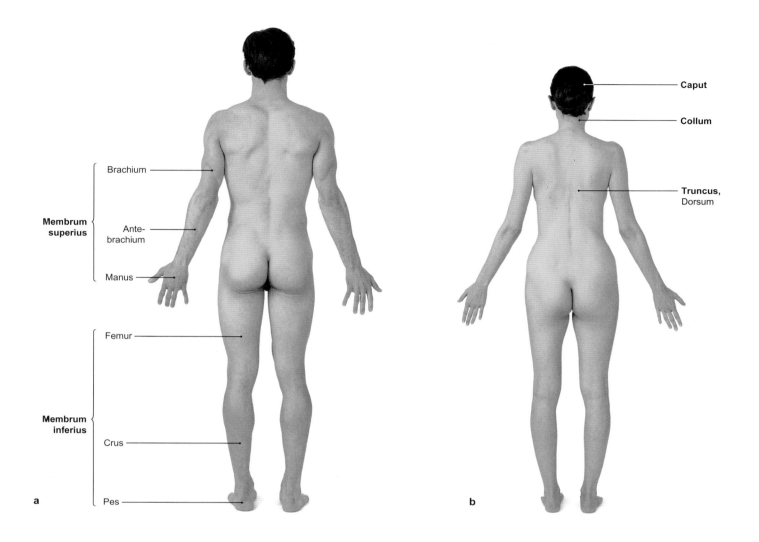

Fig. 1.2a and b **Surface anatomy;** dorsal view. [S702-J803]
a Male anatomy.
b Female anatomy.

Clinical remarks

As part of the **anamnesis** (from the ancient Greek αναμνησις, *anámnesis* = reminder), the medical history of a patient with regard to their current complaints is taken. A detailed anamnesis includes biological, psychological and social aspects. The information gathered often enables conclusions regarding risk factors and causal relationships. The anamnesis does not have a direct link to treatment, although talking about the issues may be beneficial and make things clear. The anamnesis is normally taken prior to medical examination, but in the case of an emergency requiring immediate treatment, it must be postponed. The aim of the anamnesis is to restrict as much as possible all differential diagnoses coming into question, preferably based on the main symptoms and exclusion criteria. In order to be able to make a definitive diagnosis, further examinations are usually necessary following the anamnesis.

Body proportions

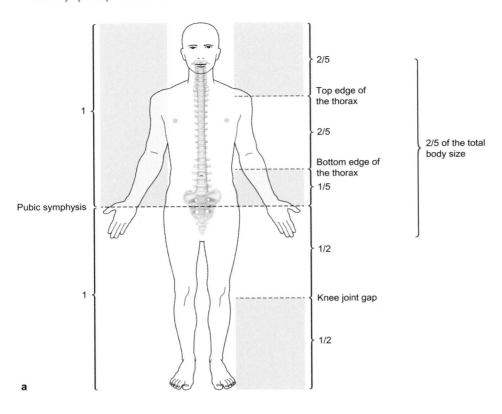

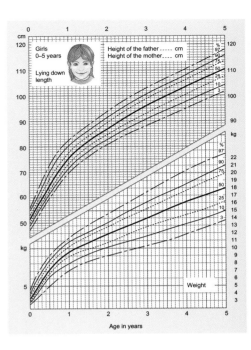

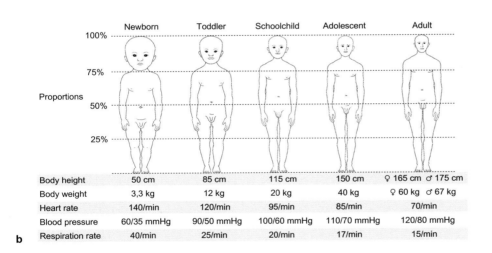

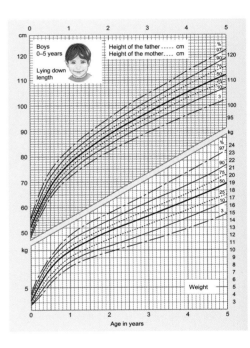

	Newborn	Toddler	Schoolchild	Adolescent	Adult
Body height	50 cm	85 cm	115 cm	150 cm	♀ 165 cm ♂ 175 cm
Body weight	3,3 kg	12 kg	20 kg	40 kg	♀ 60 kg ♂ 67 kg
Heart rate	140/min	120/min	95/min	85/min	70/min
Blood pressure	60/35 mmHg	90/50 mmHg	100/60 mmHg	110/70 mmHg	120/80 mmHg
Respiration rate	40/min	25/min	20/min	17/min	15/min

Fig. 1.3a–c Body proportions and percentile curves.
a Normal body proportions; frontal view. [S700-L127]
If an adult is divided horizontally into two equal halves, the middle is approximately at the level of the upper edge of the pubic bone. The bottom half can be divided into another two equal halves at the level of the knee. The top half can be divided into five equal sections. The spine occupies two-fifths of the total body size.
b Body proportions and vital signs at different stages of development. [R419-L190]
Body size refers to the measurement from the crown of the head to the soles of the feet (body length). In paediatrics, the postnatal period is divided into stages of development. In the different stages of development the body changes length continuously. **(1)** Neonatal period (the first two weeks of life), **(2)** infancy (up to the end of the first year of life), **(3)** early childhood (up to the end of the fifth year of life), **(4)** school age (up to the onset of puberty), **(5)** puberty (maturation into adult, duration varies), **(6)** adolescence (completion of the development and growth in length of the skeletal system up to **(7)** adulthood). Later on, the term 'old age' is sometimes used in medicine for elderly adults. At this point in time, the body length has decreased because of age-related degenerative processes.
c Percentile curves. [R306-L157]
Growth in height and weight in girls and boys in the first five years of life. The diagonal line indicates the average value each time, with all values between 3% and 97% lying within the two standard deviations.

┌─ Clinical remarks ─────────────────────────────────

In order to assess correct body growth (standard) or divergent body growth (variability) in children, body height, weight and head circumference are analysed separately in relation to age and by using percentile tables (→ Fig. 1.3c) for girls and boys.

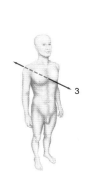
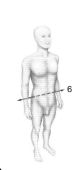
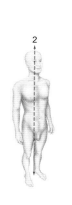
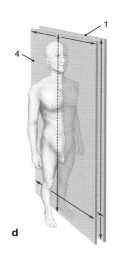

a

b

c

d

1 Sagittal plane
2 Longitudinal axis
3 Sagittal axis
4 Median sagittal plane
5 Transverse plane
6 Transverse axis
7 Frontal plane

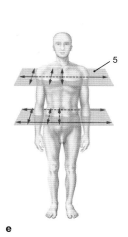
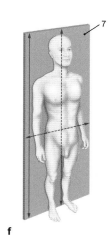
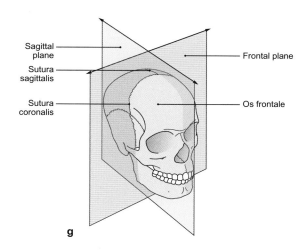

e

f

g

Sagittal plane · Sutura sagittalis · Sutura coronalis · Frontal plane · Os frontale

Main axes	
Sagittal axis	Runs vertically to the transverse and longitudinal axis
Transverse axis	Runs vertically to the longitudinal and sagittal axis
Longitudinal or vertical axis	Runs vertically to the sagittal and transverse axis

Main planes	
Median (sagittal) plane	Symmetrical plane dividing body into two equal halves
Sagittal plane	Runs parallel to the median plane (sagittal plane)
Transverse plane	All the horizontal planes of the body
Frontal plane	Parallel to the longitudinal axis

Fig. 1.4a–g Planes and axes as well as radiological terms.
[S702-L127]
a The sagittal axis.
b The transverse axis.
c The longitudinal or vertical axis.
d Sagittal plane (Planum sagittale), delineated by the sagittal and longitudinal axis.

e Transverse plane = horizontal plane (Planum transversale), delineated by the transverse and sagittal axis.
f Frontal plane = coronal plane (Planum frontale), delineated by the longitudinal and transverse axis.
g The coronal suture and sagittal suture (Sutura coronalis and Sutura sagittalis) are used especially in radiology as terms of motion: the sagittal layer corresponds to the sagittal plane, and the coronal layer corresponds to the frontal plane.

Directions of movement	
Direction	**Movement**
Extension	Extension of the trunk or extremities
Flexion	Bending of the trunk or extremities
Abduction	Moving the extremities away from the body
Adduction	Moving the extremities towards the body
Elevation	Lifting the arm above the horizontal plane
Rotation	Internal and external rotation of the extremities around the longitudinal axis
Circumduction	Gyration, composite movements made up of adduction, abduction, flexion, extension, etc.

Radiological sectional planes	
Radiological term	**Anatomical term**
Sagittal layer	Sagittal plane
Coronal layer	Frontal plane
Axial layer	Transverse plane

Radiology terminology in imaging procedures (computed tomography and magnetic resonance imaging) defines the three main anatomical planes as layers with their own nomenclature.

Anatomical planes and positions

Terms of movement

Anatomical terms of movement		
Region	**Term**	**Movement**
Limbs	Extension	Elongation
	Flexion	Bending
	Abduction	Moving extremities away from the body
	Adduction	Moving extremities towards the body
	Elevation	Lifting the arm/shoulder above the horizontal plane
	Depression	Lowering the arm/shoulder from above the horizontal plane
	Internal rotation	Inward rotation
	External rotation	Outward rotation
	Pronation	Rotational movement of hand/foot with palm of hand or sole of foot turned downwards
	Supination	Rotational movement of hand/foot with palm of hand or sole of foot turned upwards
	Radial abduction	Splaying out hand/fingers towards the radial bone
	Ulnar abduction	Splaying hand/fingers towards the ulnar bone
	Palmar flexion/volar flexion	Bending palm of hand towards surface of the palm
	Plantar flexion	Bending sole of the foot towards the sole of the foot
	Dorsiflexion	Bending back the hand/foot
	Opposition	Touching the thumb to the little finger
	Reposition	Moving the thumb back next to the index finger
	Inversion	Turning the plantar surface of the foot inwards, to face the midline of the body
	Eversion	Turning the foot outwards, away from the midline of the body
Spine	Rotation	Rotation in the longitudinal axis
	Lateral flexion	Lateral tilt
	Inclination (flexion)	Forward tilt
	Reclination (extension)	Backward tilt
Pelvis	Flexion (anterior/ventral rotation)	Forward pelvic tilt
	Extension (dorsal rotation)	Backward pelvic stretch
Temperomandibular joint	Abduction	Opening the jaw
	Adduction	Closing the jaw
	Protrusion/protraction	Pushing the lower jaw forward
	Retrusion/retraction	Pulling the lower jaw back
	Occlusion	Interlocking the teeth of the upper and lower jaw
	Mediotrusion	Lower jaw facing ventromedially on one side
	Laterotrusion	Lower jaw facing dorsolaterally on one side

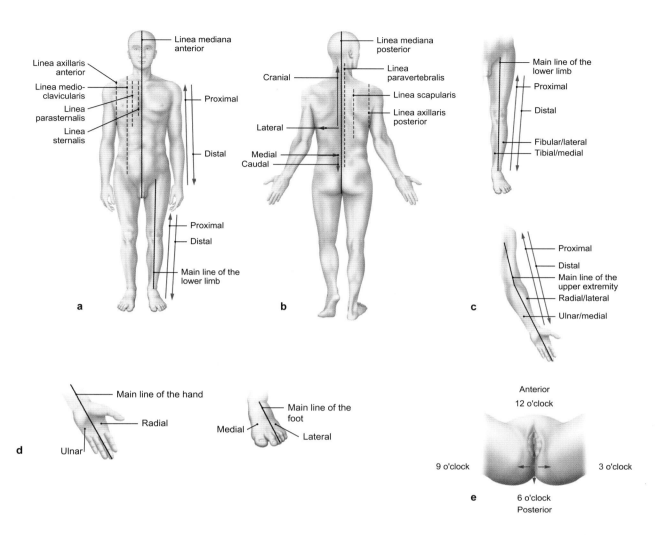

Fig. 1.5a–e Orientation lines as well as terms of movement and location. [S702-L127]
a Ventral view.
b Dorsal view.
c Ventral view of lower limb, upper limb with supinated hand.

d Palmar view of hand and view of the back of the foot.
e Lithotomy position (preferred positioning of patients for gynaecological and some proctological examinations); a clock face is traditionally used to report the location of a clinical finding.

Terms of movement and location for parts of the body			
Direction	**Meaning**	**Direction**	**Meaning**
Cranial or superior	Towards the head	Apical	Towards or belonging to the tip
Caudal or inferior	Towards the tail bone	Basal	Towards the base
Anterior or ventral	Towards the front	Dexter	Right
Posterior or dorsal	Towards the back	Sinister	Left
Lateral	Towards the side, away from the midline	Proximal	Towards the torso
Medial	In the middle, towards the midline	Distal	Towards the extremities
Median or medianus	Within the median plane	Ulnar	Towards the ulna
Intermedius	Lying in between	Radial	Towards the radius
Central	Towards the interior of the body	Tibial	Towards the tibia
Peripheral	Towards the surface of the body	Fibular	Towards the fibula
Deep or profundus	At a deeper level	Volar or palmar	Towards the palm
Superficial or superficialis	Lying on the surface	Plantar	Towards the sole
External or externus	On the outside	Dorsal	(Extremities) towards the back (Dorsum) of the hand or the foot
Internal or internus	On the inside	Frontal	Towards the front
		Rostral	Towards the mouth or tip of the nose (only for terms relating to the head)

Terms of movement

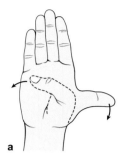

a

Opposition/reposition
of the thumb

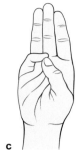

b

Abduction/adduction
of the thumb

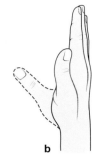

c

Opposition
(thumb/little finger test)

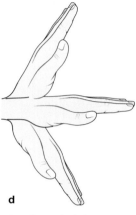

d

Dorsal extension/palmar
flexion of the hand

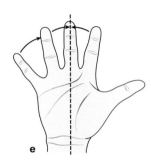

e

Adduction of the fingers

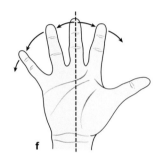

f

Abduction of the fingers

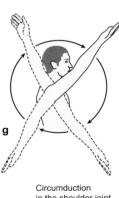

g

Circumduction
in the shoulder joint

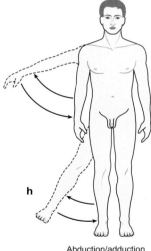

h

Abduction/adduction
of the arm and leg

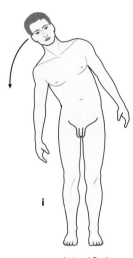

i

Lateral flexion
of the trunk

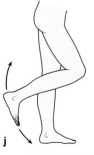

j

Flexion/extension
in the knee joint

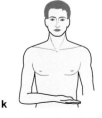

k

Internal rotation in the
shoulder joint

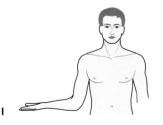

l

External rotation in the
shoulder joint

Fig. 1.6a–l   Terms of movement. [S702-L126]

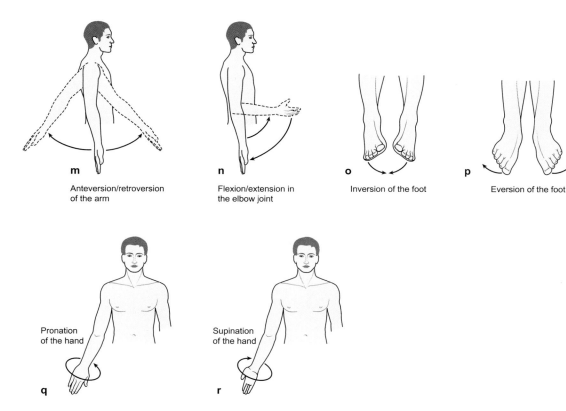

m Anteversion/retroversion of the arm

n Flexion/extension in the elbow joint

o Inversion of the foot

p Eversion of the foot

q Pronation of the hand

r Supination of the hand

Fig. 1.6m–r Terms of movement. [S702-L126]

Structure and function

Combined movements

Functional movements, including reaching over one's head and round one's back to scratch the back or apply sun screen lotion, are examples of combined movements of the upper extremity. These complex multi-axial movements frequently involve the coordinated actions of several joints:

- flexion, abduction and external rotation in the shoulder and elbow joints as well as supination of the hand (→ Fig. a)
- extension, adduction and internal rotation of the shoulder and elbow joints as well as pronation of the hand (→ Fig. b).

Open and closed kinetic (kinematic) chain

A kinetic chain represents the combination of several different joints that are connected with each other and perform a complex movement (→ Fig. c):

- An open kinetic chain is defined as a movement of a part of the body that centres around a single joint or a limb segment (e.g. extension of the knee from a sitting position). This movement is independent of movements involving other joints, such as an extension of the knee without involvement of the hip or ankle joints (1).

- A closed kinetic chain represents a body movement that is composed of the combined actions of several joints or body segments, resulting in a sequence of coordinated movements; an example is standing up from a sitting position (2).

For the knee to extend, a parallel movement in the hip joint and the upper (talocrural) ankle joint must occur. The term 'functional movements' refers to closed kinetic chain movements.

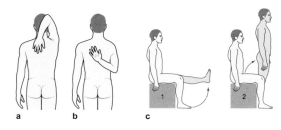

a **b** **c**

[S701-L126]

General anatomy

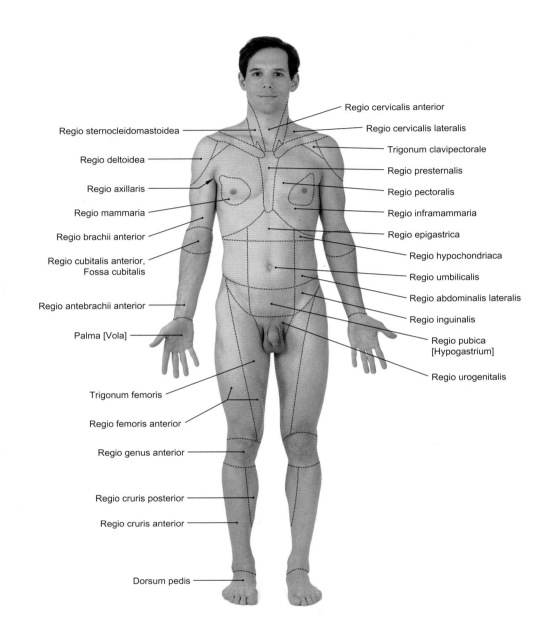

Regio cervicalis anterior

Regio sternocleidomastoidea

Regio cervicalis lateralis

Trigonum clavipectorale

Regio deltoidea

Regio presternalis

Regio axillaris

Regio pectoralis

Regio mammaria

Regio inframammaria

Regio brachii anterior

Regio epigastrica

Regio cubitalis anterior,
Fossa cubitalis

Regio hypochondriaca

Regio umbilicalis

Regio antebrachii anterior

Regio abdominalis lateralis

Regio inguinalis

Palma [Vola]

Regio pubica
[Hypogastrium]

Regio urogenitalis

Trigonum femoris

Regio femoris anterior

Regio genus anterior

Regio cruris posterior

Regio cruris anterior

Dorsum pedis

Fig. 1.7 Regions of the body; ventral view. [S702-J803]
The body surface is divided into regions to facilitate description and orientation.
Regio: region; Trigonum: triangle.

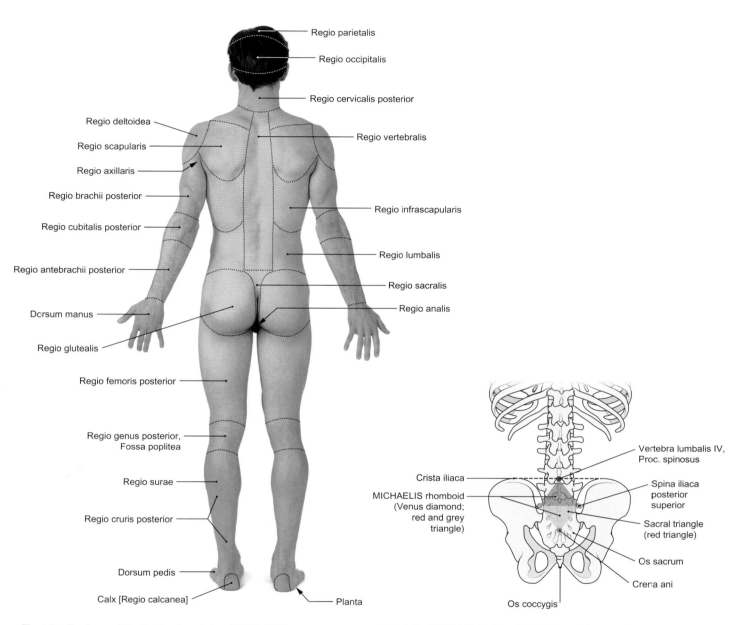

Regio parietalis

Regio occipitalis

Regio cervicalis posterior

Regio deltoidea

Regio scapularis

Regio vertebralis

Regio axillaris

Regio brachii posterior

Regio cubitalis posterior

Regio infrascapularis

Regio antebrachii posterior

Regio lumbalis

Regio sacralis

Dorsum manus

Regio analis

Regio glutealis

Regio femoris posterior

Regio genus posterior,
Fossa poplitea

Regio surae

Regio cruris posterior

Dorsum pedis

Calx [Regio calcanea]

Planta

Crista iliaca

Vertebra lumbalis IV,
Proc. spinosus

MICHAELIS rhomboid
(Venus diamond;
red and grey
triangle)

Spina iliaca
posterior
superior

Sacral triangle
(red triangle)

Os sacrum

Crena ani

Os coccygis

Fig. 1.8 Regions of the body; dorsal view. [S702-J803]
The body surface is divided into regions to facilitate description and orientation.
Regio: region.

Fig. 1.9 MICHAELIS rhomboid (Venus diamond) and sacral triangle; dorsal view. [S702-L126]
Presentation of palpable and visible corners of the MICHAELIS rhomboid (female) and sacral triangle (male).

Surface anatomy

Skin tension lines

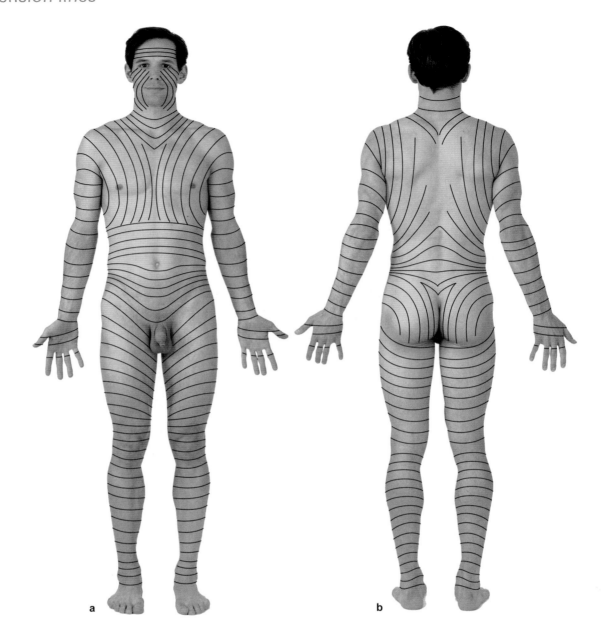

a

b

Fig. 1.10a and b   Skin tension lines. [S700-J803/L126]
a Ventral view.
b Dorsal view.

Tension lines (syn. LANGER's lines) are caused by the alignment of collagen and elastic fibres in the reticular layer of the skin. Their development is dependent on age, nutritional status, general condition and anatomical peculiarities.

Clinical remarks

Any injury to the skin leaves traces to varying degrees, e. g. a scar on the knee after a crash, or on the abdomen after removal of the appendix (appendectomy). A scar is the physiological final state of tissue repair. It consists of coarse collagenous connective tissue and differs from the surrounding skin by the lack of hair, sebaceous and/or sweat glands. If scars are in an exposed area or become hyperplastic (keloid formation), they can be aesthetically obtrusive. In order to make a scar on the body as discreet as possible in planned

surgical procedures, the incision is made along tension lines of the skin. At the edges of wounds that run perpendicularly or at an angle to the tension lines, there is significantly higher tension than at the edges of wounds that run parallel to the lines. Wherever possible, therefore, surgical incisions are made in the direction of the tension lines. This reduces the risk of the wound margins spreading (dehiscence) as well as the development of extensive scars.

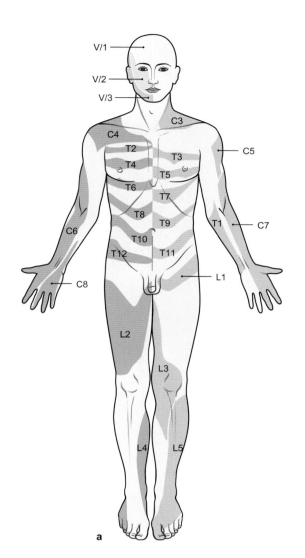
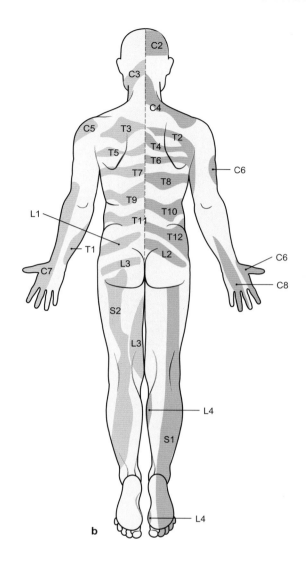

Fig. 1.11a and b Segmental innervation of the skin (dermatomes).
[S700-L126]/[F1067-001]
a Ventral view.
b Dorsal view.

A **dermatome** is an area of skin innervated autonomously by the sensory fibres of a spinal cord nerve (spinal nerves, → Fig. 1.70). Each spinal nerve can thus be assigned to an area of skin. However, the innervation areas of adjacent spinal nerves overlap and, in addition, many cutaneous nerves are composed of the sensory fibres of several spinal nerves joined together (the Rami ventrales of the spinal nerves develop branches in the neck and lumbar sacral area [plexus] → Fig. 1.72), so that the dermatomes differ from the innervation fields of the cutaneous nerves. With the exception of the midline, where the overlap is very low, the **autonomous area** of each individual spinal nerve (skin area exclusively innervated by a particular sensory nerve) is much smaller than the total skin area innervated by it. For reasons of clarity, the dermatomes are represented alternately for the

right (green) side of the body and the left (blue) side of the body. Thus, for example, T7 is visible on the left side in blue, T8 on the right side in green, and T9 again on the left side in green, etc. Regions where no colour is assigned (e.g. the area between C4, T2 and T3 around the midline), are areas in which an extraordinarily high variability and a very strong interindividual overlap occurs, so that no clear assignment is possible. Presentation of the dermatomes is based on an evidence-based dermatome card, according to LEE and co-workers (2008). In order to keep the figure clear and understandable, the dermatomes S3, S4 and S5 are not shown (they cover the area of the perineum, including the anus and the external genitalia). The skin of the face is not innervated by spinal nerves but by the cranial nerve (N. trigeminus [V]). Similar to the spinal nerves, its three branches also have autonomous sensory skin innervation areas (yellow).

Clinical remarks

Damage to a spinal nerve typically leads to loss of sensitivity in its autonomous area. **Herpes zoster** is a viral disease that is associated with an extremely painful skin rash with blisters. The virus also affects a spinal nerve. The virus triggers inflammation which spreads from the nerve to the associated dermatome and triggers the skin symptoms (colloquially: **shingles**). The disease is caused by the **var-**

icella zoster virus, belonging to the herpes virus family, which in 99 % of cases is transmitted in childhood and triggers **chickenpox** after infection, if the child has not previously been vaccinated against it. The virus persists in the body (spinal ganglion) and can be reactivated in cases of immunodeficiency.

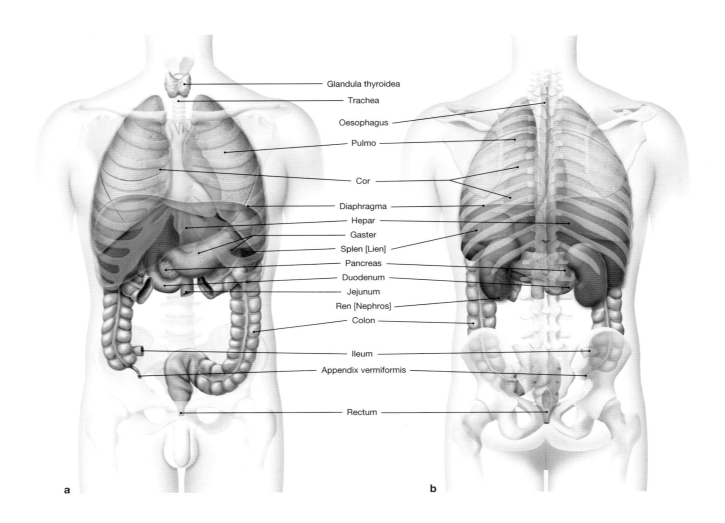

Glandula thyroidea
Trachea
Oesophagus
Pulmo
Cor
Diaphragma
Hepar
Gaster
Splen [Lien]
Pancreas
Duodenum
Jejunum
Ren [Nephros]
Colon
Ileum
Appendix vermiformis
Rectum

a

b

Fig. 1.12a and b Projection of the internal organs onto the body surface. [S700-L275]
a Surface projection of the internal organs onto the ventral trunk.
b Surface projection of the internal organs onto the dorsal trunk.

Oesophagus, thyroid gland (Glandula thyroidea), trachea, lungs (Pulmo), heart (Cor), diaphragm (Diaphragma), liver (Hepar), stomach (Gaster), spleen (Splen [Lien]), pancreas, duodenum, jejunum, kidney (Ren), colon, ileum, appendix (Appendix vermiformis) and rectum (Rectum).

Clinical remarks

Even without technical instruments, with practice it is possible to gain an insight into individual organs and their projection onto the body surface. The term **auscultation** (from Latin auscultare = listen) refers to the monitoring of the body, typically with a stethoscope. Auscultation is part of the physical examination of a patient. **Percus-**

sion (from Latin percutere = beat) refers to tapping on the body surface for diagnostic purposes. Underlying tissue is hereby set in vibration. The resulting acoustic sounds provide information about the state of the tissue. The size and position of an organ (e. g. liver) or the air content of the tissue (e. g. lung) can thus be assessed.

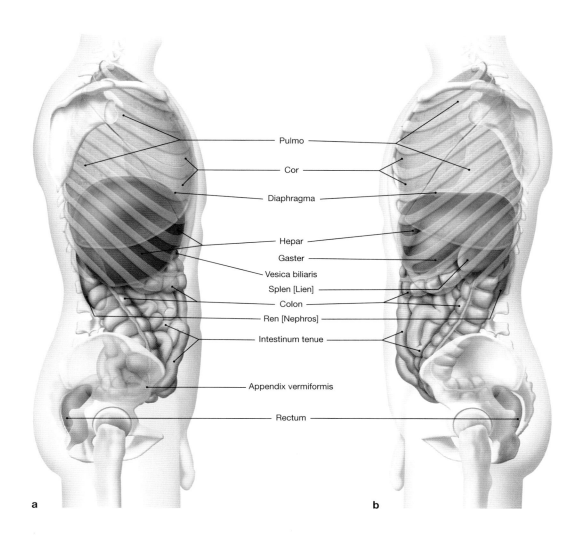

Pulmo
Cor
Diaphragma
Hepar
Gaster
Vesica biliaris
Splen [Lien]
Colon
Ren [Nephros]
Intestinum tenue
Appendix vermiformis
Rectum

a   b

Fig. 1.13a and b   Projection of internal organs onto the body surface. [S700-L275]
a Surface projection of the internal organs onto the right trunk.
b Surface projection of the internal organs onto the left trunk.

Lungs (Pulmo), heart (Cor), diaphragm (Diaphragma), liver (Hepar), stomach (Gaster), gallbladder (Vesica biliaris), spleen (Splen [Lien]), large intestine (colon), kidney (Ren), small intestine (Intestinum tenue), appendix (Appendix vermiformis) and rectum (Rectum).

Clinical remarks

Through knowledge of the **projection** of the internal organs onto the body surface, disease symptoms can be linked to specific organs during an initial physical examination and without reference to the medical history. For example, appendicitis (inflammation of the appendix [Appendix vermiformis]) is usually associated with discomfort in the lower right abdomen.

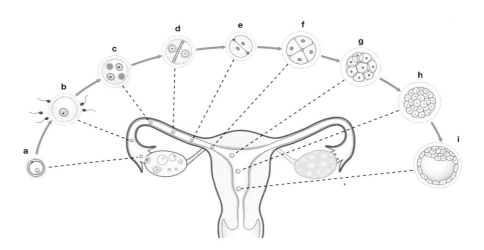

Fig. 1.14a–i First week of embryonic development: fertilisation and implantation. [E838]
a–c Normally within 24 hours after **ovulation (a), fertilisation (b)** occurs in the ampulla of the oviduct. Fusion of the nuclei of the ovum and sperm creates a **zygote (c).**

d–h Subsequent cell division **(2-, 4-, 8- and 16-cell stages)** generates a cell aggregate (morula) which is transported into the uterine cavity.
i Approximately on the fifth day after fertilisation, a fluid-filled cyst develops in the morula **(blastocyst),** which on the fifth to sixth day implants in the prepared lining of the uterus.

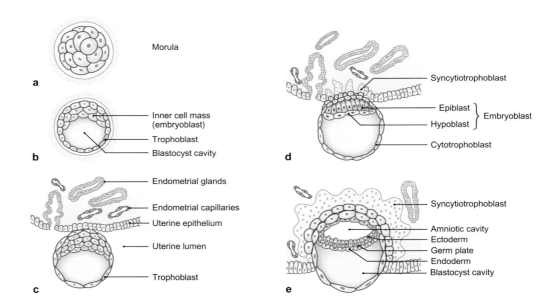

Fig. 1.15a–e First and second week of embryonic development: bilaminar germ (embryonic) disc. [E838]
a–b Upon differentiation of the morula **(a)** into the blastocyst, the latter generates an inner cell mass **(embryoblast)** and a larger fluid-filled (blastocyst cavity) outer cell layer **(trophoblast) (b).**
c–e As a result of intricate interactions of the trophoblast cell layer with the surrounding maternal endometrium, a placenta is formed. The **placenta** allows close proximity between the fetal and maternal blood circulatory systems, while a placental barrier ensures that both fetal and maternal blood circulatory systems remain separated **(uteroplacental circulation).**

The syncytiotrophoblast **(d, e)** contributes to this placental barrier. The epiblast and hypoblast are early structures in embryoblast development **(d).** The embryoblast develops into the bilaminar **embryonic disc** with **ectoderm** (columnar cells at the dorsal surface of the embryoblast) and **endoderm** (cuboidal cells at the ventral surface). The ectoderm forms a dorsal cavity, which becomes the **amniotic cavity.** The blastocyst cavity located at the front becomes the primary yolk sac, which is lined by the endoderm. On the 12th day, the ectoderm forms the actual yolk sac (not shown); the original blastocyst cavity is lined by extra-embryonic mesoderm.

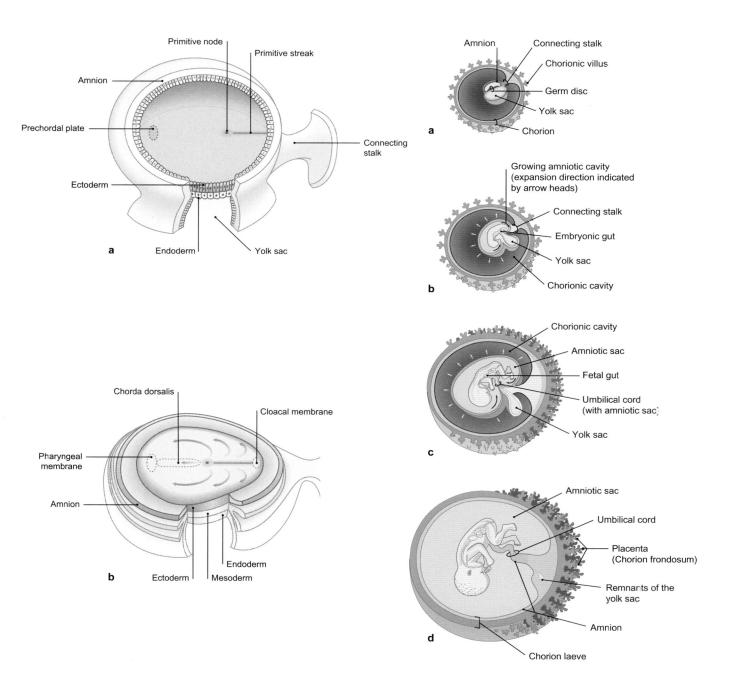

Fig. 1.16a and b   Third week of embryonic development: gastrulation. [E838]

a Development of the trilaminar germ disc begins with the appearance of the primitive streak at the dorsal surface of the ectoderm. The primitive streak is demarcated by the primitive node at the top end.

b Cells migrate out of the primitive streak and form the **intraembryonic mesoderm** between the top of the yolk sac and the ectoderm of the amniotic cavity (gastrulation). Some of the cells protrude cranially as a **chordal projection** towards the cranial part of the embryo. Here, in the ectoderm, the **prechordal plate** (adhesion surface between ectoderm and endoderm – there is no mesoderm between the two layers) evolves. The chordal projection develops a lumen and becomes a **Chorda dorsalis** (primitive stabilising structure of the embryo), which recedes later in development. Only the Nuclei pulposi of the intervertebral discs remain as relics of the Chorda dorsalis. Some mesoderm cells migrate cranially past the prechordal plate and form the heart. The **three germ layers** (ectoderm, mesoderm, endoderm) are the building blocks for the **development of all organs.** For further information on which organs emerge from which germ layer, see textbooks on embryology.

Fig. 1.17a–d   Further developmental stages. [E347-09]

a Condition as presented in → Fig. 1.16a. Third week: the amnion covers the dorsal surface of the embryo; the **chorionic cavity** is still very large at this early stage.

b In the fourth week, the **amnion** envelops the entire embryo with the exception of the umbilical cord.

c In the period that follows the amnion grows rapidly. The slower growth of the chorionic cavity and yolk sac makes these smaller.

d Finally the amnion displaces the chorionic cavity completely and forms the **amniotic sac.** The yolk sac is reduced to a remnant.

General anatomy

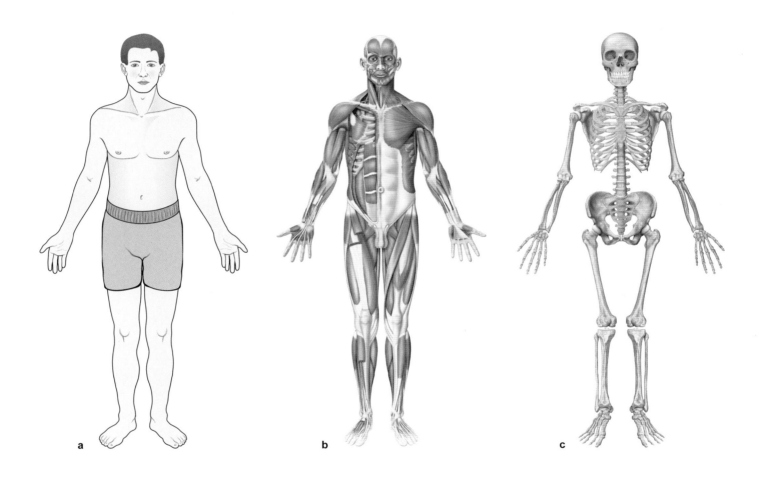

a   b   c

Fig. 1.18a–c Musculoskeletal system, Systema musculosceletale; ventral view.
a Surface anatomy. [S700-L126]
b Muscles and tendons. [S700-L275]
c Cartilage, bones and joints. [S700-L127]
The term musculoskeletal system (MSK) includes bones, muscles, tendons, joints, ligaments, cartilage and additional connective tissues which are involved in supporting, stabilising and moving the body. The major components of the MSK system are:

- **Bones:** a mineralised tissue structure to support, protect, capture and store minerals and in a broader sense (bone marrow) aid haematopoiesis.
- **Muscles:** skeletal muscles use tendons to attach to bones and move joints.
- **Tendons:** composed of mainly collagen fibres oriented in a parallel direction for added strength, tendons connect muscles with bones.
- **Joints:** enable movements of individual skeletal elements (bone and cartilage).

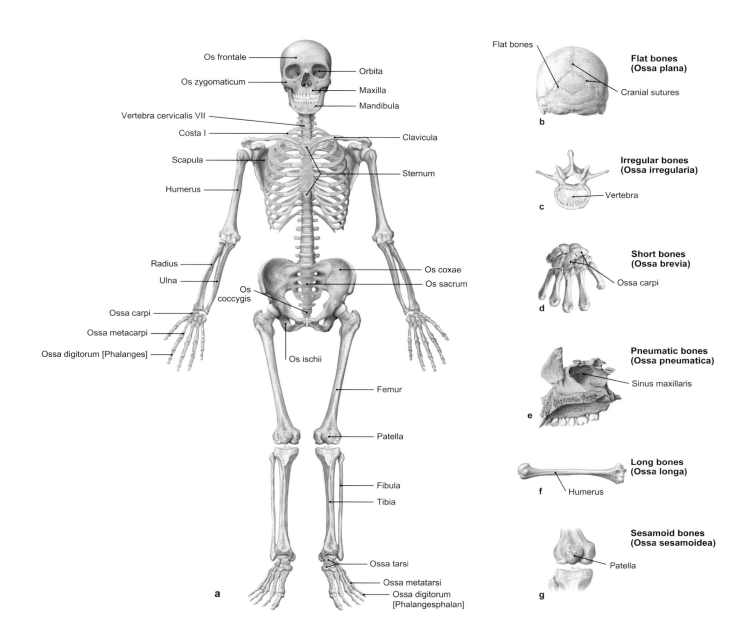

Os frontale

Os zygomaticum

Vertebra cervicalis VII

Costa I

Scapula

Humerus

Radius

Ulna

Os coccygis

Ossa carpi

Ossa metacarpi

Ossa digitorum [Phalanges]

Os ischii

Orbita

Maxilla

Mandibula

Clavicula

Sternum

Os coxae

Os sacrum

Femur

Patella

Fibula

Tibia

Ossa tarsi

Ossa metatarsi

Ossa digitorum
[Phalangesphalan]

a

Flat bones

**Flat bones
(Ossa plana)**

Cranial sutures

b

**Irregular bones
(Ossa irregularia)**

Vertebra

c

**Short bones
(Ossa brevia)**

Ossa carpi

d

**Pneumatic bones
(Ossa pneumatica)**

Sinus maxillaris

e

**Long bones
(Ossa longa)**

f Humerus

**Sesamoid bones
(Ossa sesamoidea)**

Patella

g

Fig. 1.19a–g   Skeleton, Systema sceletale, and types of bones; ventral view. [S700-L127]

a Overview of the bones of the skeleton.

b Flat bones (Ossa plana), e. g. ribs, sternum, scapula, ileum and bones of the skull.

c Irregular bones (Ossa irregularia) cannot be assigned to other bones, e. g. vertebrae and mandible.

d Short bones (Ossa brevia), e. g. carpal bone and tarsal bone.

e Pneumatic bones (Ossa pneumatica), e. g. frontal bone, ethmoid bone, sphenoid bone, maxilla and temporal bone.

f Long bones (Ossa longa), e. g. tubular bones of the extremities, such as the femur and humerus.

g Sesamoid bones (Ossa sesamoidea) are embedded in tendons, e. g. patella and pisiform bone.

Accessory bones (Ossa accessoria) are not normally found in all human skeletons, e. g. sutural bones of the skull or the cervical ribs.

Structure and composition of extremities

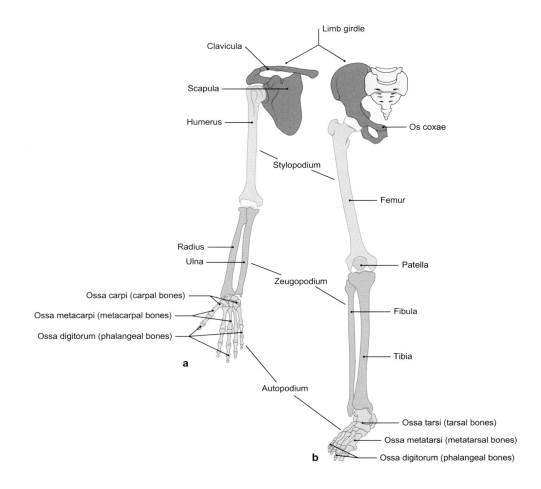

Fig. 1.20a and b   Structure and composition of the extremities; of the right side. [S700-L126]
a Upper extremity.
b Lower extremity.
The extremities are composed of a **limb girdle** (purple) and the **free limbs** (light blue, red and green). The clavicle and scapula form the shoulder girdle; the Os coxae represents the pelvic girdle. The free extremities (limbs) are composed of a **stylopodium** (blue), **zeugopodium** (red) and **autopodium** (green). The stylopodium always consists of a single bone (humerus or femur) and the zeugopodium consists of two bones (ulna and radius or tibia and fibula). The autopodium is composed of several individual bones which are divided into **basipodium** (carpal and tarsal bones), **metapodium** (metacarpal and metatarsal bones) and **acropodium** (phalangeal bones).

General anatomy

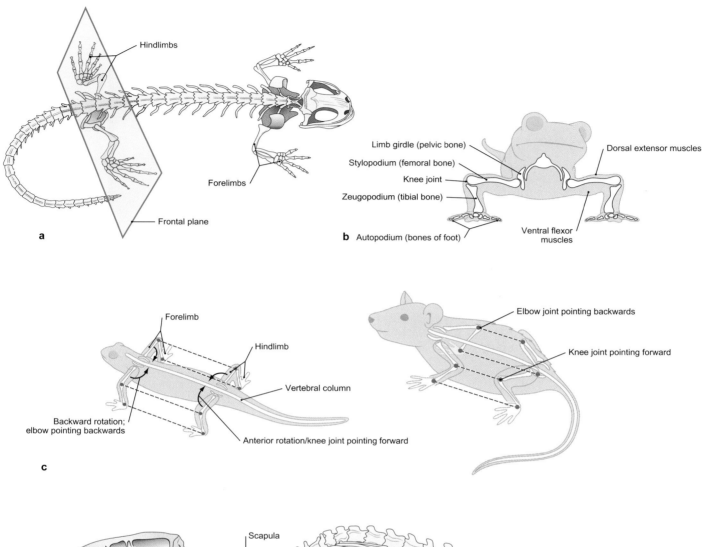

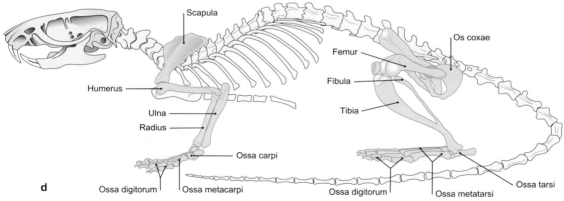

Fig. 1.21a–d Changes in limb positioning during evolution.
[S700-L126]

a Positioning of the limbs in a lizard (a lizard skeleton as an example of a primitive four-legged vertebrate), superior dorsal view.
b S‹eleton of a lizard; anterior view.
c Rotation of limb positioning during evolution from ancestors of mammals (lizards) to mammals (mouse).
d Skeleton of a rat, extremities in green.

In lower vertebrates, muscles and ligaments connect the limb girdle with the spine and the extremities are positioned almost at a right angle to the torso (**a,** green plane, and **b**). The stylopodium and zeugopodium as well as zeugopodium and autopodium are positioned almost perpendicularly to each other. Body movements thus require extensive flexibility in the spine and proportionately involve the action of many muscles. The gait appears sluggish. During the evolution from lower vertebrates to mammals, the position of the limbs rotated towards the torso **(c)**. Hereby the frontal extremities were repositioned further back and closer to the torso, while the extremities at the tail end moved further forwards towards the head. As a result, in humans, the elbow points backwards and the knee forwards **(d)**. This repositioning of the limbs in a sagittal plane close to the torso significantly reduced the lever arms of the limb muscles. This reduced the muscle mass and created a lighter and more nimble body (advantageous for flight or hunting).

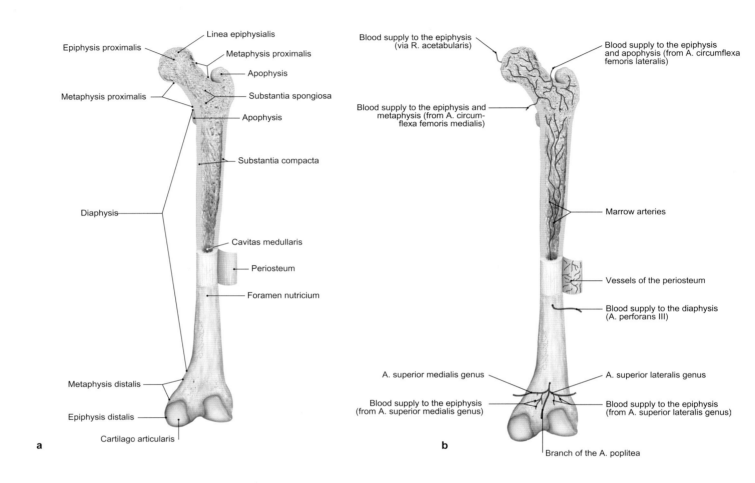

Fig. 1.22a and b   Structure and blood supply of a long bone.
a [S700], b [S701]

a Structure of a long bone, Os longum; section through the proximal part of the right thigh bone (femur) of an adult. In the diaphysis (bone shaft), the periosteum (bone membrane) is peeled away; dorsal view. Macroscopically, two different types of bone tissue can be distinguished, merging together without sharp edges:

- Substantia compacta (**compact bone** or cortical bone) is very thin in the epiphysis (end of the bone), but a strong and solid mass in the diaphysis.
- Substantia spongiosa (**Spongiosa,** spongy bone) is only well-developed in the epi- and metaphysis (bone portion between dia- and epiphysis) and forms a three-dimensional system of fine, branching rod-like bones **(trabeculae),** which are differentiated as either tensile or compressive trabeculae by the amount of stress. The special cancellous or porous structure is only clearly visible in the epi- and metaphysis. The space in-between the trabeculae is filled with blood-forming red bone marrow (young person) or fatty yellow bone marrow (old person). The trabeculae are parallel to the lines of tensile and compressive stress generated within the bone. (In the femur, these forces are proximal and eccentric, adding additional

bending stress to the bone.) In a long evolutionary process, bones have developed the greatest possible mechanical robustness with the least possible amount of material and weight.

The Foramen nutricium, to which the Canalis nutricius (running diagonally through the compact bone) is attached, is the entry point for the vessels into and out of the bone marrow (blood supply to the diaphysis). In the area of the meta- and epiphysis there are also numerous differently sized holes in the thinner cortical bone, which in particular supply blood to the epiphyses.

b Blood supply of a long bone with the femur as an example. [S700]
Only the arteries are illustrated. The blood supply to the diaphysis takes place via the **Vasa nutricia** (normally two with the femur illustrated). In the area of metaphyses and epiphyses, the cortical bone is thinner and pierced by many differently sized holes, through which the local blood vessels (supplying blood to the epiphyses in particular) enter. The entry points of these vessels are not referred to as Foramen nutricia. **Nutrient arteries** embedded in marrow are found in the centre of the diaphysis and the outer cortical bone is supplied by the **richly vascularised periosteum** (→ Fig. 1.25b). For the blood supply to the rest of the cortical bone, → Fig. 1.25a.

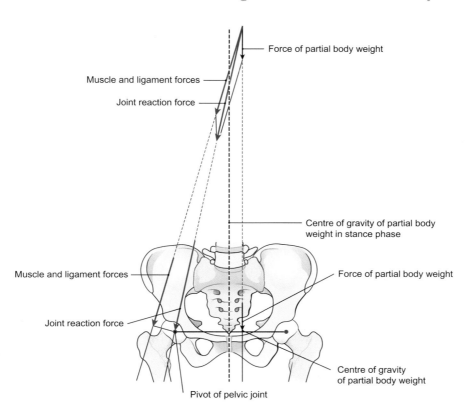

Force of partial body weight

Muscle and ligament forces

Joint reaction force

Centre of gravity of partial body weight in stance phase

Muscle and ligament forces

Force of partial body weight

Joint reaction force

Centre of gravity of partial body weight

Pivot of pelvic joint

Fig. 1.23 Vector forces projecting into the bone, demonstrated by the proximal femur in midstance. [S702-L126]
The **joint reaction force vector** (red arrow) projects through the pivot point of the hip joint and represents the true force impacting on a joint. The forces contributing to the joint reaction force vector are the partial body weight (here shown as the entire upper body from head to hip joint, black arrow) plus the forces of the muscles and ligaments stabilising the gait (blue arrow). In this vector model, forces derived from the muscles and ligaments that antagonise the force of the partial body weight stretch between hipbone and shin bone and are located on the upper leg (Tractus

iliotibialis, M. tensor fasciae latae, M. gluteus maximus and M. vastus lateralis).
In areas of higher force impact (compression load), the compact layer of the bone (Substantia compacta) is more dense. An example is the frontal plane of the femur where the higher bending forces result in a thicker cortical bone on the medial side (e.g. as Linea aspera). The joint force vector on the hip joint is higher with a one-legged versus a two-legged stance because one hip joint carries the entire body weight; this force is reduced only slightly by muscle contractions and ligaments in the stabilising leg.

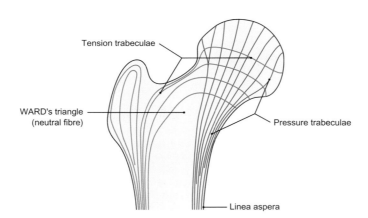

Tension trabeculae

WARD's triangle (neutral fibre)

Pressure trabeculae

Linea aspera

Fig. 1.24 Functional adjustment of bones with the proximal femur as an example. [S702-L126]/[E821]
Compact (cortical) bone and spongy (trabecular) bone adapt to the amount of stress the bone experiences. In areas of higher force (pressure), the compact bone is thicker **(quantitative adaptation).** As for the femur, the medial side has thicker cortical bone (Linea aspera) because in its frontal plane the bone is exposed to a strong bending force. Compressive and traction forces which are applied to the bone are absorbed through the

alignment of the spongy trabeculae, which form pressure trabeculae (pressure trajectories) and tension trabeculae (tension trajectories) **(qualitative adaptation).** Pressure trajectories are compressed (compression trajectories), while tension trajectories are stretched (expansion trajectories). Bone regions not subjected to any stress do not form spongy bone. This is referred to as **neutral fibre.** In the femur it does not appear as fibre but as WARD's triangle.

Clinical remarks

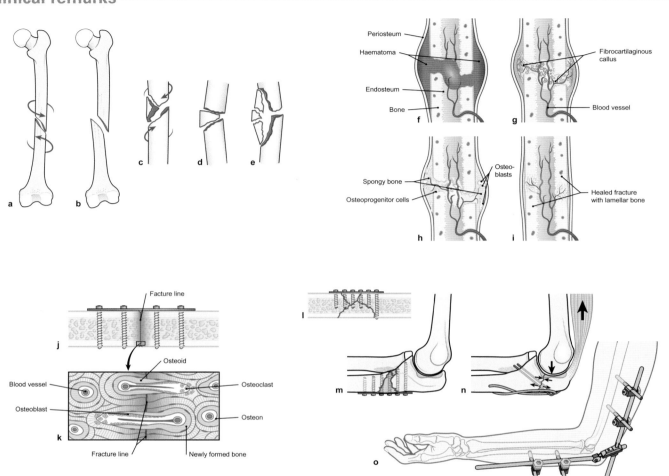

A **fracture** occurs when the bone is stressed beyond its physical limits. Two or more fragments can then be displaced. Based on the shape of the fracture, there are several fracture types:

- Spiral fracture (→ Fig. a)
- Oblique fracture +/- displacement (→ Fig. b)
- Spiral fracture with triangular bone fragment (→ Fig. c)
- Triangular 'butterfly' facture (→ Fig. d)
- Comminuted fracture (→ Fig. e).

Definite signs of a **fracture** include sudden pain, abnormal mobility, grinding sounds upon movement (crepitation), axis misalignment, initial muscle stupor (lack of muscle activity), and corresponding X-ray findings. The **healing of a fracture** ideally occurs under complete refrainment from load-bearing and movement. Under these conditions, the broken pieces will be restored to full load-bearing capacity; correspondingly also in long bones with recovery of the medullary cavity. For the healing of a fracture, the blood supply to the bone has a central role (especially in fractures in the area of articular capsules and when osteosynthesis measures are involved). **Primary** fracture-healing without callus formation can only occur when the gap between the fractured bones is small and the fracture ends are fixed in place (e. g. upon operative osteosynthesis with optimal alignment of the fracture ends using plates and screws)(→ Fig. j). During primary fracture-healing, the fracture gap is bridged by capillaries from opened HAVERSIAN canals, surrounded by osteons that stretch across the gap (→ Fig. k). **Secondary** fracture-healing frequently results in extensive **callus** formation which is then gradually converted into functional bone mass. This process is similar to wound-healing. Initially, blood enters the fracture gap (haematoma) and an inflamma-

tory reaction occurs (**inflammatory phase,** → Fig. f). This activates pluripotent mesenchymal stem cells which then differentiate into cells which can rebuild bone and interstitial tissue structures. Blood vessels sprout and enter the fracture site. This initiates the **granulation phase** resulting in the formation of a soft callus within the next four to six weeks (→ Fig. g). The replacement of soft callus with hard callus (**bony callus formation phase**) includes the gradual transformation of granulation tissue to cartilaginous tissue and then bony tissue (→ Fig. h), a process that takes approx. three to four months. Final functional remodeling of this newly formed bone occurs over a period of 6–24 months (**remodeling phase,** → Fig. i).

Osteosynthesis utilises screws, plates, wire implants and nails to stabilise and align bone fragments so they can ideally undergo primary fracture-healing. Although osteosynthesis cannot accelerate or replace the bone-healing process, optimal repositioning and stabilisation of the alignment of the bone fragments enables immediate mobilisation of patients and early onset of physiotherapy. Overall, this significantly reduces the risk of post-operative complications such as thrombosis, embolism, cutaneous ulcerations, oedema and dystrophic tissue events. Risks associated with osteosynthesis include side effects of the anaesthesia and wound infections. Examples of osteosynthesis shown are plate osteosynthesis with the use of plates in a comminuted fracture (→ Fig. l) or complex fracture of the ulna (→ Fig. m), tension band wiring osteosynthesis of Kirschner wires of a ruptured olecranon (→ Fig. n) and an external fixator osteosynthesis (a three-dimensional frame for the transcutaneous holding of broken bones in a complex ulnar fracture)(→ Fig. o). [S700-L126]

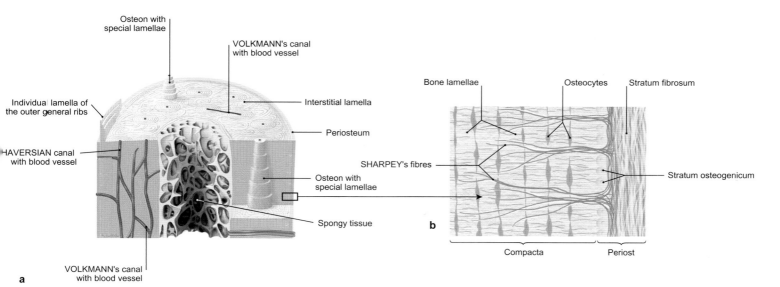

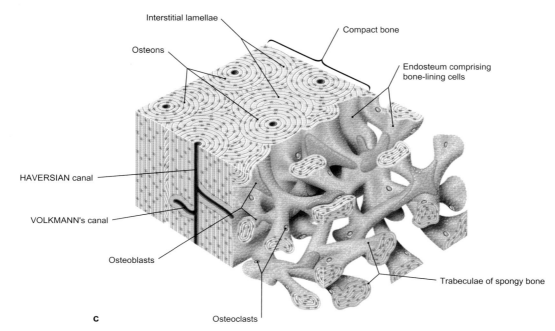

Fig. 1.25a–c Structure of a long bone, Os longum, of the bone membrane, periosteum and endosteum. [S700-L127]

a The basic histological structure of the mature bone is similar for the compact (cortical) and spongy bone and is referred to as **lamellar bone.** The building units of the mature bone are bone lamellae that form tubular systems **(osteons)** particularly in the compact bone. In the spongy bone the lamellae are predominantly parallel to the surface of the trabeculae. In the compact bone, bony lamellae can form osteons encasing blood vessels, a system (HAVERSIAN system) made up of approx. five to 20 bony lamellae **(special lamellae),** which are arranged concentrically around a HAVERSIAN canal and can be a few centimetres in length. The collagen fibrils in the **osteon lamellae** run in screw-like coils, with the direction of rotation changing in each lamella. Remains of old degraded osteons fill the space between the intact osteons **(interstitial lamellae).** The outer and inner surface of the compact bone is composed of lamellae that surround the whole bone (outer and inner **general lamellae**).

b The highly innervated **bone membrane (periosteum)** covers the outer surface of the bone and consists of the external fibrous sheath made of collagen fibrils. These collagen fibrils, named SHARPEY's fibres, radiate from the fibrous sheath into the compact bone and secure the periosteum to the bone. The inner surface of the periosteum contains the Stratum osteogenicum. It lies directly on the bone and is made from the same cells that line the inner bone surfaces as en(d)osteum. From here, reconstruction and repair processes originate.

c The lamellae of the spongy bone are also made of osteons and are covered by one to two layers of the bone-lining cells that form the **endosteum.** The surfaces of the HAVERSIAN and VOLKMANN's canals are also lined with endosteum which constitute up to 90 %, the remaining cells being quiescent osteoblasts (bone-forming cells) and osteoclasts (bone-resorbing cells). Approximately 10 % of the bone surface is covered with activated **osteoblasts** (pink layer) and **osteoclasts** (green cells) which resemble areas of active **bone remodelling.** The carpet-like assembly of activated osteoblasts generates new bone, whereas osteoclasts resorb bone. Because the larger osteoclasts quickly resorb bone, one osteoclast can resorb the same amount of bony material produced by hundreds of osteoblasts.

Musculoskeletal system

Bone marrow

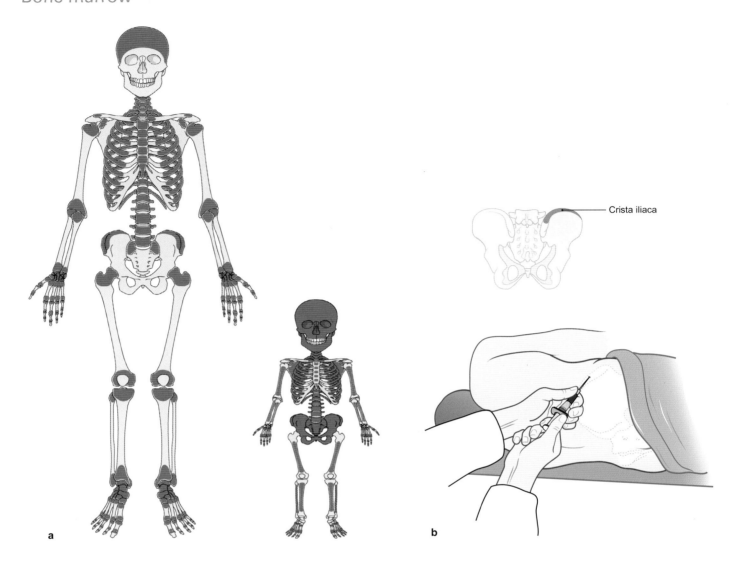

Crista iliaca

a

b

Fig. 1.26a and b   Bone marrow and bone marrow aspiration.
a Spatial distribution of, blood-forming **red none marrow** and **fatty** yellow **bone marrow.** In the fetal period, formation of the blood begins in the yolk sac and is gradually replaced by blood formation sites in the liver and spleen. From the fifth month of life, blood formation begins in the bone marrow and in a child virtually extends to all of the bone marrow. In adults, red bone marrow (Medulla ossium rubra) is found only in the epiphyses of long bones and in certain areas of the remaining bones. Otherwise, yellow bone marrow (Medulla ossium flava) is found (mainly diaphyses), which, if

necessary, can be converted into red bone marrow in a short space of time. Red bone marrow fulfils the task of blood formation; yellow bone marrow consists mainly of fatty and connective tissue. [S700-L127]
b For a **bone marrow aspiration,** the Spina iliaca posterior superior and the Crista iliaca can easily be felt under the skin. The biopsy needle is introduced into the bone at this site. The schematic drawing above shows the area of the red bone marrow that is to be punctured or aspirated. [S700-L126]

⌐ Clinical remarks

Under both physiological conditions (e. g. altitude training) and pathological conditions (e. g. significant blood loss) the yellow bone marrow in the diaphyses of adults can be converted back into red bone marrow in a short time to produce more blood for the body. If the stimulus (altitude training) disappears or the blood supply is balanced, yellow bone marrow forms again. A **bone marrow aspiration** is carried out for diagnostic reasons (e. g. a bone marrow biopsy) on

suspicion of a disorder of the haematopoietic system (e. g. leukaemia), or for therapeutic reasons (e. g. collection of healthy bone marrow from a donor for subsequent treatment of leukaemia in a recipient). The most common site for a bone marrow aspiration is the iliac crest **(iliac crest lumbar aspiration)** due to its accessibility. An aspiration at the sternum (sternal aspiration) is now only very rarely carried out.

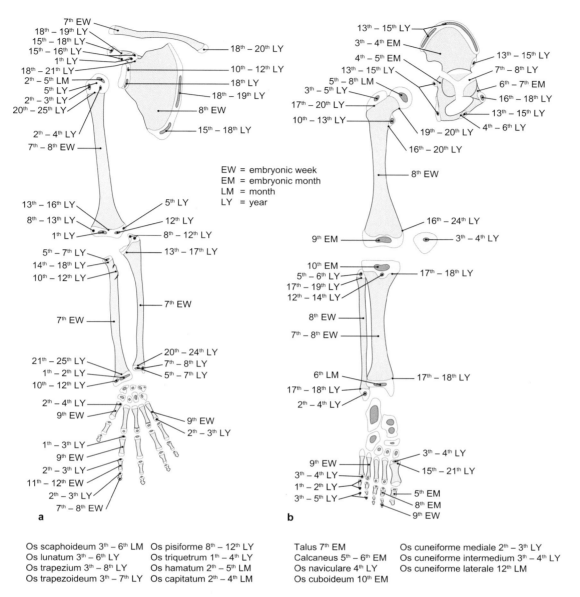

EW = embryonic week
EM = embryonic month
LM = month
LY = year

Os scaphoideum 3th – 6th LM	Os pisiforme 8th – 12th LY
Os lunatum 3th – 6th LY	Os triquetrum 1th – 4th LY
Os trapezium 3th – 8th LY	Os hamatum 2th – 5th LM
Os trapezoideum 3th – 7th LY	Os capitatum 2th – 4th LM

Talus 7th EM	Os cuneiforme mediale 2th – 3th LY
Calcaneus 5th – 6th EM	Os cuneiforme intermedium 3th – 4th LY
Os naviculare 4th LY	Os cuneiforme laterale 12th LM
Os cuboideum 10th EM	

Fig. 1.27a and b Ossification of the skeleton; location of epi- and apophysis bone cores and chronological sequence for bone core formation. [S702-L126]
a Upper limb.
b Lower limb.

Bone development **(osteogenesis) begins with consolidation of embryonic connective tissue (mesenchymal consolidation).** There are two types of bone development:

- In **desmal osteogenesis,** the mesenchymal cells are directly differentiated from the bone-forming cells (osteoblasts), which produce bone tissue (ossification). The resulting bone is also called the **connective tissue bone** (desmal bone). An example of this is the clavicle.
- In **chondral osteogenesis,** cartilage-forming cells (chondroblasts) arising from the mesenchymal cells initially create a cartilage model of the future bone (primordial skeleton out of hyaline cartilage). The cartilage model is then transformed into bone:
  - In the area of diaphysis, **perichondrium ossification** occurs with development of a perichondrium bone sleeve (the processes that occur correspond to those in desmal osteogenesis).

  - In the area of metaphysis, **enchondral ossification** occurs in the form of the development of a growth plate which is detectable until the completion of bone growth (see textbooks on histology). The resulting bone is also called **replacement bone** (cartilage bone).

The timing for the appearance of these **ossification centres** holds clues as to the stage reached in skeletal development and, thus, to the individual skeletal and bone age. A distinction is made between primary ossification centres, which during the fetal period emerge in the area of the diaphyses **(diaphyseal ossification),** and the endochondral ossification of the primordial cartilaginous epi- and apophyses as well as the marginal rims of the flat bones, which begins, with the exception of the distal epiphysis of the femur and the proximal epiphysis of the tibia (maturity signs), only after birth **(secondary or epi- and apophyseal ossification).** With the closing of the epiphyseal plates (synostosis), length growth is complete. Thereafter, isolated ossification centres are no longer visible in X-ray images.

Clinical remarks

For the planning of treatment and the prognosis of orthopaedic diseases and deformities in childhood, determining the skeletal age and any existing growth reserves is of great importance. Epiphyseal plate injuries (e.g. from fractures near joints), are feared, especially in the area of the lower extremity, because growth disorders can lead to a difference in leg length or be associated with misaligned joints.

General anatomy

Bone joints

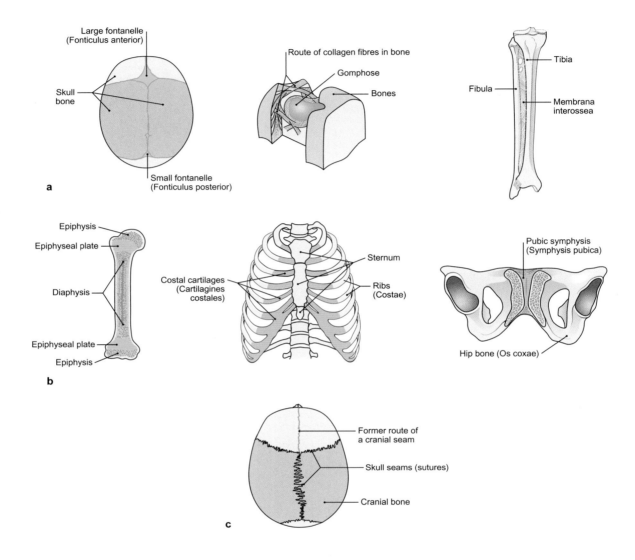

a
- Large fontanelle (Fonticulus anterior)
- Skull bone
- Small fontanelle (Fonticulus posterior)

- Route of collagen fibres in bone
- Gomphose
- Bones

- Tibia
- Fibula
- Membrana interossea

b
- Epiphysis
- Epiphyseal plate
- Diaphysis
- Epiphyseal plate
- Epiphysis

- Costal cartilages (Cartilagines costales)
- Sternum
- Ribs (Costae)

- Pubic symphysis (Symphysis pubica)
- Hip bone (Os coxae)

c
- Former route of a cranial seam
- Skull seams (sutures)
- Cranial bone

Fig. 1.28a–c   Synarthrosis (fibrous, cartilaginous and bony joints). [S702-L126]

a Fibrous joints, Junctura fibrosa (syndesmosis). Bone joints connected with connective tissue are referred to as fibrous joints. These include sutures (cranial sutures), syndesmoses (e. g. the connection between the tibia and fibula) and gomphoses (e. g. anchorage of the teeth in the dental alveoli of the maxilla and mandible).

b Cartilaginous joints, Junctura cartilaginea (synchondrosis). In cartilaginous joints, the bones are connected by **hyaline** cartilage (synchondrosis, e. g. epiphyseal plates or the connection between the ribs and the sternum) or by **fibrous cartilage** (symphysis, e. g. Symphysis pubica).

c Bony joints, Junctura ossea (synostosis). In bony joints, the bones are **fused** together, e. g. on the frontal bone of the skull. Synostoses originate from syndesmoses and synchondroses.

Clinical remarks

Laryngeal anchylosis and arthrodesis

Anchylosis may occur when two bones within an existing joint (e. g. after a joint infection or by immobilisation) become fused. The example shown is a one-sided anchylosis of neighbouring partially ossified cricoid and arytenoid cartilages, resulting from intubation damage, with consecutive hoarseness of voice on the side of the anchylosis (→ Fig. a). The normal larynx anatomy is shown on the left. In the normal larynx, cricoid and arytenoid cartilages are connected by a true joint, the Articulatio cricoarytenoidea. The partial ossification of cricoid and arytenoid cartilages is a physiological process but does not normally involve the formation of anchyloses.

Disorders in joint development can lead to the fusion of skeletal elements resulting in synostosis **(Coalitiones;** → Fig. b). Synostoses are especially common in the skeleton of the hand and foot. The stiffening of a joint for therapeutic reasons is known as **arthrodesis** (the example shown is a classical LAMBRINUDI arthrodesis for the treatment of adult drop-foot). A 'false' joint can develop as a result of unsuccessful fracture-healing and is known as a **pseudoarthrosis.** [S700-L126]

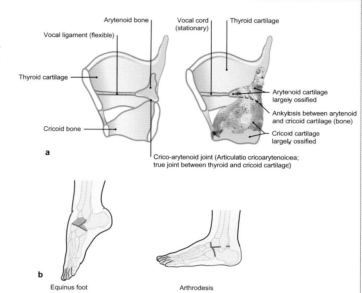

a

Crico-arytenoid joint (Articulatio cricoarytenoicea; true joint between thyroid and cricoid cartilage)

b

Equinus foot   Arthrodesis

Glossary of clinical terminology on joints	
Anchylosis	Joint stiffness due to a fibrous or bony connection of two bones across a joint
Arthritis	Inflammation of one or more joints
Arthrodesis	Surgically induced artificial induction of joint ossification between two bones
Arthrography	Radiological imaging of joints upon injection of a contrast agent
Arthroplasty	Surgical joint reconstruction or replacement
Osteoarthritis	Degenerative joint condition
Arthroscopy	Minimally invasive diagnostic and/or therapeutic inspection and/or treatment of a joint upon arthrotomy and insertion of an endoscopic device (arthroscope)
Arthrotomy	Surgical opening of a joint
Joint prosthesis	Surgical replacement arthroplasty with use of a prosthetic implant
Joint aspiration	Insertion of a needle into the joint cavity for several different medical purposes
Pseudoarthrosis	'False joint' caused by failed ossification of fractured bony ends which are joined by fibrous connections instead
Synovectomy	Arthroscopic procedure to remove inflamed synovial tissue (Membrana synovialis)

Musculoskeletal system

Bone joints

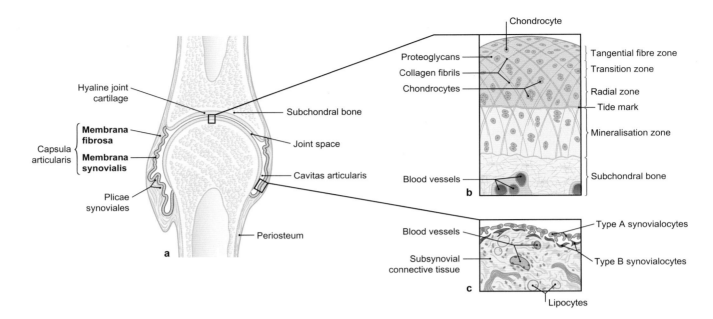

Fig. 1.29a–c   Synovial (movable) joint, Junctura synovialis [Articulatio, diarthrosis] (a) with development of joint cartilage (b) and joint capsule (c); schematic section. The joint-moving muscles and the joint capsule-strengthening ligaments are not represented.

a Structure of the joint. The bone ends are covered by hyaline articular cartilage, below which lies the subchondral bone. The joint capsule encloses the joint space and consists of an outer **fibrous membrane** and an inner **synovial membrane.** The synovial membrane secretes the joint lubrication (synovia) into the joint cavity, which serves as nourishment for the joint cartilage and parts of the intra-articular structures and lubrication (friction-free gliding of the joint surfaces), and also as a shock absorber (even distribution of compressive forces). Amphiarthroses are joints of very limited mobility due to a particularly firm joint capsule (e.g. small joints in the wrist and ankle; Articulatio sacroiliaca). [S702-L126]/ [X389~M282]

b Structure of hyaline cartilage. The joint surfaces are covered by a layer of hyaline cartilage (joint cartilage) of varying thickness. Fibrous cartilage is found only in the mandibular and sternoclavicular joints. Cartilage thickness depends on the stress (finger joints 1–2 mm, Os sacrum

4 mm, patella 6–7 mm). The cartilage cells (chondrocytes) form an extracellular matrix from proteoglycans (water-binding) and collagen fibrils. The latter are aligned in the joint cartilage and form arcades (BENNINGHOFF's arcade scheme), which can be divided into different zones (tangential fibre zone, transition zone and radial zone). The tide mark forms the border between non-mineralised and mineralised cartilage (mineralisation zone). The joint cartilage is fixed to the subchondral bone, forms a smooth surface and reduces friction between the joint bodies. It distributes the pressure on the subchondral bone. [S702-L126]

c Structure of the joint capsule. The joint capsule consists of the fibrous membrane and the synovial membrane. The **Membrana fibrosa** is made of dense connective tissue. The **Membrana synovialis** is composed of the following layers: a superficial loose layer of A cells (type A synovialocytes or M cells, specialised macrophages which take up the compounds of the joint cartilage metabolism), B cells (type B synovialocytes or F cells, active fibroblasts which produce collagen and proteoglycans, including the hyaluronic acid of the synovia) and the subsynovial connective tissue which is rich in capillaries, fibroblasts and lipocytes. [S702-L126]

Joints	
Immobile joints (synarthroses, continuous joints)	**Mobile joints (diarthroses, discontinuous joints) (→ Fig. 1.30)**
Characteristics: • Filling tissue consisting of connective tissue, cartilage or bone between the skeletal elements (plates, joints) • No joint space • Low to moderate mobility	**Characteristics:** • Articulating skeletal elements • Joint space • Joint surfaces capped with cartilage (Facies articularis) • Joint cavity (Cavitas articularis) • Surrounding joint capsule (Capsula articularis) • Joint capsule-strengthening ligaments • Depending on the ligaments, good or restricted mobility • Muscles that move and stabilise the joint
Types of synarthroses (→ Fig. 1.28) • Syndesmoses (fibrous joints) • Synchondroses (cartilaginous joints with mainly fibrous cartilage = symphysis) • Synostoses (bony joints, no movement possible)	**Types of diarthroses** based on: • Shape and form of the joints (→ Fig. 1.30) • Number of movement axes (one, two, several) • Number of articulating skeletal elements (simple joints = Articulationes simplice, composite joints = Articulationes compositates) **Amphiarthroses** (fixed joints) are rigid joints in that they have a severely limited range of motion as the joints are connected by tight ligaments.

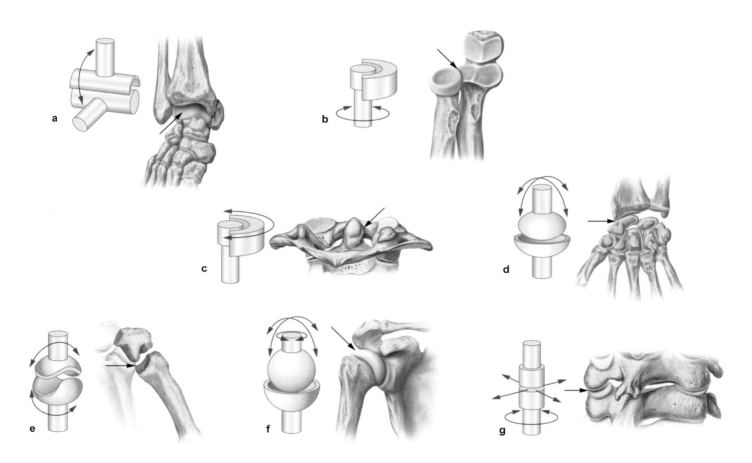

Fig. 1.30a–g   Joints, synovial joints (Articulationes, diarthroses). [S702-L127]

Joints usually have a significant range of motion. They are divided according to their shape and possible movements. A distinction is made according to the number of their main axes (corresponding to the body axes) as uniaxial, biaxial and multiaxial joints.

a Hinge joint, Articulatio cylindrica (ginglymus): uniaxial joint, with which flexion and extension is possible (e.g. Articulatio talocruralis)

b Pivot joint, Articulatio conoidea: uniaxial joint which allows rotational movements (e.g. Articulatio radioulnaris proximalis)

c Wheel joint, Articulatio trochoidea: uniaxial joint which allows rotational movements (e.g. Articulatio atlantoaxialis mediana)

d Ovoid joint, Articulatio ovoidea, Articulatio ellipsoidea: biaxial joint which allows flexion, extension, abduction, adduction and slight circumduction (e.g. proximal wrist joint)

e Saddle joint, Articulatio sellaris: biaxial joint which allows flexion, extension, abduction, adduction and slight circumduction (e.g. carpometacarpal thumb joint)

f Ball joint, Articulatio spheroidea: multiaxial joint which allows flexion, extension, abduction, adduction, medial rotation, lateral rotation and circumduction (e.g. shoulder joint)

g Plane joint, Articulatio plana: joint which allows simple gliding movements in different directions (e.g. vertebral joint)

General anatomy

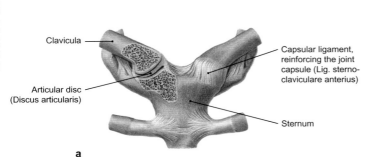

Clavicula

Articular disc
(Discus articularis)

Capsular ligament,
reinforcing the joint
capsule (Lig. sterno-
claviculare anterius)

Sternum

a

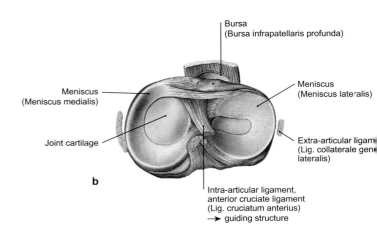

Bursa
(Bursa infrapatellaris profunda)

Meniscus
(Meniscus medialis)

Joint cartilage

Meniscus
(Meniscus lateralis)

Extra-articular ligament
(Lig. collaterale genu
lateralis)

Intra-articular ligament,
anterior cruciate ligament
(Lig. cruciatum anterius)
→ guiding structure

b

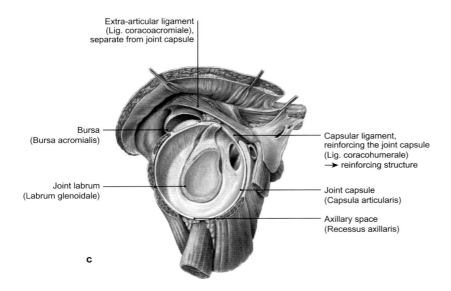

Extra-articular ligament
(Lig. coracoacromiale),
separate from joint capsule

Bursa
(Bursa acromialis)

Joint labrum
(Labrum glenoidale)

Capsular ligament,
reinforcing the joint capsule
(Lig. coracohumerale)
→ reinforcing structure

Joint capsule
(Capsula articularis)

Axillary space
(Recessus axillaris)

c

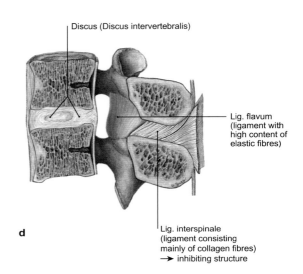

Discus (Discus intervertebralis)

Lig. flavum
(ligament with
high content of
elastic fibres)

Lig. interspinale
(ligament consisting
mainly of collagen fibres)
→ inhibiting structure

d

Fig. 1.31a–d   Auxiliary structures of joints. [S700]
Many joints have intra-articular auxiliary structures which are necessary for the biomechanical functioning and range of movement of the joints: **intra-articular discs** are used to compensate for incongruities (unevenness) between the articulating joint surfaces. They redistribute the compressive forces acting on them. Intra-articular discs occur as complete discs (**discus** = full moon, e.g. Discus articularis of the sternoclavicular joint **[a]** or Discus intervertebralis **[d]** in the spine) or as part of a disc (**meniscus** = crescent moon, e.g. Meniscus medialis and lateralis of the knee joint **[b]**). **Joint lips** (labra) are made of dense connective tissue and fibrous cartilage, are secured via a bony ring (limbus) and are used for the enlargement of the joint socket (e.g. joint **labrum** in the shoulder joint **[c]**). **Synovial bursae** (Bursae synoviales) are small fluid-filled sacs (like cushions) that occur in areas of joints with increased mechanical stress. They reduce the pressure or tension-based friction between tendons, muscles, bones or the skin. Like joint capsules, they have an outer fibrous sheath and an inner synovial sheath. The latter forms the liquid released from the inside of the little sac (synovia). According to their location they are subdi-

vided into skin bursae **(Bursa subcutanea),** tendon bursae (Bursa subtendinea, e.g. Bursa infrapatellaris profunda **[b]**) and ligament bursae (Bursa subligamentosa, e.g. Bursa subacromialis **[c]**). **Ligaments** (Ligamenta) are made of dense collagenous connective tissue and are used for connecting and fixing movable skeletal elements. They occur as **intra-articular ligaments** (e.g. **Ligamentum** cruciatum anterius **[b]**) within joints or as **extra-articular ligaments** (e.g. Lig. collaterale genus tibiale **[b]**). The extra-articular ligaments integrated in the joint capsule are called **capsular ligaments** (e.g. Lig. sternoclaviculare anterius **[a]** or Lig. coracohumerale **[c]**). They are contraposed to **extra-capsular ligaments,** which have no association with the joint capsule. Functionally **reinforcing ligaments** (e.g. Lig. sternoclaviculare anterius **[a]** or Lig. coracohumerale **[c]**) can be distinguished from **guiding ligaments** (e.g. Lig. cruciatum anterius **[b]**) and **restraining ligaments** (e.g. Lig. interspinale **[d]**). Usually ligaments have several functions or additional features. The Ligamenta flava passing through the vertebral arch **[d]** have a high proportion of elastic fibres.

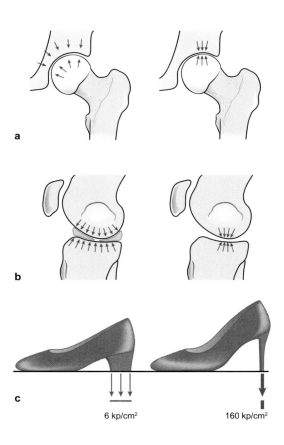

a

b

c

6 kp/cm²   160 kp/cm²

Fig. 1.32a–c   Joint stress.
The size of the load-bearing area of a joint determines the degree of joint stress. The larger the load-bearing area of a joint, the better it can distribute these forces across the wider area, with less joint stress as a result per unit of area.

a Optimal joint stress conditions with even force distribution across the whole joint (left); unfavourable joint stress associated with Coxa valga, which results in a small joint area being exposed to the majority of the mechanical force (right) with a risk of developing osteoarthritis. [S700-L126]/[G1060-001]

b Joint stress in the knee joint with menisces (left) and without (right). [S700-L126]/[G1060-001]

c An example of distribution of mechanical forces as generated by the heel parts of block-heeled (left) and spike-heeled shoes (right). [S700-L126]/[E262-1]

Clinical remarks

Degenerative changes are common in certain joints and are known as **osteoarthritis** or arthrosis (joint wear). In Germany alone, approximately 5–6 million people suffer from osteoarthritis (degenerative arthropathy). It is the most common disease seen by the family physician and is a slow degenerative process (see image). Small cartilaginous bone segments shown as cross-sections (upper row) and the cartilaginous joint surface viewed from above (lower row).

a A healthy joint cartilage.

b Initially, the joint surface becomes rough and the proteoglycan content in the extracellular matrix decreases, resulting in the degradation of collagen fibres in deeper layers of the joint cartilage.

c With advancing osteoarthritis, the cartilage acquires deep fissures, cartilage matrix is rarified, the total number of chondrocytes decreases, with some losing the ability to divide, causing clusters of chondrocytes to form, and the subchondral bone compacts (sclerosing bone). This coincides with a non-infectious joint inflammation, reactive synovialitis (also called synovitis), that can lead to synovial fluid collection in the joint.

d In late stage osteoarthritis, the cartilage has been progressively worn down, resulting in a partial to complete loss of the cartilage layer with opposing subchondral bones exposed and directly rubbing against each other during joint movements. This can result in destruction of the subchondral sclerosing bone with bone necrosis, so-called bone cysts, and the formation of osteophytes (not shown) which are bony outgrowths in response to degenerative changes in the arthritic joint.

Rheumatoid arthritis is an immunological inflammatory disease primarily of the joint capsule and can lead to the destruction of joint cartilage. Often, this leads to an irritation of the Membrana synovialis and secretion of increased synovial fluid into the joint space, resulting in an **articular effusion**. This may cause the entire joint to become strained, painful and swollen. Trauma may lead to inflammation of a bursa **(bursitis)**. The bursa becomes swollen and this can affect the function of adjacent structures, such as nerves, through increased pressure and restricted movement in neighbouring joints. The chronic irritation of certain bursae in the knee joint area is recognised as an occupational disease in professions which are carried out predominantly kneeling (e. g. carpenters).

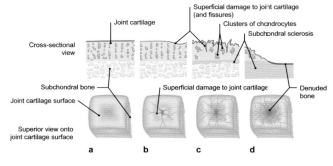

[S700-L126]/[G1060-001]

General anatomy

Range of movement in the joints

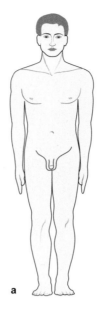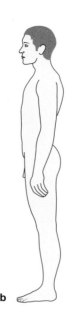

a

b

Fig. 1.33a and b Documentation for the range of movement in joints: neutral-zero-method. [S700-L126]
For a standardised documentation of the range of movement within the context of a joint examination, the neutral-zero-method is used. The joint positions are given using the stance of an upright person with arms hanging down as the neutral body starting position. The extent of movement

achieved from this neutral position is measured in angular degrees. The active range of movement away from the body is determined first, followed by the active range of movement towards the body.
a Neutral body position from the front.
b Neutral body position from the side.

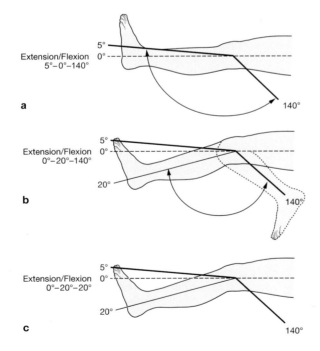

a

b

c

Extension/Flexion
5°–0°–140°

Extension/Flexion
0°–20°–140°

Extension/Flexion
0°–20°–20°

Fig. 1.34a–c Documentation for the range of movement in joints: examples. [S700-L126]
a The scope of movement of a normal healthy knee joint is a 5° extension and 140° flexion. The ankle joint is considered to be in a neutral-zero position at a right angle to the foot (90°). From this position, a 20° extension and 40° flexion is possible (not shown). The normal scope of movement for the knee joint is given as 5°–0°–140° (knee stretched, passing through the neutral-zero position, knee bent). For the ankle joint it is 20°–0°–40° (dorsiflexion, passing through the neutral-zero position, plantarflexion).
b Knee extension is not possible (text → Clinical remarks).
c Complete stiffening of the knee (text → Clinical remarks).

Clinical remarks

Limitations of joint movement are associated with a decreased range of movement. If joint movement is limited, or if the neutral-zero position of a joint is not achieved and there is contracture, this can be reproduced precisely with the neutral-zero-method.
For **limited mobility after flexion contracture,** the movement formula is, for example, 0°–20°–140° (→ Fig. 1.34b: knee extension not

possible, neutral-zero position is not achieved, knee bent at 20° and can be bent further to 140°). A **complete stiffening of the knee** due to ossification (anchylosis) results in the knee being fixed in a 20° angle of flexion. The movement formula is 0°–20°–20° (→ Fig. 1.34c: knee extension is not possible, neutral-zero position is not achieved, knee bent at 20° and cannot be bent further).

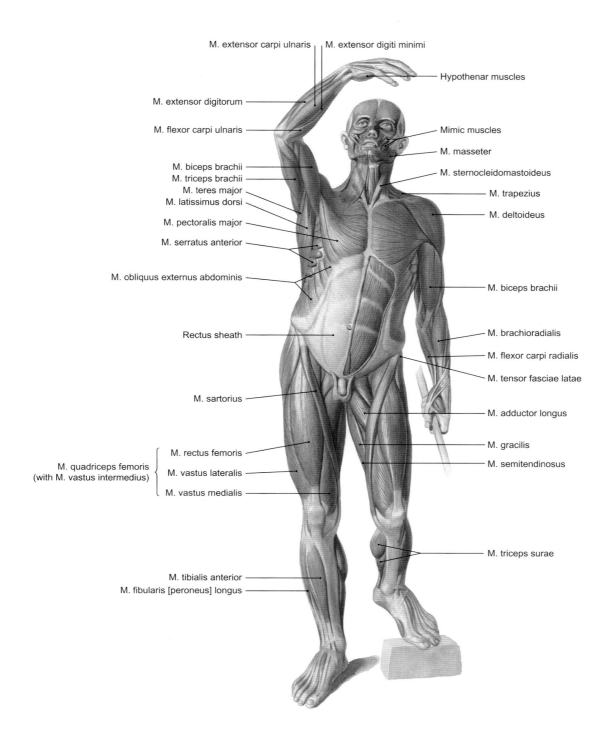

M. extensor carpi ulnaris
M. extensor digiti minimi
Hypothenar muscles
M. extensor digitorum
M. flexor carpi ulnaris
Mimic muscles
M. masseter
M. biceps brachii
M. triceps brachii
M. sternocleidomastoideus
M. teres major
M. trapezius
M. latissimus dorsi
M. deltoideus
M. pectoralis major
M. serratus anterior
M. obliquus externus abdominis
M. biceps brachii
M. brachioradialis
Rectus sheath
M. flexor carpi radialis
M. tensor fasciae latae
M. sartorius
M. adductor longus
M. gracilis
M. rectus femoris
M. semitendinosus
M. quadriceps femoris
(with M. vastus intermedius)
M. vastus lateralis
M. vastus medialis
M. triceps surae
M. tibialis anterior
M. fibularis [peroneus] longus

Fig. 1.35 Stabilising and movement muscles. [S700]

The 600+ muscles in the human body make up between 25 % (female) and 40 % (male) of the body weight, and use 20 % of the body's energy when at rest. This value can rise to 90 % during peak athletic performance. Functionally, within the working muscles also known as extrafusal muscles, a distinction is made between **stabilising muscles (tonic muscles)** and **movement muscles (phasic muscles).** The stabilising muscles **(red muscles)** are designed for continuous performance, tire slowly and have a very good blood vessel supply (e.g. Musculus adductor longus). The movement muscles **(white muscles)** are used for quick, short and powerful contractions, tire more quickly, are less well supplied with capillaries, and work primarily anaerobically (e.g. M. biceps brachii, Mm. vastus late-

ralis and medialis, M. tibialis anterior). People who do endurance sports (marathon runners) have more red muscles; people who do sports with short, sharp bursts of muscular activity (sprinters) have more white muscles.

A muscle (or muscle group) never moves alone, but is almost always dependent on one or more opponents (antagonists). Therefore, on the upper and lower extremities we have the extensors (agonists) and the flexors (antagonists). There are basically two types of muscular activity: **static and dynamic muscle.** With cycling, for example, the arm, neck and back muscles, in addition to the joint ligaments, perform static activity while keeping the torso and head steady, whereas the muscles involved in pedaling perform dynamic muscle activity.

Stabilising and movement muscles

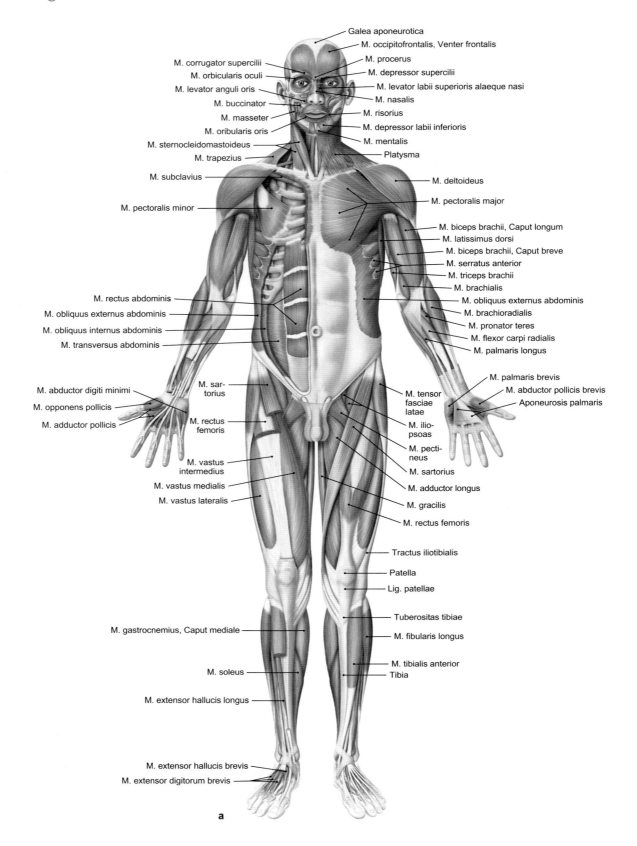

Galea aponeurotica
M. occipitofrontalis, Venter frontalis
M. corrugator supercilii
M. procerus
M. orbicularis oculi
M. depressor supercilii
M. levator anguli oris
M. levator labii superioris alaeque nasi
M. buccinator
M. nasalis
M. masseter
M. risorius
M. oribularis oris
M. depressor labii inferioris
M. sternocleidomastoideus
M. mentalis
M. trapezius
Platysma
M. subclavius
M. deltoideus
M. pectoralis minor
M. pectoralis major
M. biceps brachii, Caput longum
M. latissimus dorsi
M. biceps brachii, Caput breve
M. serratus anterior
M. triceps brachii
M. brachialis
M. rectus abdominis
M. obliquus externus abdominis
M. obliquus externus abdominis
M. brachioradialis
M. obliquus internus abdominis
M. pronator teres
M. transversus abdominis
M. flexor carpi radialis
M. palmaris longus
M. palmaris brevis
M. abductor digiti minimi
M. sar-torius
M. abductor pollicis brevis
M. opponens pollicis
Aponeurosis palmaris
M. adductor pollicis
M. rectus femoris
M. tensor fasciae latae
M. ilio-psoas
M. pecti-neus
M. vastus intermedius
M. sartorius
M. vastus medialis
M. adductor longus
M. vastus lateralis
M. gracilis
M. rectus femoris
Tractus iliotibialis
Patella
Lig. patellae
Tuberositas tibiae
M. gastrocnemius, Caput mediale
M. fibularis longus
M. tibialis anterior
M. soleus
Tibia
M. extensor hallucis longus
M. extensor hallucis brevis
M. extensor digitorum brevis

a

Fig. 1.36a Skeletal musculature; ventral view; some superficial muscles were removed on the right side to allow for a better overview. [S700-L275]

The human body contains approx. 220 fasciated skeletal muscles which can account for up to 40 % of the total body weight based on age, sex and the degree of fitness. The majority of skeletal muscles are working muscles and part of the active movement system. Some of the working muscles, particularly those located in the lower extremities, help maintain body posture (tonic or postural muscles), while other muscles enable active body movements (phasic muscles). Skeletal muscles are also found in the head-neck region. These include the skeletal muscles of facial expression, muscles of mastication, and muscles in the tongue, pharynx, larynx, eye and middle ear.

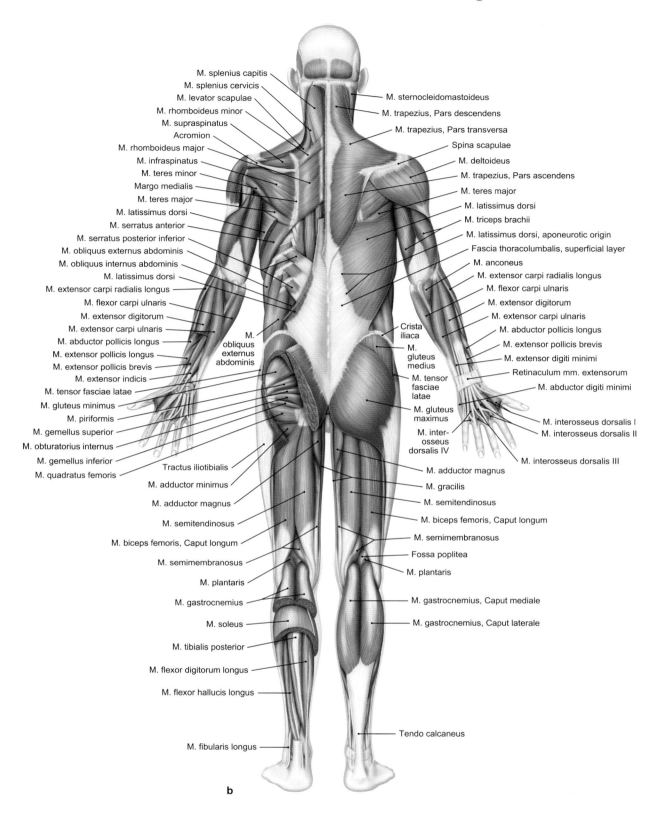

M. splenius capitis
M. splenius cervicis
M. levator scapulae
M. rhomboideus minor
M. supraspinatus
Acromion
M. rhomboideus major
M. infraspinatus
M. teres minor
Margo medialis
M. teres major
M. latissimus dorsi
M. serratus anterior
M. serratus posterior inferior
M. obliquus externus abdominis
M. obliquus internus abdominis
M. latissimus dorsi
M. extensor carpi radialis longus
M. flexor carpi ulnaris
M. extensor digitorum
M. extensor carpi ulnaris
M. abductor pollicis longus
M. extensor pollicis longus
M. extensor pollicis brevis
M. extensor indicis
M. tensor fasciae latae
M. gluteus minimus
M. piriformis
M. gemellus superior
M. obturatorius internus
M. gemellus inferior
M. quadratus femoris

M. obliquus externus abdominis

Tractus iliotibialis
M. adductor minimus
M. adductor magnus
M. semitendinosus
M. biceps femoris, Caput longum
M. semimembranosus
M. plantaris
M. gastrocnemius
M. soleus
M. tibialis posterior
M. flexor digitorum longus
M. flexor hallucis longus

M. fibularis longus

M. sternocleidomastoideus
M. trapezius, Pars descendens
M. trapezius, Pars transversa
Spina scapulae
M. deltoideus
M. trapezius, Pars ascendens
M. teres major
M. latissimus dorsi
M. triceps brachii
M. latissimus dorsi, aponeurotic origin
Fascia thoracolumbalis, superficial layer
M. anconeus
M. extensor carpi radialis longus
M. flexor carpi ulnaris
M. extensor digitorum
M. extensor carpi ulnaris
M. abductor pollicis longus
M. extensor pollicis brevis
M. extensor digiti minimi
Retinaculum mm. extensorum
M. abductor digiti minimi

Crista iliaca
M. gluteus medius
M. tensor fasciae latae
M. gluteus maximus
M. interosseus dorsalis IV

M. interosseus dorsalis I
M. interosseus dorsalis II
M. interosseus dorsalis III

M. adductor magnus
M. gracilis
M. semitendinosus
M. biceps femoris, Caput longum
M. semimembranosus
Fossa poplitea
M. plantaris
M. gastrocnemius, Caput mediale
M. gastrocnemius, Caput laterale

Tendo calcaneus

b

Fig. 1.36b Skeletal musculature; dorsal view; some superficial muscles were removed on the left side to allow for a better overview. [S700 -L275]

Musculature

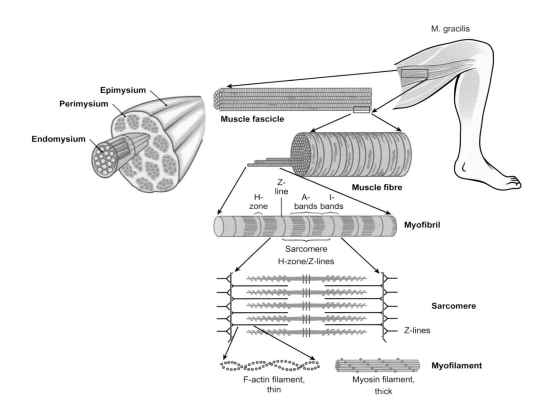

Fig. 1.37   Structure of a skeletal muscle. [S701-L126]
All skeletal muscles in the body share the same structure and are composed of muscle fibres. The smallest unit of a skeletal muscle is the sarcomere which consists of myofilaments composed of the two contractile proteins, F-actin and myosin. Sarcomeres arranged in rows (end to end) and in parallel (side by side) create a myofibril. Groups of myofibrils are wrapped in connective tissue (endomysium) to form a single muscle fibre. Many muscle fibres are surrounded by a connective tissue sheath (perimysium) and form a muscle fascicle. The fascicles are surrounded by a sheath of epimysium and form the skeletal muscle (e.g. M. gracilis).

Structure and function

A **muscle contraction** is made possible by the ability of each sarcomere to alter its length. There are also three types of muscle contractions (see image):

- Concentric contraction: the muscle becomes shorter when load-bearing and reduces the angle of the joint.
- Eccentric contraction: the muscle stretches with (external) load-bearing, thereby increasing the angle of the joint.
- Isometric contraction: the muscle contracts without changing its length and the position of the joint is unchanged.

[S701-L126]

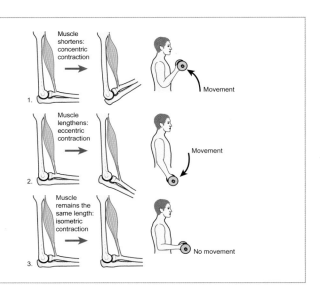

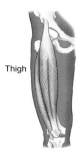
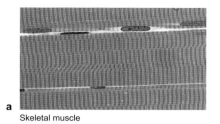

Thigh

a Skeletal muscle

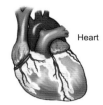

Heart

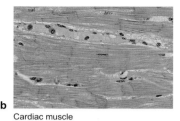

b Cardiac muscle

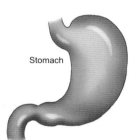

Stomach

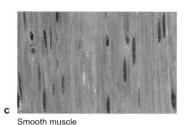

c Smooth muscle

Fig. 1.38a–c Types of muscle tissue. [E336]
There are three types of muscle tissue based on structural and functional characteristics:

a Skeletal musculature – voluntary, shows striated muscle structure in light microscopy which is based on the regular repeated arrangement of actin and myosin filaments as sarcomeres (basic contractile elements of striated muscles); shortening of sarcomeres causes isotonic muscle contraction, while muscle relaxation leads to a lengthening of the sarcomeres. Musculature of the skeletal system and other muscles. Muscle fibres can be several centimetres in length and have a diameter of 40–80 μm.

b Heart musculature – specific to the heart, with its own pacemaker and conductive system, shows fasciated or striated muscle structure in light microscopy; the same basic structure as striated skeletal musculature, muscle cells (cardiomyocytes) usually have a single nucleus, are 100 μm long and have a diameter of approx. 15 μm. Carciomyocytes connect via gap junctions (open connections to the next cell) and complex junctional structures (intercalated discs visible by light microscopy).

c Smooth musculature – involuntary, composed of thin muscle cells, that contain actin and myosin but are not classified as sarcomeres. With the exception of the heart, found as components in the walls of all hollow organs (e.g. digestive tract, urogenital tract, tracheobronchial tree, blood vessels) and in several other locations and other organs. When compared to skeletal musculature, contractions are slower but more extensive (up to a third of the original muscle length), and can maintain extended contractions at low expense of energy.

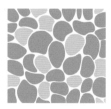
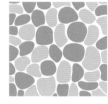
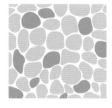

■ Slow-twitch muscle fibres   ■ Fast-twitch muscle fibres

Fig. 1.39 Types of muscle fibres in a skeletal muscle. [S701-L231]
Striated muscles are composed of two basic types of muscle fibres: fast-twitch muscle fibres and slow-twitch muscle fibres. The proportions of these fibres in a skeletal muscle is determined by genetic and external factors (e.g. how a muscle is used). Certain muscles are predominantly composed of slow-twitch muscle fibres (left), some containing equal numbers of slow- and fast-twitch muscle fibres (centre), while others consist of mainly fast-twitch muscle fibres (right). **Fast-twitch** muscles fibres (type II; particularly type IIB, white fibres) have little myoglobin, few mitochondria, mainly generate energy by glycolysis (anaerobic), are quickly fatigued, and used for short high-intensity bursts of muscle activity (e.g. 100 m sprint). **Slow-twitch muscle fibres** (type I fibres, red fibres) are rich in myoglobin, have many mitochondria, mainly generate energy through oxidative phosphorylation, resist fatigue, and are used in situations where continuous muscle contractions are required (e.g. marathon-running).

Types of muscle fibres	
Slow-twitch muscle fibres (type I)	**Fast-twitch muscle fibres (type II)**
Red fibres	White fibres
High in mitochondria	Low in mitochondria
Energy through oxidative phosphorylation	Energy through glycolysis
Resistant to fatigue	Fatigue faster
Suitable for continuous contractions	Suitable for short bursts of contractions

Structural principle and muscle fascia

Fig. 1.40 Structural principle of the skeletal muscle with the M. brachialis as an example. [S700-L126]

Skeletal muscles move bones in their joints and have a fixed point of origin (Origo) and a flexible point of insertion (Insertio). The point of origin is by definition sinewy or fleshy. It has a broader base and is less flexible than the muscle's insertion point. The origin of the extremity muscle is usually close to the body (proximal), and the insertion far from the body (distal). In the torso muscles, the origin is usually caudal and the insertion cranial. The attachment site on the stationary skeletal element is known as the fixed end and on the moving element as the mobile end. The terms fixed end and mobile end are not absolute terms. They are reversed when the limb is not moved towards the torso but the torso is moved towards the limb. The muscle belly (Venter, Gaster) is inserted via a tendon (Tendo, → Fig. 1.44) on the bone. The amount of force a muscle can transfer onto a joint depends on the length of the lever (vertical distance from the line of force of the muscle to the rotational axis of the joint = lever arm of force). The length of the lever varies depending on the joint position and is known as the virtual lever. Most muscles are enveloped on their free surface by a fascia. Fasciae are casings made of fibrous connective tissue which surround an individual muscle, several muscles (a muscle group) and tendons. The fasciae allow the muscle to contract almost invisibly without the surrounding tissue also contracting.

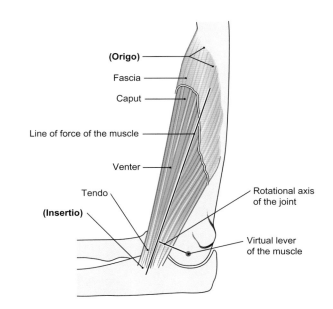

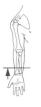

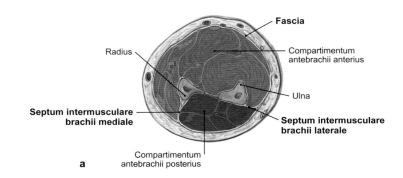

a

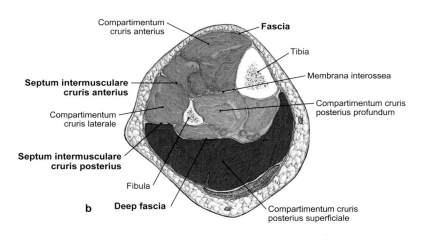

b

Fig. 1.41a and b Muscle fascia of the forearm and lower leg. [S701]
a Compartments of the forearm.
b Compartments of the lower leg.

Fasciae are collagenous tissue casings around an individual muscle or muscle groups, tendons and organs. This fascia allows muscles to contract while gliding within the fascial sheath with the skin barely moving. Apart from the fasciae surrounding the muscles, tendons and organs, the retinacula, septa and joint capsules are also considered fascial structures. The purpose of fasciae is to separate, strengthen, stabilise, and encase certain anatomical structures. Examples are the muscles of the forearm and the lower leg which are separated into several muscle compartments by a strong fascia, the **Septum intermusculare.** This anatomical architecture supports separate and different muscular functionalities in the various compartments. Muscles in the anterior compartment of the forearm are responsible for flexion and pronation, while muscles of the posterior compartment support extension and supination. The lower leg is composed of four different muscle compartments. The interstitial septa also contain the larger blood vessels and nerves.

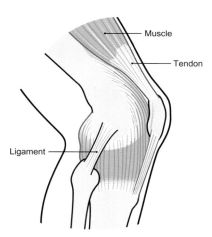

Fig. 1.42   Function of tendons, ligaments and joint capsules.
[S701-L126]
Tendons, ligaments and joint capsules ensheath, join and stabilise the joints of the musculoskeletal system. While considered to be passive structures, they are critically important for controlled and directed joint movements. **Ligaments** and **joint capsules** join, stabilise, guide movement of the joints, and prevent non-physiological and excessive joint movements. **Tendons** connect muscles with bones and transmit the mechanical forces of muscle contractions to the skeletal system, resulting in joint movements.

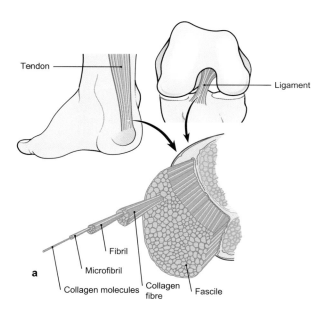

Differences in collagen fibre organisation

Fig. 1.43a–c   Structure of tendons and ligaments.
a Histologically, tendons and ligaments consist of collagenous connective tissue of high-tensile strength, which is produced by fibroblasts and deposited in the extracellular matrix. Collagen molecules are the smallest structural unit and are organised as collagen microfibrils. Several microfibrils are bundled into collagen fibrils, with several of these collagen fibrils forming a collagen fibre. Collagen fibres aggregate to generate fascicles which bundle up to form tendons and ligaments. In addition to collagen fibres, the extracellular matrix also includes a few elastic fibres, proteoglycans and glycoproteins. [S701-L126]

b Tendons transmit the mechanical force generated by muscles to the bones. Elongated tendinocytes located in-between the collagen fibres can frequently only be identified histologically by their nuclei. [G716]
c Contrary to tendons, ligaments stretch across joints and connect bones to each other. Ligaments hold bones in place and stabilise a joint to prevent excessive movements of the skeleton. The structural diversity of collagen fibres found in ligaments is more diverse than in tendons. [H061-001]

Tendon sheath

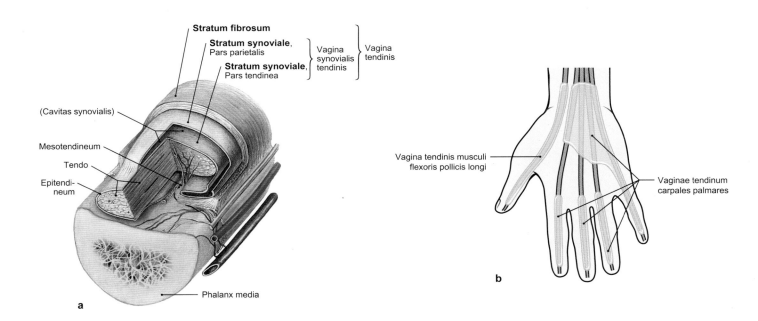

Stratum fibrosum

Stratum synoviale, Pars parietalis

Stratum synoviale, Pars tendinea

Vagina synovialis tendinis

Vagina tendinis

(Cavitas synovialis)

Mesotendineum

Tendo

Epitendineum

Phalanx media

a

Vagina tendinis musculi flexoris pollicis longi

Vaginae tendinum carpales palmares

b

Fig. 1.44a and b   Structure of the tendon sheath, Vagina tendinis, Vagina synovialis, with the finger as an example.

a Tendon sheaths enable better tendon-gliding and protect tendons from deflection by bones or ligaments. In their structure they are similar to a joint capsule or a bursa located around the tendon. The inner tendon sheath sheet (Stratum synoviale, Pars tendinea) is fused with the tendon, the outer (Stratum synoviale, Pars parietalis) with the Stratum fibrosum of the tendon sheath. In the synovial cavity (Cavitas synovialis), joint lubrication (synovia) is delivered. Small blood vessels reach the tendon via the Vincula brevia and longa (ligaments of the Mesotendineum of varying length and breadth). The Vincula can be found especially in the tendons of the finger flexors.

The muscle tendons transfer the traction of the muscles onto the bone. They consist mainly of parallel collagen fibres as well as a few elastic fi-

bres, and proteoglycans and glycoproteins stored in-between. The living cells of the tendon are called tendinocytes. The tendon is enveloped in loose connective tissue (Epitendineum). A distinction is made between traction and gliding tendons. With traction tendons, the direction of traction is identical to that of the muscle. In the case of gliding tendons, the tendon is deflected at a hypomochlion (point of deflection, e.g. bone edge, bone protrusion or sesamoid bone [bone stored in the tendon]). In the contact area, the tendon glides on the hypomochlion and is subjected here to pushing and shoving. This is the part of the tendon where fibrous cartilage occurs. [S700]

b As an example, tendon sheaths (Vagina tendinum) are shown surrounding the flexor tendons of the fingers. [S700-L126]

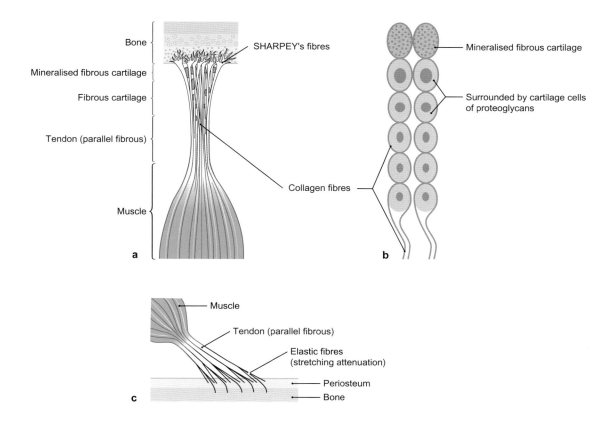

Fig. 1.45a–c   Structure of tendon insertion sites (enthesis).
[S7C2-L126]
To avoid avulsion or tearing of the tendons in the insertion area, tendon insertion sites are built-in, to enable the different elasticity modules of connective tissue, cartilage and bone to adapt to each other. There are chondral-apophyseal insertion sites and periostal-diaphyseal insertion sites.
a, b Chondral-apophyseal insertion sites are characteristic of muscles inserted in the area of formerly cartilaginous apophyses. However, these also occur with other muscles (e. g. masticatory muscles). At the insertion site, fibrous cartilage is present, of which the layer directly covering the bone is mineralised. In the insertion area there is no periosteum; the collagen fibres go directly into the bone and anchor the tendon here.
c Periostal-diaphyseal insertion sites are characteristic of the diaphyses of the long bones. The collagenous SHARPEY's fibres penetrate the bone and anchor the tendon in the cortical bone. In this way, the force is transmitted over a very large area. The SHARPEY's fibres rarely penetrate the bone directly at a site where the bone has no periosteum. On the bony skeleton, the insertion areas show as protruberances (Tuberositates).

Clinical remarks

Especially in the hands and feet, painful **tendovaginitis (tendonitis)** is common and due to excessive use. **Tendovaginitis stenosans** (stenosing tendonitis) occurs when the muscles used for bending the hand are overused. People involved in occupations or activities using job-specific movements (craftsmen, athletes, piano players – in some instances recognised as an occupational disease) are prone to this condition. In the course of the disease, minor injuries occur in the affected tendon, which the body attempts to repair with an inflammatory reaction. The inflammation is associated with swelling of the tendon, which in turn restricts the tendon sheath, leading to the formation of tendon nodules. In the case of the finger flexors, the tendons are fixed by means of annular ligaments (Ligamenta anularia). The thickened tendon area is caught in-between the individual ringshaped ligaments and gives rise to the **phenomenon of 'trigger finger'.**

Musculoskeletal system

Types of muscle

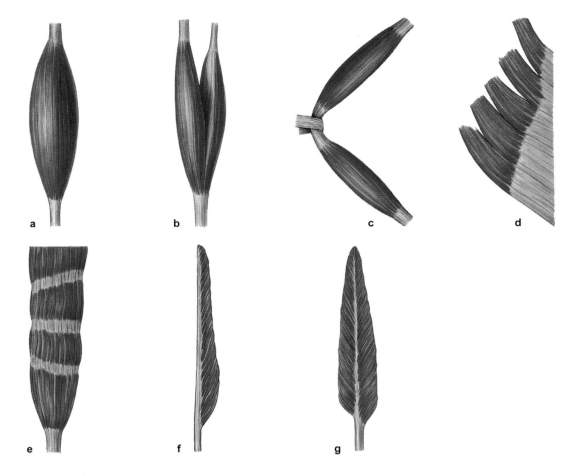

Fig. 1.46a–g   Types of muscle. [S700]
Muscles are divided according to:
* the arrangement of their muscle fibres (parallel course to the direction of traction of the tendon with substantial movements using low force, or pennate = diagonal course of muscle fibres at a particular acute angle [pennation angle] with long, wide tendons using high muscle force);
* the number of muscle heads (one, two or more);
* differences in joint involvement (depending on whether a muscle is involved in the movement in one or two joints or has no relationship to a joint: single-joint muscles, two-joint muscles or mimic muscles without joint involvement);
* muscle form, as when skeletal muscles present with transverse stripes (striation) under the microscope.

Based on their form or shape, muscles can be grouped into:
a single-headed, parallel muscles (M. fusiformis)
b two-headed, parallel muscles (M. biceps)
c two-lobed, parallel muscles (M. biventer)
d multi-lobed, flat muscles (M. planus)
e multi-lobed muscles divided by intermediate tendons (M. intersectus)
f semipennate muscles (M. semipennatus)
g multipennate muscles (M. pennatus).

Structure and function

Functionally, a distinction is made between the passive and active musculoskeletal system:
* The **passive musculoskeletal system** includes bones, joints and ligaments. The skeleton gives the body its shape, serves as an insertion point for the muscles and forms the body cavities in which the intestines are protected. Joints connect the bones in a flexible manner.
* The **active musculoskeletal system** consists of the skeletal muscles which can move the bones in the joints and are controlled voluntarily.

Clinical remarks

Stronger, unusual forms of stress (common in sports) may cause a tear in the muscle tissue (**torn muscle fibre,** or **torn muscle** if damage is greater). The muscles of the upper and lower leg are most often affected. A **muscle strain**, in contrast, is not associated with macroscopic structural change involving the destruction of muscle cells and bleeding. Often, a few hours or days after strong physical exertion of certain muscles, **muscle stiffness and ache** occurs. This is caused by small micro-tears in the muscle fibrils with a subsequent inflammatory reaction, which causes the indeterminate pain.

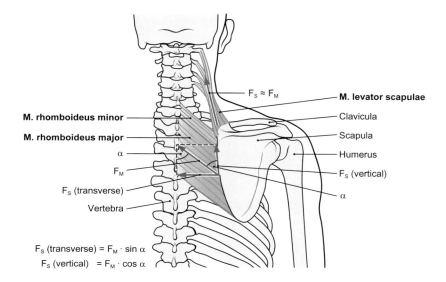

$$F_S \text{ (transverse)} = F_M \cdot \sin \alpha$$
$$F_S \text{ (vertical)} \;\; = F_M \cdot \cos \alpha$$

Fig. 1.47 Muscle and tendon force; vectors of muscle and tendon force, with the example of the Mm. levator scapulae and rhomboid muscles. [S700-L126]/[B500~M282/L132]

There is a direct proportional relationship between muscle force and the physiological cross-section of the muscle (lifting force of a muscle relative to the cross-section of all muscle fibres positioned perpendicularly to the direction of the fibres). If the tendon of the muscle runs in the direction of traction (e.g. M. levator scapulae), the complete momentum generated is

transferred to the tendon. In this case, muscle force (F_M) and tendon force (F_T) are almost equal.

If the muscle fibres are at an angle to the direction of traction of the tendon (e.g. Mm. rhomboidei major and minor), only part of their contraction force is transferred to the tendon. Here the vertical tendon force which is relative to the muscle force is reduced by the factor cos α and the transverse tendon force is reduced by the factor sin α.

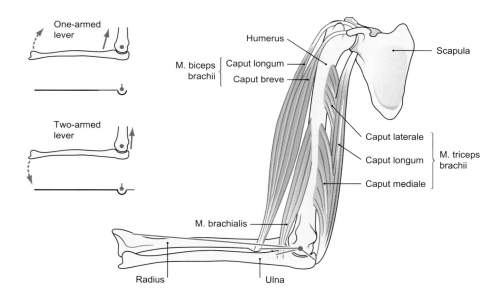

Fig. 1.48 Lever arm and muscle activity; main muscles of the elbow joint and their anatomical lever arms (red lines). [S700-L126][B500~M282/L132]

The lever arm is the part of a lever between the centre of rotation and the point where the force has an impact. For skeletal components to be moved around a rotational axis of a joint, a muscle must use an anatomical (existing) lever arm to generate torque. The length of the lever arm depends on the distance between the muscle's insertion point and the

joint's centre of rotation. For example, when the arm is moved towards the torso, the Brachioradialis muscle has a long anatomical lever arm while the Brachialis muscle has a short anatomical lever arm. If a muscle engages a one-armed lever, the skeletal element is moved in the direction of traction (e.g. Mm. brachioradialis, biceps brachii, brachialis). In the case of two-armed levers, the muscle's insertion point is moved in the direction of traction and the main part of the skeletal element is shifted in the opposite direction (e.g. M. triceps brachii).

Cardiovascular system

Fig. 1.49 Cardiopulmonary system. [S701-J803/L126]
The cardiopulmonary system is an integrated system composed of the heart and blood vessels (arteries and veins), and works with the respiratory system, consisting of the tracheobronchial tree and the lungs. The collective function of this system is to facilitate metabolic and gas transport (nutrients, oxygen) to the muscles and organs and the removal of waste products (e.g. carbon dioxide).

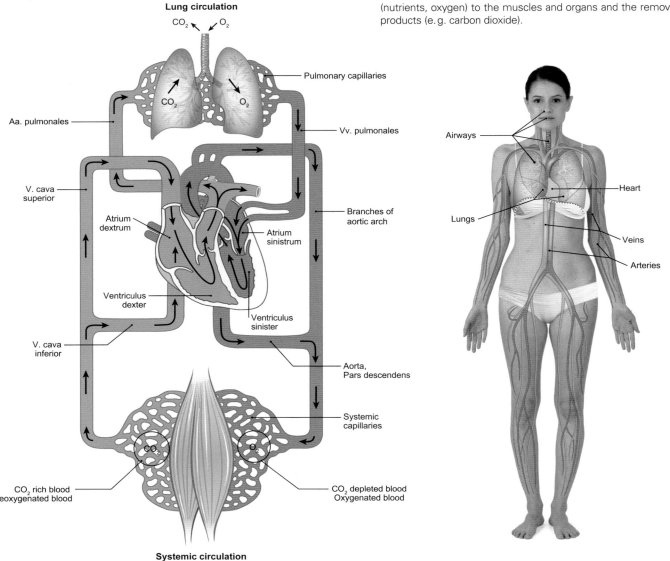

Fig. 1.50 Systemic and pulmonary circulation. [S701-L126]
The systemic and pulmonary circulatory systems together enable **blood circulation,** the continuous circulation of arterial and venous blood in the blood vessels and the heart which represent the **cardiovascular system.** Blood passes through both **circulatory systems (systemic and pulmonary)** which are sequentially connected, with the heart placed in between both circulatory systems and acting as a pump. The left side of the heart pumps oxygenated blood into the aorta, thereby supplying the arterial blood vessels of the systemic circulation. The blood enters arteries and arterioles before it reaches the capillary bed, where the exchange of gases and nutrients occurs. Deoxygenated blood collects in venules and veins to reach the right side of the heart, which pumps the venous blood into the pulmonary circulation to be oxygenated again in the pulmonary capillaries. It then returns to the left side of the heart to start a new cardiac cycle.

Based on the diameter of the blood vessels, vessels of **macrocirculation** (arteries, veins) can be differentiated from those of **microcirculation** (diameter < 100 µm; arterioles, capillaries, venules).

The perpetually active circulatory pump, the heart, is a hollow muscular organ consisting of a right and a left side, both constructed in the same way. Each side has a receiving chamber (atrium) and a discharging chamber (ventricle), which are separated by valves to facilitate directional blood flow. Both atria and ventricles are functionally synchronised. The valves between the atria and the ventricles open when the ventricular chambers relax and the atria contract to fill both ventricles. Following the relaxation of the atrial muscles, both valves between atria and ventricles close and with the contraction of the ventricular muscles, the valves open up between the right ventricle and the Truncus pulmonalis (main vessel to the lungs) and between the left ventricle and the aorta (main vessel to the systemic circulation), so that the blood flows from the ventricles into the corresponding vessels. Simultaneously, blood from the systemic veins (right atrium) and from the pulmonary veins (left atrium) enters the atria to start a new cardiac cycle.

The **high-pressure system** of the systemic arteries is distinct from the **low-pressure system** of the systemic veins and all blood vessels of the pulmonary circulation. Per definition, arteries direct blood away from the heart, and veins direct blood towards the heart. Thus, arteries of the systemic circulation transport oxygenated blood, whereas arteries of the pulmonary circulation transport deoxygenated blood. Inversely, veins of the systemic circulation transport deoxygenated blood and those in the pulmonary circulation transport oxygenated blood.

Fig. 1.51 Circulatory and blood vessel system. [B500-L238~M282/L132]

Blood transports and distributes gases, nutrients, metabolic waste products, hormones, heat and immune cells throughout the whole body. The heart serves as a pump that distributes blood via the transporting vessels. The **arteries** close to the heart (aorta and Truncus pulmonalis) divide into gradually narrowing arteries, then **arterioles,** before transitioning into the network of capillaries where an exchange of gases, nutrients and waste products occurs. Via **venules,** blood is transported through increasingly larger **veins** and finally via the V. cava superior and inferior back to the heart. The structure for both the systemic and the pulmonary circulatory system is similar. Arterioles, capillaries and venules are part of **terminal circulation** (microcirculation) (→ table). The widely distributed microcirculatory vessels account for the largest cross-sectional area of the circulatory system. Arteries are categorised as **elastic arteries** (A. elastotypica: aorta and large arteries) and **muscular arteries** (A. myotypica: smaller arteries distant from the heart). Elastic arteries facilitate the Windkessel Effect, by which the the pump function of the heart (pulsatile blood flow) converts into a continuous blood flow. This enables the pulse wave to be palpable in elastic arteries. In contrast, muscular arteries (distributing arteries) have a different muscular wall structure and are able to regulate arterial (blood) pressure. Besides these two types, there are transition types (A. mixtotypica). Instead of flowing back into the vascular system, fluid leaking from the capillaries of the microcirculation into the surrounding connecting tissue is collected by the lymphatic capillaries and lymphatic vessels (lymphatic system), which originate here, and are transported back to the venous angles close to the heart and in this way back into the blood circulation. The lymph is first filtered via numerous lymph nodes.

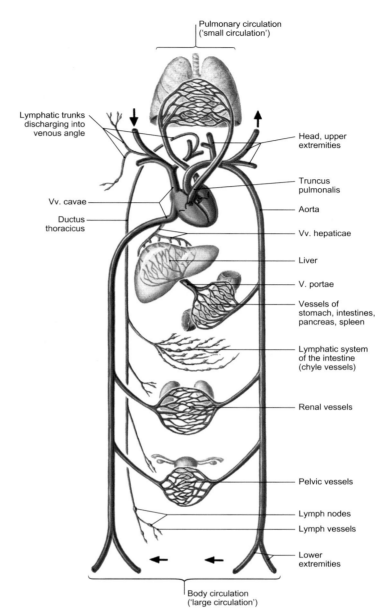

Structure of the vascular system		
System	**Components**	**Details**
Arterial system (high-pressure system)	Arteries	Arteries of the elastic type: aorta and larger arteries Arteries of the muscular type: small arteries further from the heart
Terminal vessels (microcirculation)	Terminal vessels	Arterioles Capillaries Venules
Venous system (low-pressure system)	Veins	Mid-sized and small veins Large veins

Neurovascular pathways

Cardiovascular system

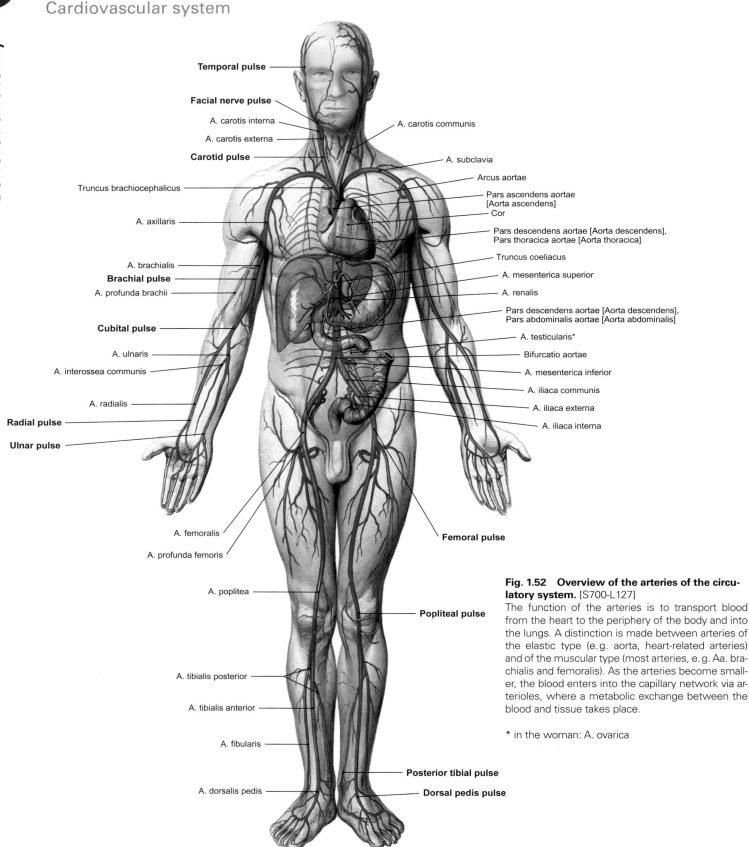

Temporal pulse

Facial nerve pulse

A. carotis interna

A. carotis externa

Carotid pulse

Truncus brachiocephalicus

A. axillaris

A. brachialis

Brachial pulse

A. profunda brachii

Cubital pulse

A. ulnaris

A. interossea communis

A. radialis

Radial pulse

Ulnar pulse

A. carotis communis

A. subclavia

Arcus aortae

Pars ascendens aortae [Aorta ascendens]

Cor

Pars descendens aortae [Aorta descendens], Pars thoracica aortae [Aorta thoracica]

Truncus coeliacus

A. mesenterica superior

A. renalis

Pars descendens aortae [Aorta descendens], Pars abdominalis aortae [Aorta abdominalis]

A. testicularis*

Bifurcatio aortae

A. mesenterica inferior

A. iliaca communis

A. iliaca externa

A. iliaca interna

A. femoralis

A. profunda femoris

Femoral pulse

A. poplitea

Popliteal pulse

A. tibialis posterior

A. tibialis anterior

A. fibularis

Posterior tibial pulse

A. dorsalis pedis

Dorsal pedis pulse

Fig. 1.52 Overview of the arteries of the circulatory system. [S700-L127]
The function of the arteries is to transport blood from the heart to the periphery of the body and into the lungs. A distinction is made between arteries of the elastic type (e.g. aorta, heart-related arteries) and of the muscular type (most arteries, e.g. Aa. brachialis and femoralis). As the arteries become smaller, the blood enters into the capillary network via arterioles, where a metabolic exchange between the blood and tissue takes place.

* in the woman: A. ovarica

Clinical remarks

In many parts of the body, large and medium-sized arteries run near the body surface. Their **pulse** can be felt by pressing the artery against a harder underlying structure. The most distal palpable pulse and thus furthest from the heart is the pulse of the Dorsalis pedis artery on the instep of the foot. Examination of the arterial pulse gives numerous indications on, for example, the frequency of the heartbeat, differences in circulation in the upper and lower extremities or, more generally, the blood flow in a section of the body. The pathological occlusion of end arteries (e.g. in the context of a hardening of the arteries) leads to the destruction of tissue normally supplied by the artery (e.g. occlusion of a coronary artery leads to a heart attack or myocardial infarction).

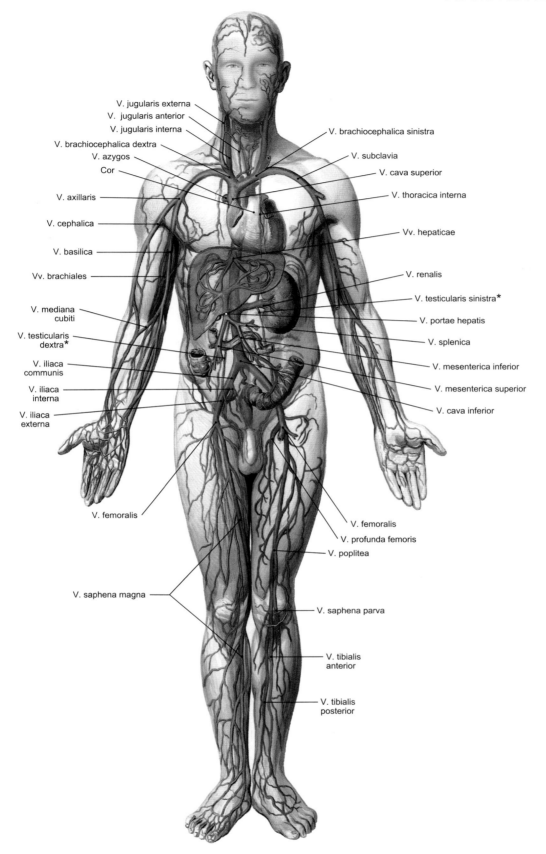

V. jugularis externa
V. jugularis anterior
V. jugularis interna
V. brachiocephalica dextra
V. azygos
Cor
V. axillaris
V. cephalica
V. basilica
Vv. brachiales
V. mediana cubiti
V. testicularis dextra*
V. iliaca communis
V. iliaca interna
V. iliaca externa
V. femoralis
V. saphena magna

V. brachiocephalica sinistra
V. subclavia
V. cava superior
V. thoracica interna
Vv. hepaticae
V. renalis
V. testicularis sinistra*
V. portae hepatis
V. splenica
V. mesenterica inferior
V. mesenterica superior
V. cava inferior
V. femoralis
V. profunda femoris
V. poplitea
V. saphena parva
V. tibialis anterior
V. tibialis posterior

Fig. 1.53 Overview of the veins of the systemic circulation.
[S700-L127]
Veins transport blood from the periphery of the body back to the heart. They are easily expandable and function as a blood reservoir. The veins of the systemic circulation transport deoxygenated blood and the veins of the pulmonary circulation transport oxygenated blood. Most veins are concomitant veins, i.e. they run parallel to corresponding arteries. Compared to the arteries, their pathways are more variable and the blood pressure is significantly lower. Together with capillaries and venules, veins belong to the **low-pressure system** of the circulatory system.

Most parts of the body contain a **superficial** venous system in the subcutaneous adipose tissue, which connects with a **deeper** venous system running parallel to the arteries (both systems are separated by venous valves so that blood can only travel in one direction from the superficial to the deep veins). Particularly the veins of the extremities are subject to large individual variation.

* in the woman: V. ovarica

Cardiovascular system

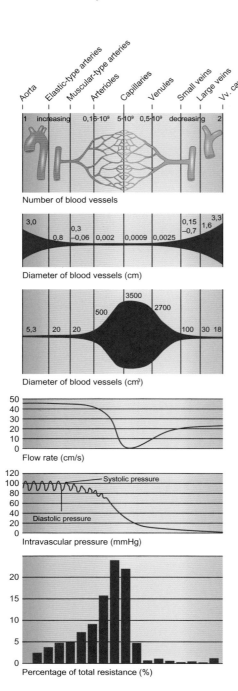

Number of blood vessels

Diameter of blood vessels (cm)

Diameter of blood vessels (cm³)

Flow rate (cm/s)

Intravascular pressure (mmHg)

Percentage of total resistance (%)

Fig. 1.54 Functions of the components of the circulatory system.
[S700-L126]/[S102-005]

An exchange of gases, nutrients and fluids occurs in the smallest vessels of the body, the capillaries. Together with pre-capillary arterioles and post-capillary venules, they form the **terminal vessels.** Capillaries are well suited for the exchange between blood and the interstitial fluid based on their thin wall structure, combined with the successively increasing cross-sectional diameter (by the factor of 800) and the substantially decelerated blood flow from approx. 50 cm/s in the aorta to 0.05 cm/s in the capillary. The time available for gas and nutrient exchange in the capillary (on average with a length of 0.5 mm) is therefore almost one second. The high friction between corpuscular components and the luminal surface of the arterioles and capillaries creates a vascular resistance which almost cancels out the blood pressure and the pulse wave.

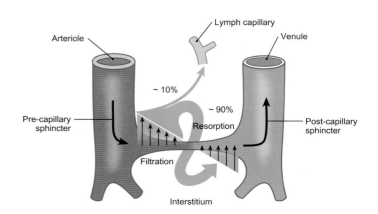

Fig. 1.55 Fluid exchange (microcirculation) at a capillary. [S700-L126]/[S102-005]

Inside the capillaries, two forces determine fluid exchange: the intravasal (or intracapillary) **colloid osmotic pressure** (based predominantly on circulating proteins, such as albumin and globulines) and the **perfusion pressure** (a hydrostatic pressure within the capillary). The **effective net filtration pressure** is the resultant difference between the two forces. At the arterial side of the capillary, the perfusion pressure (approx. 35 mmHg) is higher than the colloid osmotic pressure (approx 25 mmHg) by approx. 10 mmHg, resulting in extravasation of vascular fluid into the surrounding interstitial tissue (high effective filtration pressure; **filtration**). During capillary flow, the perfusion pressure reduces and the colloid osmotic pressure remains almost constant. Thus, in the centre of the capillary, the effective net filtration pressure equals nill, gradually becoming negative towards the venous side of the capillary, resulting in a fluid shift with dissolved particles into the capillary lumen (**resorption**).

However, the capillaries are constructed in such a way that of the 20 l blood that passes through and is filtered from the capillary bed every day (100 %), only 18 l (90 %) will be resorbed at the venous side. Thus, 2–3 l (10 %) of the remaining interstitial fluid is drained as lymph (lymph fluid) via the lymph vessel system and finally reaches the systemic circulation via the large lymph ducts (Ductus thoracicus on the left side and Ductus lymphaticus dexter on the right side), entering the venous angle of V. jugularis and V. subclavia (→ Fig. 1.60). By being drained through the lymphatic vessels, the lymph flows through numerous lymph nodes, which puts it under the 'control' of the immune system.

Clinical remarks

Insufficient lymphatic drainage causes **lymphoedema** with visible and palpable interstitial fluid accumulation (contrary to an oedema caused by extravasated interstitial fluid that leaves a dent upon focal pressure, the lymphoedema is firm). Lymphoedema can be caused by the transection of lymphatic vessels during surgery or the remov-

al of lymph nodes may cause a **postoperative lymphoedema.** Tumours or tissue damage following injuries, infection or radiation can cause **secondary lymphoedemas** which are distinct from the **primary lymphoedemas** that result from a defect in the embryological development of lymphatic vessels or lymph nodes.

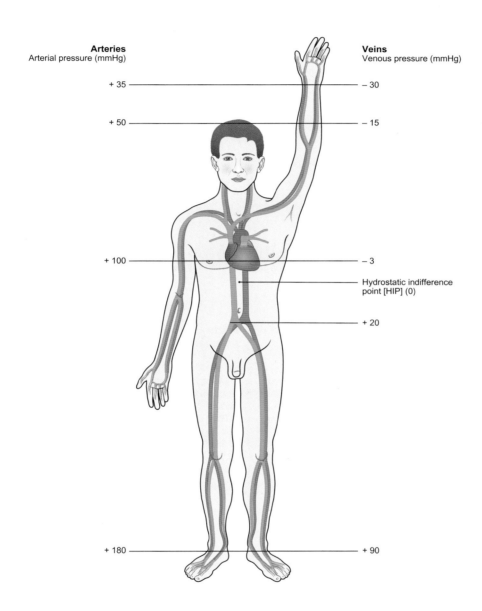

Arteries
Arterial pressure (mmHg)

Veins
Venous pressure (mmHg)

+ 35 ——————————— − 30

+ 50 ——————————— − 15

+ 100 ——————————— − 3

Hydrostatic indifference
point [HIP] (0)

+ 20

+ 180 ——————————— + 90

Fig. 1.56   Vessel pressure in arteries and veins in the upright position. [S700-L126]
The **high-pressure system** of the arteries in the systemic circulation is distinct from the **low-pressure system** that comprises the veins of the systemic circulation and the blood vessels of the pulmonary system. Arteries are defined to transport blood away from the heart, while veins bring blood back to the heart. Thus, arteries of the systemic circulation carry oxygenated blood whereas arteries of the pulmonary circulation carry deoxygenated blood. Similarly, veins of the systemic circulation carry deoxygenated blood whereas pulmonary veins bring oxygenated blood back to the heart. **Blood pressure** is defined as the pressure (force/area) of the blood within a vessel and normally describes the **arterial blood pressure.** It is dependent on both the cardiac output and the arterial resist-ance, thus the blood pressure decreases gradually when flowing from the aorta through the blood vessel system to reach the heart again. Measuring the blood pressure with the sphygmomanometer and the stethoscope yields a systolic pressure (depending, for example, on the cardiac output) and a diastolic pressure (depending, for example, on ventricular filling, cardiac relaxation, and the elasticity and capacity of the large vessels) and is usually given in mmHg (millimeter mercury column). 'Normal' blood pressure is usually 120/80 mmHg. This measurement also depends on which arteries were used. Veins have a lower blood pressure than arteries. However, the venous pressure in the lower extremities is higher than in the upper body and have a different wall structure as well as valves. The figure depicts the systolic blood pressure for arteries and veins in the upright position.

General anatomy

Venous blood flow

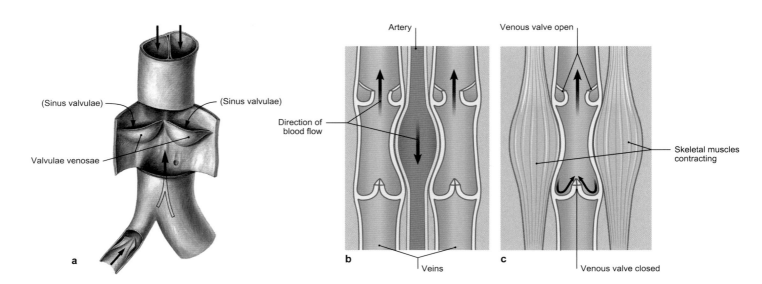

Fig. 1.57a–c   Venous valves and mechanisms of venous blood flow to the heart.
a Venous valves. Veins which move blood against gravity, such as the larger veins of the extremities and the lower neck, have valves that support the directional flow of blood towards the heart. In addition, the action of muscles and the arterial pulse support venous blood flow (only if valves are present). The upward pointing arrows depict the direction of the blood flow. The backflow of blood (arrows pointing downwards) closes the valves. [S700]

b Arteriovenous coupling. Arteries in the lower extremities are usually accompanied by two adjacent veins. The arterial pulse intermittently compresses the adjacent veins. With the blood flowing in the veins via the valves, the venous blood drains towards the heart. [S700-L126]
c Muscular pump. The involvement of the muscles surrounding the blood vessels leads to compression of the veins and contributes to transporting the blood via the venous valves in the direction of the heart. [S700-L126]
Besides the mechanisms described, the heart's suction effect contributes to the reverse flow of blood in the venous system.

Clinical remarks

A **deep vein thrombosis (DVT)** can occur when a blood clot **(thrombus)** forms in one or more of the deep veins of the body. A DVT may cause swelling and pain in the lower extremity but may not have any symptoms. Diagnostic ultrasound imaging is done to confirm a DVT (→ figure). If a part or the whole of the thrombus dislodges from the

venous wall, the resulting **embolus** travels through the blood vessel and may cause occlusion of a pulmonary artery resulting in a **pulmonary embolism**. As a result, the deoxygenated blood cannot reach the lungs, with life-threatening consequences. a [E708], b [G704]

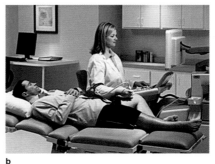

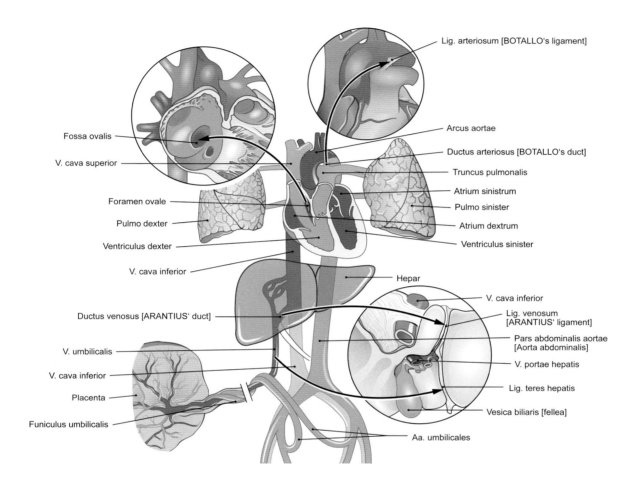

Lig. arteriosum [BOTALLO's ligament]

Fossa ovalis

V. cava superior

Arcus aortae

Ductus arteriosus [BOTALLO's duct]

Truncus pulmonalis

Atrium sinistrum

Foramen ovale

Pulmo sinister

Pulmo dexter

Atrium dextrum

Ventriculus dexter

Ventriculus sinister

V. cava inferior

Hepar

V. cava inferior

Ductus venosus [ARANTIUS' duct]

Lig. venosum [ARANTIUS' ligament]

Pars abdominalis aortae [Aorta abdominalis]

V. umbilicalis

V. portae hepatis

V. cava inferior

Placenta

Lig. teres hepatis

Vesica biliaris [fellea]

Funiculus umbilicalis

Aa. umbilicales

Fig. 1.58 Organisation of the prenatal cardiovascular system; schematic drawing. [S700-L126]

Arrows indicate the direction of blood flow. The prenatal circulation is different from the circulation after the birth.

Oxygenated blood moves from the placenta via the umbilical vein to the liver, where it is mostly fed directly into the V. cava inferior via the venous duct (Ductus venosus, ARANTIUS' duct). The main bloodstream flows from the V. cava inferior via the right atrium through the open Foramen ovale in the atrial septum directly into the left atrium. From here it flows into the left chamber, where it is distributed via the aorta in the systemic circulation.

Venous blood from the upper half of the body enters the right atrium via the V. cava superior and is directed largely into the right ventricle. Upon contraction of the heart, the blood is led from here mostly via the Ductus arteriosus (BOTALLO's duct) directly to the Aorta descendens. Both of the shunts (open Foramen ovale and open Ductus arteriosus) are necessary because the lungs are not yet developed in the fetus. From the systemic circulation of the fetus, the blood reaches the two umbilical arteries (Aa. umbilicales) largely via the iliac vessels and from here the placenta via the umbilical cord.

Interruption of the placental circulation shortly after birth, with the development of the lungs and the onset of breathing, leads to **closure** of the:

• venous duct
• Foramen ovale
• Ductus arteriosus between the pulmonary trunk and Arcus aortae
• Aa. umbilicales and V. umbilicalis.

At this point, the cardiovascular system still only consists of the heart, as well as the systemic circulation (supply of body tissues) and the pulmonary circulation (gas exchange) (→ Fig. 1.50). The cardiac output for an adult at rest is 70 ml.

Approximately 64 % of blood resides in the venous system at any given moment and this can increase to approximately 80 % (blood reservoir).

The small arteries and arterioles of the muscles mainly determine the vascular resistance. In the arterial system (high pressure system) the average blood pressure is approx. 100 mmHg (= mm mercury column), whereas in the venous system it is approx. 20 mmHg. Between the two systems lies the capillary region in which the metabolic exchange takes place.

Portal vein circulation

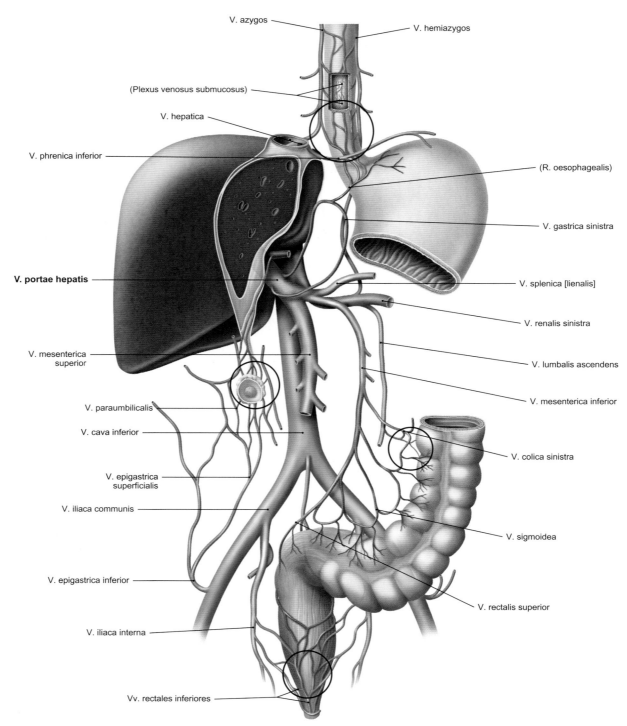

V. azygos

V. hemiazygos

(Plexus venosus submucosus)

V. hepatica

(R. oesophagealis)

V. phrenica inferior

V. gastrica sinistra

V. portae hepatis

V. splenica [lienalis]

V. renalis sinistra

V. mesenterica
superior

V. lumbalis ascendens

V. mesenterica inferior

V. paraumbilicalis

V. cava inferior

V. colica sinistra

V. epigastrica
superficialis

V. iliaca communis

V. sigmoidea

V. epigastrica inferior

V. rectalis superior

V. iliaca interna

Vv. rectales inferiores

**Fig. 1.59 Portal vein, V. portae hepatis, and inferior vena cava,
V. cava inferior;** semi-schematic representation; tributaries into the
V. cava inferior in blue; tributaries into the V. portae hepatis in purple. Pos-
sible portocaval anastomoses are highlighted by black circles.
[S700-L275]
The portal vein circulation has a special status within the systemic circula-
tion. Here two capillary areas (intestine, liver) are successively connected.

Prior to reaching the systemic circulation, venous blood from most un-
paired abdominal organs (stomach, parts of the intestines, pancreas,
spleen) is drained into the portal vein and from here into the liver. In this
way, many nutritional substances absorbed in the abdominal digestive
organs reach the liver and are metabolised here. Only after passing
through the liver does the blood reach the systemic circulation via the
hepatic veins (Vv. hepaticae) by flowing into the cava inferior vein.

Clinical remarks

In patients with, for example, liver cirrhosis, the liver is more highly
resistant, resulting in increased **portal vein pressure** which means
significantly less blood flowing through the liver. Bypassing the liver,
the remainder of the blood flows through portocaval anastomoses
directly into the systemic system. The veins in the anastomosis area
are not adapted to the increasing blood flow and may expand (devel-

opment of **varicose veins**). This allows varices to form in the area of
the gastroesophageal transition, a so-called Caput medusae in the
area of the paraumbilical veins (rare) or varicose veins in the anal canal. Particularly **oesophageal varices** can be easily damaged during
food intake and lead to life-threatening bleeding.

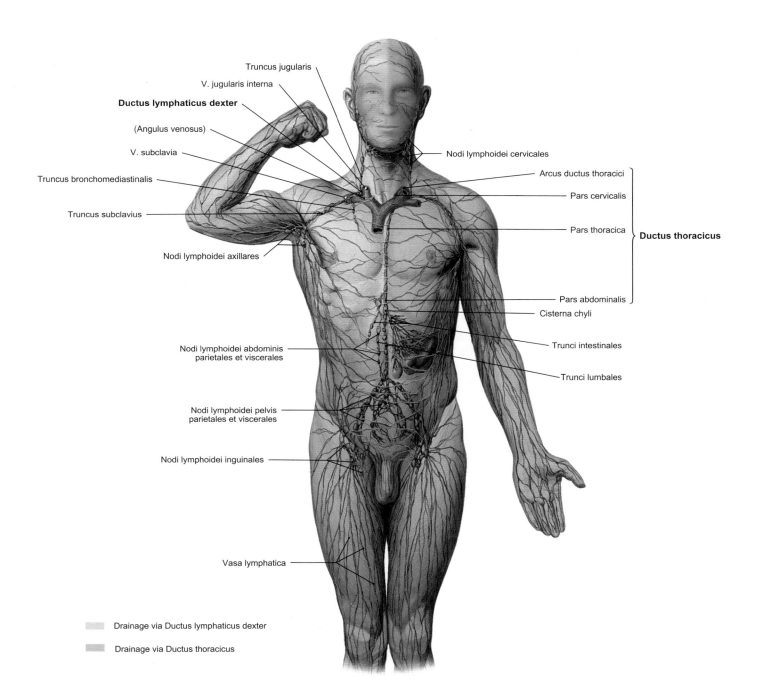

Truncus jugularis

V. jugularis interna

Ductus lymphaticus dexter

(Angulus venosus)

V. subclavia

Truncus bronchomediastinalis

Truncus subclavius

Nodi lymphoidei axillares

Nodi lymphoidei abdominis
parietales et viscerales

Nodi lymphoidei pelvis
parietales et viscerales

Nodi lymphoidei inguinales

Vasa lymphatica

Nodi lymphoidei cervicales

Arcus ductus thoracici

Pars cervicalis

Pars thoracica

Pars abdominalis

Cisterna chyli

Trunci intestinales

Trunci lumbales

Ductus thoracicus

Drainage via Ductus lymphaticus dexter

Drainage via Ductus thoracicus

Fig. 1.60 Overview of the lymphatic vessel system. [S700-L127]
The **lymph capillaries** incipient in the periphery absorb the fluid (lymph) from the interstitium and lead it via lymph collectors to the **lymphatic vessels** and the intermediate **lymph nodes.** Lymph nodes responsible for the collection and filtration of a particular body region are called regional lymph nodes. Lymph nodes which receive lymph from various other lymph nodes are called lymph-collecting nodes.

Finally, the lymph reaches the major **lymphatic ducts** (Ductus thoracicus and Ductus lymphaticus dexter) and then passes to the venous blood vessel system of the systemic circulation. Most of the lymph is drained through the **Ductus thoracicus** into the left venous angle (between the

Vv. jugularis interna sinistra and subclavia sinistra); only the right upper quadrant of the body is drained through the **Ductus lymphaticus dexter** into the right venous angle (between the Vv. jugularis interna dextra and subclavia dextra). The transport mechanism within the lymph vessels is similar to the directed flow of venous blood: **lymphatic valves,** muscular pump.

Besides the lymphatic vessels and lymph nodes, the lymphatic system also includes **lymphatic organs** (thymus, bone marrow, spleen, tonsils, mucosa-associated lymphatic tissue). Functionally, it serves the immune system and fat absorption.

General anatomy

Lymph nodes

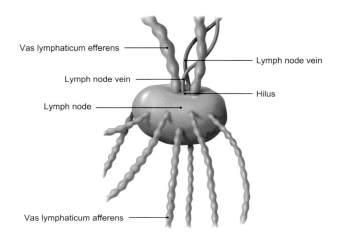

Vas lymphaticum efferens

Lymph node vein

Lymph node vein

Lymph node

Lymph node vein

Hilus

Vas lymphaticum afferens

Fig. 1.61 Lymph nodes with inbound and outbound lymphatic vessels; semi-schematic representation. [S700-L127]
The lymph nodes are the **secondary lymphatic organs** and are part of the lymphatic system. They come in various shapes (mostly lens- or bean-shaped with a diameter of 5–20 mm). The body contains approx. 1,000 lymph nodes and of those, 200 to 300 are located in the neck alone. Functionally, lymph nodes are part of the immune system and play an important role in fighting infection. Besides the lymph nodes, the following all belong to the secondary lymphatic organs: parts of the spleen, the tonsils (pharyngeal tonsils [Tonsilla pharyngea], palatine tonsils [Tonsilla palatina], lingual tonsil [Tonsilla lingualis], as well as the additional lymphatic tissue of the pharyngeal lymphoid ring [WALDEYER tonsillar ring]), the mucosa-associated lymphatic tissue (MALT), which includes the appendix (Appendix vermiformis), and the PEYER's patches of the small intestine. The **primary lymphatic organs,** on the other hand, include the thymus and the bone marrow which produce naïve immature immune cells.

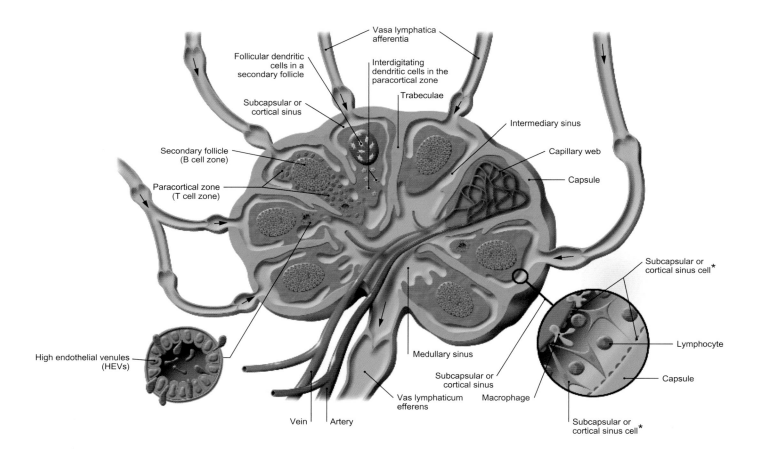

Vasa lymphatica afferentia

Follicular dendritic cells in a secondary follicle

Interdigitating dendritic cells in the paracortical zone

Subcapsular or cortical sinus

Trabeculae

Intermediary sinus

Secondary follicle (B cell zone)

Capillary web

Paracortical zone (T cell zone)

Capsule

Subcapsular or cortical sinus cell*

High endothelial venules (HEVs)

Lymphocyte

Medullary sinus

Capsule

Subcapsular or cortical sinus

Macrophage

Vas lymphaticum efferens

Vein   Artery

Subcapsular or cortical sinus cell*

Fig. 1.62 Lymph nodes; schematic section. [S700-L127]/[M109/L319])
Besides the inbound and outbound lymphatic vessels (Vasa afferentia and Vasa efferentia), the blood vessel supply and the compartmentalisation of the lymph node into a B-region (secondary follicle), T-region (paracortical zone) with high endothelial venules, follicular and interdigitating dendritic cells, medullary sinus, intermediary sinus and subcapsular or cortical sinus (with cellular structure) are represented.

* Sinus wall cells (reticular cells) line the sinus as well as crossing through it.

Clinical remarks

Examination of the lymph nodes is an important aspect of the physical examination of a patient. The examination includes the palpable lymph nodes of the neck, axilla and groin. Lymph node enlargement can be a sign of inflammatory processes (lymphadenitis) or malignant disease (e.g. metastasis of a malignant tumour or a generalised disease of the lymphatic system, such as HODGKIN's disease).

Sentinel lymph nodes are the lymph nodes into which a malignant tumour (especially breast and prostate cancer as well as malignant melanoma) drains first. If this already contains tumour cells, it is highly likely to find further lymphogenic metastases in the surrounding area. If it is tumour-free, additional lymph node metastases are unlikely. The sentinel lymph node status is therefore crucial for further therapeutic procedures.

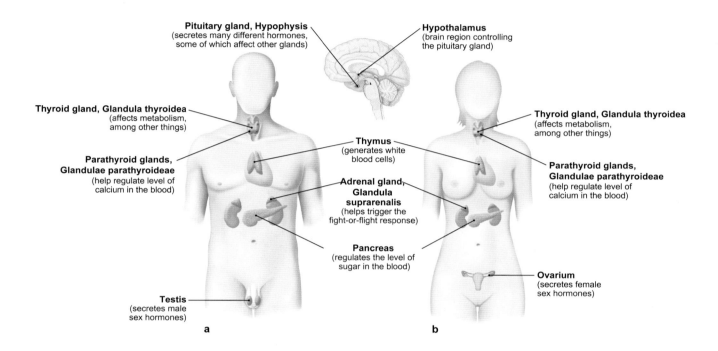

Pituitary gland, Hypophysis
(secretes many different hormones,
some of which affect other glands)

Hypothalamus
(brain region controlling
the pituitary gland)

Thyroid gland, Glandula thyroidea
(affects metabolism,
among other things)

Thyroid gland, Glandula thyroidea
(affects metabolism,
among other things)

Thymus
(generates white
blood cells)

**Parathyroid glands,
Glandulae parathyroideae**
(help regulate level of
calcium in the blood)

**Parathyroid glands,
Glandulae parathyroideae**
(help regulate level of
calcium in the blood)

**Adrenal gland,
Glandula
suprarenalis**
(helps trigger the
fight-or-flight response)

Pancreas
(regulates the level of
sugar in the blood)

Ovarium
(secretes female
sex hormones)

Testis
(secretes male
sex hormones)

a

b

Fig. 1.63a and b   Organs and basic functions of the endocrine system. [S701-L275]
a Male endocrine system.
b Female endocrine system.
The endocrine system is composed of different organs that have the ability to produce hormones and release them into the circulatory system to regulate the activity of certain other target tissues. The hypothalamus located in the basal part of the diencephalon is the superior integration centre for most endocrine organs. Downstream of the hypothalamus, the pituitary (hypophysis) regulates the hormonal production in the thyroid gland, the parathyroid glands, the adrenals, the pancreas, and organs of reproduction (ovaries in women and testes in men). Additionally, thymus functions are under endocrine control. The key functions of the endocrine system are:

* metabolic regulation
* acid-base homeostasis and pH regulation
* stress regulation
* regulation of body growth, development and reproduction
* production of hormones.

Reproductive system

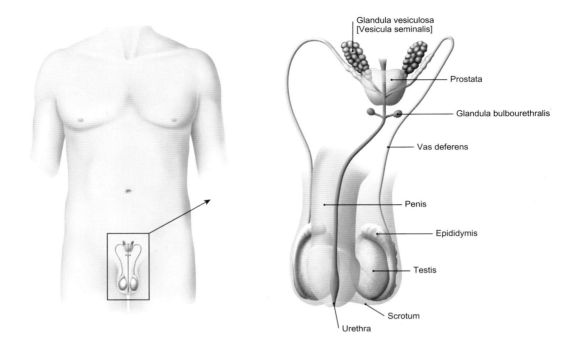

Fig. 1.64   Male reproductive organs. [S701-L275]
The male reproductive organs include the paired **testicles** (testes), with paired epididymis and paired Ductus deferens, the **accessory genitalia** (prostate, paired seminal vesicles (Glandula vesiculosa), paired bulbo-urethral glands (COWPER's glands), multiple small LITTRÉ glands (Glandulae urethrales), and the **external genitalia** with the penis and penile urethra. The testes are located outside the body within the scrotal sac (scrotum). They produce the sperm and contain endocrine cells which produce **male sex hormones** (androgens, particularly testosterone). These

male sex hormone-producing cells are under the control of the pituitary gland (hypophysis) and are part of the male endocrine system. Sperm cells mature in the epididymis and are ejaculated via the Ductus deferens and urethra. Fluids produced in the prostate and seminal vesicles are added to protect the viability of sperm cells and generate a cell suspension **(semen).** COWPER's and LITTRÉ glands condition the **urethra,** the passageway for both urine and semen, to allow smooth transport of the ejaculate.

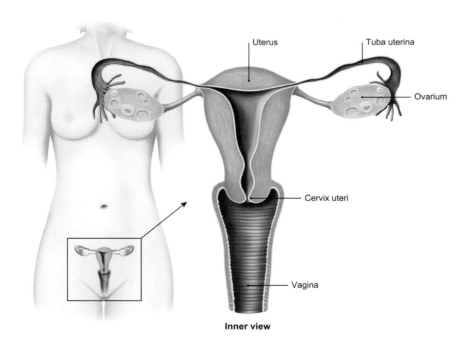

Inner view

Fig. 1.65   Female reproductive organs. [S701-L275]
The female reproductive organs include the paired **ovaries,** the paired **oviducts** (Tubae uterinae), the **uterus,** the **vagina,** and the **external genitalia** (vulva) with the clitoris, Labia minora and majora, lesser vestibular glands (SKENE's glands; Glandulae vestibulares minores [equivalent of the male Glandulae urethrales]), and the Glandulae vestibulares majores (BARTHOLIN's glands, which produce mucus). During sexual maturity,

the ovaries produce egg cells (ova) and **female sex hormones** under the control of the hypothalamus and pituitary. The endocrine system regulates the **ovarian cycle** (on average 28 days) which prepares the oviducts and uterine mucosal layers for **implantation** of the fertilised egg. Upon successful implantation, the fertilised egg develops further into an embryo and **placenta.** The penis enters the vagina during sexual intercourse.

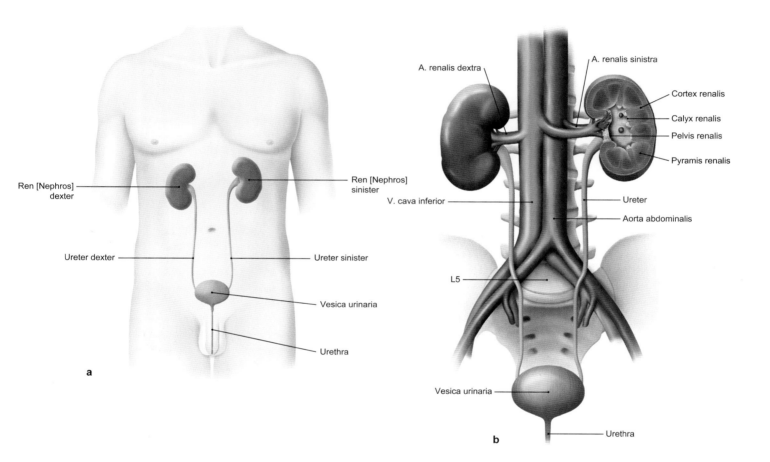

Fig. 1.66a and b Organs of the urinary tract. [S701-L275]
a The organs of the urinary tract include the paired **kidneys** (Ren), the paired **ureters,** the **urinary bladder** (Vesica urinaria) and the **urethra** (passageway for both urine and semen; → Fig. 164).
b The urinary bladder collects and stores urine; the tubular ureter and urethra discharge the urine. The **kidneys** are essential excretory organs, are vascularised intensively, and serve key functions in the regulation of min-
eral and water homeostasis. Additionally, the kidneys have endocrine functions and produce certain hormones (erythropoietin, thrombopoietin, renin, calcitriol). The urine produced by the kidneys, along with the bile, are the two most important excretory pathways for water-soluble metabolic waste products of the body. Urine collected in the renal pelvis and drained via the urinary bladder, the ureter and the urethra is temporarily stored in the urinary bladder.

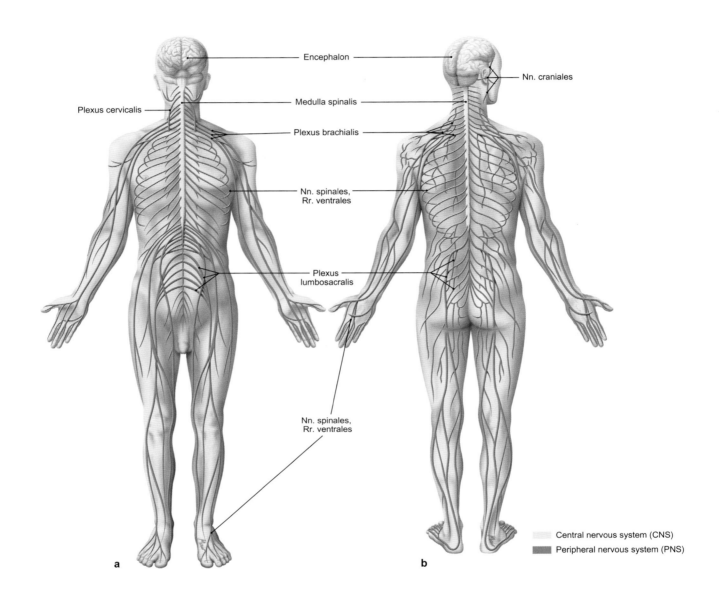

Encephalon

Nn. craniales

Plexus cervicalis

Medulla spinalis

Plexus brachialis

Nn. spinales,
Rr. ventrales

Plexus
lumbosacralis

Nn. spinales,
Rr. ventrales

Central nervous system (CNS)
Peripheral nervous system (PNS)

a

b

Fig. 1.67a and b Structure of the nervous system. [S701-L127]
a Ventral view.
b Dorsal view.
The nervous system is composed of the central (**CNS;** brain, spinal cord) and peripheral nervous system **(PNS).** The PNS is mainly composed of spinal nerves (with connections to the spinal cord) and cranial nerves (with connections to the brain).
The nervous system:
- controls the activity of muscles and intestines
- is used for communication between the environment and the human body, helping the entire organism to adapt quickly to changes in the environment and the body itself

- meets complex functions, such as storage of experience (memory), development of ideas (thinking) as well as emotions.

Functionally, the nervous system is divided into the **autonomic** (vegetative, visceral, to control intestinal activity, mostly involuntary) and **somatic** (animalistic, innervation of skeletal muscles, conscious sensory perception, communication with the environment) **nervous system.** Both systems are closely interlaced and interact with each other. Besides the nervous system, the endocrine system also participates in the regulation of the entire organism.

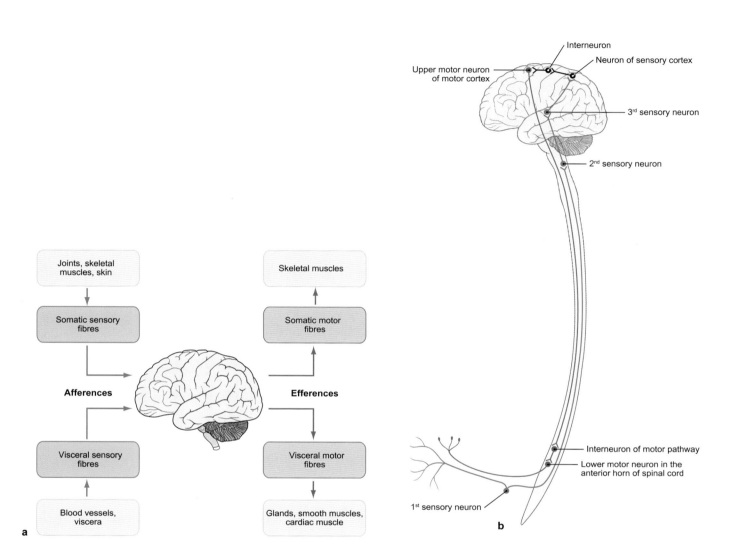

Fig. 1.68a and b   Information flow in the nervous system.
a Afferents and efferents. Afferent nerve fibres (**afferents,** green) of the peripheral nervous system (PNS) send information directly to the central nervous system (CNS) for further processing. Information derived from joints, skeletal muscles or skin represent somatic sensory afferents of corresponding **somatic sensory nerve fibres. Visceral sensory nerve fibres** carry information from blood vessels and the intestines. Information directed outward from the CNS to the body periphery are **efferents** (red; they can be seen as 'commands'). For example, if a skeletal muscle should contract, efferent information reaches the PNS via corresponding **somatic motor nerve fibres** for this muscle; when the heart is to beat faster or the secretory activity of a gland increases, this information is relayed via **visceral motor nerve fibres** of the PNS to the target organ. [S700-L126]

b Information flow in the PNS and CNS. The information flow via afferents from the body periphery to the CNS and back through efferents from the CNS to the periphery are interconnected at different levels. For example, the information (e.g. touching a metal plate with a flat hand) is transmitted via afferent nerve fibres from the PNS to the CNS (green), where this information is synapsed at multiple sites and processed via several interneurons (black) before the reaction is sent via efferent nerve fibres (red). The sensation of a hand touching the metal plate will not be particularly pleasant and the CNS directs the hand to pull back, requiring the activation of certain muscle groups. Here, the information flow involves somatic sensory afferents (green) to the brain and somatic motor efferents (red) to the arm/hand (the schematic shown is an extreme simplification of the complex processes occurring in the CNS). [S700-L126]/[G1060-001]

Nervous system

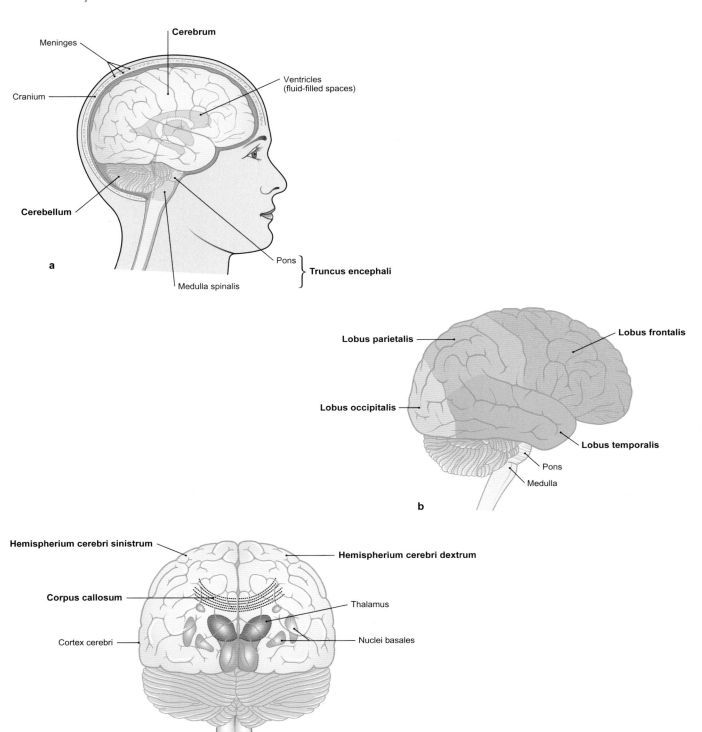

Fig. 1.69a–c   Topography of the brain; lateral view from the right **(a, b)** and from occipital **(c)**. [S701-L126]

a Parts of the brain. A lateral view shows parts of the **cerebrum** (encephalon), the **cerebellum,** and the **brainstem** (Truncus cerebri, Truncus encephali).

b Cerebral hemispheres. Four different cerebral hemispheres are visible: the **frontal lobe** (Lobus frontalis), the **parietal lobe** (Lobus parietalis), the **temporal lobe** (Lobus temporalis), and the **occipital lobe** (Lobus occipitalis). Each of these lobes has different functions. The frontal lobe is not only responsible for deliberate motor functions, but also important for executive functions. The parietal lobe is the integration centre for sensory information: it assists in the visual control of movements, spatial acuity, spatial perception, arithmetic and reading. The most important function of the temporal lobe is auditory perception (hearing), but also understanding

speech and written text. The most important role of the occipital lobe is visual perception and the processing of visual impressions.

c Hemispheres. The cerebrum is composed of two hemispheres (right and left hemisphere) which are connected via several different structures. One of these structures is the **Corpus callosum** (also called the callosal commissure) which relays information from one hemisphere to the other. Despite the fact that both hemispheres are structurally similar, functions related to control of speech, conceptual perception, or arithmetic- and writing-related skills are located in one hemisphere only, while the other hemisphere controls other activities, such as creativity, musical talent, and spatial and/or artistic capabilities. Located deeper in the brain are important nuclei (**basal ganglia**) which have roles in filtering information.

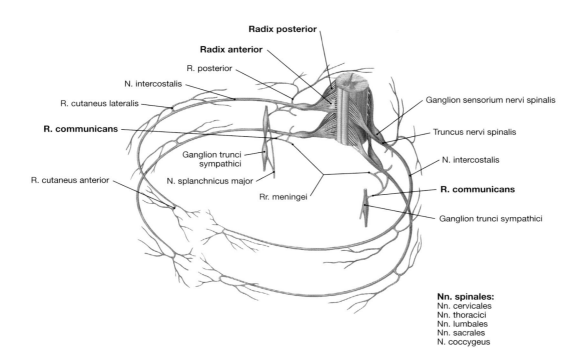

Radix posterior

Radix anterior

R. posterior

N. intercostalis

R. cutaneus lateralis

R. communicans

Ganglion trunci
sympathici

R. cutaneus anterior

N. splanchnicus major

Rr. meningei

Ganglion sensorium nervi spinalis

Truncus nervi spinalis

N. intercostalis

R. communicans

Ganglion trunci sympathici

Nn. spinales:
Nn. cervicales
Nn. thoracici
Nn. lumbales
Nn. sacrales
N. coccygeus

Fig. 1.70 Diagram of the spinal nerve (spinal cord segment) illustrated by two thoracic nerves; view from above at an oblique lateral angle. [S700]
The human body has 31 pairs of spinal nerves (eight cervical, 12 thoracic, five lumbar, five sacral and one coccygeal). Each spinal nerve consists of a front root (Radix anterior) and a rear root (Radix posterior). The cell bodies (perikarya) of the motor neurons are located in the gray matter of the spinal cord and exit via the anterior root; the perikarya of sensory nerve cells are located in the dorsal root ganglion (Ganglion sensorium nervi spinalis). They continue through the posterior root into the spinal cord. Via communicating branches, connections are made between the spinal cord and the sympathetic trunk (Ganglia trunci sympathici). All dorsal branches of the spinal nerves as well as the ventral branches of the thoracic spinal nerves T2 to T11 have a segmental arrangement. The remaining ventral branches usually come together to form the plexus (Plexus cervicalis, brachialis, lumbosacralis).

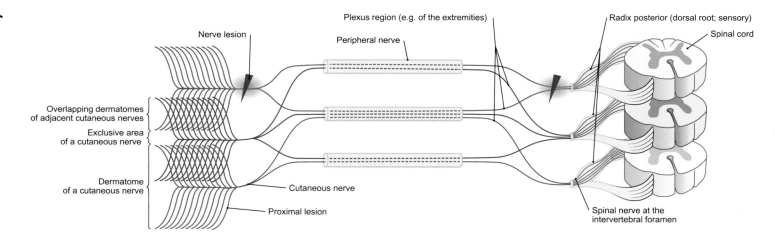

Fig. 1.71 labels:
- Nerve lesion
- Plexus region (e.g. of the extremities)
- Peripheral nerve
- Radix posterior (dorsal root; sensory)
- Spinal cord
- Overlapping dermatomes of adjacent cutaneous nerves
- Exclusive area of a cutaneous nerve
- Dermatome of a cutaneous nerve
- Cutaneous nerve
- Proximal lesion
- Spinal nerve at the intervertebral foramen

Fig. 1.71   Pathway of the peripheral sensory afferents from the dermatome to the spinal dorsal (sensory) root; three dermatomes are shown (green, red, blue). [S700-L126]

A **dermatome** is a defined area of skin with sensory fibres of a single spinal nerve root. These sensory fibres, together with other afferent and efferent fibres (see spinal nerve), reach the Foramen intervertebrale as a peripheral nerve. Here, the sensory fibres form the spinal dorsal root and their pseudo-unipolar nerve bodies are contained within the Ganglion spinale (dorsal root ganglion; see Histology textbooks). The dorsal root of each spinal nerve enters the posterior horn of the spinal cord in a segmental order. A simple segmental arrangement of sensory afferents is typical for the trunk region. However, the migration of primordial skin and muscle with the corresponding formation of a nerve plexus cause them to be raised or altered on the extremities (→ Fig. 1.72 and → Fig. 1.73). As a result, the segmental structure has been altered or lost. In most cases, dermatomes of neighbouring spinal cord segments are located close to each other and show some overlap at their borders. Hence, the autonomous area innervated exclusively by a single spinal nerve is rather small. Loss of a single segment (indicated by pale red oval area with arrowhead) leads to a complete sensory loss only within the area of autonomic innervation, whereas overlapping regions still receive innervation via the neighbouring dermatomes.

Clinical remarks

Superficial nerves and those close to bones are at risk of **peripheral nerve injury** as part of a trauma or surgical procedure (→ Fig. a), resulting in motor and sensory deficits (see illustration). Shortly after an injury (→ Fig. b), the axon distal to the injury degenerates (WALLER's degeneration). A few weeks later, sprouting of the proximal end of the severed axon as well as neighbouring axons occurs. At this point, the muscle fibres affected by the peripheral nerve lesion have already atrophied (→ Fig. c). The regeneration process takes several months. The newly generated axons re-innervate the skeletal muscle cells, and physical rehabilitation and training enable the musculature to regain their original strength. Axons and axon collaterals that fail to reach their corresponding muscle cells perish (→ Fig. d). Excessive alcohol consumption, Diabetes mellitus, vitamin B deficiency, poisoning with heavy metals and drugs as well as impaired blood circulation can result in disorders of the peripheral nerves. This can lead to the malfunction or excessive excitation of the nerve cells (neurons). When many nerves are affected, this is referred to as **polyneuropathy.**
[S700-L126]

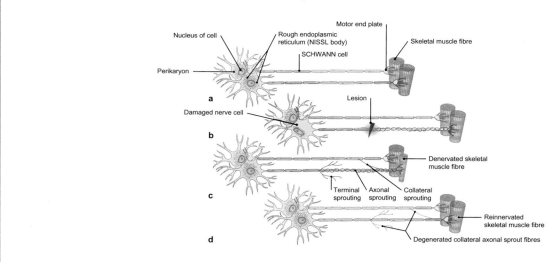

Clinical figure labels:
- Nucleus of cell
- Rough endoplasmic reticulum (NISSL body)
- Motor end plate
- Skeletal muscle fibre
- SCHWANN cell
- Perikaryon
- a
- Damaged nerve cell
- Lesion
- b
- Denervated skeletal muscle fibre
- c
- Terminal sprouting
- Axonal sprouting
- Collateral sprouting
- Reinnervated skeletal muscle fibre
- d
- Degenerated collateral axonal sprout fibres

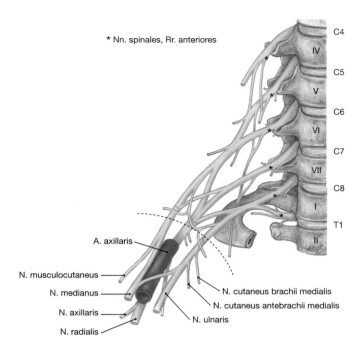

* Nn. spinales, Rr. anteriores

C4
IV
C5
V
C6
VI
C7
VII
C8
I
T1
II

A. axillaris

N. musculocutaneus

N. medianus

N. axillaris

N. radialis

N. cutaneus brachii medialis

N. cutaneus antebrachii medialis

N. ulnaris

Fig. 1.72   Diagram of a plexus with the example of the brachial plexus; ventral view. [S700]

A plexus refers to a network of nerve fibres. The human body contains two plexuses, the Plexus cervicobrachialis and lumbosacralis. Because the cervical plexus has no connection with the brachial plexus, the plexuses are referred to individually, in contrast to the Plexus lumbosacralis where there is a connection between the Plexus lumbalis and Plexus sacralis. The brachial plexus is responsible for innervation of the muscles and sen-

sitivity of the shoulder and arm. It forms the Rami ventrales of the spinal nerve roots C5 to T1 and belongs to the somatic plexuses, as with the other plexuses mentioned. They stand in contrast to the autonomic nervous plexuses. These include, for example, the Plexus coeliacus and the Plexus mesentericus superior in the upper abdomen, which are known collectively as the Plexus solaris. They contain sympathetic and parasympathetic fibres (→ Fig. 1.75).

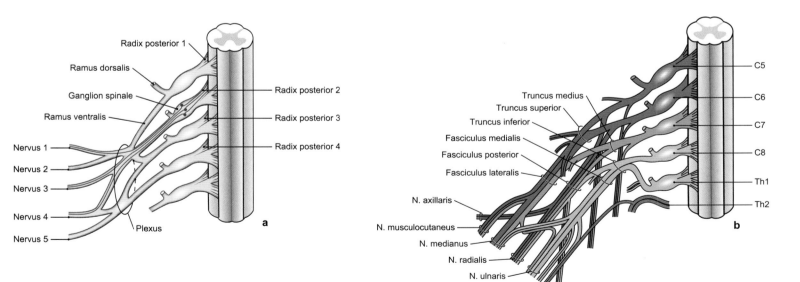

Fig. 1.73a and b   Formation of a plexus; ventral view. [S700-L126]

a Around a plexus, axons of a root (radix) are mostly distributed to several peripheral nerves.

b This figure shows the Plexus brachialis and the complex diverse distribution of axons from several radices (C5-Th2) with different peripheral nerves for the upper extremity (→ Fig. 1.11, segmental skin innervation).

General anatomy

Autonomic nervous system

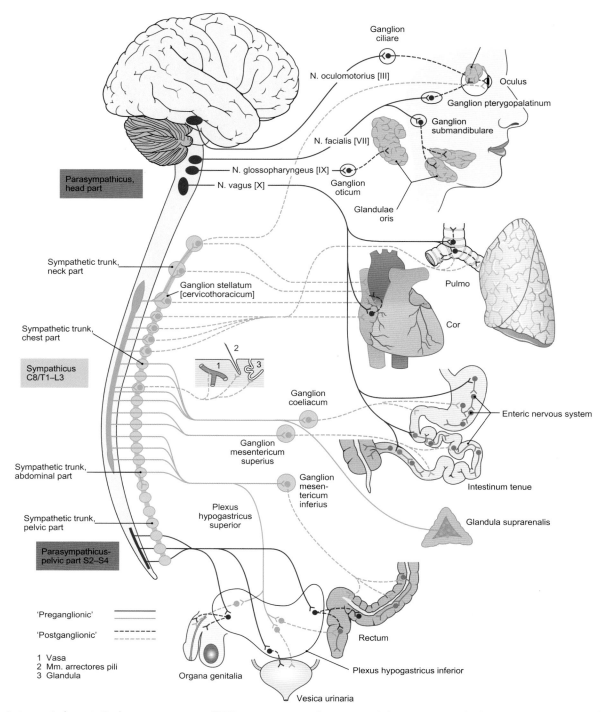

Ganglion
ciliare

N. oculomotorius [III]

Ganglion pterygopalatinum

Oculus

N. facialis [VII]

Ganglion
submandibulare

Parasympathicus,
head part

N. glossopharyngeus [IX]

N. vagus [X]

Ganglion
oticum

Glandulae
oris

Sympathetic trunk,
neck part

Pulmo

Ganglion stellatum
[cervicothoracicum]

Cor

Sympathetic trunk,
chest part

Sympathicus
C8/T1–L3

1 2 3

Ganglion
coeliacum

Enteric nervous system

Ganglion
mesentericum
superius

Sympathetic trunk,
abdominal part

Ganglion
mesen-
tericum
inferius

Intestinum tenue

Sympathetic trunk,
pelvic part

Plexus
hypogastricus
superior

Glandula suprarenalis

Parasympathicus-
pelvic part S2–S4

'Preganglionic'

'Postganglionic'

Rectum

1 Vasa
2 Mm. arrectores pili
3 Glandula

Organa genitalia

Plexus hypogastricus inferior

Vesica urinaria

Fig. 1.74   Autonomic (vegetative) nervous system. [S700-
L126~S130-L106]
The autonomic nervous system consists of the sympathetic, parasympathetic and enteric nervous system.
The nerve cells of the **sympathetic nervous system** are located in the
lateral horn of the thoracolumbar segments of the spinal cord. Their axons
project onto the sympathetic trunk ganglia and the ganglia of the digestive
tract, where they synapse onto postganglionic neurons that project to the
effector organs. Sympathetic excitation takes place to mobilise the body
during activity and also in emergency situations. The trunk also consists of
the adrenal medulla, which can release adrenaline and noradrenaline.

Core areas of the **parasympathetic nervous system** are found in the
brainstem and the sacral spinal cord. Their axons reach ganglia near the
effector organs in the head, thorax and abdominal cavity. Here the switch
is made to postganglionic neurons, which reach the effector organs via
short axons. The parasympathetic nervous system is used for food intake
and processing as well as sexual arousal, and is in opposition to the sympathetic nervous system.
The **enteric nervous system** regulates intestinal activity and is influenced
by the sympathetic and parasympathetic nervous systems.

Clinical remarks

Disorders of the autonomic nervous system play a role in almost
all medical disciplines. They can occur as independent diseases (e.g.
inherited autonomic neuropathy), as a result of other diseases (e.g.
autonomic neuropathy in Diabetes mellitus or PARKINSON's disease), or in response to external influences or other disorders (e.g.

autonomic dysregulation accompanying stress, severe pain or psychiatric disorders). Depending on the affected region of the autonomic nervous system, disorders of the circulatory system, diges-
tion, sexual function or other functions may prevail.

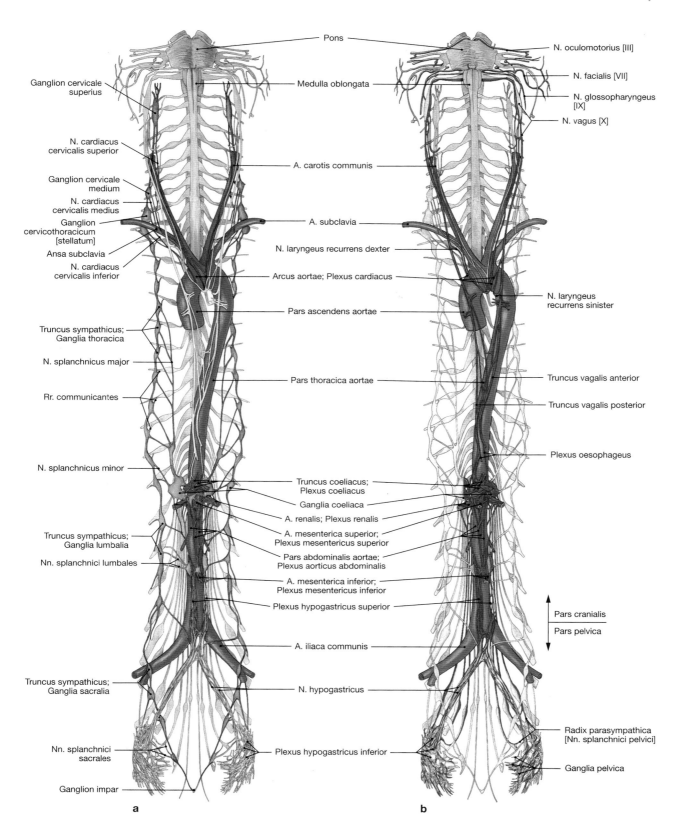

Pons
Ganglion cervicale superius
Medulla oblongata
N. oculomotorius [III]
N. facialis [VII]
N. glossopharyngeus [IX]
N. vagus [X]
N. cardiacus cervicalis superior
A. carotis communis
Ganglion cervicale medium
N. cardiacus cervicalis medius
Ganglion cervicothoracicum [stellatum]
A. subclavia
Ansa subclavia
N. cardiacus cervicalis inferior
N. laryngeus recurrens dexter
Arcus aortae; Plexus cardiacus
N. laryngeus recurrens sinister
Pars ascendens aortae
Truncus sympathicus; Ganglia thoracica
N. splanchnicus major
Pars thoracica aortae
Truncus vagalis anterior
Truncus vagalis posterior
Rr. communicantes
Plexus oesophageus
N. splanchnicus minor
Truncus coeliacus; Plexus coeliacus
Ganglia coeliaca
A. renalis; Plexus renalis
A. mesenterica superior; Plexus mesentericus superior
Truncus sympathicus; Ganglia lumbalia
Nn. splanchnici lumbales
Pars abdominalis aortae; Plexus aorticus abdominalis
A. mesenterica inferior; Plexus mesentericus inferior
Plexus hypogastricus superior
Pars cranialis
Pars pelvica
A. iliaca communis
Truncus sympathicus; Ganglia sacralia
N. hypogastricus
Radix parasympathica [Nn. splanchnici pelvici]
Nn. splanchnici sacrales
Plexus hypogastricus inferior
Ganglia pelvica
Ganglion impar

a   b

Fig. 1.75a and b   Representation of the autonomic sympathetic and parasympathetic nervous system. [S700]
a Sympathetic system, Pars sympathica. The complete set of sympathetic ganglia positioned near the spine and their connections with each other is referred to as the sympathetic trunk (Truncus sympathicus) (green).

b Parasympathetic system, Pars parasympathica. The parasympathetic fibres (purple) normally run alongside other nerve fibres. The fibres of the autonomic nervous system form the autonomic plexus.

X-ray

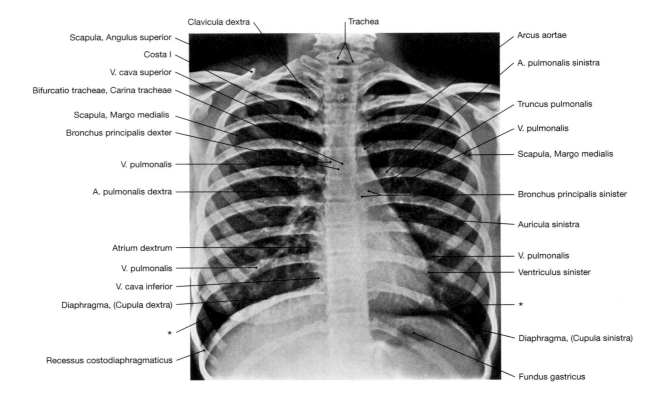

Clavicula dextra
Scapula, Angulus superior
Costa I
V. cava superior
Bifurcatio tracheae, Carina tracheae
Scapula, Margo medialis
Bronchus principalis dexter
V. pulmonalis
A. pulmonalis dextra
Atrium dextrum
V. pulmonalis
V. cava inferior
Diaphragma, (Cupula dextra)
*
Recessus costodiaphragmaticus

Trachea
Arcus aortae
A. pulmonalis sinistra
Truncus pulmonalis
V. pulmonalis
Scapula, Margo medialis
Bronchus principalis sinister
Auricula sinistra
V. pulmonalis
Ventriculus sinister
*
Diaphragma, (Cupula sinistra)
Fundus gastricus

Fig. 1.76   Conventional X-ray, thorax overview image. [R316-007]
Normal X-rays are undoubtedly one of the most frequently produced images in hospitals and practices. Before evaluation takes place, one should establish clearly which technique has been used and whether it is a standard image. Chest X-rays are the most frequent X-ray images requested by a physician. The image is taken with the patient standing upright and X-rays passing through the thorax in a postero-anterior (PA) direction (patient faces radiographic film) and with the patient lying down to generate a supine antero-posterior (AP) chest X-ray image. A good radiographic image of the thorax displays the major bronchi and blood vessels of the lungs, the cardiomediastinal contour, the diaphragm, ribs and peripheral soft tissue.

* mammary shadow (contour)

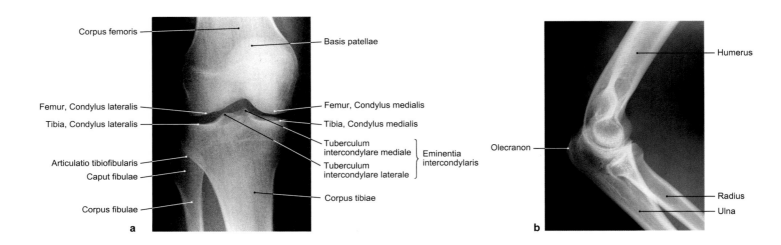

Corpus femoris
Femur, Condylus lateralis
Tibia, Condylus lateralis
Articulatio tibiofibularis
Caput fibulae
Corpus fibulae

Basis patellae
Femur, Condylus medialis
Tibia, Condylus medialis
Tuberculum intercondylare mediale
Tuberculum intercondylare laterale
} Eminentia intercondylaris
Corpus tibiae

a

Humerus
Olecranon
Radius
Ulna

b

Fig. 1.77a and b   Conventional X-ray images. [S700-T902]
a Antero-posterior X-ray images of the right knee joint.
b X-ray image with lateral view of the right elbow joint.
Conventional X-ray radiography is one of the most frequent and cost-effective medical imaging techniques. X-rays pass through a segment of the body and are captured on X-ray-sensitive film which darkens when exposed to the rays. Different tissues absorb X-rays in different ways which results in characteristic shades of grey to black in the X-ray image. Bones appear whitish in an X-ray image because they strongly absorb the X-ray energy. X-rays are electromagnetic waves and considered to be ionising radiation. Conventional X-rays are used particularly frequently in orthopoedics and emergency surgery.

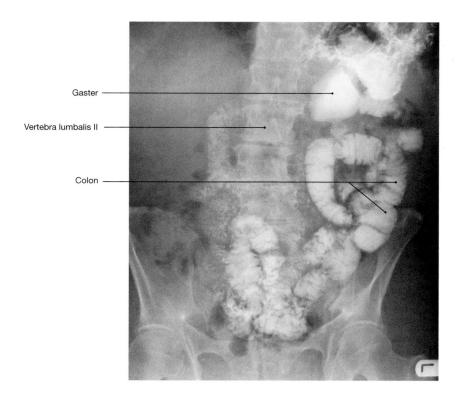

Gaster

Vertebra lumbalis II

Colon

Fig. 1.78   Conventional X-ray, contrast agent imaging of the large intestine. [E402]

In order to display arteries, veins, intestinal loops or other hollow organs, these must be filled with substances that absorb the X-rays to a greater extent than under normal circumstances. The substance administered must however not be toxic. A frequently used contrast agent is barium sulphate, an insoluble, non-toxic salt of high density. For vessels, iodinated molecules are normally used as a contrast agent. They are safe and well tolerated by most patients. Because they are then excreted via the urogenital tract, the kidneys, ureters and bladder (intravenous [IV] urography, IV urogram) can also be displayed.

General anatomy · **1**

Scintigraphy and ultrasound

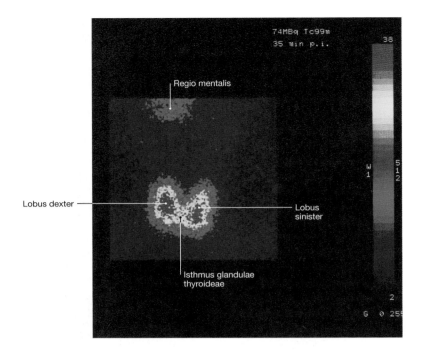

Regio mentalis

Lobus dexter

Lobus sinister

Isthmus glandulae thyroideae

Fig. 1.79 Scintigraphy, scintogram of the thyroid gland. [R316-007]
In scintigraphy, gamma rays (a form of electromagnetic rays) are used to generate an image. Gamma rays are produced as a result of the decay of unstable atomic nuclei, whereas X-rays are excess energy released during the bombardment of atoms with electrons. The gamma ray emitter has to be administered to the patient. The radioisotope technetium-99 m (^{99m}Tc) is most frequently used. It is usually injected in combination with other molecules. Following injection, and depending on how the radioactive pharmaceutical is absorbed, distributed, metabolised and excreted by the body, images are generated by a gamma camera.

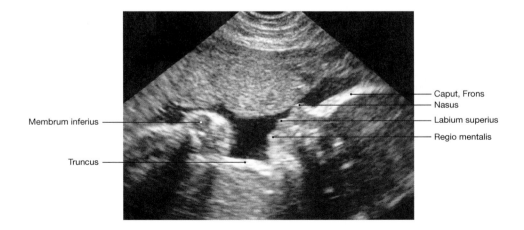

Caput, Frons
Nasus
Labium superius
Regio mentalis

Membrum inferius

Truncus

Fig. 1.80 Ultrasound image of a fetus in the 28th week of pregnancy; lateral view. [S700-T909]
Ultrasound examination of the body is used in all fields of medicine. Ultrasound is a very high frequency sound wave (no electromagnetic radiation) generated by piezoelectric materials that produce a series of sound waves. These sound waves are reflected from the inner organs and their contents (fetus in the uterus), registered by the same piezoelectric material, and evaluated in a computer. This creates a live image on the connected monitor, so that with a fetus, for example, the movements of the extremities and the opening of the mouth can be tracked.

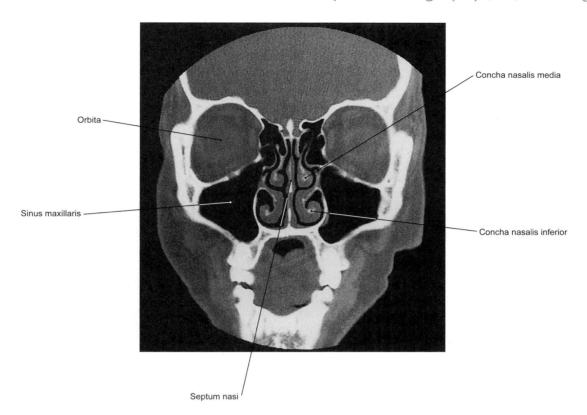

Orbita

Concha nasalis media

Sinus maxillaris

Concha nasalis inferior

Septum nasi

Fig. 1.81 Computed tomography, coronal computed tomography (CT) of the sinuses. [R331]

Computed tomography (CT) was developed by Sir Godfrey Hounsfield in the 1970s. Since then, the use of constantly updated CT scanners has meant continual further development. The computed tomography generates a series of cross-sectional images through the body in the transverse or, as shown here, coronal plane. The patient lies on a table and an X-ray tube takes one sectional image after the other while circling the body. Then a computer generates a sectional image using complex mathematical image analysis technology from the extensive data recorded.

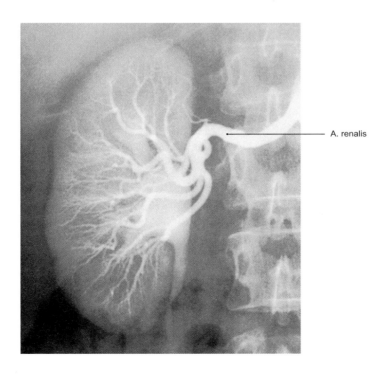

A. renalis

Fig. 1.82 Renal angiogram. [G570]

An **angiogram** is the specific radiological imaging technique for vessel structures (mostly blood vessels) using X-ray imaging. The image here shows a typical **renal angiogram** with the inner spaces of the vascular tree filled with the contrast agent. The contrast agent is excreted through the kidneys, which allows physicians to also examine the urinary tract, the ureter, urinary bladder and urethra for abnormalities.

General anatomy

3-D CT angiography

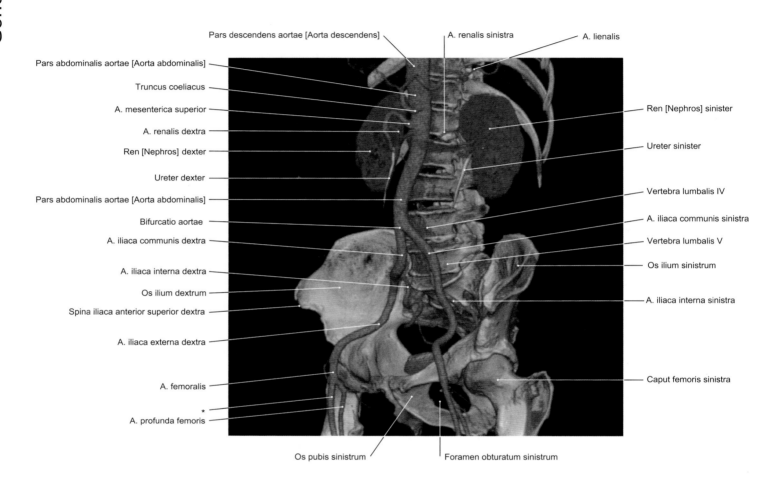

Pars descendens aortae [Aorta descendens]

A. renalis sinistra

A. lienalis

Pars abdominalis aortae [Aorta abdominalis]

Truncus coeliacus

A. mesenterica superior

A. renalis dextra

Ren [Nephros] dexter

Ureter dexter

Pars abdominalis aortae [Aorta abdominalis]

Bifurcatio aortae

A. iliaca communis dextra

A. iliaca interna dextra

Os ilium dextrum

Spina iliaca anterior superior dextra

A. iliaca externa dextra

A. femoralis

*

A. profunda femoris

Ren [Nephros] sinister

Ureter sinister

Vertebra lumbalis IV

A. iliaca communis sinistra

Vertebra lumbalis V

Os ilium sinistrum

A. iliaca interna sinistra

Caput femoris sinistra

Os pubis sinistrum

Foramen obturatum sinistrum

Fig. 1.83 3-D CT angiography, 3-D CT angiogram of different structures of the abdomen and pelvis (volume-rendering technique, VRT) derived from multidetector CT slices. [R316-007]
Modern computed tomography technology (e.g. 64-line volume spiral multilayer CT) provides new dimensions and indications for CT diagnostics. State-of-the-art equipment technology guarantees an individual, lowest-dose treatment for the patient.

A CT angiogram is based on such a multi-layer CT. The relevant blood vessel regions are scanned during rapid intravenous (IV) injection of an iodinated contrast agent. The resulting image slices of the vascular tree are then processed by a computer to generate a 3-D image.

* clin.: superficial femoral artery

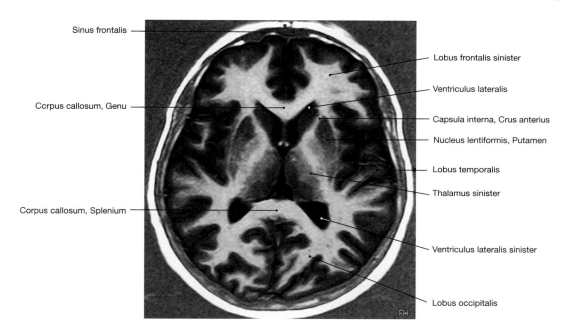

Sinus frontalis

Corpus callosum, Genu

Corpus callosum, Splenium

Lobus frontalis sinister

Ventriculus lateralis

Capsula interna, Crus anterius

Nucleus lentiformis, Putamen

Lobus temporalis

Thalamus sinister

Ventriculus lateralis sinister

Lobus occipitalis

Fig. 1.84 Magnetic resonance imaging, axial (transverse) magnetic resonance image (MRI) of the brain (T1-weighted). [R316-007]
In magnetic resonance imaging (MRI), the patient is exposed to a very strong magnetic field. All hydrogen protons in the body are aligned to the magnetic field. If the patient is exposed in the short term to a radio wave pulse, the magnets are deflected. When returning to the target position, the magnets emit small radio waves. Strength, frequency and the time needed by the protons to return to the original position influence the signal emitted. This signal is analysed and processed by a computer, which generates an image.

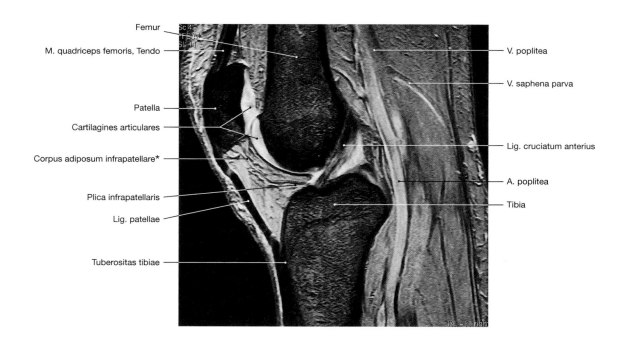

Femur

M. quadriceps femoris, Tendo

Patella

Cartilagines articulares

Corpus adiposum infrapatellare*

Plica infrapatellaris

Lig. patellae

Tuberositas tibiae

V. poplitea

V. saphena parva

Lig. cruciatum anterius

A. poplitea

Tibia

Fig. 1.85 Magnetic resonance imaging, sagittal magnetic resonance image (MRI) of a knee (T2-weighted). [R316-007]
By changing the sequence of pulses with which the protons are stimulated, different characteristics of the protons can be assessed. This is known as scan **weighting.** By changing the pulse sequence and the scanning parameters, T1-weighted images (liquids dark, fat pale, e.g. articular effusion dark) and T2-weighted images (liquids pale, fat medium tone, e.g. HOFFA's fat pad between the patella and tibia clearly visible) are produced, emphasising different tissue properties. An MRI can also be used to generate angiograms of the peripheral and central circulation.

* HOFFA's fat pad

Skin and its derivatives

Skin

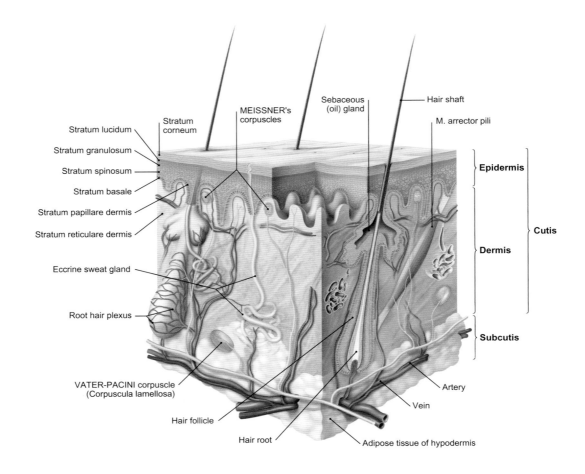

Stratum lucidum

Stratum corneum

MEISSNER's corpuscles

Sebaceous (oil) gland

Hair shaft

Stratum granulosum

M. arrector pili

Stratum spinosum

Stratum basale

Epidermis

Stratum papillare dermis

Stratum reticulare dermis

Cutis

Dermis

Eccrine sweat gland

Root hair plexus

Subcutis

VATER-PACINI corpuscle (Corpuscula lamellosa)

Artery

Vein

Hair follicle

Hair root

Adipose tissue of hypodermis

Fig. 1.86 Structure of the skin. [S701-L275]
The skin (**cutis**) is composed of a superficial, multilayered epithelial lining (**epidermis;** keratinised squamous epithelium) with underlying interstitial tissue (**dermis**) and an innermost layer containing fat cells (**subcutis,** hypodermis, Tela subcutanea). In everyday speech, we refer to skin as all three parts combined (cutaneous covering). Cutis and subcutis are a functional unit. They harbour **epidermal derivatives** (also called epidermal appendages), including hair, glands (eccrine and apocrine sweat glands, sebaceous glands). Additionally, the skin contains **somatic vis-ceral sensory organs** (mechanoreceptors: MERKEL cell-axon complexes, RUFFINI corpuscles (also named bulbous corpuscles or RUFFINI endings), MEISSNER's corpuscles and VATER-PACINI corpuscles.
The skin is an essential organ and covers an area of approx. 2 m². The skin protects the body from water loss and potentially hazardous external substances, serves as a thermoregulator (by altering cutaneous blood flow, sweat production), and detects external mechanical stimuli through the help of mechanoreceptors.

Structure and function

The majority of the exterior surface of the body (approx. 96 %) is covered in **hairy skin** with glands. It is characterised morphologically by its triangular and polygonal surface areas, which are separated from each other by ridges. It contains hair and glands and differs in thickness depending on the body region.
Hairless skin of the palms (Palmae manus) and the soles of the feet (Plantae pedes) has a distinct surface structure and constitutes approx. 4 % of the total body surface area. Genetically determined parallel ridges (unique fingerprints) form arches, loops and whorls for a better mechanical grip. Hairless skin contains a high number of eccrine sweat glands. Hair, sebaceous glands and apocrine sweat glands are absent in the hairless skin but present in hairy skin.

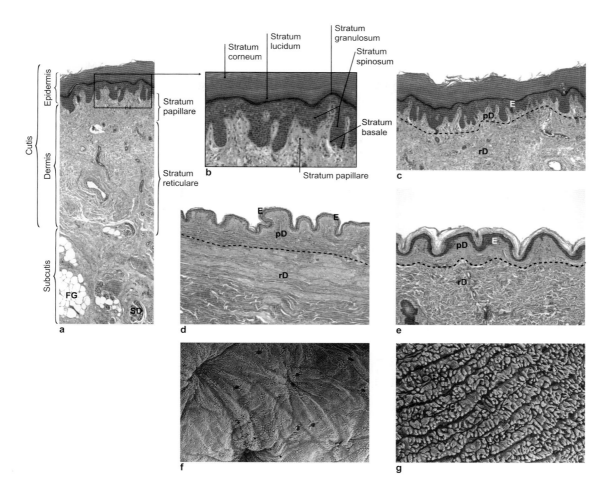

Fig. 1.87a–g   Layers of the cutaneous covering, Integumentum commune, and skin types (**a–c** hairless skin, **f** backs of the fingers) **and hairy skin** (**d** upper body, **e** upper arm, **g** finger pads). FG: fatty tissue; SD: eccrine sweat glands; E: epidermis; pD: papillary dermis; rD: reticular dermis. HE-staining, enlarged **a** 80-fold, **b** 200-fold, **c–e** 135-fold. [S700-P310]

a The skin (cutis) is composed of the **epidermis** (outer skin; epithelium) and underlying **dermis** (fibro-elastic connective tissue layer with capillary plexus, specialised receptors, nerves, immune cells, melatonin-producing cells, sweat glands, hair follicles, sebaceous glands, smooth muscle cells of which the thickness varies depending on the body region). Beneath the dermis lies the **subcutis** (subcutaneous fatty tissue). As the largest organ (ca. 2 m²), the skin functions to protect the body from mechanical damage, as a thermoregulator, as a sensory organ, and to prevent loss of water.

b The epidermis consists of the Stratum basale, Stratu spinosum, Stratum granulosum, Stratum lucidum (only in the hairless skin) and Stratum corneum **(b)**. The dermis consists of the Stratum papillare (compare scanning electron microscope (SEM) images, **f, g**) and Stratum reticulare.

c–e The dotted lines indicate the demarcations between those dermis layers which have been mentioned (Stratum papillare and Stratum reticulare). The epidermis of the hairy skin is visibly thinner than that of the hairless skin. The SEM images in **f** and **g** show the surface of the Stratum papillare of the dermis after removal of the epidermis.

f Scanning electron microscope (SEM) image of the dermal papillary layer (Stratum papillare) of the back of the finger after removal of the epidermis.

g SEM image of the dermal papillary layer (Stratum papillare) of the fingertip after removal of the epidermis.

Clinical remarks

Different proteins and structural features ensure dermo-epidermal connectivity. Genetic diseases can result in a dysfunction or loss of selected proteins and impaired structural integrity that diminishes adhesion mechanisms between the two zones. This can make the affected skin prone to shear forces which leads to tearing associated with **blistering** (bullae) and, in extreme cases, extensive detachment of the epidermis. Epidermal detachment can also occur as a result of autoantibodies directly binding components of the dermo-epidermal adhesion structures (bullous pemphigoid; pemphigus).

Skin and its derivatives

Hair

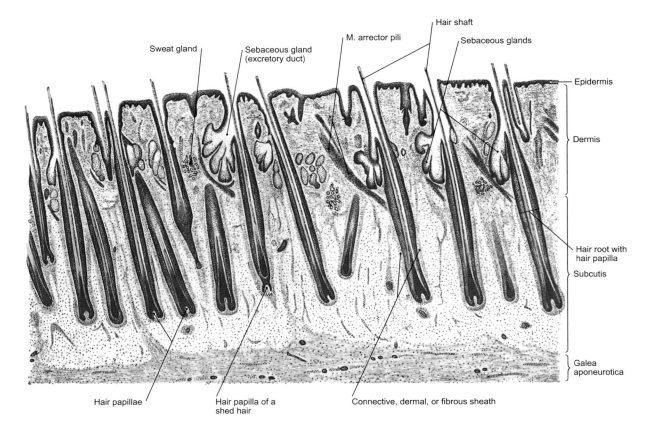

Fig. 1.88 labels: Sweat gland · Sebaceous gland (excretory duct) · M. arrector pili · Hair shaft · Sebaceous glands · Epidermis · Dermis · Hair root with hair papilla · Subcutis · Galea aponeurotica · Hair papillae · Hair papilla of a shed hair · Connective, dermal, or fibrous sheath

Fig. 1.88 Hair, Pili; longitudinal section through the scalp. [R170-5]
Hair is the product of keratinisation of the epidermis. It originates from invaginations of the epidermis which form follicles that contain mitotically active cells (matrix cells) at the base. The cells emerging from matrix cells diversify into horn cells, which form the hair shaft. Postnatally, a distinction is made between two basic types of hair:
- **vellus hair** (downy hair), which is soft, short (the follicles are in the dermis), thin and virtually unpigmented with no centre; it corre-

sponds to the fetal lanugo and covers most of the body in children and women
- **terminal hair** (long hair), which is strong, long (the follicles reach the subcutis), thick and pigmented with a centre; it occurs as scalp hair, eyelashes, eyebrows, pubic hair, armpit hair and beard hair (in men) and usually differs considerably in different ethnic groups.

Hair serves to protect against UV light and heat as well as to provide tactile sensation.

Fig. 1.89 Structure of a hair follicle; longitudinal section. [R170-5]
Hair arises in cylindrical epithelial depressions which reach down to the dermis or subcutis and are referred to as hair follicles. The **hair follicle** consists of the hair bulb and papilla. It is nourished by blood vessels and is the point of origin of hair growth. Each hair follicle has a sebaceous gland **(pilosebaceous gland unit)** and a smooth muscle **(Musculus arrector pili)** associated with it. The latter is responsible for elevating the hair (sympathetic activation), simultaneously retracting the epidermis, forming small depressions (goose bumps).
A distinction is made between:
- the fully keratinised **hair shaft** with an epithelial hair root sheath
- the non-keratinised **hair root,** separated by the keratogenous zone (keratinisation of hair cells) from the keratinised hair shaft
- the **hair bulb** (Bulbus pili), the distended epithelial initial part of the hair, which contains cell division-enabling **matrix cells**
- the **hair papilla,** a cell-rich connective tissue process of the dermis, which extends up into the hair bulb
- the **hair funnel;** represents the outlet of the follicle to the skin surface which is accompanied by the sebaceous gland
- the **epithelial root sheath,** subdivided into the inner and outer root sheaths: the layers of the **inner** root sheath, from the inside to the outside, consist of: the cuticle, the HUXLEY's and HENLE's layers; the **outer** root sheath is composed of several layers of bright, non-keratinised cells, which are only keratinised in the area of the hair funnel and from there continue into the epidermis of the skin.
The hair colour depends not only on genetic predisposition but also on the pigment content (melanin) of the hair. Once production of melanin ceases, the hair turns to grey or white.

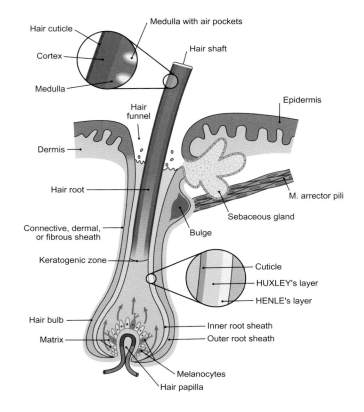

Fig. 1.89 labels: Hair cuticle · Medulla with air pockets · Cortex · Hair shaft · Medulla · Hair funnel · Epidermis · Dermis · Hair root · M. arrector pili · Sebaceous gland · Bulge · Connective, dermal, or fibrous sheath · Keratogenic zone · Cuticle · HUXLEY's layer · HENLE's layer · Hair bulb · Inner root sheath · Matrix · Outer root sheath · Melanocytes · Hair papilla

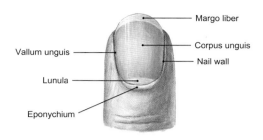

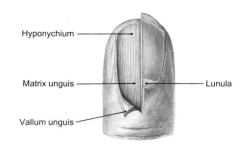

Fig. 1.90   Finger phalanx with nail. [S700]
The nail (Unguis) is a convex-shaped, translucent keratin plate (nail plate) on the upper side of the distal phalanx of the fingers and toes. It provides protection for the toe- and fingertips and supports the gripping function. It lies laterally in skin pockets (nail bed, Vallum unguis) which are surrounded by a slightly raised skin fold (nail fold). The epithelium, located beneath the nail plate at the dorsal end of the nail bed, is known as the eponychium (cuticle, cuticula). The nail plate is anchored here to the nail bed.

Fig. 1.91   Finger phalanx; nail partially removed. [S700]
The epithelium, on which the nail rests, is called the hyponychium. Beneath this lies the nail bed, composed of loose connective tissue, which is firmly fused with the periosteum of the distal phalanx. Proximally, the hyponychium turns into the nail matrix (Matrix unguis), from which the nail plate emerges (visible from the outside as the lunula).

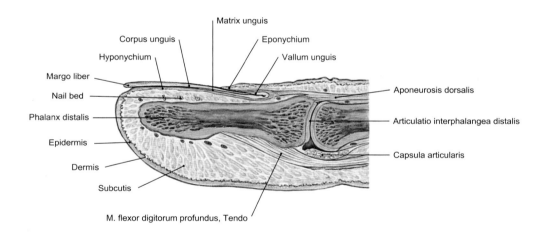

Fig. 1.92   Finger phalanx, Phalanx distalis; sagittal section. [S700]
The nail bed comprises the region between the nail and the distal phalanx. It consists of the epithelium (Hyponychium and Matrix unguis) and the underlying dermis.

Clinical remarks

White spots under nails are due to defective fusion of the nail plate with the nail bed. Changes in light reflection at these points cause the nail plate to appear milky-white (similar to the lunula). Defective fusion can have different causes, e.g. it can be triggered by impact, medication or various illnesses. **Brittle nails** can be a sign of a lack of biotin (vitamin H). Biotin is required for the formation of keratin, the main component of the nail plate. Numerous systemic diseases are accompanied by nail changes. Psoriasis, for example, leads to the formation of **dents** (small pits), **oil stains** and sometimes **crumbling nails** or extreme **nail dystrophy**. Skin and nail injuries can be followed by colonisation by fungi **(nail mycosis),** for which the treatment, especially in toenails, can often be lengthy.

Sample exam questions

To check that you are completely familiar with the content of this chapter, sample questions from an oral anatomy exam are listed here.

Explain the structure of a bone:

- How do you distinguish bones according to their form and structure?
- How can you classify a long tubular bone?
- What happens in fracture-healing?
- What types of bone joints do you know?
- How can bone adapt functionally to increased stress?

Describe the structure of a joint:

- What specific joint types do you know?
- What is the structure of the joint capsule?
- What is meant by the neutral-zero-method?
- What is an amphiarthrosis?
- What auxiliary structures do you know in joints?
- How is a bursa structured?

Explain the structure of a skeletal muscle:

- What types of muscle do you know and how can you classify muscles?
- How is a tendon sheath structured?
- What is meant by muscle activity?
- What is a lever arm?
- What is meant by dynamic muscle activity?

Explain different circulatory systems:

- Where can the pulse be palpated on the upper and lower extremities?
- What is the low-pressure system within the circulatory system?
- What mechanisms are there for the return of venous blood to the heart?
- What types of shunts are there in fetal circulation?

What is meant by portal vein circulation?

- What pathway does the lymph take from the periphery of the body?
- Can you describe the general structure of a lymph node?

Explain the lymphatic drainage pathways in the neck:

- How many lymph nodes are there in the neck area?
- What lymph node groups exist in the neck area?
- Why is the throat area divided into lymphatic drainage regions (compartments)?
- What structures drain their lymph into the cervical lymph nodes?

Explain the structure of the nervous system:

- How is the nervous system divided up?
- What is a dermatome?
- What is meant by the autonomic nervous system?
- What is the enteric nervous system?

Explain imaging methods:

- Name some imaging methods used in routine clinical practice.
- How does computer tomography differ from magnetic resonance imaging?
- What is contrast agent imaging?
- What advantage does ultrasound imaging offer compared to conventional X-ray imaging?

Explain the skin and its derivatives:

- What layers of the skin do you know? How is a fingernail structured?
- How is a hair structured?
- Which basic types of hair do you know?

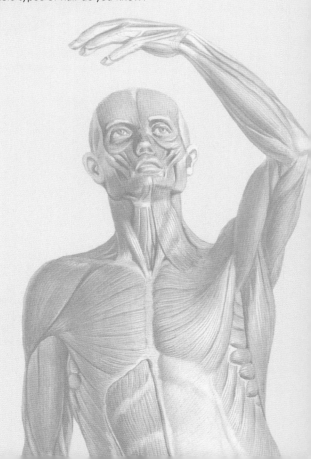

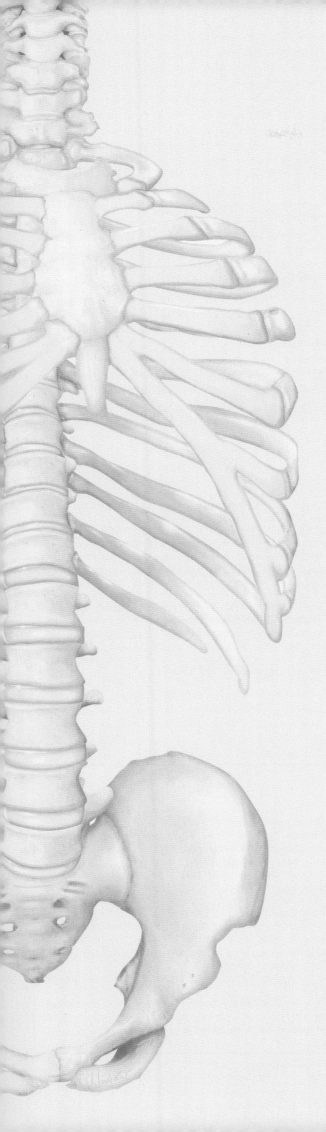

Trunk

Surface   84

Development   88

Skeleton   90

Imaging methods 124

Musculature 132

Neurovascular pathways 160

Topography, dorsal trunk wall 170

Female breast 182

Topography, ventral trunk wall 186

2

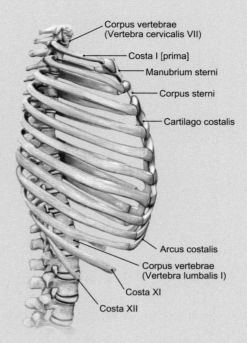

Corpus vertebrae
(Vertebra cervicalis VII)

Costa I [prima]

Manubrium sterni

Corpus sterni

Cartilago costalis

Arcus costalis

Corpus vertebrae
(Vertebra lumbalis I)

Costa XI

Costa XII

Overview

The torso supports the head and upper extremities, which are secured in a flexible manner. The **spine** is the support structure of the torso, with its vertebrae increasing in size from top to bottom to support the weight of the body. To cushion any impact there are **intervertebral discs** (Disci intervertebrales) between the individual vertebrae which consist of a fibrous ring and a central gelatinous core. For protection against injuries, the spinal cord is encased by the vertebral arches in the vertebral canal. In the lower section, the vertebra is fused to the **sacrum** (Os sacrum) and forms the stable pelvic ring together with the pelvic bone. The characteristic curvature of the spine in humans is caused by the biped walk and the upright torso. There are numerous muscles mainly on the back and sides of the vertebrae (autochthonous muscles). This enables the individual vertebrae to move against each other. The viscera chambers of the torso lie in front of the spine, consisting of the thoracic cavity (Cavitas thoracis), **abdominal cavity** (Ca-

vitas abdominalis) and **pelvic cavity** (Cavitas pelvis). The thoracic cavity is framed by the thorax, which includes the twelve pairs of ribs and the sternum as well as the vertebrae. The musculature is located between the ribs. In contrast, the wall of the abdomen consists solely of muscles and their tendons (aponeurosis). The thoracic and abdominal cavities are separated by the **midriff or diaphragm.** The **mammary gland** (Mamma) is situated on the outer anterior side of the thoracic wall and can move freely on the M. pectoralis major. During pregnancy, it produces milk which is important for the nutrition of the baby. In males, there is a passageway **(inguinal canal)** in the lower section of the abdominal wall between the **scrotum** and the abdominal cavity which connects the spermatic cord and the structures contained in it to the corresponding organs and structures in the abdominal cavity, e.g. the urethra. Females also have an inguinal canal.

Main topics

After working through this chapter, you should be able to:

- show and name palpable surface structures, allocate the regions of the torso and get your bearings topographically using anatomical lines on the torso;
- explain the difference between dermatomes and the HEAD's zone;
- know the principles of abdominal wall development, including the development of ribs, sternum and spine, and associated clinically relevant variations and malformations;
- describe the structure of the bony spine and thorax along with the corresponding joints, name the various associated ligaments, show them on the skeleton or specimen and outline the movement capabilities of the individual joints and as a whole;
- describe the autochthonous musculature in the back and the corresponding fascia as well as the posture and movement functions of the head and torso;
- describe the layered structure of the abdominal wall, in particular the musculature of the abdominal wall, thoracic and abdominal

  area, including the muscles inside the thoracic and abdominal cavity, as well as the muscles in the neck;
- name the base and origin of the straight and oblique abdominal muscles and explain the weak points of the abdominal wall as predilection sites for abdominal wall ruptures;
- describe the structure and the innervation of the diaphragm, explain the penetration points in addition to the penetrating structures and name possible weak points;
- name the types of bypass circulation;
- describe the lymph catchment areas of the superficial axillary and inguinal lymph nodes;
- outline the morphological principles of lumbar puncture, epidural anaesthesia and pleurocentesis;
- describe the female breast from a topographical and oncoplastic perspective;
- explain the inguinal canal from an evolutionary and clinical perspective;
- explain the structure of the Plexus lumbosacralis.

Clinical relevance

In order not to lose touch with prospective everyday clinical life with so many anatomical details, the following describes a typical case that shows why the content of this chapter is so important.

Inguinal hernia

Case study
A 27-year-old man noticed a swelling in his right inguinal area which became larger when pressed, while doing sports or with coughing. Initially the swelling was very small, but over the last two months it has grown. Sometimes, he now also has a dull pain in the right lower abdomen and in the inguinal area. The young man feels well otherwise, has no additional complaints or illnesses, and does not take medication.

Result of examination
In a standing position, a slight swelling of the skin in the right inguinal area is apparent, which is absent on the opposite side. This protrusion can easily be pushed back manually (repositioning). There is no tenderness in the inguinal area, and the repositioning is painless. If the examiner pushes an index finger from a caudal direction lightly towards the inner inguinal ring and asks the young man to cough while pushing the inguinal skin inwards, they can feel a protrusion with the fingertip, pointing in the direction of the right scrotum. This is a clear indication of an inguinal hernia. The neck of the hernia sac seems to lie lateral of the Vasa epigastrica inferiora and above the Tuberculum pubicum.

Diagnostic procedure
This diagnosis of an inguinal hernia does not require additional clinical examination. The diagnosis is ideally made on a standing patient, as is the case with the young man. When using the index or little finger to gently push scrotal or inguinal skin inwards through the outer hernia ring, the fingertip should come to rest on the inner inguinal ring (→ Fig. a). The patient is asked to cough and/or contract their abdominal muscles to push the intestines downwards. This way, even small hernias can be palpated. The young man is diagnosed as having an indirect inguinal hernia. The hernial sac had extended into the Fossa inguinalis lateralis via the inner inguinal ring, through the inguinal canal, and into the scrotum. The hernial orifice is the inner inguinal ring. The three finger rule can help to differentiate between direct inguinal hernias and femoral hernias in the inguinal region.

 Femoral hernias (Herniae femorales) are more common in older women.

The palm of the right or left hand is placed on the Spina iliaca anterior superior with fingers pointing at the inguinal region. The middle finger marks the pathway of the indirect hernia, the index finger the direct hernia, and the ring finger points at the location of the femoral hernia (→ Fig. b).

Diagnosis
Hernia inguinalis.

Treatment
Inguinal hernias have to be treated surgically **every time.** The patient is informed about a minimally invasive TEPP (total extraperitoneal patch plasty) and prepared for surgery. As part of the TEP, an endoscopy is conducted on the abdominal wall through two to three small cuts in the abdominal skin. In this procedure the hernial sac was exposed and dissected, the content of the hernial sac (an intestinal loop, which caused the swelling and mild pain) was repositioned into the abdominal cavity and finally the hernial sac was removed. During the operation a thin plastic mesh is laid between the layers of the abdominal wall (behind the M. transversus and below the Peritoneum parietale).

Further developments
The great advantage of this surgical procedure is the immediate ability to sustain pressure, which generally makes it possible to do even intense sport within one week. The young man was able to go home on the same day of the operation and within a week was active again playing volleyball completely pain-free and with no protrusion in the inguinal area.

Dissection lab
Examine the walls and the content of the inguinal canal (→ Fig. 2.164) in the dissection lab.

 Regardless of gender, the R. genitalis of the N. genitofemoralis and the N. ilioinguinalis run through the inguinal canal.

In the male inguinal canal, note the N. ilioinguinalis in addition to the spermatic cord (consisting of A. testicularis, Plexus pampiniformis, Ductus deferens, A. ductus deferentis, R. genitalis of the N. genitofemoralis). In females, the Lig. teres uteri, the R. genitalis of the N. genito-femoralis, the N. ilioinguinalis and the lymphatic vessels pass through this area from the uterus.

Back in the clinic
The inguinal canal is a predilection site for hernias. A distinction is made between indirect and direct inguinal hernias depending on the hernial ring.

 Direct inguinal hernias lie medial.

In the case in question, the patient had an indirect inguinal hernia, which was not hereditary but acquired. Such acquired indirect hernias are the most common abdominal wall ruptures in adults and are predominant in men. Direct inguinal hernias penetrate through the muscle-free Trigonum inguinale (HESSELBACH's triangle) into the Fossa inguinalis medialis. The triangle is a weak point, because in this area the abdominal wall only consists of the Fascia transversalis and Peritoneum parietale. In this case, the hernial ring lies medial of the Vasa epigastrica inferiora.

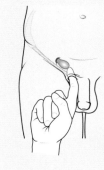

Fig. a Diagnosis of an inguinal hernia using the finger. [S700-L126]

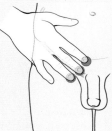

Fig. b Three-finger rule to demarcate direct inguinal hernias and femoral hernias in the inguinal area. [S700-L126]

Surface anatomy

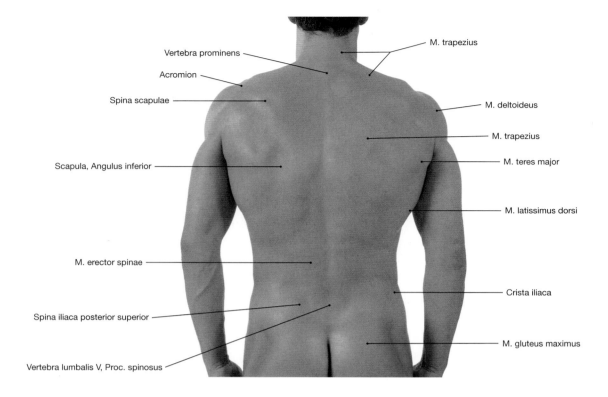

Vertebra prominens

Acromion

Spina scapulae

Scapula, Angulus inferior

M. erector spinae

Spina iliaca posterior superior

Vertebra lumbalis V, Proc. spinosus

M. trapezius

M. deltoideus

M. trapezius

M. teres major

M. latissimus dorsi

Crista iliaca

M. gluteus maximus

Fig. 2.1   Back, dorsum, surface anatomy. [S700]
The surface anatomy of the back provides useful landmarks to define different regions of the spine, muscles, the approximate position of the end of the spinal cord or the position of the organs (e. g. kidneys). Par-

ticularly easily palpable bone points include the Proc. spinosus of the seventh cervical vertebra (Vertebra prominens), the acromion, the Spina scapulae, the Angulus inferior of the scapula and the Proc. spinosus of the fifth lumbar vertebra.

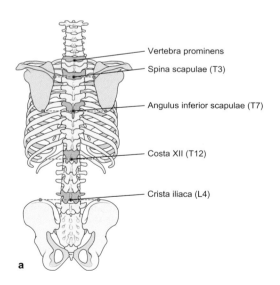

Vertebra prominens

Spina scapulae (T3)

Angulus inferior scapulae (T7)

Costa XII (T12)

Crista iliaca (L4)

a

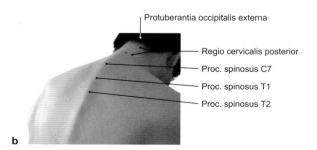

Protuberantia occipitalis externa

Regio cervicalis posterior

Proc. spinosus C7

Proc. spinosus T1

Proc. spinosus T2

b

Fig. 2.2a and b   Skeleton and back with bony landmarks.
a Bony landmarks are easy to palpate, e. g. the Vertebra prominens (C7). Several other vertebrae can be located because of their spatial relationship with easily palpable anatomical structures, e. g. T3 at the level of the Spina scapulae, T7 at the level of the Angulus inferior scapulae, T12

at the level of the 12th rib pair, and L4 at the level of the Crista iliaca. [S701-L126]
b By bending the head forward so the chin rests on the chest and rolling the shoulders forward, the bony dorsal spines of several cervical and upper thoracic vertebrae are easily palpable. [S701-L271]

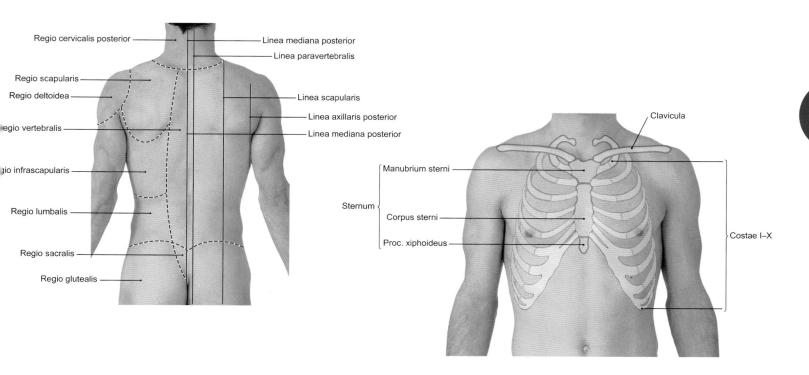

Fig. 2.3 Regions and orientation lines on the back. [S701-J803/L126] A distinction is made between the following topographical regions on the back and in the neck area: Regio cervicalis posterior (Regio nuchalis), Regiones vertebralis, scapularis, infrascapularis, deltoidea, lumbalis, sacralis and glutealis. The Lineae mediana posterior, paravertebralis, scapularis and axillaris posterior serve as orientation lines.

Fig. 2.4 Projection of the sternum onto the chest wall. [S700-J803/L126]

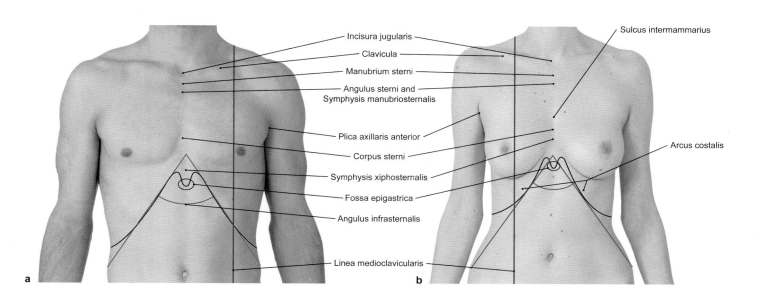

Fig. 2.5a and b Surface anatomy of the anterior chest wall. [S700-J803]

a View of a man.
b View of a woman.

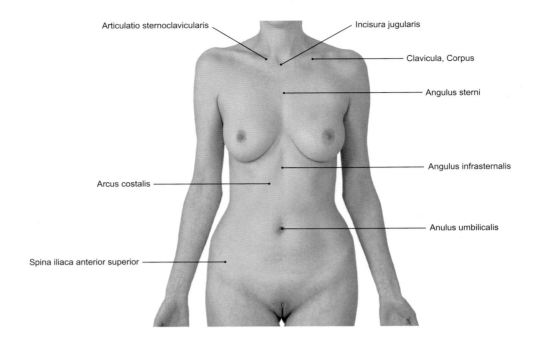

Fig. 2.6 **Surface anatomy of the chest and abdominal wall of a young woman.** [S701-J803]

Landmarks are useful to get one's bearings on the ventral wall, such as the costal arch (Arcus costalis), the navel (Anulus umbilicalis) and the Spina iliaca anterior superior. Other landmarks are depicted.

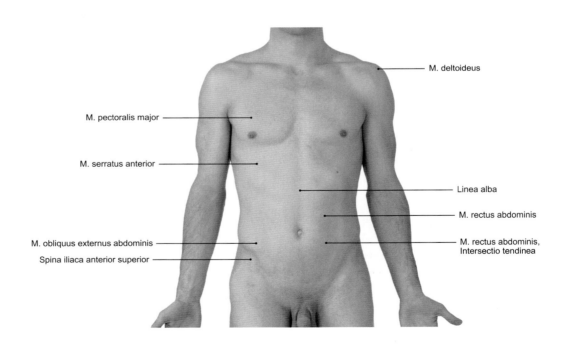

Fig. 2.7 **Surface anatomy of the chest and abdominal wall in a young man.** [S701-J803]

Landmarks on the ventral abdominal wall.

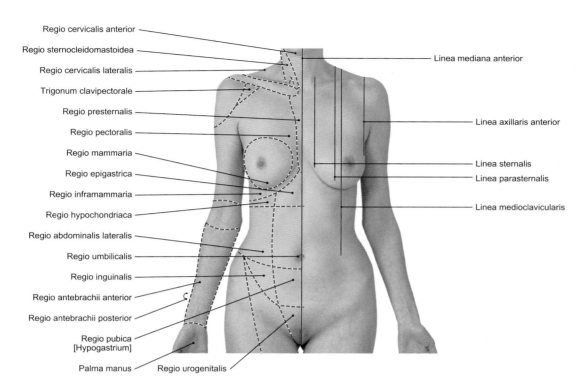

Regio cervicalis anterior
Regio sternocleidomastoidea
Regio cervicalis lateralis
Trigonum clavipectorale
Regio presternalis
Regio pectoralis
Regio mammaria
Regio epigastrica
Regio inframammaria
Regio hypochondriaca
Regio abdominalis lateralis
Regio umbilicalis
Regio inguinalis
Regio antebrachii anterior
Regio antebrachii posterior
Regio pubica [Hypogastrium]
Palma manus
Regio urogenitalis

Linea mediana anterior
Linea axillaris anterior
Linea sternalis
Linea parasternalis
Linea medioclavicularis

Fig. 2.8 Regions and orientation lines on the chest and abdominal wall in a young woman. [S700-J803/L126]
A distinction is made between the following topographic regions in the base of the neck and on the thoracic and abdominal wall: Regio cervicalis lateralis (Trigonum cervicale lateral), Regio sternocleidomastoidea, Regio cervicalis anterior (Trigonum cervicale anterius), Trigonum clavipectorale, Regiones presternalis, mammaria, inframammaria, deltoidea, epigastrica, hypochondriaca, umbilicalis, abdominalis lateralis,

pubica and urogenitalis. The Lineae anterior, sternalis, parasternalis, medioclavicularis and axillaris anterior serve as orientation lines. The Regio pectoralis is overlapped in females by the Mamma and correspondingly by the Regiones mammaria and inframammaria. The Lineae mediana anterior, sternalis, parasternalis medioclavicularis and axillaris anterior serve as orientation lines: mediana anterior, sternalis, parasternalis medioclavicularis and axillaris anterior.

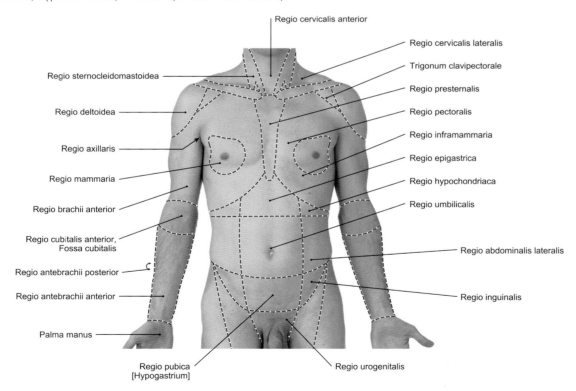

Regio cervicalis anterior
Regio sternocleidomastoidea
Regio deltoidea
Regio axillaris
Regio mammaria
Regio brachii anterior
Regio cubitalis anterior, Fossa cubitalis
Regio antebrachii posterior
Regio antebrachii anterior
Palma manus
Regio pubica [Hypogastrium]

Regio cervicalis lateralis
Trigonum clavipectorale
Regio presternalis
Regio pectoralis
Regio inframammaria
Regio epigastrica
Regio hypochondriaca
Regio umbilicalis
Regio abdominalis lateralis
Regio inguinalis
Regio urogenitalis

Fig. 2.9 Regions and orientation lines on the chest and abdominal wall in a young man. [S700-J803/L126]
A distinction is made between the following topographical regions in the base of the neck and on the thoracic and abdominal wall: Regio cervicalis lateralis (Trigonum cervicale lateral), Regio sternocleidomastoidea, Regio cervicalis anterior (Trigonum cervicale anterius), Trigonum

clavipectorale, Regiones presternalis, mammaria, inframammaria, deltoidea, epigastrica, hypochondriaca, umbilicalis, abdominalis lateralis, pubica and urogenitalis. In the same way as in females (→ Fig. 2.5), the Lineae mediana anterior, sternalis, parasternalis, medioclavicularis and axillaris anterior serve as orientation lines.

Development

Walls of the trunk

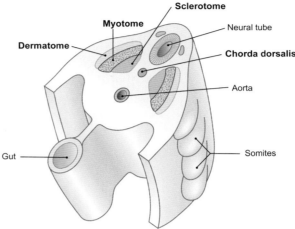

Week 4

Fig. 2.10 Development of the walls of the trunk: division of the somites in the fourth week. [E838]

The elements of the musculoskeletal system of the ventral and dorsal trunk wall originate exclusively from the middle germ layer **(mesoderm)**. The mesoderm condenses itself on both sides of the Chorda dorsalis and of the neural tube to the somites and the unsegmented lateral plate mesoderms. Within the somites, a ventromedial section, the **sclerotome,** can be differentiated in the fourth week. The cells of the sclerotome generally circulate around the neural tube and the Chorda dorsalis, and differentiate into primitive vertebrae. The **myotome** and the **dermatome,** which supply the muscle and skin cells, emerge from the lateral section of the somites.

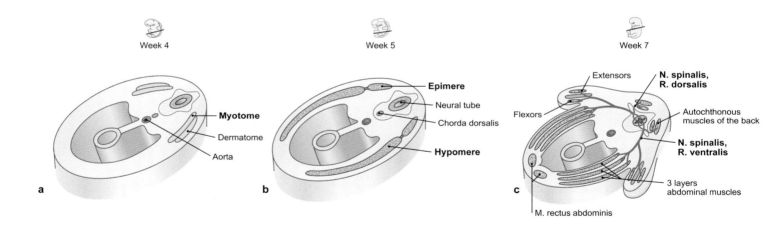

Fig. 2.11a–c Development of the walls of the trunk: formation of epimere and hypomere from the myotomes. [E838]

a Developmental stage at week 4: The striated muscles of the trunk develop from lateral sections of the somites, the dermatomyotomes, which differentiated in the fourth week.

b Developmental stage at week 5: During the fifth week, a larger ventral group of mesenchymal cells, the **hypomere** (supplying the Mm. scaleni, the prevertebral neck muscles, the infrahyoid muscles, the Mm. intercostales, subcostales, transversus thoracis, the oblique abdominal muscles, the Mm. rectus abdominis, quadratus lumborum, the pelvic floor muscles and the sphincters of the anus and urethra), separates from a smaller dorsal group, the epimere (supplying the autochthonous muscles – M. erector spinae).

c Developmental stage at week 7: in the seventh week the oblique and straight abdominal muscles differentiate from the hypomere in the area of the abdominal wall; the **epimere** forms parts of the autochthonous muscles of the back. The epimere and the hypomere get a separate nerve supply: the Rr. ventrales of the spinal nerves are responsible for the hypomere; the epimere is innervated by the Rr. dorsales of the spinal nerves.

Clinical remarks

Certain muscles are sometimes absent, but often without any clinical relevance. Movement disorders with varying degrees of severity are however associated with uni- or bilateral absence of the M. pectoralis or the Mm. trapezius and serratus anterior, respectively.

In the case of the very rare **prune belly syndrome,** the abdominal musculature is completely absent. The organs are palpable through the skin. Larger muscle defects can lead to hernias pushing through the abdominal wall.

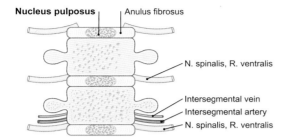

Fig. 2.12 Development of the walls of the trunk: Nuclei pulposi as remnants of the Chorda dorsalis in the adult spine. [E838]
From the fourth week of development, cells migrate from the sclerotome and settle around the neural tube. A part of the cells encloses the Chorda dorsalis and differentiates into vertebral bodies. The Chorda regresses to become the small base of the gelatinous Nucleus pulposus in the centre of the intervertebral discs.

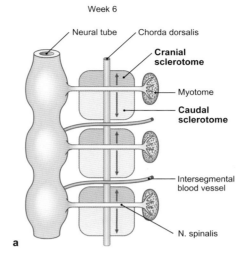

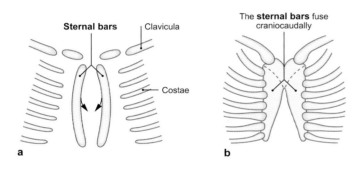

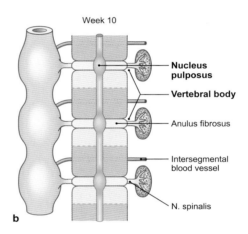

Fig. 2.13a and b Development of the ribs and the sternum. [E838]
a The sternum develops from two sternal bars which develop at a distance from each other as vertical mesenchymal concentrations in the chest wall. The ribs of the thoracic region and the Procc. costales in the cervical and lumbar spine are formed by sclerotome cells which migrated ventrolaterally.
b The sternal bars fuse in a cranio-caudal direction. The Proc. xiphoideus only ossifies between 20 to 25 years of age. The ribs connect dorsally with the spine and ventrally in part with the sternum (ribs I–VII; **real ribs, Costae verae**). The VIIIth–X[th] ribs fuse ventrally with each other and make indirect contact with the sternum via the cartilaginous costal arch **(false ribs, Costae spuriae).** Ribs XI and XII are exclusively connected with the vertebrae and end as floating ribs **(Costae fluctuantes)** in the ventral thoracic wall.

Fig. 2.14a and b Formation of the vertebral body from two adjacent sclerotomes. [E838]
a Week 6. The sclerotomes are divided into a cranial and caudal section. Assigned to a sclerotome, the myotome is always innervated by a spinal nerve. Intersegmental vessels run between the sclerotomes and myotomes.
b Week 10. Each of the individual vertebrae are created through a fusion of the caudal sclerotome section with a cranial sclerotome section of the adjacent (successive) sclerotomes. The spinal nerve associated with the myotome is enclosed between the cranial and caudal sclerotome sections as part of the fusion and exits from the Foramen intervertebrale. Intervertebral discs develop between the Corpus vertebrae. Muscles that are only created from parts of a myotome (e.g. M. rotatoris brevis, → Fig. 2.86) can move two adjacent vertebrae against each other. The functional unit of all structures participating in the respective movement between two adjacent vertebrae is called a motion segment.

Clinical remarks

A **spina bifida** is a split, dorsal open spine, in which single or multiple vertebral arches have not grown together. If not only the vertebral arches are open but also the neural folds, this is referred to as **rachischisis.** If the spinal cord is also affected, this can be associated with paralysis. If the cleft in the vertebral arches is covered with skin, it is called a spina bifida occulta. If only one instead of two cartilage centres emerge in a vertebral body, the result is a **wedge vertebra** (hemivertebra). If two vertebrae fuse with each other, because the intervertebral discs have degenerated, the result is a **block vertebra.**

Merger disorders of the sternum often occur as a fissure formation of the Corpus sterni or the Proc. xiphoideus. Clinically, these types of columns or holes are usually meaningless.
Accessory ribs are common in the cervical and lumbar region (cervical and lumbar ribs). In the lumbar region, they are usually clinically insignificant (Clinical remarks → Fig. 2.41). However, in the neck region they may lead to a compression of the brachial plexus or the subclavian artery (Clinical remarks → Fig. 2.17).

Skeleton of the trunk

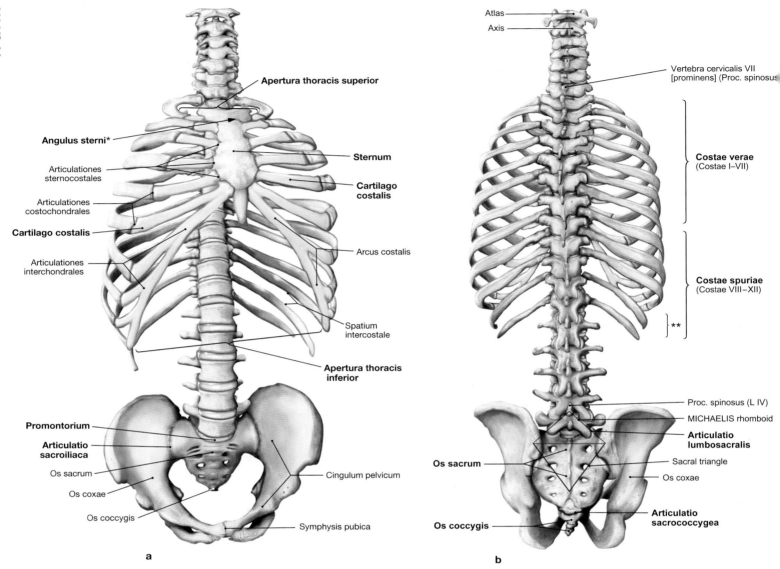

Fig. 2.15a and b Bone and cartilage of the skeleton of the trunk; the bones of the chest (Ossa thoracis), spine (Columna vertebralis) and pelvic girdle (Cingulum pelvicum) are shown. [S700-L127]
a Ventral view.
b Dorsal view.
All ribs articulate with the spine but only the first seven ribs are directly connected to the sternum via their rib cartilage (Cartilago costalis). They are therefore referred to as real ribs **(Costae verae).** The remaining five rib pairs are considered false ribs **(Costae spuriae);** ribs XI and XII. Ribs have no contact with the cartilaginous costal arch **(Costae fluctuantes).**

The diamond-shaped connection of the Proc. spinous of the fourth lumbar vertebra with the Spinae iliacae posteriores superiores and the start of the Crena ani on the back of the female is called the **MICHAELIS rhomboid** (lumbar rhombus, venus diamond). In the case of the male, the sacral triangle (the connection between Spinae iliacae posteriores superiores and the start of the Crena ani) is visible.

*   clin.: Angulus LUDOVICI
** Costae fluctuantes (Costae XI–XII)

Clinical remarks

As a part of the clinical examination, the easily palpated **Angulus sterni** (Angulus LUDOVICI) is an important landmark for orientation on the thorax. It is located at the level of the IInd rib. The shape of the sacral triangle (male) or the MICHAELIS rhomboid (lumbar rhombus) in women provides information on the form of the pelvis. In the case of deformed pelvises, for example due to rickets (vitamin D deficien-

cy), the transverse axis is extended; in the case of scoliosis it becomes asymmetric.
The **Proc. spinous of the fourth lumbar vertebra** lies at the same level as the iliac crest. It serves as a reference point for the lumbar puncture, as well as for intrathecal or epidural (peridural) anaesthesia.

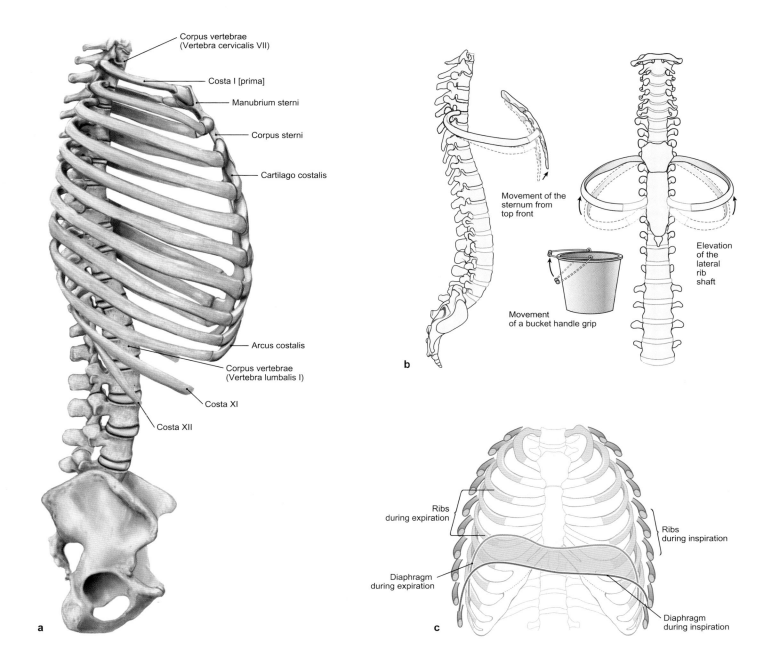

Fig. 2.16a–c   Skeleton of the trunk and movements of the thoracic wall.

a Skeletal bones and cartilage of the trunk. A lateral view from the right side shows the thorax (Cavea thoracis) with the twelve ribs on the right side. The XIth rib with its Corpus costae still extends far ventrally and lies in a continued line with the costal arch. The XIIth rib is usually significantly shorter. [S702-L266]

b Upon inspiration, the movements in the sternocostal and costovertebral joints lead to an expansion of the rib cage through the raising of the arch-shaped ribs, as illustrated in the bucket handle grip. [S702-L126]
c When at rest, inspiration results from the joint contraction of the diaphragm (lower red line) and the thoracic inspiration muscles, leading to an expansion of the thoracic cavity (red). Expiration reduces the volume of the thoracic cavity (blue), leading to the relaxation of the diaphragm, coupled with an upward movement (upper blue line). [S700-L126]

Clinical remarks

The rib cartilage ossifies with ageing, the ribs are lowered and the sternum moves closer to the spine. As a result, the entire chest becomes flatter and the lower ribcage opening contracts. Rib fractures can therefore often occur, for example during resuscitation, even if a small amount of pressure is applied to the thorax of people aged over 50. In contrast, the chests of young people (especially children) can be forcefully compressed without the occurrence of rib fractures.

Trunk

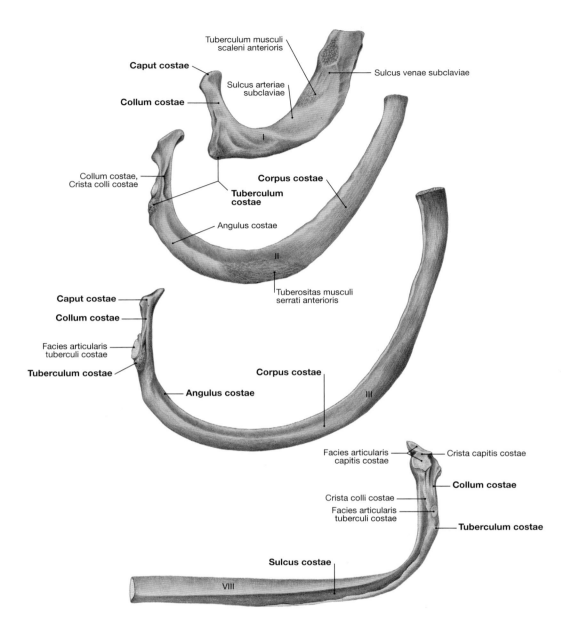

Fig. 2.17 Ribs, Costae; ribs I to III: view from cranial; rib VIII: caudal view. [S700]

Ribs III to X have a typical rib shape. The rib head (Caput costae) is wedge-shaped and bears two joint facets (Facies articulares capitis costae). The Tuberculum costae presents a joint surface (Facies articularis tuberculi costae). V., A. and N. intercostalis are deposited on the Sulcus costae. An invagination at the ventral end of the body of the rib (Corpus costae) facilitates contact with the rib cartilage.

Ribs I, II, XI and XII deviate from the typical rib structure. Rib I is short, broad and has the strongest curve; its tiny head has only one joint facet. The IInd rib only has an implied Sulcus costae and a Tuberositas musculi serrati anterioris for the origin point of the M. serratus anterior. The heads of the XIth and XIIth ribs have only one articular surface. These ribs do not connect with the costal arch; its front end is pointed. They also do not have any Tuberculum costae.

Clinical remarks

Rib anomalies are common:
- A **cervical rib** can be found in approximately 1 % of the population. As a result, the rib system on the seventh cervical vertebra is enlarged. Apart from isolated enlargements of the Proc. transversus, additional ribs which may be in contact with the sternum may occur uni- or bilaterally. The pressure of a cervical rib on the lower roots of the Plexus brachialis can cause sensory loss and motor deficits in the N. ulnaris.

- In the case of **two-headed ribs,** two ribs have been partially fused.
- A **bifid rib** is a variant in which the rib bifurcates at the front end into two parts.
- Extensions of the intercostal arteries which run in the Sulcus costae in the case of aortic isthmus stenosis cause pressure atrophy of the bone. This is referred to as **rib erosion.**

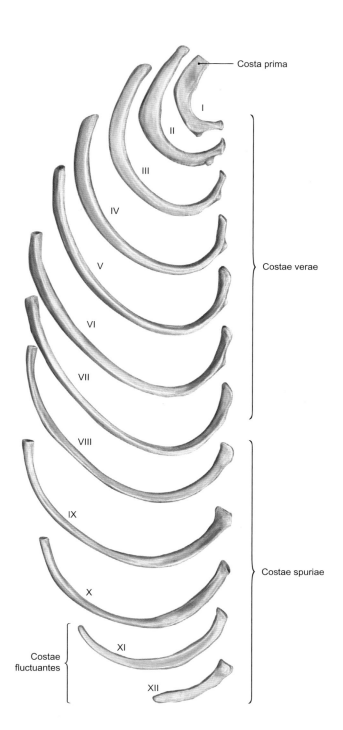

Costa prima

I

II

III

IV

V

VI

VII

VIII

IX

X

Costae
fluctuantes

XI

XII

Costae verae

Costae spuriae

Fig. 2.18 Ribs, Costae; bony part of the ribs I–XII on the left side; superior view. [S702-L266]
Usually, there are twelve rib pairs. Depending on whether the ribs (via the rib cartilage) make contact with the sternum or (cartilaginous) costal arch or remain without making contact with the sternum or costal arch, a distinction is made between **true ribs** (Costae verae, ribs I-VII, which are connected directly and flexibly to the sternum), **false ribs** (Costae spuriae, ribs VIII–XII, which are not directly connected to the sternum) and **floating ribs** (Costae fluctuantes: ribs XI–XII, which end freely between the thoracic wall muscles).

Clinical remarks

Lumbar ribs are a common rib abnormality, affecting approximately 7–8 % of the population. This involves additional ribs, which end freely between the thoracic wall muscles, as do the rib pairs XI and XII. In contrast to ribs XI and XII, they do not come from the thoracic spine, but insert on the first or second lumbar vertebrae. They can occur in close topographical proximity to the kidneys and can cause pain in this area.

Skeleton

Spine

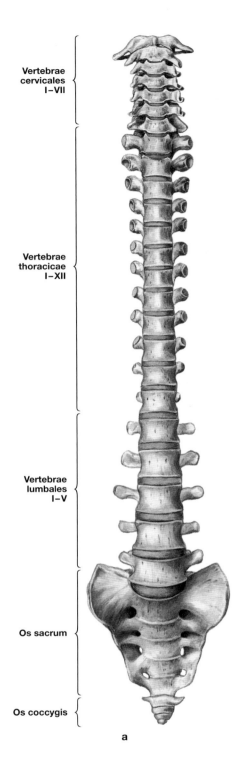

Vertebrae
cervicales
I–VII

Vertebrae
thoracicae
I–XII

Vertebrae
lumbales
I–V

Os sacrum

Os coccygis

a

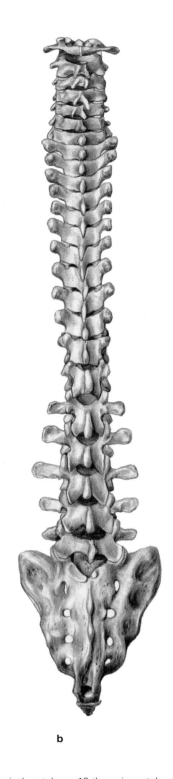

b

Fig. 2.19a and b   Spine, Columna vertebralis. [S700]
a Ventral view.
b Dorsal view.
The spine is two-fifths of the size of a human. A quarter of this can be attributed to the intervertebral discs. The spine consists of 24 presacral vertebrae (seven cervical vertebrae, 12 thoracic vertebrae, five lumbar vertebrae) as well as two synostotic sections, the sacrum (Os sacrum) and the
coccyx (Os coccygis). The thoracic vertebrae are in contact with the 12 rib
pairs; the sacrum articulates with the Ossa coxae. Within the spine, the
stress in a standing position increases from cranial to caudal.

Clinical remarks

If the fifth lumbar vertebra merges with the Os sacrum (only 23 presacral vertebrae), this is referred to as **sacralisation.** If the top vertebra of the Os sacrum remains separated from the remainder of the
sacrum and does not fuse with them (25 presacral vertebrae), the
condition is called **lumbalisation.** In this case, an X-ray will show six

lumbar vertebrae and four sacral vertebrae. If the Os sacrum exhibits
five vertebrae, there is an additional sacralisation of the first Coccyx
vortex. If the first cervical vertebra (atlas) merges with the skull, it is
referred to as **assimilation of the atlas.**

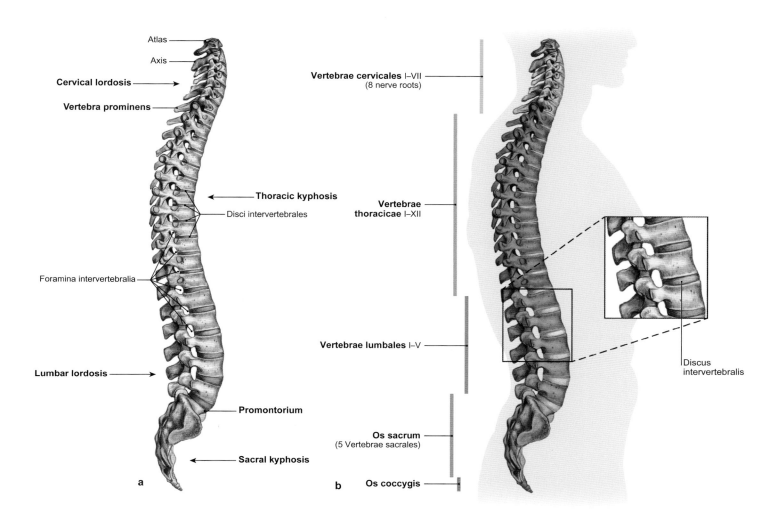

Atlas
Axis
Cervical lordosis
Vertebra prominens
Thoracic kyphosis
Disci intervertebrales
Foramina intervertebralia
Lumbar lordosis
Promontorium
Sacral kyphosis
a

Vertebrae cervicales I–VII
(8 nerve roots)
Vertebrae thoracicae I–XII
Vertebrae lumbales I–V
Os sacrum
(5 Vertebrae sacrales)
b **Os coccygis**
Discus intervertebralis

Fig. 2.20a and b   Spine, Columna vertebralis; curvatures. a [S700], b [S700-L127]
a View from the right.
b In the sagittal plane, the spine shows characteristic curves:
* Cervical lordosis (curved forward, convex, yellow)
* Thoracic kyphosis (curved backwards, concave, blue)

* Lumbar lordosis (curved forward, convex, orange)
* Sacral kyphosis (curved backwards, concave, green)
* The coccyx, which is composed of up to five synostotic (fused) coccygeal vertebrae, extends the sacral kyphosis.
Lordosis is the medical term for a ventrally facing convex curvature of the spine, kyphosis for a dorsally facing curvature.

Spine

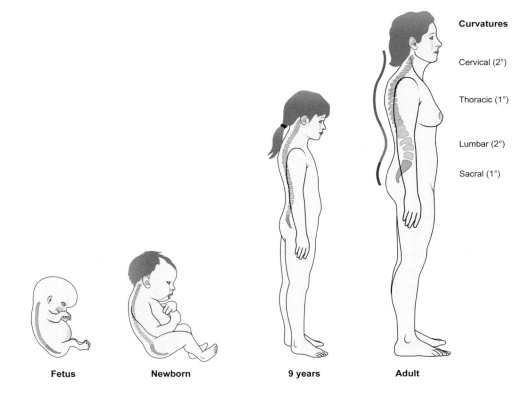

Curvatures

Cervical (2°)

Thoracic (1°)

Lumbar (2°)

Sacral (1°)

Fetus   Newborn   9 years   Adult

Fig. 2.21   Spine, Columna vertebralis; curvatures. View from the right side. [S701-L126]
In the first few months after birth, all sections of the spine show a dorsal convex curvature. The cervical lordotic curve begins to form with the body's ability to sit upright, while the lumbar lordotic curve develops with the start of bipedal walking at 1–2 years of age.

Clinical remarks

The dorsal convex curvature of the spine is called a kyphosis (→ Fig. 2.20). A slight kyphosis is considered physiological in the thoracic part of the spine. By contrast, any kyphosis in the cervical or lumbar segment of the spine is pathological. A severe kyphosis **(hyperkyphosis)** with excessive primary convex curvature of the thoracic spine is also pathological. A kyphosis disorder can make a person look as if they have a 'hunchback' and this so-called gibbus deformity presents in different forms (e.g. **postural kyphosis** in young children, adolescent or **juvenile kyphosis** [SCHEUERMANN kyphosis], and **senile kyphosis** at advanced age due to a loss in elasticity and degeneration of the intervertebral disks). Clinically generally referred to as kyphosis, these deformities qualify as hyperkyphosis.
A **lordosis** denotes a secondary ventrally facing convex curvature of the spine (→ Fig. 2.20), which is physiological in the cervical and lumbar segment of the spine. **Hyperlordosis** is a severe form of non-physiological lordosis and occurs most frequently in the lumbar spine.
Excessive curvature of the spine in the frontal plane **(scoliosis)** is always pathological. This is a growth deformity of the spine with fixed lateral curvature, torsion of the spine and rotation of the axial organs. These can no longer be straightened by the musculature. Scoliosis is one of the longest-known pathological conditions in or-thopaedics. Despite intense scientific and clinical efforts, many problems associated with scoliosis remain unresolved. Almost everyone has a minimal degree of scoliosis since most people do not have legs of the same length.

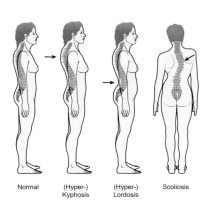

Normal   (Hyper-)   (Hyper-)   Scoliosis
                 Kyphosis   Lordosis

[S701-L126]

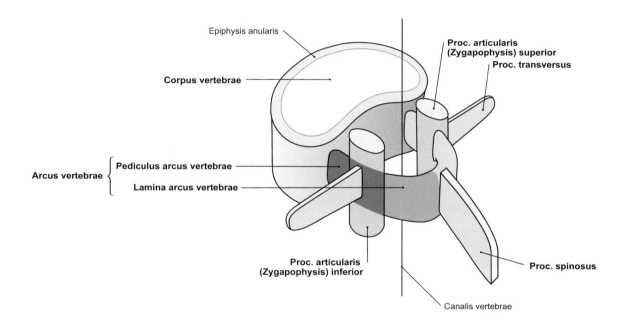

Epiphysis anularis

Corpus vertebrae

Proc. articularis
(Zygapophysis) superior

Proc. transversus

Arcus vertebrae {
Pediculus arcus vertebrae

Lamina arcus vertebrae

Proc. articularis
(Zygapophysis) inferior

Proc. spinosus

Canalis vertebrae

Fig. 2.22   Schematic depiction of a vertebra, Vertebra; dorsolateral view from the left side. [S700-L126]
A vertebra consists of a body, the Corpus vertebrae, and a bony arch, the Arcus vertebrae, connecting to the dorsal side of the vertebrae, and forming a vertebral canal, Canalis vertebrae. Paired transverse process-es, the Procc. transversus, originate from both sides of the vertebrae as well as dorsally from the spinous process, the Proc. spinosus. The ver-tebral arch also possesses articular facets as contact sides for verte-brae located above and below it or other structures (skull, coccyx), the Procc. articulares superiores and inferiores. On each side, the vertebral arch is divided into an anterior part, Pediculus arcus vertebrae (dark red) and a posterior part, Lamina arcus vertebrae (light red).

Atlas, axis and atlanto-occipital joints

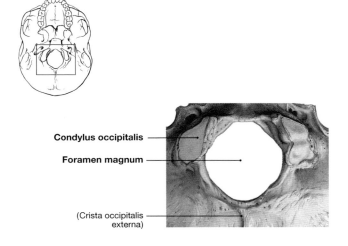

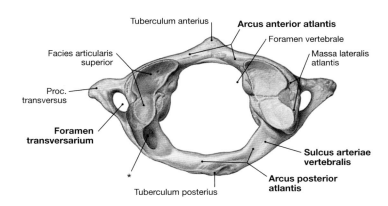

Fig. 2.23 Occipital bone, Os occipitale, section with Foramen magnum and occipital (upper) articular surfaces of the atlanto-occipital joint; caudal view. [S700]
The condyles of the skull are located at the front lateral of the Foramen magnum.

Fig. 2.24 First cervical vertebrae, atlas; cranial view. [S700]
The atlas has no vertebrae. During development, the latter fuses with the axis to form the dens. The front atlas arch (Arcus anterior atlantis) is located in front of the dens and articulates with it. The rear atlas arch (Arcus posterior atlantis) has a Tuberculum posterius instead of a Proc. spinosus. The upper articular surfaces of the atlas are often divided. Compared to other vertebrae, the atlas has a slightly longer transverse process.
* variant: Canalis arteriae vertebralis

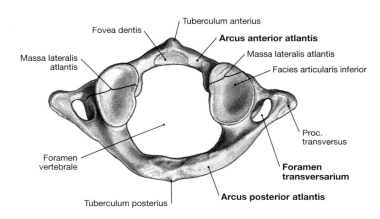

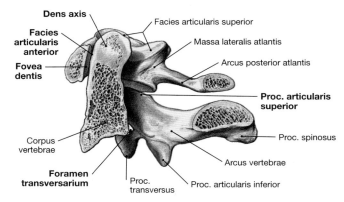

Fig. 2.25 First cervical vertebrae, atlas; caudal view. [S700]
The Fovea dentis for articulation with the dens axis is located on the inside of the Arcus anterior atlantis. The Facies articulares inferiores are shallow, concave and curved at an angle of approximately 30° to the transverse level. The Foramen transversarium, characteristic for the cervical vertebrae, serves as the passage for the A. vertebralis.

Fig. 2.26 First and second cervical vertebrae, atlas and axis; median section; view from the left side. [S700]
The median section reveals the vertebral canal. The atlas and axis articulate with the Fovea dentis and the Facies articularis anterior in the Articulatio atlantoaxialis mediana. The Arcus posterior atlantis is significantly smaller in relation to the Arcus vertebrae of the axis.

Clinical remarks

Degenerative changes of the cervical vertebrae become more frequent with age. They also manifest themselves as **osteochondrosis intervertebralis** with dorsal spondylophytes, which can lead to narrowing of the vertebral canal, resulting in compression of the spinal cord. **Osteoarthritis** in the vertebral joints and the uncovertebral gaps (→ Fig. 2.31) with formation of osteophytes results in narrowing of the Foramen intervertebrale and/or the Foramen transversarium, with symptoms resembling spinal nerve compression as well as pressure on the A. vertebralis and the sympathetic nerve plexus.

Isolated fractures of the atlas arch are particularly common following car accidents, but have decreased in the past few years due to improved safety measures in vehicles (airbags). Fractures must be distinguished from atlas variants. In contrast to variations such as the occurrence of a Canalis arteriae vertebralis, or abnormalities such as the **assimilation of the atlas** (fusion with the internal surface of the cranial base), **cleft formations in the region of the vertebral arches** are common (Clinical remarks → Fig. 2.41).

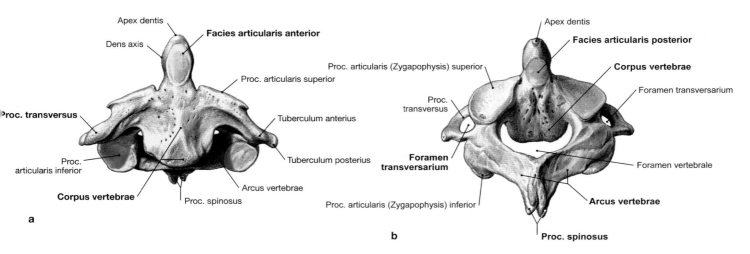

Fig. 2.27a and b   Second cervical vertebrae, axis. [S700]
a Ventral view.
b Dorsocranial view.
A distinct feature setting apart the axis from the other cervical verte-brae is the Dens axis. The dens possesses a joint facet on both its ante-rior and posterior sides (Facies articulares anterior and posterior). The

joint surfaces of the Procc. articulares superiores are tilted sideways and those of the Procc. articulares inferiores incline to the frontal plane. From the third cervical vertebra onwards all joint surfaces of the Procc. articulares superiores incline to the frontal plane. The transverse pro-cess (Proc. transversus) is small and the spinous process (Proc. spino-sus) is often split into two parts.

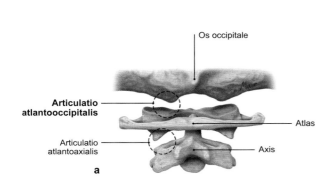

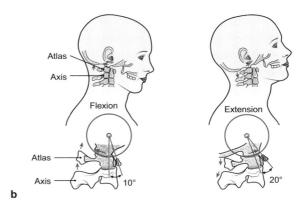

Fig. 2.28a and b   Atlanto-occipital joint, Articulatio atlantooccipi-talis.
a Ventral view. The paired Articulatio atlantooccipitalis is a true diarthro-sis (synovial joint) which connects the occipital base of the skull (C0) with the atlas (C1). The semi-ellipsoid shape of the condyles of this joint enables nodding movements of the head in the transverse plane and

some small sideways head movements. No vertebral disk separates the opposing joint surfaces! [S701-L127]
b Range of motion. This joint supports mainly nodding movements (flex-ion and extension over a maximal range of 30°; 10° flexion and 20° ex-tension). Sideways movements (not shown) of maximally 15° are possi-ble; 7–8° to each side, left and right. [S701-L126]

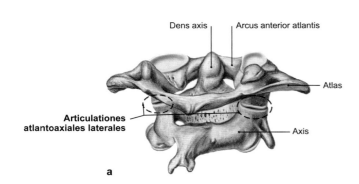

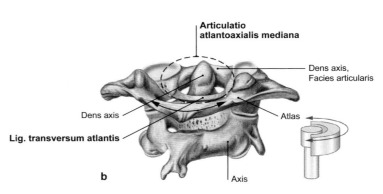

Fig. 2.29a and b   Atlantoaxial joint, Articulatio atlantoaxialis; dorsal view. [S701-L127]
Three synovial joints allow movements between the atlas (C1) and the axis (C2). As between C0 and C1, the complex atlantoaxial joint does not contain vertebral disks!
a The paired **Articulatio atlantoaxialis lateralis** are planar-type syno-vial joints located between the upper and lower transverse processes of the atlas and axis, respectively.

b The **Articulatio atlantoaxialis mediana** is a synovial pivot joint with its vertical axis projecting through the dens. At the dorsal side, the dens is secured via the Lig. transversum atlantis to the anterior arch of the atlas, which enables rotational movements of approximately 25° to the left and right side.

Cervical vertebrae

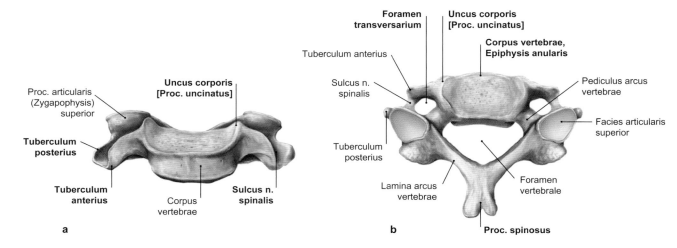

Proc. articularis
(Zygapophysis)
superior

Uncus corporis
[Proc. uncinatus]

**Tuberculum
posterius**

**Tuberculum
anterius**

Corpus
vertebrae

**Sulcus n.
spinalis**

a

Foramen
transversarium

Uncus corporis
[Proc. uncinatus]

Tuberculum anterius

**Corpus vertebrae,
Epiphysis anularis**

Sulcus n.
spinalis

Pediculus arcus
vertebrae

Facies articularis
superior

Tuberculum
posterius

Lamina arcus
vertebrae

Foramen
vertebrale

b

Proc. spinosus

Fig. 2.30a–c   Fifth cervical vertebrae, Vertebra cervicalis V.
[S702-L266]
a Ventral view.
b Cranial view.
c View from the left.
The fifth cervical vertebra shows a structure which is typical for the third to sixth cervical vertebrae. With the exception of the seventh cervical vertebra, the Proc. spinosus of the other cervical vertebrae is short and bifurcated. The Proc. transversus is short, includes the Foramen transversarium and ends in a lateral Tuberculum anterius and Tuberculum posterius, with the Sulcus nervi spinalis lying in-between them. The Foramen vertebrale is large and triangular. The vertebral body is longer in the transverse axis than in the sagittal axis and equally wide at the front and the back. Within the spine, the vertebrae articulate with their upper and lower counterparts via the Facies articularis superior and inferior (facet joints), respectively.

Proc. articularis (Zygapophysis)
superior

Proc. transversus

Facies articularis
superior

Corpus
vertebrae

Proc. spinosus

**Foramen
transversarium**

**Sulcus n.
spinalis**

Proc. articularis
inferior

c

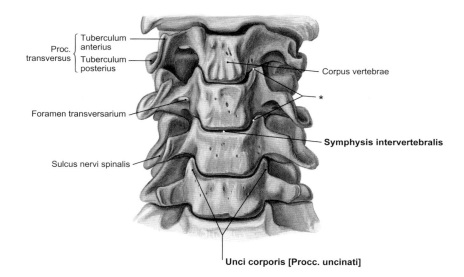

Proc.
transversus

Tuberculum
anterius

Tuberculum
posterius

Corpus vertebrae

*

Foramen transversarium

Symphysis intervertebralis

Sulcus nervi spinalis

Unci corporis [Procc. uncinati]

Fig. 2.31   Second to seventh cervical vertebrae, Vertebrae cervicales II–VII; ventral view. [S700]
The third to the sixth cervical vertebrae have a typical structure, whereas the first, second and seventh cervical vertebrae deviate from this structure. The end plates of the superior body surface turn upwards (Unci corporis). These, also named Procc. uncinati, articulate with the lateral and caudal parts of the Corpus vertebrae of the vertebra which lies above it in the Articulatio (hemiarthrosis) uncovertebralis.

* so-called uncovertebral gaps

Clinical remarks

An **Os odontoideum** is a combined congenital malformation with dens hypoplasia. It consists of a separate odontoid process which replaces the dens above the the body of the axis. It is attached to the axis primarily via connective tissue. This area is therefore obviously more flexible. In MRI images, the separate odontoid process appears to hover above the axis, free of a dens.

The **dens fracture** or the fracture of the vertebral body (the so-called hangman's fracture) presents the risk of cervical cord compression and occurs mostly as a result of motor vehicle accidents. A dens fracture can also affect small children and is difficult to diagnose.

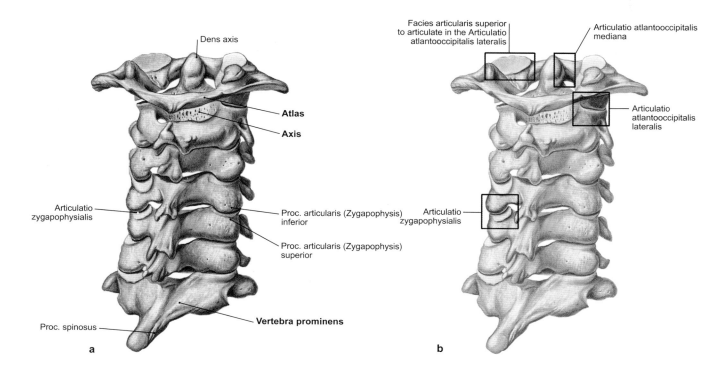

Dens axis

Atlas

Axis

Articulatio
zygapophysialis

Proc. articularis (Zygapophysis)
inferior

Proc. articularis (Zygapophysis)
superior

Proc. spinosus

Vertebra prominens

a

Facies articularis superior
to articulate in the Articulatio
atlantooccipitalis lateralis

Articulatio atlantooccipitalis
mediana

Articulatio
atlantooccipitalis
lateralis

Articulatio
zygapophysialis

b

Fig. 2.32a and b   First to seventh cervical vertebrae, Vertebrae cervicales I–VII; dorsal lateral view.

a The long and non-bifid spinous process of the seventh cervical vertebra (which is also referred to as the **Vertebra prominens**) can be easily palpated at the back of the neck. However, it can be confused with the even more protruding spinous process of the first thoracic vertebra. The respective joint surfaces (Facies articularis superior or inferior) of a vertebral articular process (Proc. articularis superior or inferior) articulate with the respective partner in the Articulatio zygapophysialis. [S700]

b The first cervical vertebra, the atlas, utilises the paired Articulatio atlantooccipitalis to articulate with the condyles of the occipital skull bone. The atlas articulates with the dens axis of the second cervical vertebra, the axis, in the Articulatio atlantoaxialis mediana, with which it also articulates in the paired Articulatio atlantoaxialis lateralis. The rest of the vertebrae, the axis and the third to seventh cervical vertebrae articulate via the respectively paired Articulatio zygapophysialis with the cervical vertebrae located below them. [S700-L127]

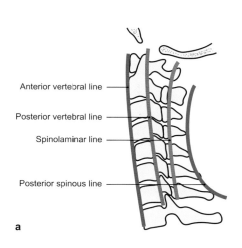

Anterior vertebral line

Posterior vertebral line

Spinolaminar line

Posterior spinous line

a

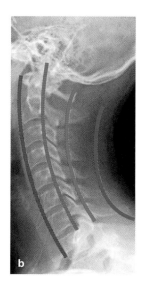

b

Fig. 2.33a and b   Normal cervical spine. a [S701-L126], b [G724]
a Schematic.

b Lateral X-ray image. Lateral view of the cervical spine frequently serve to diagnose potential injuries to this area. Various lines are used for orientation and to check the normal anatomy:

- The line at the anterior margin of the vertebral bodies (red; **anterior vertebral line**) should show a slightly curved shape.
- The **posterior vertebral line** demarcates the posterior vertebral body (brown) and, along with the anterior vertebral line, indicates the parallel alignment and distance between the individual vertebral bodies. A narrowing of these lines may suggest a vertebral disk prolapse.

- The **spinolaminar line** outlines the posterior margin of the cervical vertebral canal (green) and serves as an important indicator of possible displacement of vertebrae.

- A discontinuous **posterior spinous line** (blue), which connects the tips of the spinous processes, is a sign of vertebral disk injury and/or fractures.

Facet joints and motion segment

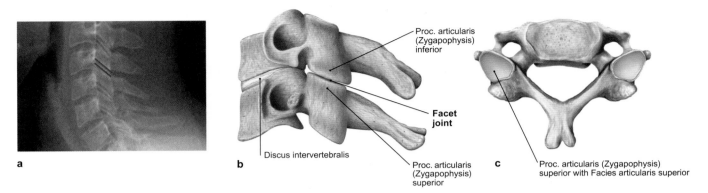

a **b** **c**

Proc. articularis (Zygapophysis) inferior

Facet joint

Discus intervertebralis

Proc. articularis (Zygapophysis) superior

Proc. articularis (Zygapophysis) superior with Facies articularis superior

Fig. 2.34a–c   Facet joint, Articulatio zygapophysialis, and motion segment.
a Lateral X-ray image of the cervical spine, Columna vertebralis cervicalis. The red line indicates the location of the facet joints. [G723]
b Cervical motion element, view from the right. [S701-L127]
c Cervical motion element, view from cranial. [S701-L127]
The paired **zygapophyseal joint,** Articulatio zygapophysialis (also called the **facet joint**), is a true diarthrosis (synovial joint) and an integral part of every motion segment in the spine. Vertebrae within the spine use the facet joints to articulate with each other (including L5 with the Os sacrum), whereby these facet joints guide and limit the range of motion of each motion segment. The tilt of the facet joints differs in the various regions of the spine (see Structure and Function box) which determines the range of motion of each regional segment.
The **motion segment** is the smallest physiological motion unit of the spine and includes all that which can be accomplished by two neigh-

bouring vertebrae. The motion segment encompasses the vertebra (including the vertebral body, arch, transverse and spinal process), the vertebral disk in-between both vertebrae, the paired zygapophyseal joints, the corresponding ligaments and muscles, the paired Foramen intervertebrale with exiting spinal nerve, spinal nerve ganglion, afferent and efferent nerve fibres and associated blood and lymph vessels. Some authors divide the motion segment into an anterior and posterior column or region:
- The anterior column provides stability and surrounds the vertebral body with the vertebral disc and associated ligaments. It only allows limited movements and alleviates load-bearing affecting the motion segment.
- The posterior column facilitates mobility and surrounds the vertebral arches with the transverse and spinal processes, associated ligaments and the zygapophyseal joints.

Structure and function

Zygapophyseal joints (facet joints)
The variations in form, size and positioning of the joint facets (Facies articulares superior and inferior of the Articulatio zygapophysiales) are characteristic structural features specific to the individual regions of the spine.
In the **cervical spine**, with the exception of the atlanto-occipital joint, the facets are positioned almost parallel in the frontal plane and at a 45° angle to the transverse plane. The superior facets point backward and up, while the inferior facets point forward and down. This facilitates flexion and extension as well as lateral flexion and rotation.
In the **thoracic spine**, the facets all have a concave shape with the centre of this articulation surface located far ventrally to enable an unobstructed rotation and lateral flexion in all segments of the thoracic spine. With the facets positioned at a 60° angle to the transverse plane and a 20° angle to the frontal plane with the upper facets tilting backward and lateral (and slightly upward) and the lower facets forward and medial (and slightly downward), flexion and extension movements are restricted.
At their medial aspect, the joints in the **lumbar spine** without exception contain a small surface anatomy that aligns with the frontal

plane. This region is load-bearing for ventrally projecting shear forces and ensures the stability of the lumbar spine segment. The majority of the facets aligns almost perfectly with the sagittal plane (although caudally they diverge slightly). The superior and inferior facets point medially and laterally, respectively. This positioning facilitates flexion and extension movements but restricts rotational movements.
The **lumbosacral joint L5/S1** (not shown) is consistently positioned at a 60° angle to the sagittal plane and manifests the enormous physical stress of shifting the weight from one leg to the other when walking, running or jumping. In the other lumbosacral joints, the small facets aligned with the frontal plane take on the stress of the thrusts, but the larger transitional region at the Os sacrum experiences far greater shear forces.
The musculoskeletal system, with particular emphasis on dynamic loads, adapts to the smallest of anatomical details. The images provide a better understanding of the anatomy.
a, b Positioning of the zygapophyseal joints. [S702-L126]
c Range of motion in different sections (motion segments) of the spine. [S701-L126]

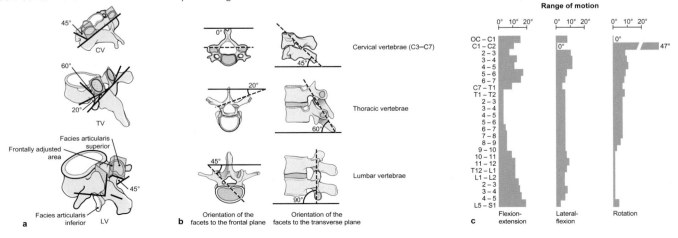

a CV TV Facies articularis superior Frontally adjusted area Facies articularis inferior LV

b Orientation of the facets to the frontal plane   Orientation of the facets to the transverse plane

Range of motion

c   Cervical vertebrae (C3–C7)   Thoracic vertebrae   Lumbar vertebrae

OC – C1, C1 – C2, 2 – 3, 3 – 4, 4 – 5, 5 – 6, 6 – 7, C7 – T1, T1 – T2, 2 – 3, 3 – 4, 4 – 5, 5 – 6, 6 – 7, 7 – 8, 8 – 9, 9 – 10, 10 – 11, 11 – 12, T12 – L1, L1 – L2, 2 – 3, 3 – 4, 4 – 5, L5 – S1

Flexion-extension   Lateral-flexion   Rotation   47°

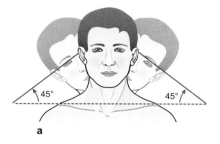

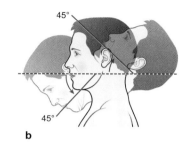

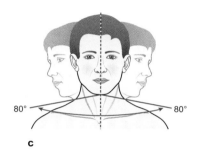

Fig. 2.35a–c Range of movements in the cervical spine.
[S700-L126]
a Lateral flexion.
b Flexion and extension.
c Rotation.
The cervical spine is commonly divided into an upper segment composed of the atlanto-occipital (C0/C1) and atlanto-axial (C1/C2) joints and a lower segment of cervical vertebrae C3–C7. The C3–C7 vertebrae share a common structure which consists of intervertebral discs and zygapophyseal joints. The combined actions of all motion segments and structures of the cervical spine allow extensive lateral flexion, forward flexion and extension, as well as rotational movements of the head.

Structure and function

The lordosis of the cervical spine enables controlled movements and the optimal transfer of forces from the muscles and soft tissue that attach at the cervical spine.
a The cervical lordosis is lost during flexion of the head. In this position, the cervical spine is more vulnerable to dislocations and fractures.
b In the extended neck position, the lordotic curvature of the spine increases even further.
[G724]

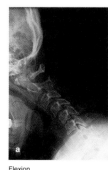

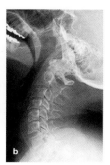

Flexion   Extension

Thoracic vertebrae

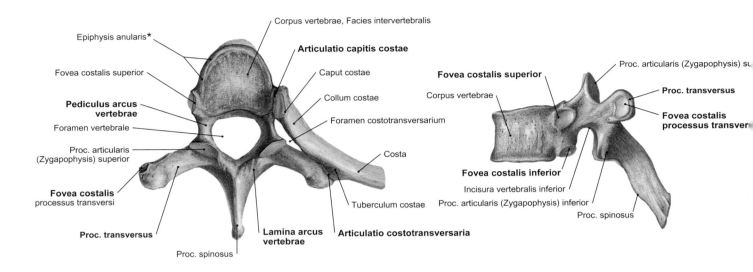

Fig. 2.36 Vertebra(-ae): structural features using the fifth thoracic vertebra as an example; cranial view. [S700]
The vertebral arch (Arcus vertebrae) is divided into the Pediculus arcus vertebrae and the Lamina arcus vertebrae. The Procc. transversi originates laterally and the Proc. spinosus dorsally from the arch. Joint surfaces (Procc. articulares) are located cranially and caudally for the vertebral joints (zygapophyseal joints). Cranially and caudally, the spine has a joint surface on each side for the rib heads (Foveae costales superior and inferior). At the Proc. transversus, the Fovea costalis articulates with the Articulatio costotransversaria with the joint surface of the Tuberculum costae of the corresponding rib.

* also: annular rim

Fig. 2.37 Sixth thoracic vertebra, Vertebra thoracica VI; view from the left side. [S700]
The joint surfaces of the costal heads (Foveae costales superior and inferior) can be seen here, as well as the articular processes of the zygapophyseal joints (at the Procc. articulares superior and inferior) which are positioned almost in the frontal plane, the joint surfaces (Fovea costalis) for articulation with the Tuberculum costae of the ribs, the Incisura vertebralis inferior and the steeply inclining Proc. spinosus.

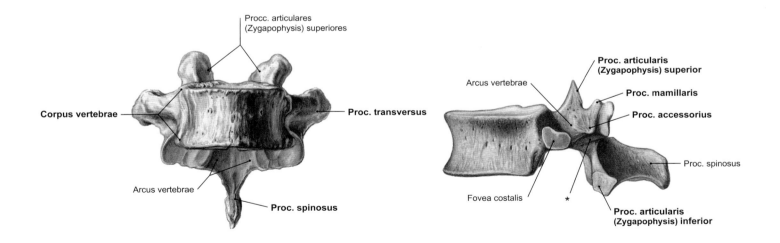

Fig. 2.38 10th Thoracic vertebra, Vertebra thoracica X; ventral view onto the spine with superior and inferior end plates. [S700]
The joint surfaces of the Procc. articulares protrude over the vertebral body cranially and caudally.

Fig. 2.39 12th Thoracic vertebra, Vertebra thoracica XII; view from the left side. [S700]
The 12th thoracic vertebra only has one Fovea costalis located at each side and already displays characteristics of the lumbar spine: the inferior joint processes point laterally. The Procc. mamillares and accessorii are also already in evidence.

* region of the vertebral arch between the superior and inferior joint processes (so-called isthmus = interarticular portion)

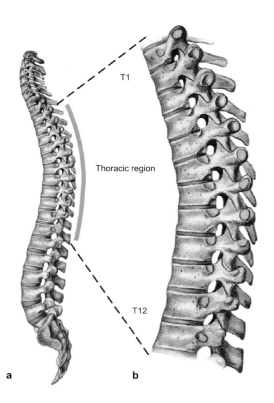

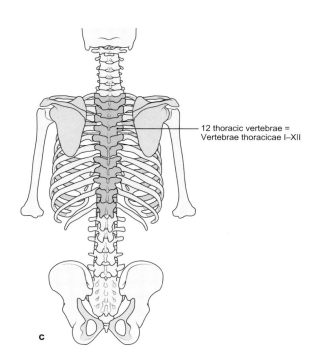

12 thoracic vertebrae =
Vertebrae thoracicae I–XII

Fig. 2.40a–c   Thoracic spine, Columna vertebralis thoracica.
a View of the entire spine from the left side. The thoracic segment is outlined. [S701]
b View of the thoracic spine from the left side. [S701]
c View of the entire spine with a dorsal view of the thoracic spine. [S701-L126]

The thoracic spine is composed of 12 characteristic thoracic vertebrae and corresponding intervertebral discs. The thoracic spine follows on from the cervical spine and extends up to the lumbar spine. Together with the 12 paired ribs and the sternum, the thoracic spine forms the bony thorax which protects and stabilises the organs within it (heart and lungs).

Trunk

Thoracic and lumbar vertebrae

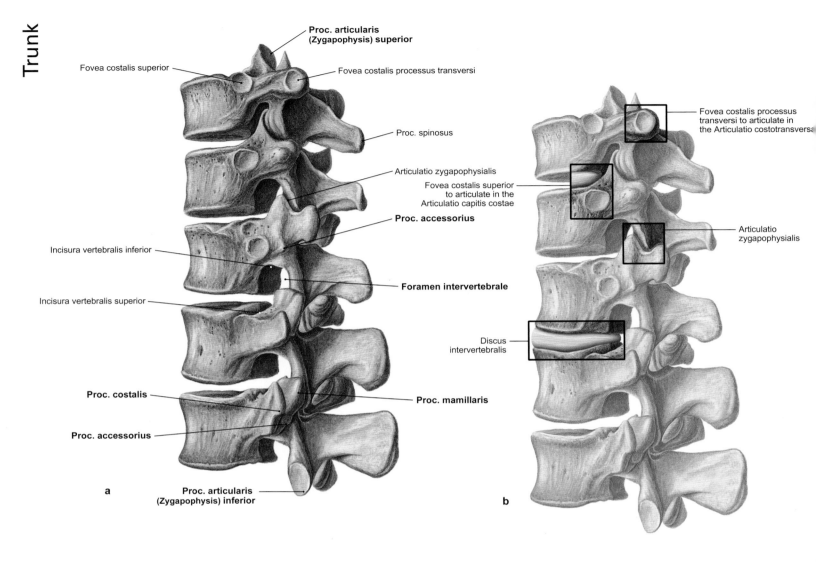

Proc. articularis
(Zygapophysis) **superior**

Fovea costalis superior

Fovea costalis processus transversi

Proc. spinosus

Articulatio zygapophysialis

Fovea costalis processus
transversi to articulate in
the Articulatio costotransversaria

Fovea costalis superior
to articulate in the
Articulatio capitis costae

Proc. accessorius

Articulatio
zygapophysialis

Incisura vertebralis inferior

Foramen intervertebrale

Incisura vertebralis superior

Discus
intervertebralis

Proc. costalis

Proc. mamillaris

Proc. accessorius

a

Proc. articularis
(Zygapophysis) **inferior**

b

Fig. 2.41a and b   10th–12th Thoracic vertebrae, Vertebrae thoracicae X–XII, and first to second lumbar vertebra, Vertebrae lumbales I–II; dorsal view from the left side.

a The size of the thoracic vertebrae increase gradually from cranial to caudal, continuing into the lumbar vertebrae. Due to the higher pressure, the bodies of the lumbar vertebrae are much more powerful than the rest of the vertebrae. In the lumbar spine, the Procc. spinosi are short and plump and aligned almost horizontally. Emanating from the vertebral arches of the lumbar spine are the Procc. costales (originating from the rib system and fused with the vertebrae), the variable large Procc. accessorii, the Procc. articulares superiores (which support the

upper joint surfaces, the Facies articulares) and the Procc. mamillares (rest of the transverse process) as well as the Procc. articulares inferiores with the lower joint surfaces (Facies articulares). [S700]

b The thoracic and lumbar vertebrae can be differentiated as the thoracic vertebrae have facets for the articulation of the ribs (paired Articulatio capitis costae and paired Articulatio costo-transversaria). The Articulatio zygapophyseales appear along the entire spine, including the thoracic and lumbar spine, in exactly the same way as intervertebral discs are intercalated between all vertebrae (with the exception of the atlanto-occipital joint). [S700-L127]

Clinical remarks

- Posterolateral disc problems or osteophytes of arthrotically modified vertebra joints can lead to the **narrowing of the Foramen intervertebrale** and to compression of the spinal nerve roots which can lead to nerve paralysis.
- **Lumbar ribs** can cause kidney pain due to being closely linked topographically.

- **Lateral vertebral arch columns** can lead to the separation of the Procc. articulares inferiores from the rear part of the arcus and of the Proc. spinosus from the rest of the vertebral section (the so-called **spondylolysis**).
- The bony separation of the isthmus (→ Fig. 2.39) can primarily cause slipping of the vertebrae **(spondylolisthesis).**

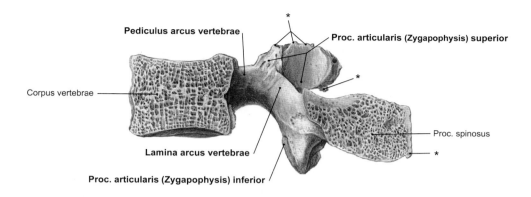

Fig. 2.42   Third lumbar vertebra, Vertebra lumbalis III, of an older person; median section; view from the left side. [S700]

The joint surfaces of the Procc. articulares superiores face each other (that is the reason they are not clearly visible from the side) and grip the lower joint processes of the vertebra above it between them.

* ossification of ligament origins

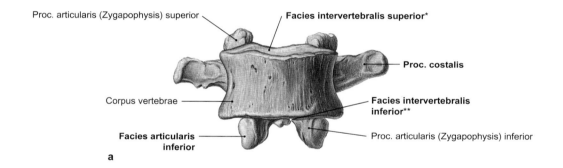

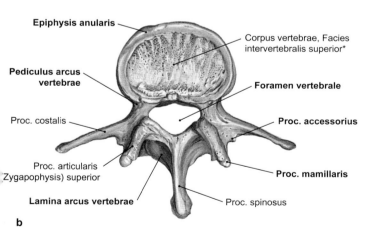

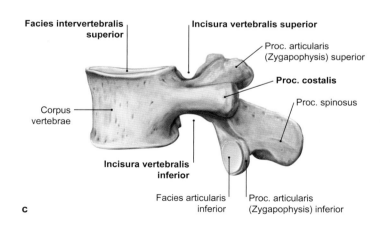

Fig. 2.43a–c   Fourth lumbar vertebra, Vertebra lumbalis IV.
a Ventral view. The lumbar vertebra has a powerful body (Corpus vertebrae) with distinctive end plates (Facies intervertebrales superior and inferior). The joint surfaces of the zygapophyseal joints protrude from the corpus cranially and caudally. [S700]
b Cranial view. Due to the size of a lumbar vertebra, the Pediculus arcus vertebrae is very powerful. On the side of the arch, you can see the

different processes (Procc. costales, accessorii, mamillares and articulares superiores and inferiores), with behind it the strong Proc. spinosus. [S700]
c View from the left side. [S700-L266]

* also: superior end plate
** also: inferior end plate

Sacrum

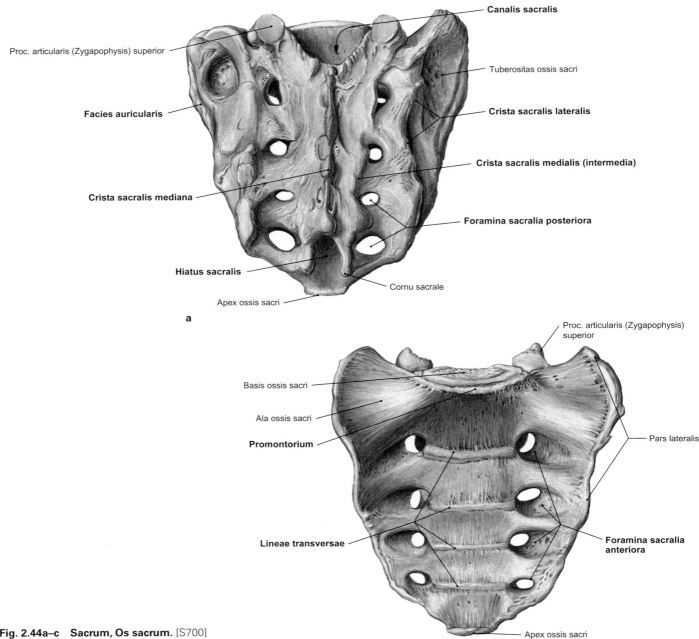

Canalis sacralis

Proc. articularis (Zygapophysis) superior

Tuberositas ossis sacri

Facies auricularis

Crista sacralis lateralis

Crista sacralis medialis (intermedia)

Crista sacralis mediana

Foramina sacralia posteriora

Hiatus sacralis

Cornu sacrale

Apex ossis sacri

a

Proc. articularis (Zygapophysis) superior

Basis ossis sacri

Ala ossis sacri

Pars lateralis

Promontorium

Lineae transversae

Foramina sacralia anteriora

Apex ossis sacri

b

Fig. 2.44a–c Sacrum, Os sacrum. [S700]
a Dorsal view. The **Facies dorsalis** has five distinct horizontal ridges which are formed during the fusion of the corresponding processes. The fusion of the Procc. spinosi corresponds to the **Crista sacralis mediana,** the fusion of its joint processes to the **Crista sacralis medialis** and the fusion of its rudimentary lateral processes to the **Crista sacralis lateralis.** The Crista sacralis mediana terminates above the Hiatus sacralis, which represents the caudal opening of the vertebral canal. It is used as a gateway to sacral anaesthesia in children.
b Ventral view. The **Facies pelvina** shows the fused borders on the sacral vertebral body (Lineae transversae) and the paired Foramina sacralia anteriora, which represent the outlet openings for the ventral spinal nerve branches. The part of the Os sacrum located laterally from the Foramina sacralia anteriora is referred to as the Pars lateralis.
c Cranial view. The **Basis ossis sacri,** which is visible from above, is the contact surface point for the intervertebral disc with the fifth lumbar vertebra. This spinal disc bulges further into the pelvis and, together with the front edge of the Basis ossis sacri, is called the **Promontorium.** The Alae ossis sacri spreads laterally from the base as the cranial part of the Partes laterales. The triangular sacral channel lies behind the base with the Procc. articulares superiores to the side, making contact with the fifth lumbar vertebra.

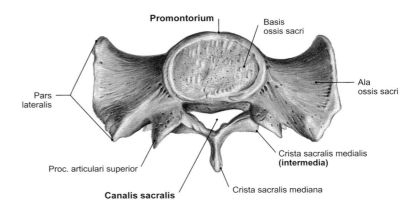

Promontorium

Basis ossis sacri

Pars lateralis

Ala ossis sacri

Proc. articulari superior

Crista sacralis medialis **(intermedia)**

Canalis sacralis

Crista sacralis mediana

c

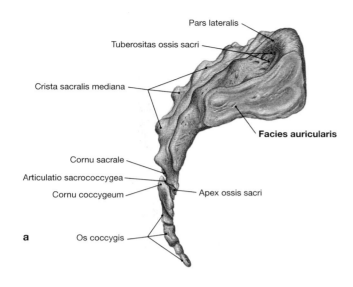

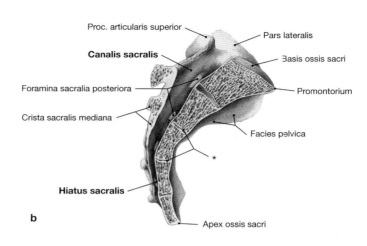

Fig. 2.45a and b   Sacrum, Os sacrum. [S700]
a View from the right side. The side view shows the Facies auricularis, which is used for the joint connection with the Os coxae (Articulatio sacroiliaca). The Tuberositas ossis sacri is located on the dorsal side, where the ligaments attach.

b Median section, view from the right side. The median section shows the entrance to the Hiatus sacralis and the transition to the Canalis sacralis.

* Remnants of intervertebral disc tissue can remain in adults. In addition, an incomplete fusion of the sacral vertebra is common.

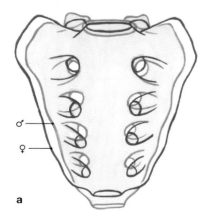

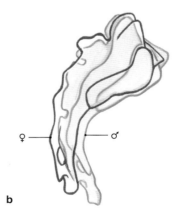

Fig. 2.46a and b   Sacrum, Os sacrum; gender differences. [S700]
a Ventral view.
b Lateral view.

The sacrum of the male is slightly longer but not as wide as that of the female. The different shape of the female sacrum is advantageous when giving birth due to the wider shape of the female pelvis.

Coccyx

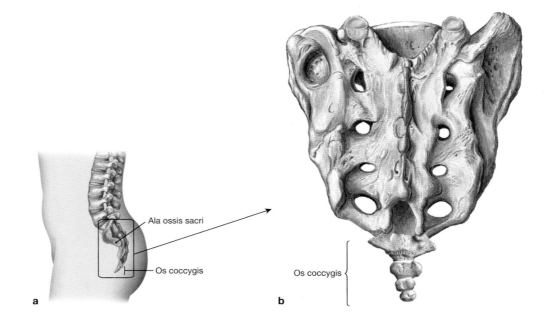

a

Ala ossis sacri

Os coccygis

b

Os coccygis {

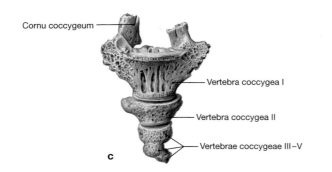

Cornu coccygeum

Vertebra coccygea I

Vertebra coccygea II

Vertebrae coccygeae III–V

c

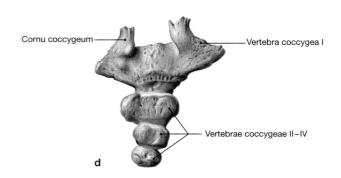

Cornu coccygeum

Vertebra coccygea I

Vertebrae coccygeae II–IV

d

Fig. 2.47a–d Coccyx, Os coccygis.
a View from the lateral left side. [S701-L127]
b Dorsal view. [S700]
c Ventral cranial view. [S700]
d Dorsal caudal view. [S700]
The coccyx (tailbone) is the caudal end of the spine. The coccyx developed mostly from three to four vertebrae synostotically melded to each other but can also – as shown here – develop from five rudimentary vertebrae. The coccyx is connected to the Os sacrum via the Cornua coccygea and the rudimentary vertebrae. The size of the coccygeal vertebrae decreases from cranial to caudal. Only the first coccygeal vertebra is still structurally similar to a typical vertebra.

Clinical remarks

Injuries to the coccyx (bruising, dislocation or fracture) are mostly caused by traumata, like a fall onto the coccyx in a seated position when slipping on the stairs or repeated stress or friction to the coccygeal region during cycling or rowing. Despite a protracted healing process, most injuries respond well to rest and conservative treatment.

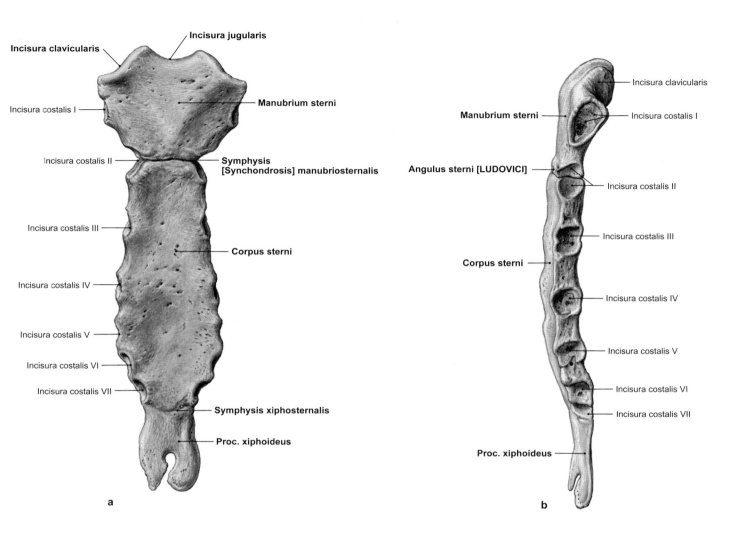

a Ventral view.

b Lateral view.

Fig. 2.48a and b Sternum. [S700]
a Ventral view.
b Lateral view.
The sternum has a handle (manubrium), a body (corpus) and a xiphoid process (Proc. xiphoideus). It forms the Incisura jugularis which is the ventral upper margin of the upper thoracic aperture and articulates with the clavicles via the Incisurae claviculares as well as with the ribs I–VII

via the Incisurae costales. The manubrium and the corpus are connected to each other via the **symphysis (Synchondrosis) manubriosternalis,** and the corpus and the Proc. xiphoideus are linked via the **Symphysis xiphosternalis.** The Proc. xiphoideus can be split.

* LUDOVICI

Clinical remarks

Bone taps (punctures) can be conducted on the sternum, and the pelvic and iliac crest. Rarely conducted today, the **sternal tap** is a diagnostic bone marrow tap to assess bone marrow cells for diseases of the blood. The puncture site is located in the median line in the Corpus sterni between the roots of the IInd and IIIrd rib. **A sternal tap is conducted on obese patients, since it is easier to puncture the sternum here than at the more commonly used iliac crest.**

Areas that should not be tapped include the area of the rib-sternum connections, as there may be synchondrosis in this region, and likewise in the lower two thirds of the Corpus sterni, because there may be a **Fissura sterni congenita** (opening within the sternum) due to the bone apposition, and the puncture needle could penetrate the heart (Clinical remarks → Fig. 2.13).

Sternum

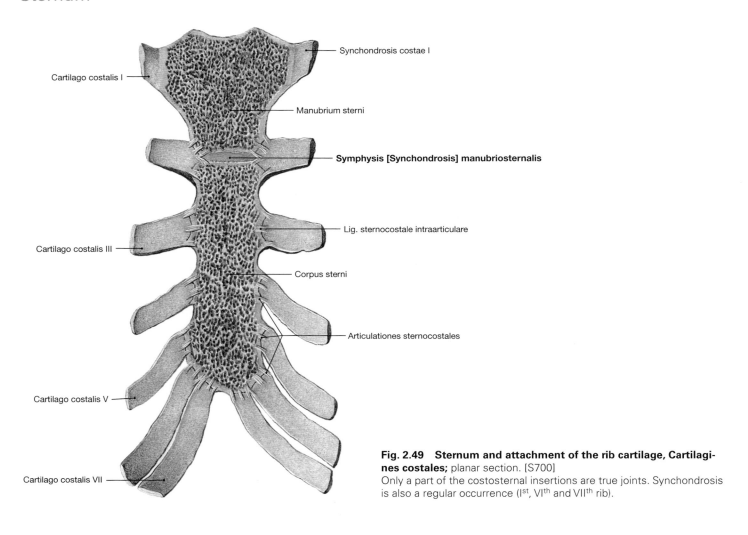

Synchondrosis costae I

Cartilago costalis I

Manubrium sterni

Symphysis [Synchondrosis] manubriosternalis

Lig. sternocostale intraarticulare

Cartilago costalis III

Corpus sterni

Articulationes sternocostales

Cartilago costalis V

Cartilago costalis VII

Fig. 2.49   Sternum and attachment of the rib cartilage, Cartilagines costales; planar section. [S700]
Only a part of the costosternal insertions are true joints. Synchondrosis is also a regular occurrence (I^st, VIth and VIIth rib).

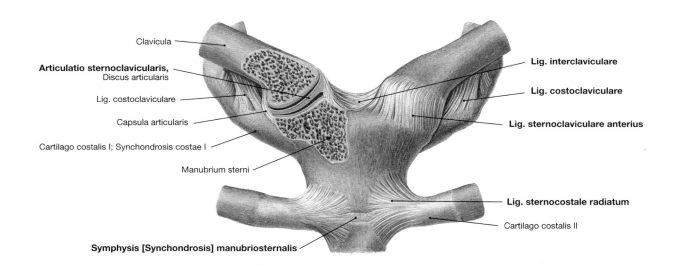

Clavicula

Articulatio sternoclavicularis,
Discus articularis

Lig. costoclaviculare

Capsula articularis

Cartilago costalis I; Synchondrosis costae I

Manubrium sterni

Lig. interclaviculare

Lig. costoclaviculare

Lig. sternoclaviculare anterius

Lig. sternocostale radiatum

Cartilago costalis II

Symphysis [Synchondrosis] manubriosternalis

Fig. 2.50   Sternoclavicular joints, Articulationes sternoclaviculares; ventral view; right frontal section through the joint. [S700]
The sternoclavicular joint is a functional **ball and socket joint** with three degrees of freedom. It contains a fibrocartilaginous **Discus articularis,** dividing the joint into two chambers **(dithalamic joint).** The

shape of this joint is a reflection of the demands of multiaxial mobility and very diverse mechanical stresses in different joint positions. Because the disc is able to absorb high shear forces, the joint surfaces can be kept small. The Ligg. sternoclavicularia anterius and posterius, and Ligg. interclaviculare and costoclaviculare reinforce the joint capsule.

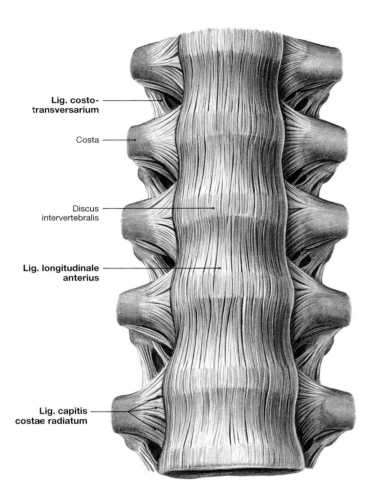

Lig. costo-
transversarium

Costa

Discus
intervertebralis

Lig. longitudinale
anterius

Lig. capitis
costae radiatum

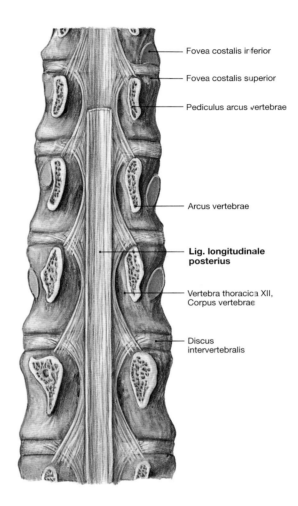

Fovea costalis inferior

Fovea costalis superior

Pediculus arcus vertebrae

Arcus vertebrae

Lig. longitudinale
posterius

Vertebra thoracica XII,
Corpus vertebrae

Discus
intervertebralis

Fig. 2.51 Ligaments of the spine with the lower thoracic spine as an example; ventral view. [S700]

The anterior longitudinal ligament **(Lig. longitudinale anterius)** extends from the Tuberculum anterius of the atlas to the Os sacrum. Here it is firmly fused with the front surfaces of the vertebral body and also affixed to the Disci intervertebrales. The ligament increases the strength of the spinal column when **extending.**

Fig. 2.52 Ligaments of the spine with the lower thoracic and upper lumbar spine as an example; dorsal view. [S700]

The posterior longitudinal ligament **(Lig. longitudinale posterius)** originates from the Membrana tectoria and extends into the Canalis sacralis. It is firmly connected to the intervertebral discs and the edges of the superior end plates, securing the Disci intervertebrales. The ligament increases the strength of the spinal column when **flexed.**

Ligaments of the spine

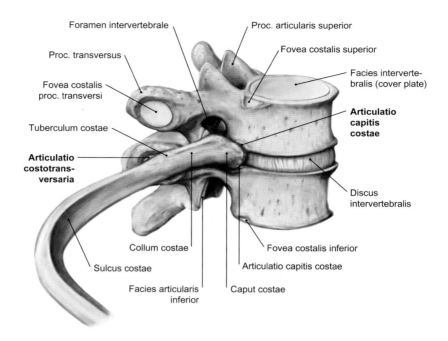

Foramen intervertebrale

Proc. transversus

Fovea costalis proc. transversi

Tuberculum costae

Articulatio costotransversaria

Proc. articularis superior

Fovea costalis superior

Facies interverte-bralis (cover plate)

Articulatio capitis costae

Discus intervertebralis

Collum costae

Sulcus costae

Facies articularis inferior

Fovea costalis inferior

Articulatio capitis costae

Caput costae

Fig. 2.53 Costovertebral joints, Articulationes costovertebrales; costovertebral joint at the level of the seventh and eighth thoracic vertebrae; view from the right side. [S702-L266]

The heads of the ribs articulate via the Articulatio capitis costae with the thoracic vertebra/e. With the exception of the Ist, XIth and XIIth rib, they are each seen as a two-chamber joint (dithalamic joint), as each head articulates with the top and bottom edge of two adjacent vertebrae.

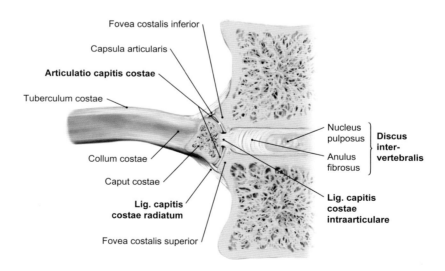

Fovea costalis inferior

Capsula articularis

Articulatio capitis costae

Tuberculum costae

Collum costae

Caput costae

Lig. capitis costae radiatum

Fovea costalis superior

Nucleus pulposus

Anulus fibrosus

Discus inter-vertebralis

Lig. capitis costae intraarticulare

Fig. 2.54 Head of rib joint, Articulatio capitis costae; lateral view from the right side. [S702-L266]
Each head of the ribs II–X articulates with the upper and the lower edges of the two adjacent vertebrae and with the intervertebral disc via a

ligament (Lig. capitis costae intraarticulare), which is secured to the Crista capitis costae (not visible). The joint cavity is divided into two chambers (dithalamic joint).

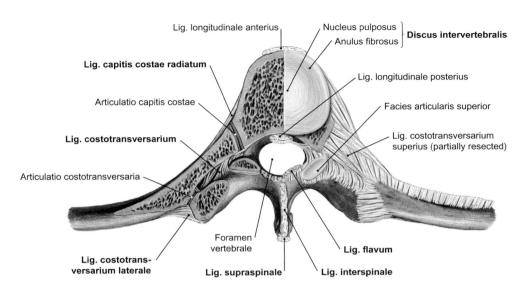

Lig. longitudinale anterius

Lig. capitis costae radiatum

Articulatio capitis costae

Lig. costotransversarium

Articulatio costotransversaria

Lig. costotrans-
versarium laterale

Nucleus pulposus ⎫
Anulus fibrosus ⎭ **Discus intervertebralis**

Lig. longitudinale posterius

Facies articularis superior

Lig. costotransversarium
superius (partially resected)

Foramen
vertebrale

Lig. supraspinale

Lig. flavum

Lig. interspinale

Fig. 2.55 Costovertebral joints, Articulationes costovertebrales; on the left, cross-section at the level of the lower portion of a head of a rib joint (Articulatio costovertebralis); on the right, depiction of the disc covering the vertebral body and the capsule ligament apparatus of the corresponding rib with the thoracic vertebra; cranial view. [S702-L127]

The ribs articulate in the **Articulatio costotransversaria** with the Proc. transversus of the corresponding thoracic vertebra, for example rib I with the first thoracic vertebra or the Vth rib with T5 (exception XIth and XIIth rib). Thereby the Facies articularis tuberculi costae and the Fovea costalis proc. transversi articulate. The joint capsules are weak and are strengthened by different ligaments (→ Fig. 2.56).

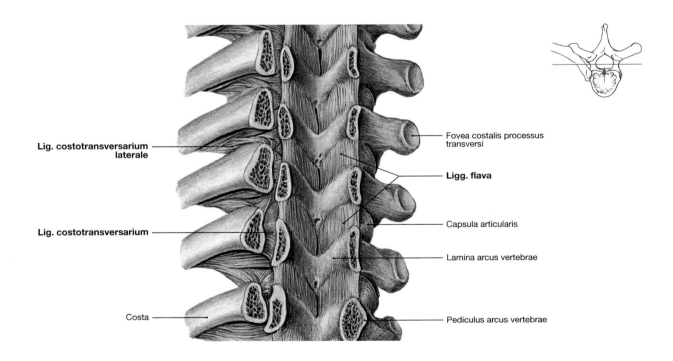

Lig. costotransversarium
laterale

Lig. costotransversarium

Costa

Fovea costalis processus
transversi

Ligg. flava

Capsula articularis

Lamina arcus vertebrae

Pediculus arcus vertebrae

Fig. 2.56 Compounds of the vertebral arches; ventral view. [S700] Between the vertebral arches, the **Ligg. flava** stretch segmentally (yellowish colour, caused by a very high number of elastic fibres arranged

like the folds of a concertina). They border the Foramina intervertebralia dorsally. The Ligg. flava are stretched in every direction and support the muscles of the back when erecting the spine from all flexed positions.

2

Trunk

Ligaments of the spine

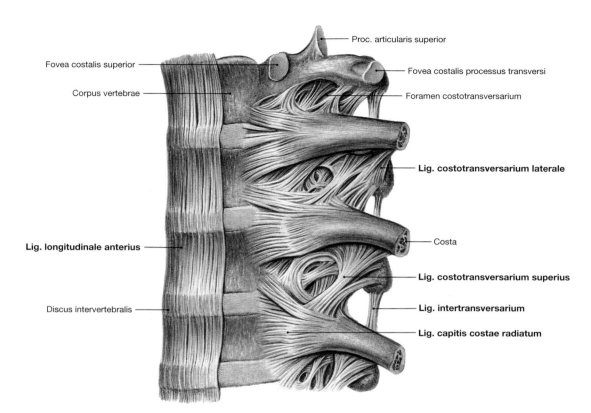

Proc. articularis superior

Fovea costalis superior

Fovea costalis processus transversi

Corpus vertebrae

Foramen costotransversarium

Lig. costotransversarium laterale

Lig. longitudinale anterius

Costa

Lig. costotransversarium superius

Lig. intertransversarium

Discus intervertebralis

Lig. capitis costae radiatum

Fig. 2.57   Ligaments of the spine and the costovertebral joints, Articulationes costovertebrales; view from the left side; lateral parts of the front longitudinal ligament removed. [S700]
The joint capsules of the Articulationes capitis costae are reinforced respectively by a Lig. capitis costae radiatum; the joint capsules of the

Articulationes costotransversariae are secured by the Ligg. costotransversaria (Lig. costotransversarium lateral and Lig. costotransversarium superius).

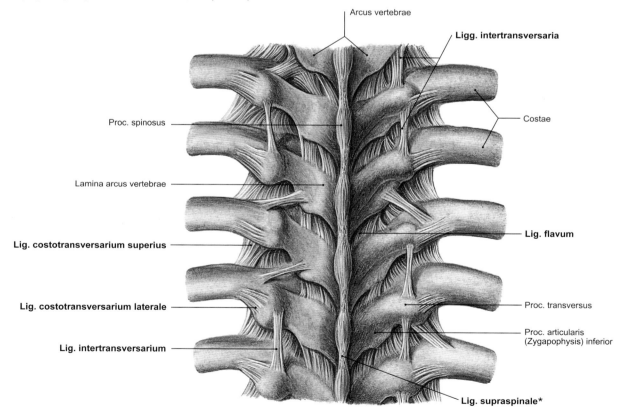

Arcus vertebrae

Ligg. intertransversaria

Proc. spinosus

Costae

Lamina arcus vertebrae

Lig. flavum

Lig. costotransversarium superius

Lig. costotransversarium laterale

Proc. transversus

Lig. intertransversarium

Proc. articularis (Zygapophysis) inferior

Lig. supraspinale*

Fig. 2.58   Ligaments of the vertebral arches and the costovertebral joints, Articulationes costovertebrales; dorsal view. [S700]
The joint capsules of the Articulationes costotransversariae are dorsally reinforced by the Ligg. costotransversaria lateralia and superiora. The Ligg. intertransversaria guarantee additional stability.

* The median portion of the Fascia thoracolumbalis is referred to as the Lig. supraspinale.

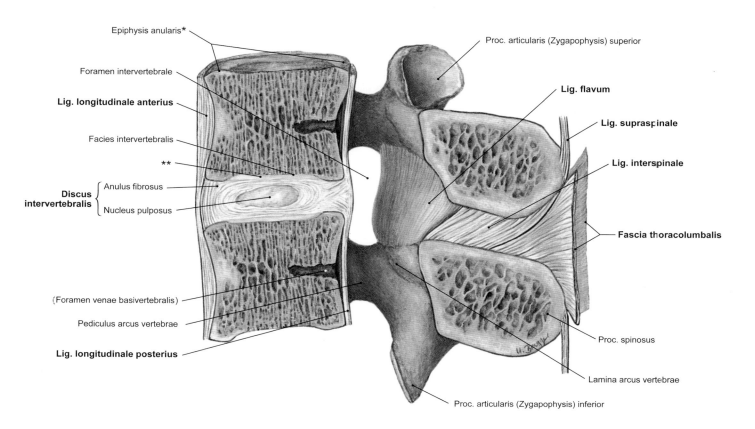

Epiphysis anularis*
Foramen intervertebrale
Lig. longitudinale anterius
Facies intervertebralis
**
Discus intervertebralis { Anulus fibrosus / Nucleus pulposus
(Foramen venae basivertebralis)
Pediculus arcus vertebrae
Lig. longitudinale posterius

Proc. articularis (Zygapophysis) superior
Lig. flavum
Lig. supraspinale
Lig. interspinale
Fascia thoracolumbalis
Proc. spinosus
Lamina arcus vertebrae
Proc. articularis (Zygapophysis) inferior

Fig. 2.59 Ligamentous apparatus of the lumbar motion segment;
median section; view from the left side. [S700]
The intervertebral disc (Discus intervertebralis) consists of a central gelatinous nucleus (Nucleus pulposus), originating from the Chorda dorsalis, and a connective tissue ring (Anulus fibrosus) surrounding the nucleus pulposus without a sharp margin. The Anulus fibrosus is largely
affixed via a bony rim and a cartilaginous hyaline covering (**) of the
end plate as non-ossified remains of the vertebral body epiphyses (*) on
the Corpus vertebrae as well as via the Lig. longitudinale posterius, and

to a lesser extent via the Lig. longitudinale anterius. A Discus intervertebralis connects two adjacent vertebrae as the Symphysis intervertebralis. The tension between the Ligg. flava, interspinale and supraspinale is guaranteed in the area of the vertebral arches. The Lig. interspinale
radiates into the Fascia thoracolumbalis into the thoracolumbar area.

* also: annular rim
** cartilagenous hyaline covering on the inferior end plate

Clinical remarks

The genetically determined (HLA-B27-positive) Spondylitis ankylosans **(BECHTEREW disease)** is associated with a progressive ossification of the Anulus fibrosus of the ligaments, the vertebral joints,
the Ligg. capitum costarum radiata and costotransversaria and the
Ligg. longitudinale anterius and interspinalia. In the early stages, it is

mostly only the sacroiliac joints that are affected. In spite of a limited
ability to flex, the shape of the back initially looks normal. When the
disease progresses, the back appears flat as a board (as if smoothly
ironed). In addition, there is a significant restriction of thoracic wall
excursions and a lessening of the respiratory capacity.

Ligamentous head joints

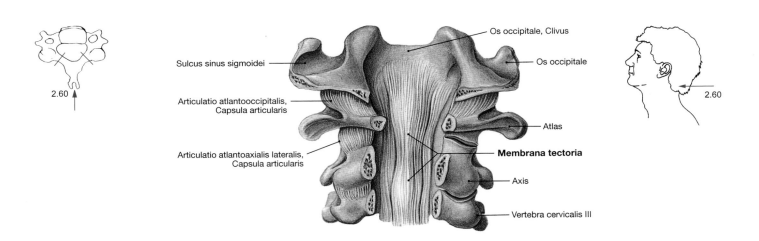

Fig. 2.60 Head joints with deep ligaments; dorsal view. [S700]
The **Membrana tectoria** is the extension of the **Lig. longitudinale posterius** to the cranial. It covers the ligaments and the joint capsule of the Articulatio atlantoaxialis mediana (not visible). The joint capsule of the Articulatio atlantooccipitalis can be recognised laterally between the occipital bone and the atlas, and the joint capsule of the Articulatio atlantoaxialis lateralis is visible between the atlas and the axis.

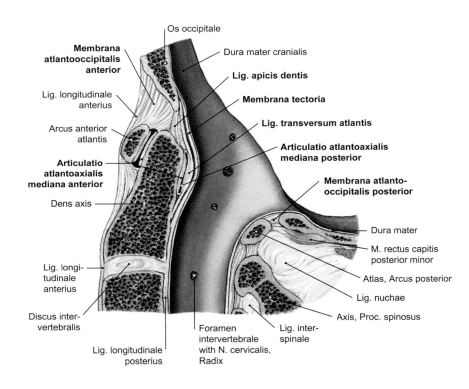

Fig. 2.61 Cervico-occipital transition region with intermediate atlantoaxial joint and ligaments; median-sagittal section; view from the left side. [S700]
As part of the so-called lower head joint (consisting of the Articulationes atlantoaxiales laterales and Articulatio atlantoaxialis mediana, which opposes the upper head joint consisting of the Articulationes atlantooccipitales), the flexible connection can be seen in the median section between the Dens axis and the front atlas arch (Articulatio atlantoaxialis mediana). The joint capsule is reinforced above the atlas of the **Membrana atlantooccipitalis anterior** and by the **Lig. longitudinale anterius** (→ Fig. 2.64). At the back, the Fasciculi longitudinales and the Lig. transversum atlantis (collectively the **Lig. cruciforme atlantis**) form a reinforcement of the joint capsule as well as the 'cruciate ligament'-covering **Membrana tectoria,** which in turn is covered with hard meninges (Dura mater spinalis). On the dorsal side of the vertebral canal, the **Membrana atlantooccipitalis posterior** stretches between the Os occipitale and the atlas, and in the neck the **Ligamentum nuchae** stretches from the axis to the occiput.

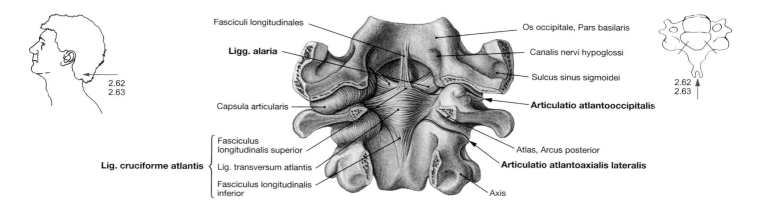

Fasciculi longitudinales
Ligg. alaria
Capsula articularis
Lig. cruciforme atlantis {
Fasciculus longitudinalis superior
Lig. transversum atlantis
Fasciculus longitudinalis inferior

Os occipitale, Pars basilaris
Canalis nervi hypoglossi
Sulcus sinus sigmoidei
Articulatio atlantooccipitalis
Atlas, Arcus posterior
Articulatio atlantoaxialis lateralis
Axis

Fig. 2.62 Head joints with deep ligaments; dorsal view; after removal of the Membrana tectoria. [S700]
Centrally, one can recognise the **Lig. cruciforme atlantis,** which consists of the Lig. transversum atlantis and both the two Fasciculi longitudinales. Behind it, the alar ligaments **(Ligg. alaria)** are visible, originat-

ing at the tip and the sides of the dens axis (→ Fig. 2.63) and reaching diagonally upwards. On the one side, the joint capsules of the Articulatio atlantooccipitalis and the Articulatio atlantoaxialis can be identified; on the other side, the joint capsules have been removed and the joint opening is visible.

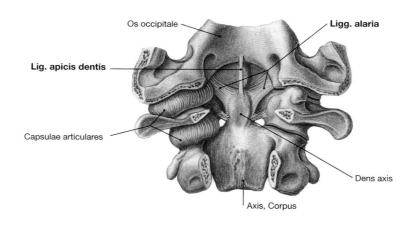

Lig. apicis dentis
Capsulae articulares

Os occipitale
Ligg. alaria
Dens axis
Axis, Corpus

Fig. 2.63 Head joints with deep ligaments; dorsal view; after removal of Membrana tectoria and Lig. cruciatum atlantis. [S700]

One can see the **Ligg. alaria** (→ Fig. 2.62) which frequently project to the Massae laterales of the atlas as well as the thin **Lig. apicis dentis.**

Clinical remarks

In the case of a rupture of the Lig. transversum atlantis or the Lig. cruciforme atlantis, there may be a dislocation of the Dens axis in the vertebral canal, causing contusion or separation of the structures **(neck fracture)** in the Medulla oblongata and spinal cord. The nerve

centres for respiration and blood circulation are hereby destroyed, immediately resulting in death.
Occasionally, a missing dens or incomplete formation of the Dens axis may cause an **atlantoaxial subluxation.**

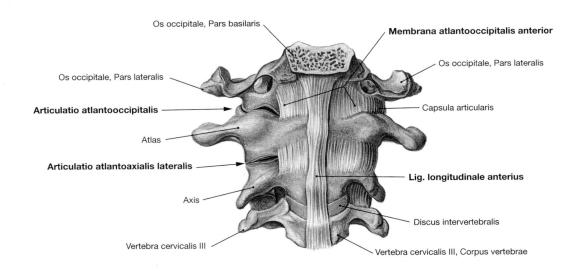

Os occipitale, Pars basilaris

Membrana atlantooccipitalis anterior

Os occipitale, Pars lateralis

Os occipitale, Pars lateralis

Articulatio atlantooccipitalis

Capsula articularis

Atlas

Articulatio atlantoaxialis lateralis

Lig. longitudinale anterius

Axis

Discus intervertebralis

Vertebra cervicalis III

Vertebra cervicalis III, Corpus vertebrae

Fig. 2.64   Head joints with ligaments and upper cervical spine; ventral view. [S700]
In the midline, the **Lig. longitudinale anterius** can be seen. The **Membrana atlantooccipitalis anterior** stretches between the occipital bone and the atlas. Lateral thereof, you can see the joint capsule of the Articulatio atlantooccipitalis, which has been removed on the opposite side.

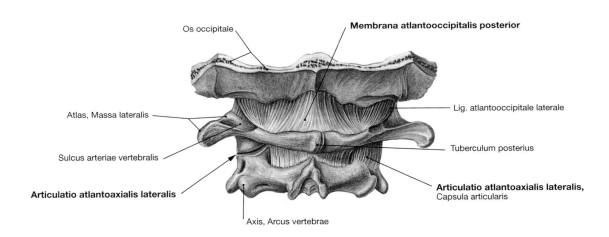

Os occipitale

Membrana atlantooccipitalis posterior

Lig. atlantooccipitale laterale

Atlas, Massa lateralis

Sulcus arteriae vertebralis

Tuberculum posterius

Articulatio atlantoaxialis lateralis

Articulatio atlantoaxialis lateralis, Capsula articularis

Axis, Arcus vertebrae

Fig. 2.65   Head joints; dorsal view. [S700]
Dorsally, between the Os occipitale and the Arcus posterior atlantis, the Membrana atlantooccipitalis posterior and the Lig. atlantooccipitale lateral are visible. On the right, between the atlas and the axis, the joint capsule of the Articulatio atlantoaxialis lateralis is visible; it has been removed on the left.

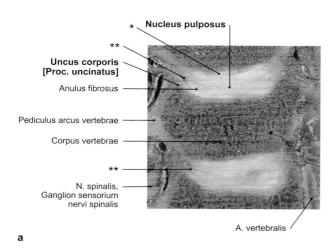

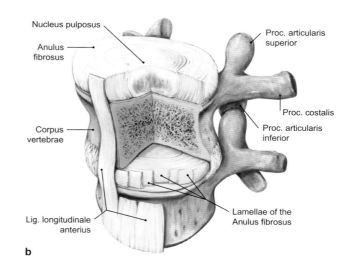

Fig. 2.66a and b   Intervertebral discs, Disci intervertebrales.
a Cervical intervertebral discs, Disci intervertebrales cervicales; frontal section; ventral view. As early as in the first decade of life, so-called uncovertebral gaps start forming in the lateral areas of the cervical intervertebral discs. Approximately between the fifth and 10th year of life, there are cleft formations in the Disci intervertebrales of the cervical spine, which assume a joint-like character. They are called uncovertebral joints, which initially provide functional benefits in terms of the movement of the cervical spine, but can tear completely later in life and can have negative effects. [S700]
b Structure of the intervertebral discs, Disci intervertebrales lumbales, shown for the lumbar vertebral column; view from the front diagonally. An intervertebral disc consists of an outer fibrous ring (Anulus fibrosus),

which is structured from opposing blades (herringbone pattern) made of collagen fibres. It is fused at the front and rear with Ligg. longitudinalia anterius and posterius, respectively. It is further divided into an external zone, an internal zone and a transition zone. The latter establishes the connection to the gelatinous Nucleus pulposus. The Nucleus pulposus borders the cartilage of the deck and floor plates of the adjacent vertebrae and the sides of the Anulus fibrosus (transition zone), cranially and caudally. If the Anulus fibrosus tears, the disc prolapses (Clinical remarks → Fig. 2.68). [S700-L266]/[R449]

*   hyaline cartilaginous coverage of the end plates of the vertebral body as non-ossified portions of the vertebral body epiphyses
** so-called uncovertebral gap

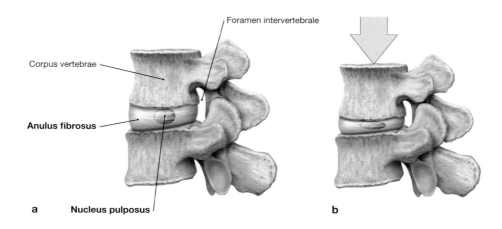

Fig. 2.67a and b   Intervertebral disc, Discus intervertebralis, in a motion segment of the lumbar spine; view from left lateral.
[S701-L127]
a Status in the morning. Intervertebral discs are located between all vertebrae of the cervical (except atlanto-occipital joints), thoracic and lumbar spine (as well as L5 and Os sacrum). The intervertebral disc is composed of an Anulus fibrosus and a Nucleus pulposus and forms a flexible symphyseal joint between the vertebral bodies. The disc en-

ables minimal movement between the vertebral bodies and acts as a shock absorber.
b Status in the evening. The height of the intervertebral disc reduces slightly during the day (arrow shows force applied to vertrebral spine) due to loss of water. This water is replenished and the height of the disc increases again when lying down during sleep. This is why people are almost a centimetre shorter in the evening than in the morning. Rudimentary intervertebral discs can be found between the upper synostotically fused vertrebral bodies of the Os sacrum.

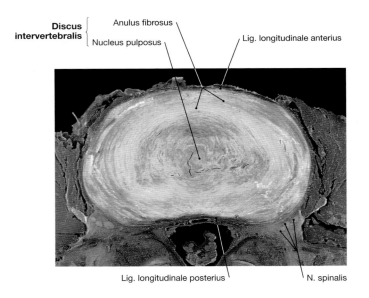

Discus intervertebralis — Anulus fibrosus / Nucleus pulposus

Lig. longitudinale anterius

Lig. longitudinale posterius

N. spinalis

Fig. 2.68 Lumbar intervertebral disc, Discus intervertebralis lumbalis; cranial view. [S700]
The intervertebral disc (Discus intervertebralis) consists of a central gelatinous nucleus **(Nucleus pulposus),** originating from the Chorda dorsalis, and a connective tissue ring **(Anulus fibrosus)** surrounding the Nucleus pulposus.

Clinical remarks

a Approximately 25 % of people under the age of 40 and approximately 60 % of people over the age of 40 suffer from degenerative changes to the intervertebral discs. Most frequently affected are the lumbar and cervical spine. This can lead to a prolapse/bulge and protrusions/herniation of vertebral discs **(herniated disc).** The intervertebral disc tissue protrudes either posterolaterally (more frequent) or mediodorsally (less frequent) into the spinal canal (→ Fig. b**). The result is a compression of the spinal nerve root **(radicular syndrome).** The segments S1, L5 and L4 are most frequently affected. Starting at the uncovertebral fissures, rupture of an intervertebral disc causing disc herniation can also occur in the cervical spine. [S701-L127]
b Depiction of a laterodorsal prolapse with compression of the N. spinalis as well as of a mediodorsal prolapse with narrowing of the vertebral canal. [S702-L266]/[R449]

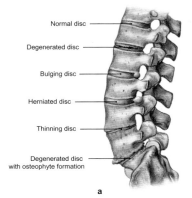

Normal disc
Degenerated disc
Bulging disc
Herniated disc
Thinning disc
Degenerated disc with osteophyte formation

a

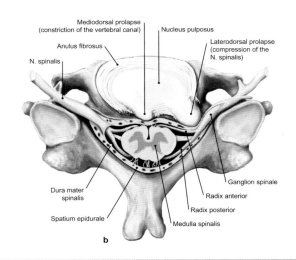

Mediodorsal prolapse (constriction of the vertebral canal)
Anulus fibrosus
N. spinalis
Nucleus pulposus
Laterodorsal prolapse (compression of the N. spinalis)
Dura mater spinalis
Ganglion spinale
Radix anterior
Radix posterior
Spatium epidurale
Medulla spinalis

b

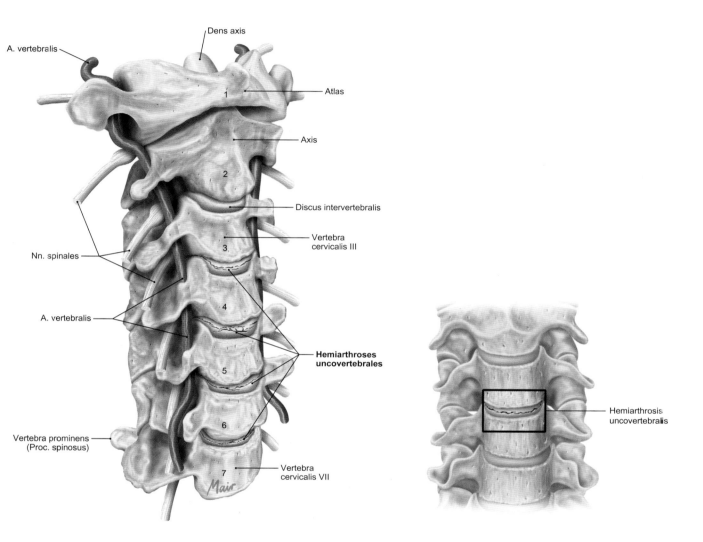

Fig. 2.69 Uncovertebral joints, Hemiarthroses uncovertebrales; ventral view, lateral right side. [S700-L127]
The formation of uncovertebral joints weakens the stability of the spine but strong ligaments compensate for this instability. Although the functional role of the uncovertebral joints is unclear, they may allow for increased ventral and dorsal movements while restricting lateral range of motion.

Fig. 2.70 Cervical intervertebral disc, Discus intervertebralis cervicalis, with uncovertebral joint; ventral view. [S700-L127]
The lateral parts of the intervertebral discs of the cervical spine are constricted and shielded by the Procc. uncinati (Unci corporis). From the age of approximately 10 years onwards, the intervertebral discs between the third and sixth vertebral bodies develop a physiological gap, which creates a new joint-like structure composed of connective tissue. These uncovertebral joints are exclusively observed in the discs of the cervical spine (Hemiarthroses uncovertebrales; LUSCHKA's joints). An uncovertebral joint in the cervical intervertebral segment C4/C5 is shown (Hemiarthrosis uncovertebralis; LUSCHKA's joint).

Imaging methods

Cervical spine, X-ray

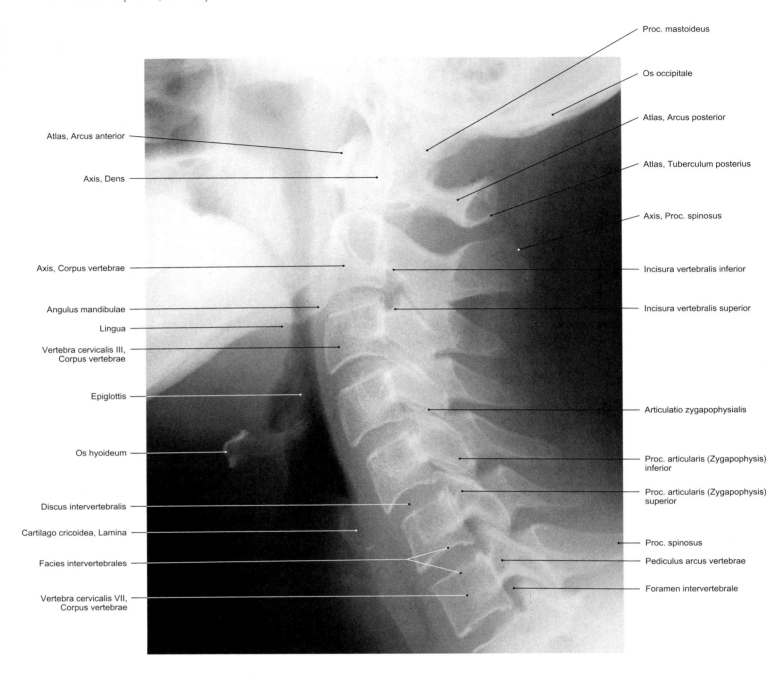

Proc. mastoideus

Os occipitale

Atlas, Arcus posterior

Atlas, Tuberculum posterius

Axis, Proc. spinosus

Incisura vertebralis inferior

Incisura vertebralis superior

Articulatio zygapophysialis

Proc. articularis (Zygapophysis) inferior

Proc. articularis (Zygapophysis) superior

Proc. spinosus

Pediculus arcus vertebrae

Foramen intervertebrale

Atlas, Arcus anterior

Axis, Dens

Axis, Corpus vertebrae

Angulus mandibulae

Lingua

Vertebra cervicalis III, Corpus vertebrae

Epiglottis

Os hyoideum

Discus intervertebralis

Cartilago cricoidea, Lamina

Facies intervertebrales

Vertebra cervicalis VII, Corpus vertebrae

Fig. 2.71 Cervical vertebrae, Vertebrae cervicales; X-ray image in lateral projection; setting: upright position; central beam set at the third cervical vertebrae; shoulders pulled down. [S700-T904]

Clinical remarks

A convex and dorsally curved spine is referred to as a **kyphosis.** In the thoracic spine, this slight curvature is physiological, but in the cervical and lumbar spine it is always pathological. A reinforcement of the kyphosis leads to the formation of a hunchback (gibbus) and appears in various forms (e.g. in early childhood as a **hunchback,** in juveniles as **adolescent kyphosis** [SCHEUERMANN disease], in more advanced years with loss of elasticity and disc degeneration as senile or **age-related kyphosis**). Congenital kyphosis is usually caused by hemi or block vertebrae.

A strong non-physiological lordosis is called **hyperlordosis** and occurs particularly in the lumbar spine.
[G725]

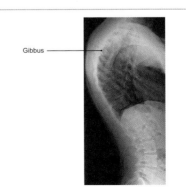

Gibbus

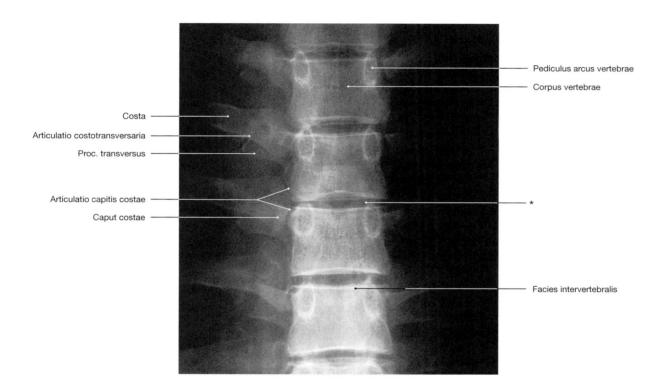

Pediculus arcus vertebrae

Corpus vertebrae

Costa

Articulatio costotransversaria

Proc. transversus

Articulatio capitis costae

Caput costae

*

Facies intervertebralis

Fig. 2.72 Thoracic vertebrae, Vertebrae thoracicae; X-ray in anteroposterior (AP) projection; setting: upright position, thorax in inhalation position; central beam on the sixth thoracic vertebra. [S700-T902]

* intervertebral disc space

The spine is more frequently a **metastasis site** for malignant tumours because of the dense capillary net within the vertebrae. The normal bone matrix of affected vertebrae together with the mechanical bone properties are destroyed. This can lead to even smaller loads causing vertebral collapses. Often vertebral fragments enter the vertebral canal or the Foramen intervertebrale and result in injuries and compression of the spinal cord and the spinal nerves.

Lumbar spine, X-ray

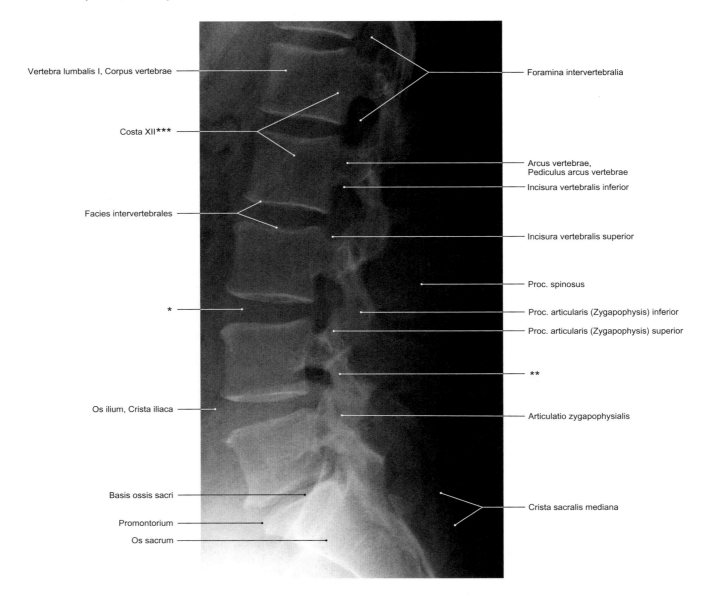

Vertebra lumbalis I, Corpus vertebrae

Costa XII***

Facies intervertebrales

*

Os ilium, Crista iliaca

Basis ossis sacri

Promontorium

Os sacrum

Foramina intervertebralia

Arcus vertebrae,
Pediculus arcus vertebrae

Incisura vertebralis inferior

Incisura vertebralis superior

Proc. spinosus

Proc. articularis (Zygapophysis) inferior

Proc. articularis (Zygapophysis) superior

**

Articulatio zygapophysialis

Crista sacralis mediana

Fig. 2.73 Lumbar vertebrae, Vertebrae lumbales; X-ray in lateral projection; setting: upright position; central beam on the second lumbar vertebra. Tapering at the front edges of the lower lumbar vertebrae is an initial sign of degenerative changes and thus of pathological changes. [S700-T902]

*   intervertebral disc space
**   vertebral arch area between the superior and inferior joint process (so-called isthmus = interarticular portion)
*** The terminal points indicate the pathway of rib XII, which is poorly visible in this copy of the X-ray.

Clinical remarks

Osteoporosis is a metabolic bone disease with largely unknown aetiology which is characterised by a localised or general decrease of bony mass or density without changing the external shape of the bone. This condition primarily affects women over 55 and men over 70. Genetic predisposition, lack of physical activity, poor nutritional state and unfavourable oestrogen levels contribute to the development of osteoporosis. As a result of the weakened bone structure, fractures such as vertebral fractures, distal radius fractures, and femoral neck fractures occur frequently.

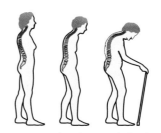

Osteoporosis causes progressive changes in body posture with ageing. [S701-L126]

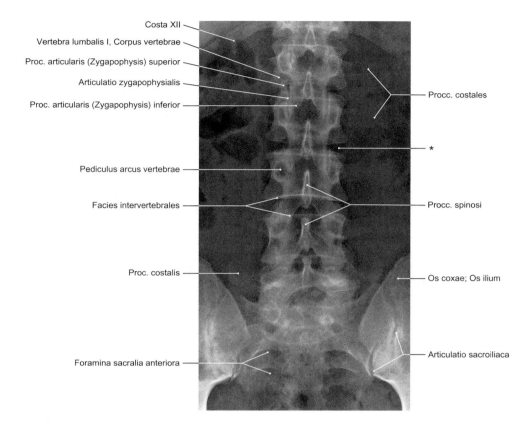

Costa XII
Vertebra lumbalis I, Corpus vertebrae
Proc. articularis (Zygapophysis) superior
Articulatio zygapophysialis
Proc. articularis (Zygapophysis) inferior

Pediculus arcus vertebrae

Facies intervertebrales

Proc. costalis

Foramina sacralia anteriora

Procc. costales

*

Procc. spinosi

Os coxae; Os ilium

Articulatio sacroiliaca

Fig. 2.74 Lumbar vertebrae, Vertebrae lumbales, and sacrum, Os sacrum; X-ray image in anteroposterior (AP) projection; setting: upright position; central beam on the second lumbar vertebra. [S700-T902]

* intervertebral disc space

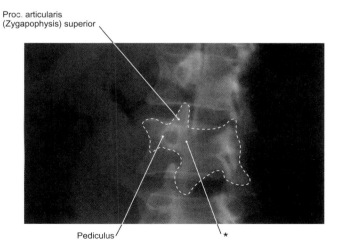

Proc. articularis
(Zygapophysis) superior

Pediculus

*

Fig. 2.75 Lumbar vertebrae, Vertebrae lumbales; X-ray in oblique projection; setting: upright position. [E402]
The experienced radiologist will recognise a dog-like figure ('Scottie dog', dotted line) in this oblique X-ray image. The central area is the interarticular part. The purely clinical term refers to the vertebral section between the superior and inferior joint facets of the zygapophyseal joints (→ Fig. 2.39).

* interarticular portion

Clinical remarks

Fractures in the area of the interarticular part (isthmus) cause a change in the Scottie dog figure, e.g. dog with collar (white arrow in →Fig. a), caused by spondylolysis. The fracture can occur on one or both sides and mostly as a result from sports injuries. This can lead to damage at the level of L4 and L5 and particularly at the interarticular part (isthmus).

In the case of a spondylolysis (→Fig. b), it is possible to develop a **spondylolisthesis**. However, even without a fracture of the interarticular part, the cranial vertebra can slip ventrally over the vertebrae below. Usually inherited or degenerative changes in the joint facets are to blame. All the above-mentioned conditions (including a fracture of the interarticular part) are termed spondylolisthesis. The slippage is measured over a range of four grades, from grade 1 (25 %) to grade 4 (100 %). The more severe the slippage, the more pronounced the lordosis of the spine in the affected spinal segment.

a [E329], b [S701-L126]

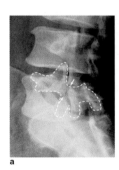

a

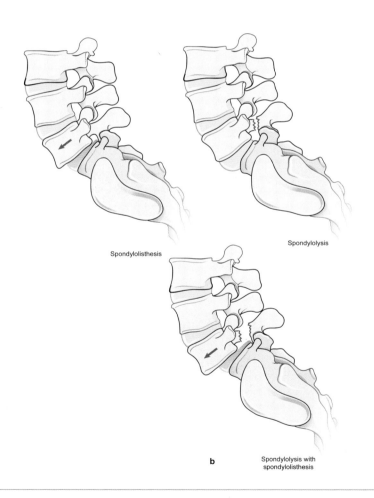

Spondylolisthesis

Spondylolysis

Spondylolysis with spondylolisthesis

b

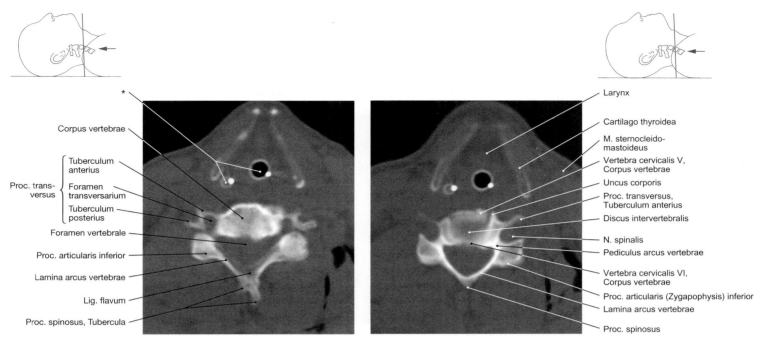

Fig. 2.76 **Cervical spine;** computed tomographic (CT) cross-section at the level of the intervertebral disc between the fourth and fifth cervical vertebrae. [S700-T902]
* artificial respiration tube and endoscopic instrument

Fig. 2.77 **Cervical spine;** computed tomographic (CT) cross-section at the level of the fifth cervical vertebra. [S700-T902]

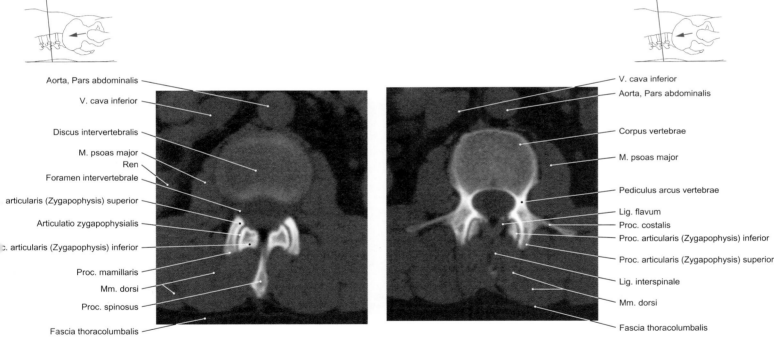

Fig. 2.78 **Lumbar spine;** computed tomographic (CT) cross-section at the level of the intervertebral disc between the second and third lumbar vertebrae. [S700-T902]

Fig. 2.79 **Lumbar spine;** computed tomographic (CT) cross-section at the level of the pediculi of the third lumbar vertebra. [S700-T902]

Clinical remarks

Some genetic disorders are associated with variations of the number of vertebrae. The **KLIPPEL-FEIL syndrome** for example is a hereditary development disorder of the cervical spine with spinal fusion during the early embryonic stage (usually of the atlas and axis or of the fifth and sixth cervical vertebrae). The characteristics of this dis-

order, caused by the fusion, are a short neck and often shoulder elevation. Spina bifida, lower placement of ears, and abnormalities of heart and other organs can also accompany this disease.
When a vertebra only emerges on one side from the corresponding sclerotome, it is referred to as a semi-vertebra **(hemivertebra).**

Spine, CT, MRI

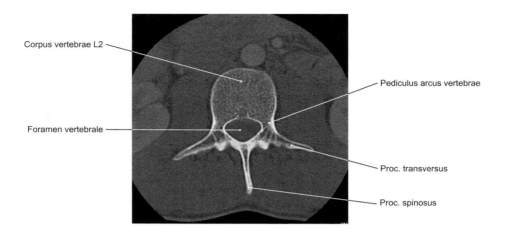

Corpus vertebrae L2

Foramen vertebrale

Pediculus arcus vertebrae

Proc. transversus

Proc. spinosus

Fig. 2.80 Lumbar spine; computed tomography (CT) cross-section at the level of the second lumbar vertebra. [E458]

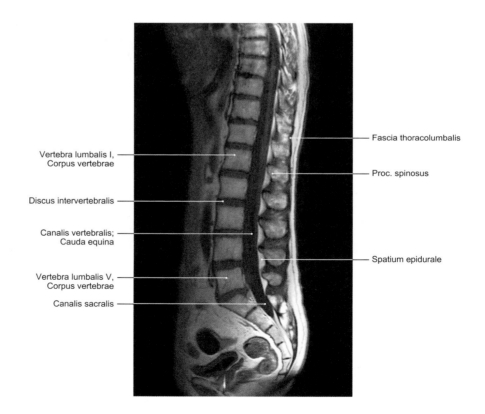

Vertebra lumbalis I, Corpus vertebrae

Discus intervertebralis

Canalis vertebralis; Cauda equina

Vertebra lumbalis V, Corpus vertebrae

Canalis sacralis

Fascia thoracolumbalis

Proc. spinosus

Spatium epidurale

Fig. 2.81 Lumbar spine; magnetic resonance tomographic median section (MRI) of the thoracic and lumbar spine as well as the Os sacrum. [S700-T906]

MRI is a suitable imaging technique to view intervertebral discs, the spinal cord, and the epidural space (Spatium epidurale).

Clinical remarks

Ageing decreases the ability of the Anulus fibrosus and Nucleus pulposus to retain water which, among other symptoms, leads to the formation of small cracks in the Anulus fibrosus **(chondrosis).** This can be detected radiologically by a reduction in height and pathologically by an instability with increased mobility in the motion segment. In due course, gradual height reduction of the disc and the resulting reduction in mechanical buffer function lead to increased strain on the superior and inferior end plates of the vertebral bodies. Radiologically, this manifests itself in a **sclerotisation** with increased radiation density **(osteochondrosis).** Furthermore, it causes the formation of **spondylophytes** (bony osteophytes) on the vertebral bodies, which are also radiologically visible. If the radial cracks in the Anulus fibrosus increase, intervertebral disc tissue can emerge from the intervertebral space **(disc prolapse;** → Fig. a, → Fig. b).

a Median disc prolapse (arrow); T2-weighted magnetic resonance imaging (MRI) of a sagittal median section in the lumbar spine. The overlying segments also show prolapsing discs that inflict pressure on the spinal cord. [E684]

b Median disc prolapse; T2-weighted magnetic resonance imaging (MRI) of a cross-section (MRI) in the lumbar spine. The arrows show disc prolapse compressing the spinal cord. [E684]

A **spinal canal stenosis** is an abnormal narrowing of the vertebral canal or of a Foramen intervertebrale which causes pressure or compression of the spinal cord and/or the root of a spinal nerve. Degenerative changes to the spine are the most frequent cause for spinal stenosis (→ Fig. c, → Fig. d) (e. g. osteoarthritis of the zygapophyseal joints). Clinical symptoms include pain, numbness, paraesthesia, and the loss of motor control. The location of the spinal stenosis determines the affected body region. Approximately 75 % of all spinal stenosis cases are located in the lumbar region and affect the sciatic nerve (tingling sensations, muscle weakness or numbness, which can radiate into the back and leg areas). In severe cases, an operation is the only choice to widen the spinal canal or Foramen intervertebrale and again make sufficient space for the spinal cord or affected spinal nerve.

Degenerative changes of the cervical spine:

c The formation of small osteophytes, particularly on the vertebral body and Procc. uncinati. [S700-L127]

d Degenerative changes on the cervical spine with pronounced osteophytes and narrowing of the spinal canal and Foramina intervertebralia. [S700-L127]

Canalis vertebralis with Liquor cerebrospinalis

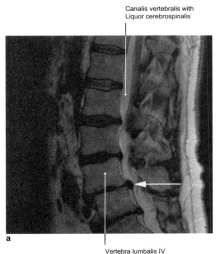

a

Vertebra lumbalis IV

M. psoas major   Corpus vertebrae

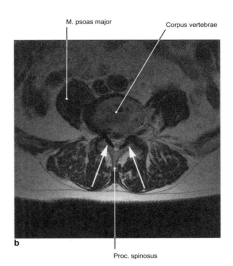

b

Proc. spinosus

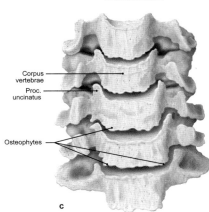

Corpus vertebrae
Proc. uncinatus

Osteophytes

c

Corpus vertebrae
Foramen transversarium
Proc. uncinatus
Osteophytes
Facies articularis superior

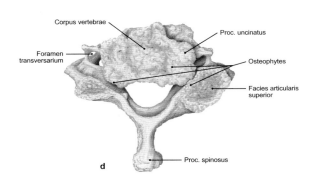

Proc. spinosus

d

Superficial muscles of the back

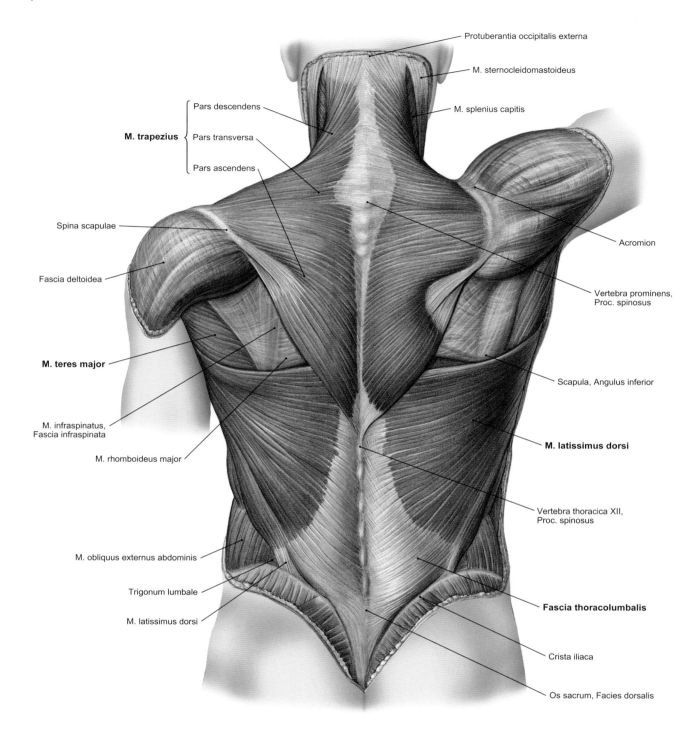

Protuberantia occipitalis externa

M. sternocleidomastoideus

M. splenius capitis

M. trapezius {
Pars descendens
Pars transversa
Pars ascendens

Spina scapulae

Fascia deltoidea

Acromion

Vertebra prominens, Proc. spinosus

M. teres major

Scapula, Angulus inferior

M. infraspinatus, Fascia infraspinata

M. rhomboideus major

M. latissimus dorsi

M. obliquus externus abdominis

Vertebra thoracica XII, Proc. spinosus

Trigonum lumbale

Fascia thoracolumbalis

M. latissimus dorsi

Crista iliaca

Os sacrum, Facies dorsalis

Fig. 2.82 Superficial layer of the trunk-arm and trunk-shoulder girdle muscles; dorsal view. [S700]
The Mm. trapezius and latissimus dorsi form the largest part of the superficial layer of muscles of the back. The **M. trapezius** secures the scapula and thus the shoulder girdle. It also allows the scapula and with it the clavicle to pull backwards medially to the spine. The Partes descendens and ascendens turn the Angulus inferior of the scapula medially. In addition, the Pars descendens adducts and supports the M. serratus anterior in shoulder elevation.

In terms of surface area, the **M. latissimus dorsi** is the widest muscle of the human body. It lowers the elevated arm, adducts it, can pull it backward from the adduction position medially, rotates it inwardly and can support expiration. It is often referred to as the 'lats muscle'. On an evolutionary level, the M. latissimus dorsi connects with the **M. teres major.** It pulls the arm to the rear medially, is involved in the adduction, and rotates it inwardly.

→ T 29, T 30

Clinical remarks

Units of the **M. latissimus dorsi** are used to **cover defects of the trunk wall,** as well as for the reconstruction of the breast after resection in breast cancer. To this end, a so-called pedicle flap is formed, on which the A. and V. thoracodorsalis are prepared and displaced. The **M. pectoralis major** (ventral trunk wall) is often used as a pedicle flap graft to cover **facial defects.**

Trunk

2

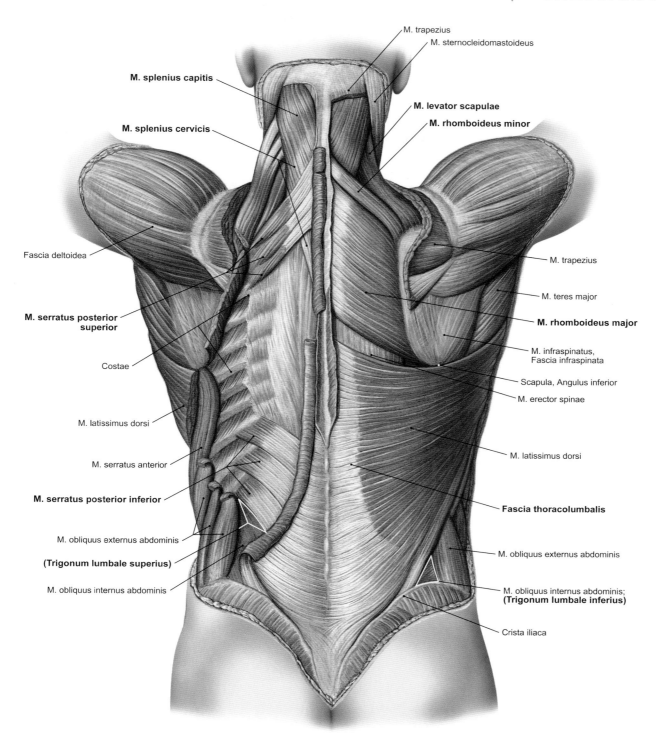

M. trapezius
M. sternocleidomastoideus
M. splenius capitis
M. levator scapulae
M. splenius cervicis
M. rhomboideus minor
Fascia deltoidea
M. trapezius
M. teres major
M. serratus posterior superior
M. rhomboideus major
Costae
M. infraspinatus, Fascia infraspinata
Scapula, Angulus inferior
M. erector spinae
M. latissimus dorsi
M. latissimus dorsi
M. serratus anterior
M. serratus posterior inferior
Fascia thoracolumbalis
M. obliquus externus abdominis
M. obliquus externus abdominis
(Trigonum lumbale superius)
M. obliquus internus abdominis
M. obliquus internus abdominis; **(Trigonum lumbale inferius)**
Crista iliaca

Fig. 2.83   Deep layer of the trunk/arm and the trunk/shoulder girdle muscles; dorsal view. [S700]

The Mm. levator scapulae, rhomboideus minor and major are visible on the right side after removal of the M. trapezius. The **M. levator scapulae** can lift the scapula and simultaneously turn its Angulus inferior medially.

The **M. rhomboideus minor** and **M. rhomboideus major** secure the scapula to the thorax and pull it towards the spine.

After removal of the three muscles and the M. latissimus dorsi, the **Mm. serrati posteriores superior and inferior** become visible. The M. serratus posterior superior lifts the upper ribs and acts as a respiratory muscle with inspiration. The M. serratus posterior inferior broadens the lower thoracic aperture and stabilises the lower ribs during contraction of the Pars costalis of the diaphragm. It is therefore also a respiratory muscle for inspiration.

The **Fascia thoracolumbalis** is designed as a rough aponeurosis. In a fibrous context it completes the osteofibrous channel formed by the spine and the dorsal surfaces of the ribs, and wraps around the autochthonous muscles of the back. Its superficial lamina serves as the origin for the M. latissimus dorsi and the M. serratus posterior inferior. The lamina is firmly fused with the tendon of the M. erector spinae. Cranially it separates the M. splenius cervicis from the M. trapezius and the Mm. rhomboidei and unites with the Fascia nuchae. The deep lamina is shown in → Fig. 2.85.

In the area of the **Trigonum lumbale superius** (GRYN-FELT-LESSHAFT-LUSCHKA triangle) and the **Trigonum lumbale inferius** (PETIT triangle) it may lead to the formation of **GRYNFELT and PETIT lumbal hernias.**

→ T 18, T 29

Deep (autochthonous) muscles of the back

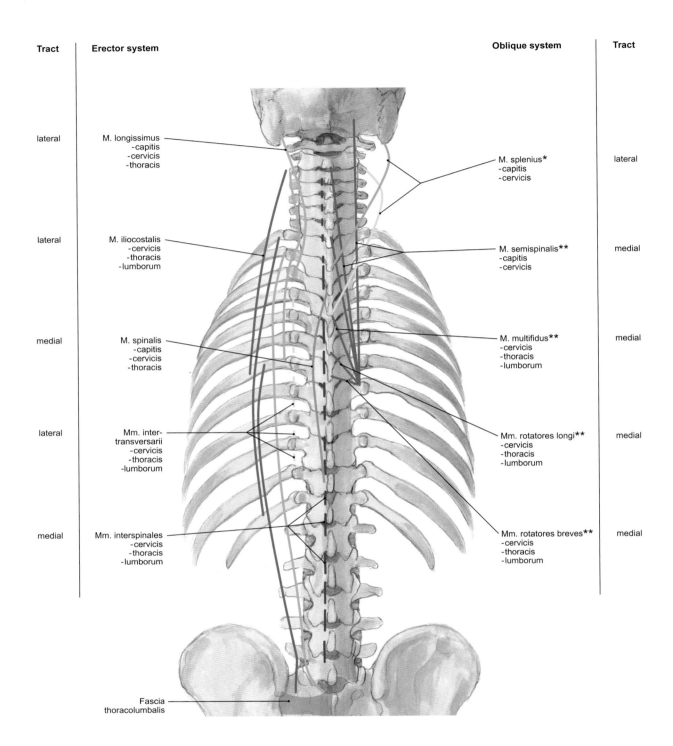

Tract	Erector system		Oblique system	Tract
lateral	M. longissimus -capitis -cervicis -thoracis		M. splenius* -capitis -cervicis	lateral
lateral	M. iliocostalis -cervicis -thoracis -lumborum		M. semispinalis** -capitis -cervicis	medial
medial	M. spinalis -capitis -cervicis -thoracis		M. multifidus** -cervicis -thoracis -lumborum	medial
lateral	Mm. inter- transversarii -cervicis -thoracis -lumborum		Mm. rotatores longi** -cervicis -thoracis -lumborum	medial
medial	Mm. interspinales -cervicis -thoracis -lumborum		Mm. rotatores breves** -cervicis -thoracis -lumborum	medial
	Fascia thoracolumbalis			

Fig. 2.84 Deep (autochthonous) back muscles; orientation scheme of the muscle groups. [S700]

The autochthonous muscles of the back, collectively named the M. erector spinae, can be divided into a longitudinal 'erector system' and an 'oblique system', as well as into a lateral and medial tract.

The **lateral tract** is divided into an intertransverse system (Mm. intertransversarii), a sacrospinal system (M. iliocostalis, M. longissimus) and a spinotransverse system (M. splenius cervicis, M. splenius capitis):

- The **intertransverse system** is used for stabilisation as well as the lateral flexion and extension between the transverse processes.
- The **sacrospinal system** stretches the spine, leads to the extension of and is used for the lateral flexion and the rotation of the torso on the ipsilateral side.

- The **spinotransverse system** acts as a stabiliser according to the bow-tendon principle and, together with the short neck muscles, supports all movements of the cervical spine and the atlanto-occipital joints.

The **medial tract** is divided into a spinal system (Mm. interspinales, M. spinalis) and into a transversospinal system (Mm. rotatores breves, Mm. rotatores longi, M. multifidus, M. semispinalis). Functionally, the **spinal system** is important for extension and torsion; the **transversospinal system** stabilises and rotates to the contralateral side.

* spinotransverse
** transversospinal

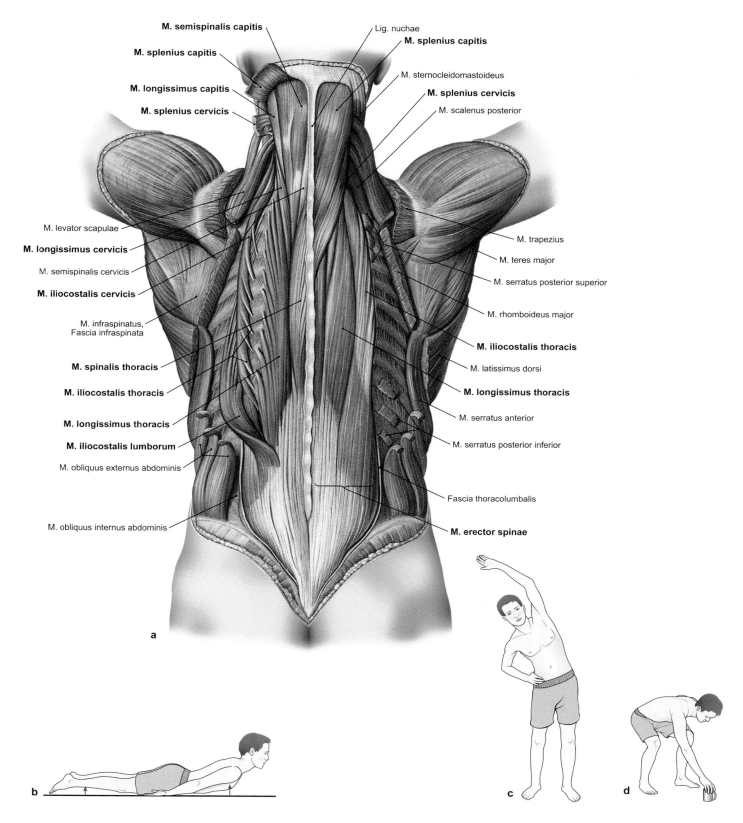

M. semispinalis capitis
M. splenius capitis
M. longissimus capitis
M. splenius cervicis

Lig. nuchae
M. splenius capitis
M. sternocleidomastoideus
M. splenius cervicis
M. scalenus posterior

M. levator scapulae
M. longissimus cervicis
M. semispinalis cervicis
M. iliocostalis cervicis
M. infraspinatus, Fascia infraspinata
M. spinalis thoracis
M. iliocostalis thoracis
M. longissimus thoracis
M. iliocostalis lumborum
M. obliquus externus abdominis
M. obliquus internus abdominis

M. trapezius
M. teres major
M. serratus posterior superior
M. rhomboideus major
M. iliocostalis thoracis
M. latissimus dorsi
M. longissimus thoracis
M. serratus anterior
M. serratus posterior inferior
Fascia thoracolumbalis
M. erector spinae

a

b   c   d

Fig. 2.85a-d   Superficial layer (lateral tract) of the deep (autochthonous) back muscles.

a Dorsal view. The autochthonous muscles of the back are collectively named the **M. erector spinae.** It is divided into a medial (deep) and a lateral (superficial) tract. Each tract is composed of different systems (→ Fig. 2.84). The M. erector spinae extends from the sacrum to the occipital bone. The abdominal muscles and the M. erector spinae form a functional unit (bowstring principle). The superficial layer is composed of three different muscle columns: M iliocostalis (lateral column), M. longissimus (middle column), and M. spinalis (median column). [S700]

b The three muscular columns form a functional unit. Upon bilateral contraction, they extend the spine. [S700-L126]
c Upon unilateral contraction, these muscles support lateral flexion to the side of the contracted muscles. [S700-L126]
d These muscles also serve to counteract gravity during forward movements. The M. erector spinae keeps the spine erect and prevents and/or enables the slow movement of the trunk when bending over to pick something up from the ground. [S700-L126]

→ T 19

Deep (autochthonous) muscles of the back

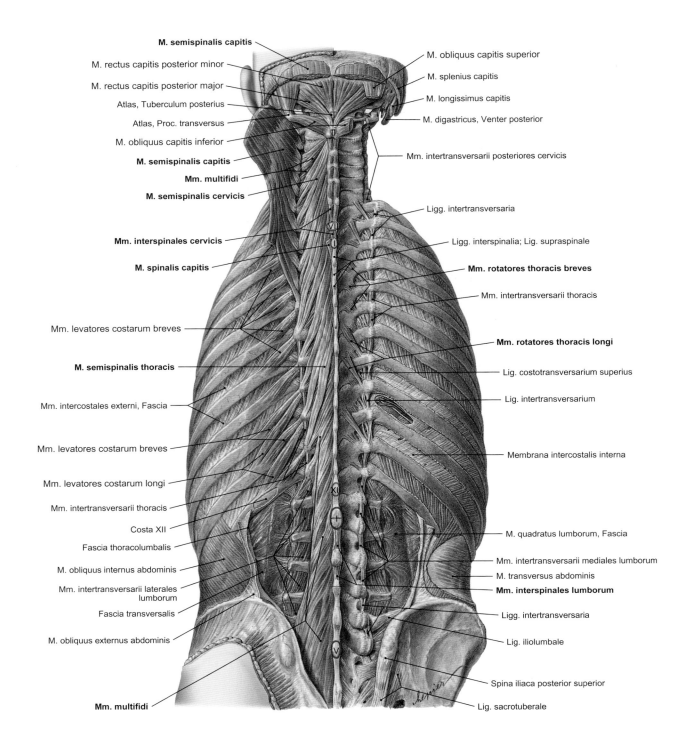

M. semispinalis capitis

M. rectus capitis posterior minor

M. rectus capitis posterior major

Atlas, Tuberculum posterius

Atlas, Proc. transversus

M. obliquus capitis inferior

M. semispinalis capitis

Mm. multifidi

M. semispinalis cervicis

Mm. interspinales cervicis

M. spinalis capitis

Mm. levatores costarum breves

M. semispinalis thoracis

Mm. intercostales externi, Fascia

Mm. levatores costarum breves

Mm. levatores costarum longi

Mm. intertransversarii thoracis

Costa XII

Fascia thoracolumbalis

M. obliquus internus abdominis

Mm. intertransversarii laterales lumborum

Fascia transversalis

M. obliquus externus abdominis

Mm. multifidi

M. obliquus capitis superior

M. splenius capitis

M. longissimus capitis

M. digastricus, Venter posterior

Mm. intertransversarii posteriores cervicis

Ligg. intertransversaria

Ligg. interspinalia; Lig. supraspinale

Mm. rotatores thoracis breves

Mm. intertransversarii thoracis

Mm. rotatores thoracis longi

Lig. costotransversarium superius

Lig. intertransversarium

Membrana intercostalis interna

M. quadratus lumborum, Fascia

Mm. intertransversarii mediales lumborum

M. transversus abdominis

Mm. interspinales lumborum

Ligg. intertransversaria

Lig. iliolumbale

Spina iliaca posterior superior

Lig. sacrotuberale

Fig. 2.86 Deep layer (medial tract) of the deep (autochthonous) back muscles, Mm. dorsi, and neck muscles, Mm. suboccipitales; dorsal view. [S700]

Upon removal of the Mm. splenius capitis and semispinalis capitis, the short neck muscles (Mm. rectus capitis posterior minor, rectus capitis posterior major, obliquus capitis superior, obliquus capitis inferior) become visible. → Fig. 2.89, → Fig. 2.90 and → Fig. 2.91 show these muscles and describe their functions in detail.

For classification of other depicted authochtonous back muscles see → Fig. 2.84.

The depicted 12 paired Mm. levatores costarum are back muscles which are not assigned to a specific muscle group. They are innervated by the Rr. posteriores of the spinal nerves and additionally by small branches of the intercostal nerves. It is assumed that these muscles originated from the transverse processes and then migrated to the ribs. In the literature, these are therefore partly seen as secondary migrated back muscles. Contraction of the Mm. levatores costarum results in a rotation on the contralateral side and side flexion on the ipsilateral side of the spine. Their role in inspiration is discussed.

→ T 19

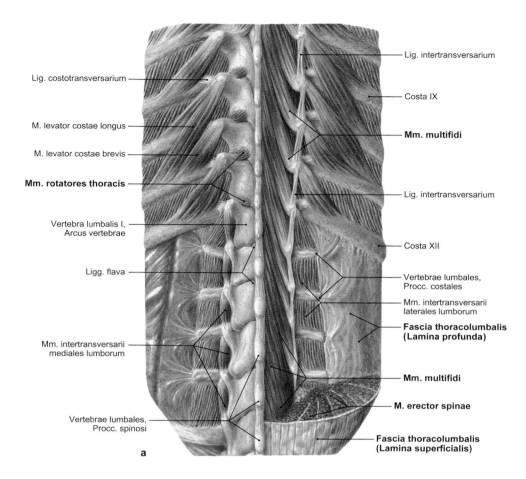

Lig. costotransversarium

M. levator costae longus

M. levator costae brevis

Mm. rotatores thoracis

Vertebra lumbalis I,
Arcus vertebrae

Ligg. flava

Mm. intertransversarii
mediales lumborum

Vertebrae lumbales,
Procc. spinosi

a

Lig. intertransversarium

Costa IX

Mm. multifidi

Lig. intertransversarium

Costa XII

Vertebrae lumbales,
Procc. costales

Mm. intertransversarii
laterales lumborum

**Fascia thoracolumbalis
(Lamina profunda)**

Mm. multifidi

M. erector spinae

**Fascia thoracolumbalis
(Lamina superficialis)**

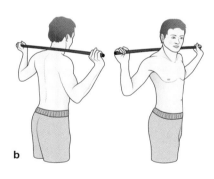

b

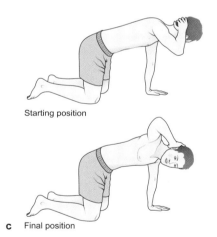

Starting position

c   Final position

Fig. 2.87a–c   Deep layer (medial tract) of the deep autochthonous muscles of the back, Mm. dorsi, in the region of the lower thoracic and the lumbar spine.
a Dorsal view. On the right is a cross-section through the M. erector spinae in the caudal region. Located medially are the Mm. multifidi which belong to the medial tract and the superficial, deep layer of the Fascia thoracolumbalis. On the left side, the Mm. rotatores thoracis are visible. [S700]

b The transversospinal system (Mm. semispinalis, Mm. multifidi, Mm. rotatores) of the M. erector spinae functions as a muscle that facilitates rotations and extensions of the spine. [S700-L126]
c Additionally, the M. erector spinae controls and enables precise rotation and extension movements in specific spinal regions (e. g. as shown for the thoracic region of the spine). [S700-L126]

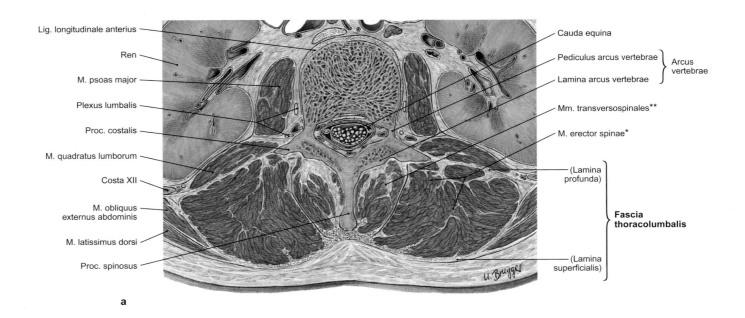

Lig. longitudinale anterius

Ren

M. psoas major

Plexus lumbalis

Proc. costalis

M. quadratus lumborum

Costa XII

M. obliquus externus abdominis

M. latissimus dorsi

Proc. spinosus

Cauda equina

Pediculus arcus vertebrae ⎫ Arcus
Lamina arcus vertebrae ⎭ vertebrae

Mm. transversospinales**

M. erector spinae*

(Lamina profunda)

Fascia thoracolumbalis

(Lamina superficialis)

a

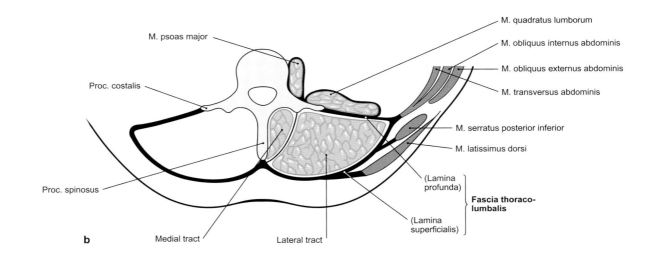

M. psoas major

Proc. costalis

Proc. spinosus

M. quadratus lumborum

M. obliquus internus abdominis

M. obliquus externus abdominis

M. transversus abdominis

M. serratus posterior inferior

M. latissimus dorsi

(Lamina profunda) **Fascia thoraco-lumbalis**

(Lamina superficialis)

Medial tract

Lateral tract

b

Fig. 2.88a and b   Deep (autochthonous) back muscles and Fascia thoracolumbalis; cross-section at the level of the second lumbar vertebra; caudal view.
a The lateral (*) and medial tract (**) of the deep autochthonous back muscles are located within an osteofibrous sheath, with its inner and

outer margins formed by the dorsal vertebrae parts and the Fascia thoracolumbalis, respectively. [S700]
b The Fascia thoracolumbalis is divided into strong superficial and deep fascial layers called Lamina superficialis and Lamina profunda, respectively. [S702-L126]

→ T 19

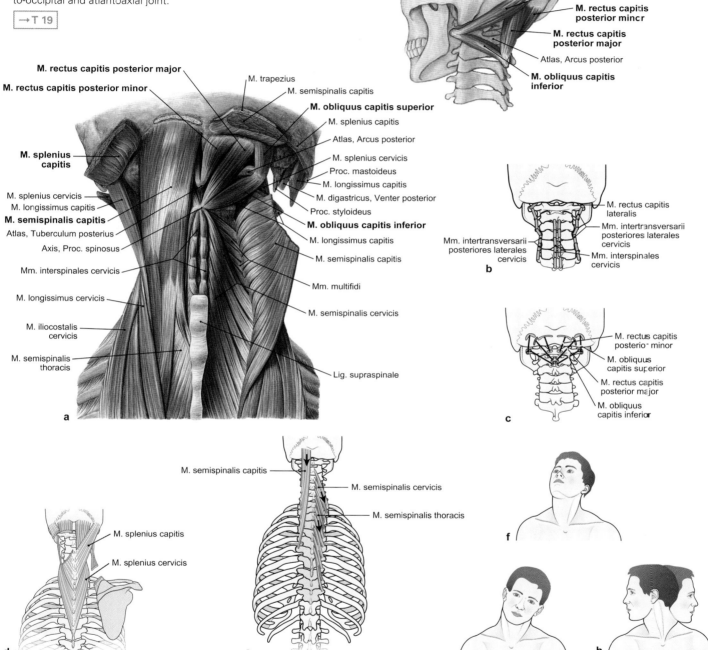

Fig. 2.89   Short neck muscles, Mm. suboccipitales; oblique dorsal view. [S700]

Together, the Mm. rectus capitis posterior major, obliquus capitis superior, and obliquus capitis inferior create a triangle **(vertebralis triangle).** The M. rectus capitis posterior minor is located medially to the M. rectus capitis posterior major. Functionally, the four muscles direct precise movements of the head joints (Articulationes atlantooccipitalis and atlantoaxialis) and perform minute adjustments of the head in the atlanto-occipital and atlantoaxial joint.

→ T 19

Fig. 2.90a–h   Back muscles, Mm. dorsi, and neck muscles, Mm. suboccipitales; dorsal view.

a To view the short muscles of the neck, the Mm. splenius capitis and semispinalis capitis were removed on the right side. The M. rectus capitis posterior minor has its origin at the Tuberculum posterius of the atlas and inserts medially at the Linea nuchalis inferior. The M. rectus capitis posterior major originates at the Proc. spinosus of the axis and starts laterally next to the M. rectus capitis posterior minor at the inferior nuchal line. The M. obliquus capitis superior originates at the Proc. transversus of the atlas and inserts above and laterally to the M. rectus capitis posterior major. The M. obliquus capitis inferior comes from the Proc. spinosus of the axis and inserts at the Proc. transverse of the atlas. [S700]

b Position of the short neck muscles (diagram). [S702-L126]

c Position of the short suboccipital muscles (Mm. suboccipitales) with origin and insertion points [diagram]. [S702-L126]

d Position of the M. splenius capitis and M. splenius cervicis which belong to the muscles of the upper back (diagram). Bilateral contraction of these muscles and the shorter suboccipital muscles enables the extension of the neck. [S701-L126]

e Position of the M. semispinalis capitis, M. semispinalis cervicis, and M. semispinalis thoracis as part of the upper back muscles (diagram). Unilateral contraction of these muscles together with the neck muscles enables side and rotational movements. [S701-L126]

f–h Upper back muscles and neck muscles enable head movements such as looking up at the ceiling (f), leaning the head towards the shoulder (g), or looking over the shoulder (h). [S700-L126]

→ T 19

Neck muscles

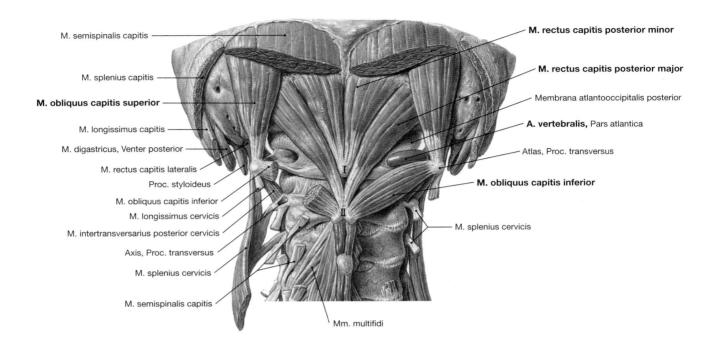

M. semispinalis capitis

M. splenius capitis

M. obliquus capitis superior

M. longissimus capitis

M. digastricus, Venter posterior

M. rectus capitis lateralis

Proc. styloideus

M. obliquus capitis inferior

M. longissimus cervicis

M. intertransversarius posterior cervicis

Axis, Proc. transversus

M. splenius cervicis

M. semispinalis capitis

Mm. multifidi

M. rectus capitis posterior minor

M. rectus capitis posterior major

Membrana atlantooccipitalis posterior

A. vertebralis, Pars atlantica

Atlas, Proc. transversus

M. obliquus capitis inferior

M. splenius cervicis

Fig. 2.91 Neck muscles, Mm. suboccipitales; dorsal view. [S700]
The Mm. rectus capitis posterior major, obliquus capitis superior, and
M. obliquus capitis inferior all border the vertebralis triangle (**Trigonum
arteriae vertebralis,** → Fig. 2.89). The A. vertebralis crosses the Arcus
posterior atlantis at the base of this triangle.

I = Tuberculum posterius of the atlas
II = Proc. spinosus of the axis

→ T 19

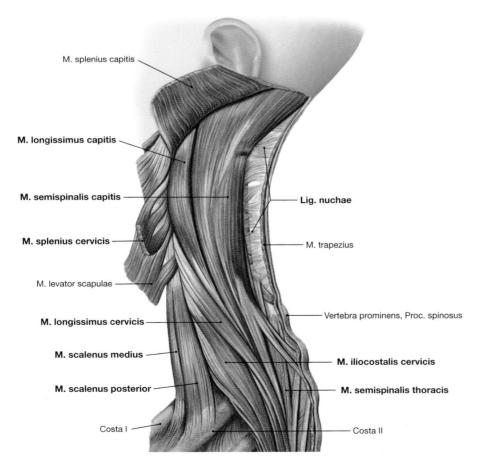

M. splenius capitis

M. longissimus capitis

M. semispinalis capitis

M. splenius cervicis

M. levator scapulae

M. longissimus cervicis

M. scalenus medius

M. scalenus posterior

Costa I

Lig. nuchae

M. trapezius

Vertebra prominens, Proc. spinosus

M. iliocostalis cervicis

M. semispinalis thoracis

Costa II

**Fig. 2.92 Neck muscles, Mm. suboccipitales,
and cervical muscles, Mm. colli;** view from the
left side. [S700]
Upon dissection of the M. splenius capitis (the
rest turned over cranially), the lateral view of the
neck reveals from anterior to posterior the Mm.
scalenus medius and posterior as well as autochthonous muscles of the back with the lateral
(Mm. iliocostalis cervicis, longissimus cervicis,
splenius cervicis, longissimus capitis) and medial
(Mm. semispinalis thoracis, semispinalis capitis)
tract. After removal of the superficial back muscles in the neck area, the Lig. nuchae and remnants of the M. trapezius can be seen in the midline.

→ T 19

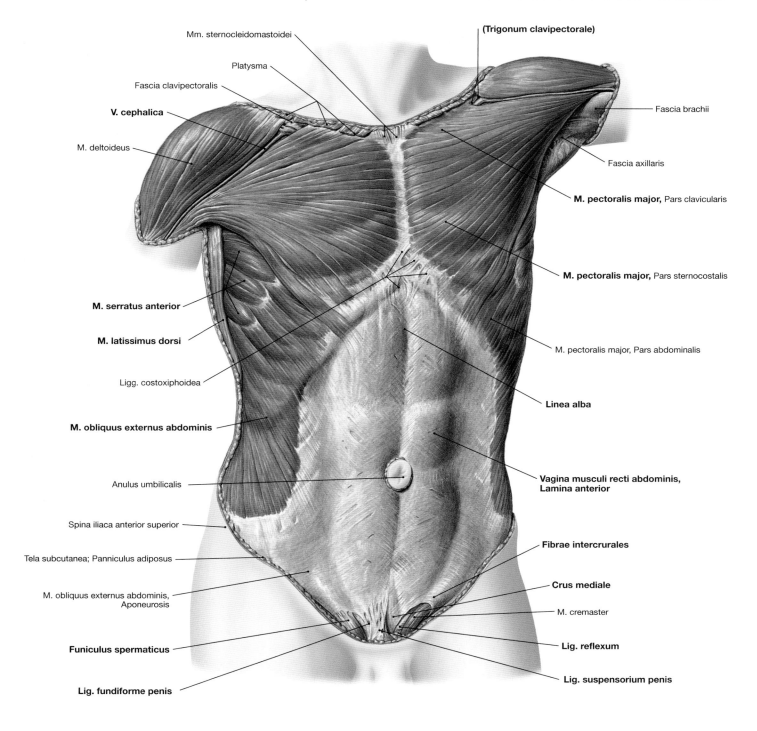

Mm. sternocleidomastoidei

(Trigonum clavipectorale)

Platysma

Fascia clavipectoralis

V. cephalica

M. deltoideus

Fascia brachii

Fascia axillaris

M. pectoralis major, Pars clavicularis

M. pectoralis major, Pars sternocostalis

M. serratus anterior

M. latissimus dorsi

M. pectoralis major, Pars abdominalis

Ligg. costoxiphoidea

Linea alba

M. obliquus externus abdominis

Anulus umbilicalis

**Vagina musculi recti abdominis,
Lamina anterior**

Spina iliaca anterior superior

Tela subcutanea; Panniculus adiposus

Fibrae intercrurales

Crus mediale

M. obliquus externus abdominis,
Aponeurosis

M. cremaster

Funiculus spermaticus

Lig. reflexum

Lig. suspensorium penis

Lig. fundiforme penis

Fig. 2.93 Superficial layer of muscles of the thoracic and abdominal wall, Mm. thoracis and Mm. abdominis; ventral view. [S700]
The V. cephalica runs along the border between the M. deltoideus and M. pectoralis major to the Trigonum clavipectorale (MOHRENHEIM fossa) where it enters deeply to flow into the V. axillaris. The lower margin of the M. pectoralis major forms the anterior axillary fold, and the anterior margin of the M. latissimus dorsi forms the posterior axillary fold, while the M. serratus anterior forms the floor of the axilla.
The **M. pectoralis major** functionally participates in the anteversion (= flexion) of the arm in the shoulder joint and is also a strong adductor and rotates inwardly. It can also pull the shoulder forward and lower it when the arm is secured. In addition, it is an auxiliary muscle for inspiration.

In the abdominal region, the rectus sheath is formed by the aponeurosis of the oblique abdominal muscles. On the exterior we see the **M. obliquus externus abdominis,** which forms the outer surface of the rectus sheath with its aponeurosis.
In the midline, the aponeuroses merge in the Linea alba. The caudal suspensory ligaments for the penis, Ligg. fundiforme and suspensorium penis, are shown. To the side, the Funiculus spermaticus is visible with the Anulus inguinalis superficialis, with the Crus medial, Fibrae intercrurales and Lig. reflexum on the opposite side.

→ T 26

141

2

Superficial muscles of the thoracic and abdominal wall

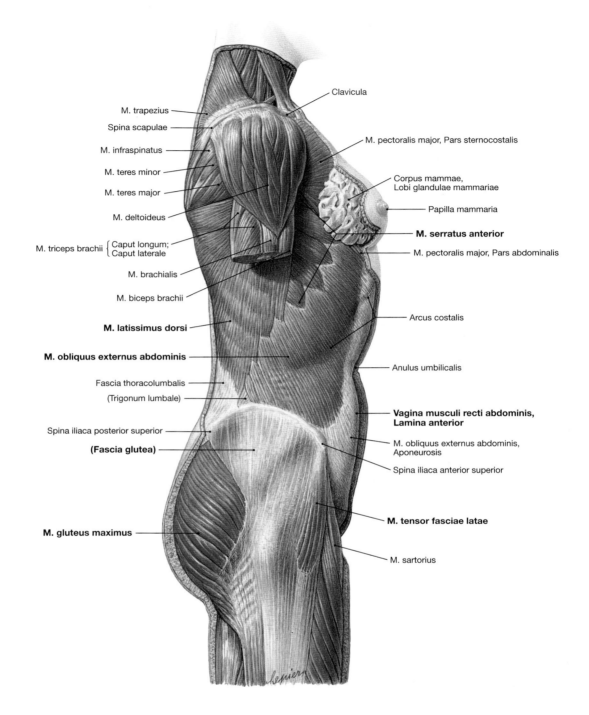

M. trapezius

Spina scapulae

M. infraspinatus

M. teres minor

M. teres major

M. deltoideus

M. triceps brachii { Caput longum; Caput laterale }

M. brachialis

M. biceps brachii

M. latissimus dorsi

M. obliquus externus abdominis

Fascia thoracolumbalis

(Trigonum lumbale)

Spina iliaca posterior superior

(Fascia glutea)

M. gluteus maximus

Clavicula

M. pectoralis major, Pars sternocostalis

Corpus mammae, Lobi glandulae mammariae

Papilla mammaria

M. serratus anterior

M. pectoralis major, Pars abdominalis

Arcus costalis

Anulus umbilicalis

Vagina musculi recti abdominis, Lamina anterior

M. obliquus externus abdominis, Aponeurosis

Spina iliaca anterior superior

M. tensor fasciae latae

M. sartorius

**Fig. 2.94   Surperficial layer of muscles of the thoracic and ab-
dominal wall, Mm. thoracis and Mm. abdominis;** view from the
right side. [S700]
The lateral view shows the female breast (Mamma) which supports the
M. pectoralis major. The lateral abdominal wall shows the muscular origins of the M. obliquus externus abdominis interlaced with those of the
M. serratus anterior. Dorsally, the M. latissimus dorsi covers it.
The **M. obliquus externus abdominis** extends from the lateral upper
back to the medial front lower. The fibres coming from the lower ribs

run almost perpendicular to the Labium externum of the Crista iliaca.
The remaining fibres pass to the ventral trunk wall into a sheet-like layer
of aponeurosis, which is involved in the structuring of the rectus sheath
(Vagina musculi recti abdominis). On the upper thigh, you can see the
Fascia glutea, as well as the **Mm. gluteus maximus** and **tensor fasci-
ae latae** radiating into the iliotibialis tract.

→ T 26

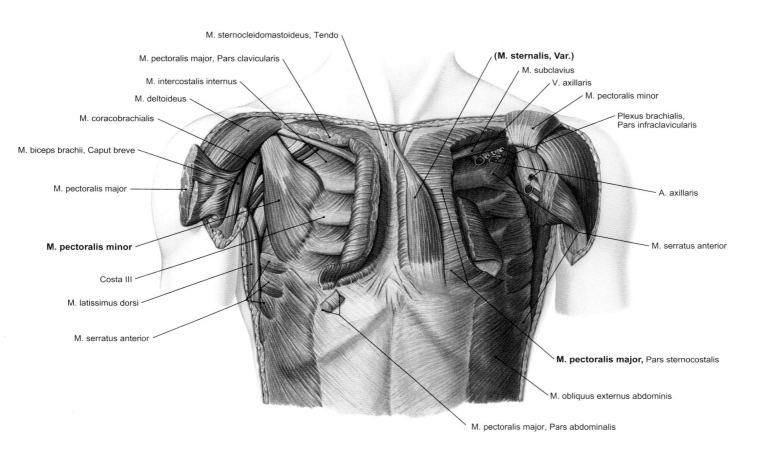

M. sternocleidomastoideus, Tendo

M. pectoralis major, Pars clavicularis

M. intercostalis internus

M. deltoideus

M. coracobrachialis

M. biceps brachii, Caput breve

M. pectoralis major

M. pectoralis minor

Costa III

M. latissimus dorsi

M. serratus anterior

(M. sternalis, Var.)

M. subclavius

V. axillaris

M. pectoralis minor

Plexus brachialis, Pars infraclavicularis

A. axillaris

M. serratus anterior

M. pectoralis major, Pars sternocostalis

M. obliquus externus abdominis

M. pectoralis major, Pars abdominalis

Fig. 2.95 Deep layer of muscles of the thoracic wall, Mm. thoracis; ventral view. [S700]
The M. pectoralis major was removed on both sides, as well as the M. pectoralis minor on the left side. On the right side of the body, the pathway of the neurovascular bundle to the upper extremity is visible below the M. pectoralis minor. Although the **M. pectoralis minor** is considered a muscle of the shoulder, it does not start at the upper extremity but at the Proc. coracoideus. The M. pectoralis minor originates from ribs III to V and participates in lowering and rotation of the scapula. It is not at all uncommon for a very variable M. sternalis to appear on the M. pectoralis major.

→ T 14

Thoracic wall and thoracic wall muscles

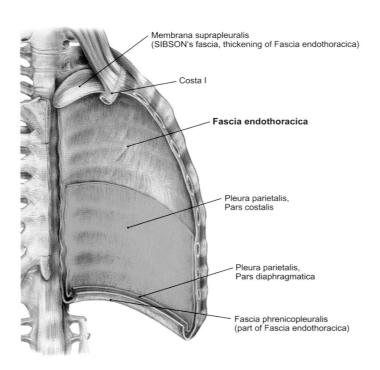

Membrana suprapleuralis
(SIBSON's fascia, thickening of Fascia endothoracica)

Costa I

Fascia endothoracica

Pleura parietalis,
Pars costalis

Pleura parietalis,
Pars diaphragmatica

Fascia phrenicopleuralis
(part of Fascia endothoracica)

Fig. 2.96 Fascia endothoracica as part of the inner lining of the thoracic wall; the dorsal part of the thoracic wall is shown, view at the inner lining of the thoracic wall upon removal of the left lung. [S701-L285]
The inner thoracic wall is covered with the Fascia endothoracica. The Pleura parietalis lies on top and is firmly attached to the Fascia endothoracica.

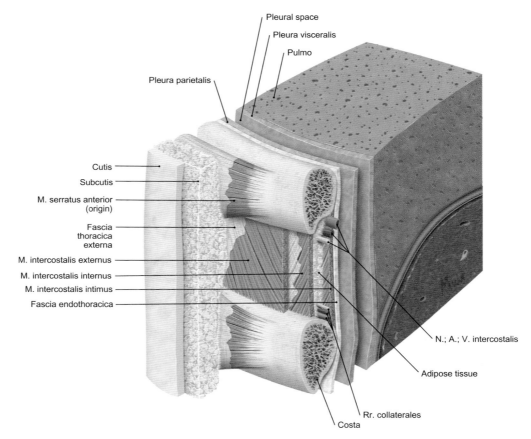

Pleural space

Pleura visceralis

Pulmo

Pleura parietalis

Cutis

Subcutis

M. serratus anterior
(origin)

Fascia
thoracica
externa

M. intercostalis externus

M. intercostalis internus

M. intercostalis intimus

Fascia endothoracica

N.; A.; V. intercostalis

Adipose tissue

Rr. collaterales

Costa

Fig. 2.97 Muscles and structure of the thoracic wall, Mm. thoracis; depiction of an intercostal space. [S702-L127]
The thoracic wall is formed by the following structures from outside to inside:
- Cutis/subcutis
- Fascia musculi serrati
- M. serratus anterior
- Fascia thoracica externa
- M. intercostalis externus
- M. intercostalis internus, M. intercostalis intimus (as part of the M. intercostalis internus)

- Fascia intercostalis interna (not shown, →Fig. 2.98)
- Fascia endothoracica
- Pleura parietalis.

The pleural space and the Pleura visceralis connect to the Pleura parietalis, which covers the lungs. The N., A. and V. intercostalis run below the ribs into the Sulcus costae from the outside to the inside, with the much smaller Rr. collaterales running above the ribs.

→ T 14, T 26

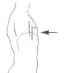

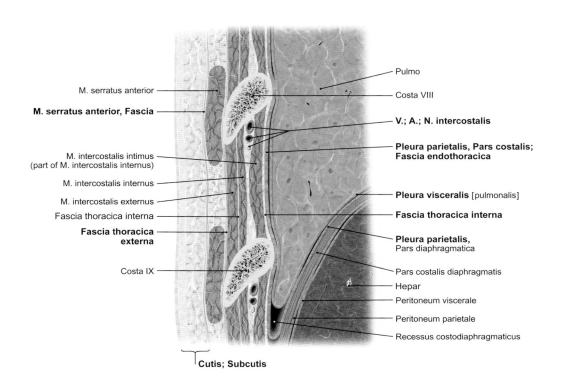

M. serratus anterior

M. serratus anterior, Fascia

M. intercostalis intimus
(part of M. intercostalis internus)

M. intercostalis internus

M. intercostalis externus

Fascia thoracica interna

**Fascia thoracica
externa**

Costa IX

Pulmo

Costa VIII

V.; A.; N. intercostalis

**Pleura parietalis, Pars costalis;
Fascia endothoracica**

Pleura visceralis [pulmonalis]

Fascia thoracica interna

Pleura parietalis,
Pars diaphragmatica

Pars costalis diaphragmatis

Hepar

Peritoneum viscerale

Peritoneum parietale

Recessus costodiaphragmaticus

Cutis; Subcutis

Fig. 2.98 Muscles of the thoracic wall, Mm. thoracis; frontal cross-section of two intercostal spaces. [S701-L127]
The M. intercostalis internus together with its innermost part (M. intercostalis intimus) are enveloped in a true muscle fascia, known as the

Fascia thoracica interna. Towards the inside of the thoracic cavity, this fascia borders the Fascia endothoracica, located in-between the Fascia thoracica interna and the Pleura parietalis.

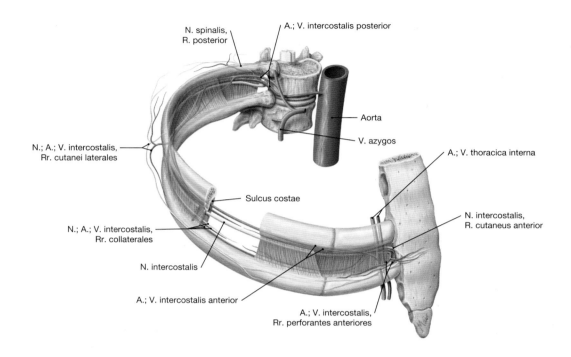

Fig. 2.99 **Vasa intercostalia and N. intercostalis;** image shows an intercostal space with blood vessels and the intercostal nerve. [S701-L127]
The N. intercostalis and Vasa intercostalia run between the M. intercostalis internus and M. intercostalis intimus (as part of the M. intercostalis internus). The typical topography from superior to inferior is: **veins – artery –** **nerve (VAN).** Of these three structures, the intercostal nerve is the structure least protected by the inferior margin of the rib. Located within adipose tissue on top of the rib, collateral blood vessels derived from the Vasa intercostalia and small branches of the N. intercostalis run between the M. intercostalis internus and M. intercostalis intimus as Rr. collaterales.

Clinical remarks

A pleural effusion denotes an accumulation of fluid in the pleural space between the two pleural layers, which covers the ribs (Pleura parietalis) and lungs (Pleura visceralis). A **pleural puncture** taps this pleural space. A differentiation is made between a diagnostic puncture (for obtaining material, e.g. in the case of inflammation) and a therapeutic puncture (e.g. for relief and recovery of good ventilation). In a pleural puncture, the following structures are pierced: the cutis/subcutis, Fascia musculi serrati, M. serratus anterior, Fascia thoracica externa, M. intercostalis externus, M. intercostalis internus, Fascia thoracica interna, Fascia endothoracica and Pleura parietalis. The pleural puncture is always carried out at the top edge of the rib, because the neurovascular pathways run just below the rib (V., A. and N. intercostalis). [S701-L127]

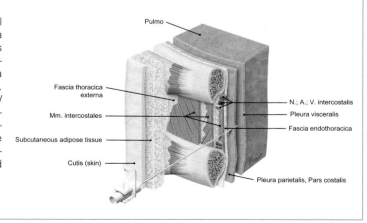

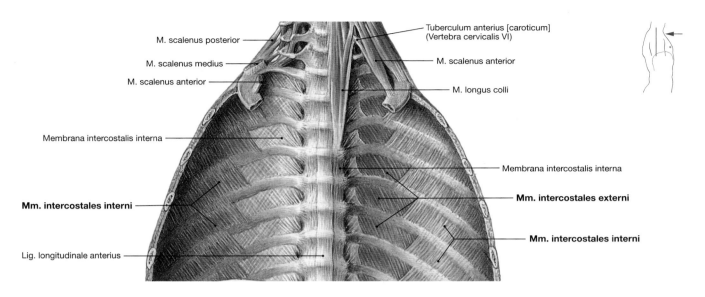

M. scalenus posterior

M. scalenus medius

M. scalenus anterior

Membrana intercostalis interna

Mm. intercostales interni

Lig. longitudinale anterius

Tuberculum anterius [caroticum]
(Vertebra cervicalis VI)

M. scalenus anterior

M. longus colli

Membrana intercostalis interna

Mm. intercostales externi

Mm. intercostales interni

Fig. 2.100 Posterior wall of the thoracic cavity, Cavea thoracis; ventral view. [S700]
The **Mm. intercostales externi** run from behind and above to the front and below. They start at the Tubercula costarum and extend forwards parasternally to where the cartilage transitions (not visible). These muscles act together with the Mm. intercartilaginei (not shown) by **raising the ribs** during inspiration.
The **Mm. intercostales interni** pull from behind and below towards the top and the front. They start at the Angulus costae and run to the ster-

num (not visible). They act by **lowering the ribs** in expiration. One exception is the sections running between the cartilaginous sections of the ribs (Mm. intercartilaginei), which support inspiration. The muscular elements of the Mm. intercostales interni stretching across multiple segments, known as the Mm. subcostales and serving the same function as the Mm. intercostales interni, are not shown.

→ T 14

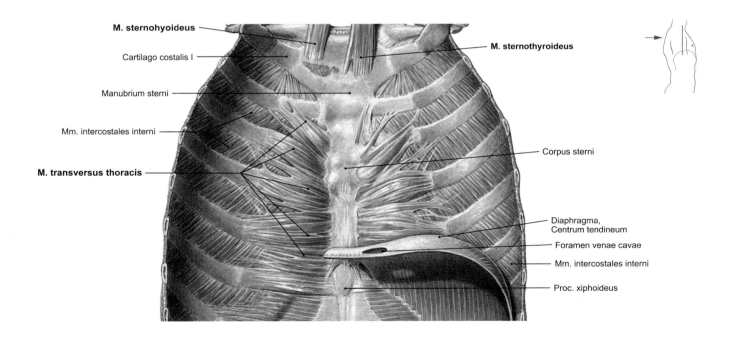

M. sternohyoideus

Cartilago costalis I

Manubrium sterni

Mm. intercostales interni

M. transversus thoracis

M. sternothyroideus

Corpus sterni

Diaphragma,
Centrum tendineum

Foramen venae cavae

Mm. intercostales interni

Proc. xiphoideus

Fig. 2.101 Anterior wall of the thoracic cavity, Cavea thoracis; dorsal view. [S700]
The view of the inner wall of the front thoracic cavity next to the sternum shows the cluster of the **M. transversus thoracis.** They originate at the lateral side of the sternum and of the Proc. xiphoideus and start

on the inside of the second to sixth rib cartilage. They act as **expirators.** The M. sternothyroideus and the M. sternohyoideus originate on the back of the Manubrium sterni.

→ T 14

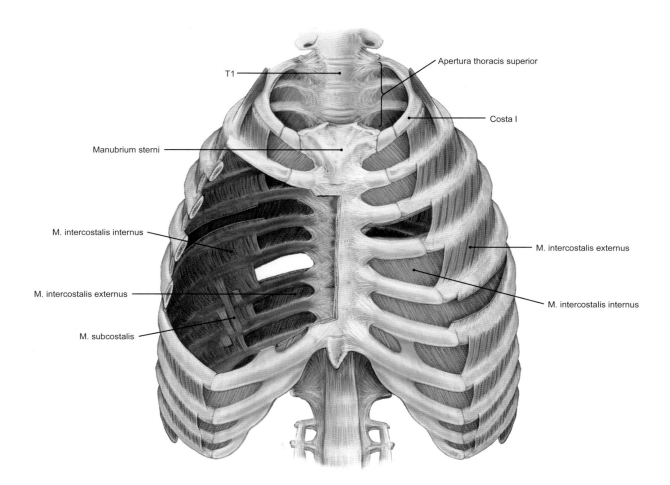

T1

Apertura thoracis superior

Costa I

Manubrium sterni

M. intercostalis internus

M. intercostalis externus

M. intercostalis externus

M. intercostalis internus

M. subcostalis

Fig. 2.102 Upper thoracic aperture, Apertura thoracis superior, and muscles of the thoracic wall, Mm. thoracis; dorsal view. [S701-L285]

The upper thoracic aperture is delineated by the first thoracic vertebra (T1), die paired first rib, and the upper margin of the Manubrium sterni. The figure also demonstrates the course of the intercostal muscles at the posterior thoracic wall (right) and the anterior thoracic wall (left).

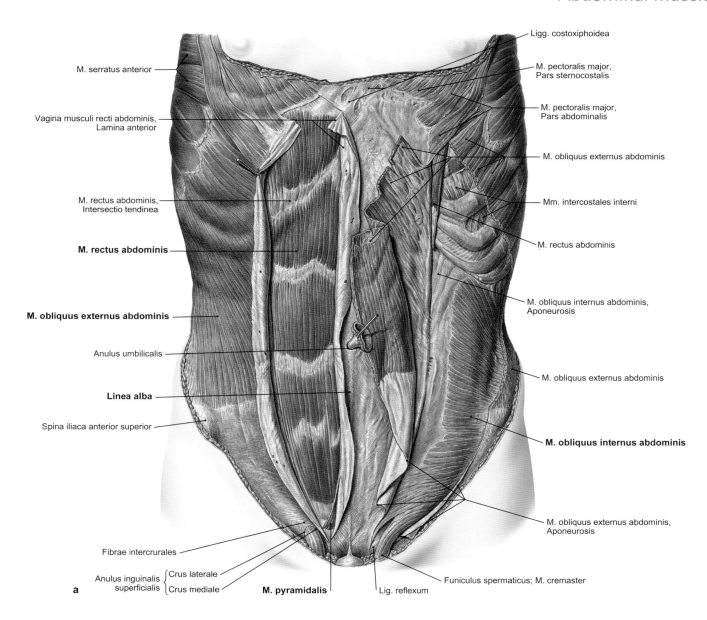

M. serratus anterior

Vagina musculi recti abdominis,
Lamina anterior

M. rectus abdominis,
Intersectio tendinea

M. rectus abdominis

M. obliquus externus abdominis

Anulus umbilicalis

Linea alba

Spina iliaca anterior superior

Fibrae intercrurales

Anulus inguinalis { Crus laterale
superficialis { Crus mediale

M. pyramidalis

Lig. reflexum

a

Ligg. costoxiphoidea

M. pectoralis major,
Pars sternocostalis

M. pectoralis major,
Pars abdominalis

M. obliquus externus abdominis

Mm. intercostales interni

M. rectus abdominis

M. obliquus internus abdominis,
Aponeurosis

M. obliquus externus abdominis

M. obliquus internus abdominis

M. obliquus externus abdominis,
Aponeurosis

Funiculus spermaticus; M. cremaster

Fig. 2.103a–c Superficial and middle layer of the abdominal muscles, Mm. abdominis.

a Ventral view. On the right side, the superficial layer (Lamina anterior) of the rectus sheath (Vagina musculi recti abdominis) has been opened. The underlying **M. rectus abdominis** is visible. It is interrupted by three to four Intersectiones tendinei, which as a result of extensive abdominal exercises can result in the so-called six-pack. The muscle located in the rectus sheath is used for trunk flexion and lateral flexion. In the caudal part of the rectus sheath we see the small triangular **M. pyramidalis,** which originates from the Os pubis and projects into the Linea alba. The M. pyramidalis is a rudimentary pouch muscle (anatomically, the kangaroo possesses a strongly developed M. pyramidalis).

On the left side, the **M. obliquus externus abdominis** has been folded back medially over the rectus sheath. The largest part passes into an aponeurosis, which helps form the superficial layer (Lamina anterior) of the rectus sheath. It plays a functional part when bending forward, to the side and when twisting the upper body, and acts as an oblique brace and as abdominal wall tension. Together with the muscle on the opposite side, as well as the Mm. obliqui interni and transversi abdominis, it functions collectively. [S700]

b Bilateral contraction of the oblique abdominal muscles stabilises the lateral abdominal wall and performs a lateral pressure on internal abdominal organs. [S700-L126]

c Unilateral contraction of the oblique abdominal muscles during a side plank position lifts the trunk off the floor. [S700-L126]

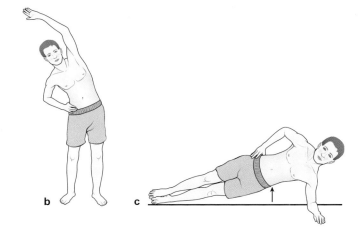

b   c

→ T 15, T 16

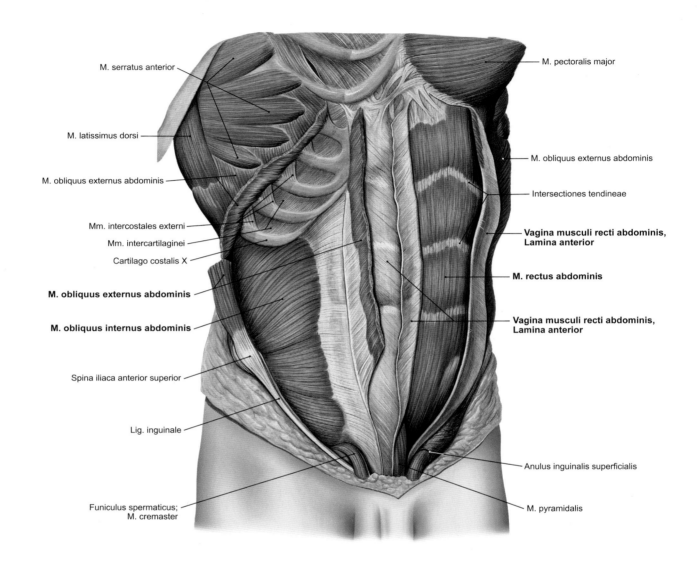

M. serratus anterior

M. latissimus dorsi

M. obliquus externus abdominis

Mm. intercostales externi

Mm. intercartilaginei

Cartilago costalis X

M. obliquus externus abdominis

M. obliquus internus abdominis

Spina iliaca anterior superior

Lig. inguinale

Funiculus spermaticus;
M. cremaster

M. pectoralis major

M. obliquus externus abdominis

Intersectiones tendineae

**Vagina musculi recti abdominis,
Lamina anterior**

M. rectus abdominis

**Vagina musculi recti abdominis,
Lamina anterior**

Anulus inguinalis superficialis

M. pyramidalis

Fig. 2.104   Middle layer of the abdominal muscles, Mm. abdominis; ventral view. [S700]
On the right side, the M. obliquus externus abdominis has mostly been removed. Underneath you can see the **M. obliquus internus abdominis.** Its aponeurosis is involved in the construction of both the superficial (Lamina anterior) as well as the deep (Lamina posterior) layer of the rectus sheath. The M. obliquus internus abdominis extends from lateral caudal to medial cranial. As in the M. obliquus externus abdominis it acts as an oblique brace and provides abdominal wall tension, and plays a functional part when bending forward, to the side and when twisting the upper body.

→ T 16

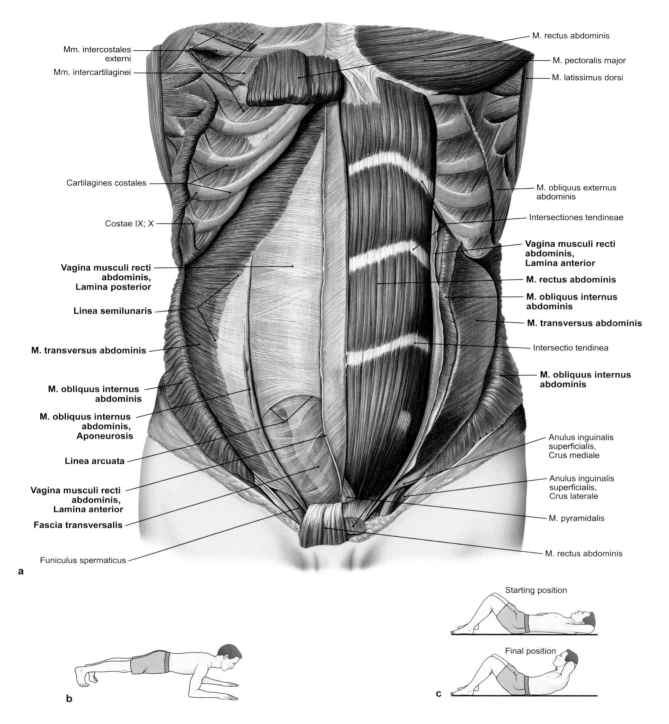

Mm. intercostales externi

Mm. intercartilaginei

Cartilagines costales

Costae IX; X

Vagina musculi recti abdominis, Lamina posterior

Linea semilunaris

M. transversus abdominis

M. obliquus internus abdominis

M. obliquus internus abdominis, Aponeurosis

Linea arcuata

Vagina musculi recti abdominis, Lamina anterior

Fascia transversalis

Funiculus spermaticus

a

M. rectus abdominis

M. pectoralis major

M. latissimus dorsi

M. obliquus externus abdominis

Intersectiones tendineae

Vagina musculi recti abdominis, Lamina anterior

M. rectus abdominis

M. obliquus internus abdominis

M. transversus abdominis

Intersectio tendinea

M. obliquus internus abdominis

Anulus inguinalis superficialis, Crus mediale

Anulus inguinalis superficialis, Crus laterale

M. pyramidalis

M. rectus abdominis

b

Starting position

Final position

c

Fig. 2.105a–c   Deep layer of the abdominal muscles, Mm. abdominis.

a Ventral view. [S700]

On the right side of the abdomen, the M. transversus abdominis is visible. In addition, the front layer (Lamina anterior) of the rectus sheath (Vagina musculi recti abdominis) has been removed and the M. rectus abdominis has been separated from the rectus sheath.

In the area of a crescent-shaped line (Linea semilunaris), the muscle fibres of the **M. transversus abdominis** pass into the muscle aponeurosis, which for the most part forms the posterior wall of the deep layer (Lamina posterior) of the rectus sheath. Caudally of the Linea (Zona) arcuata, the aponeurosis participates in the formation of the Lamina anterior of the rectus sheath (→ Fig. 2.108). The aponeurosis radiates into the Linea alba.

The main functions of the M. transversus abdominis include the increase in abdominal pressure, raising the upper trunk and forced expiration.

The deep layer (Lamina posterior) of the rectus sheath is formed in the upper section (from the sternum to the Linea [Zona] arcuata) from a part of the aponeurosis of the M. obliquus internus abdominis and the aponeurosis of the M. transversus abdominis. Underneath (from the Linea arcuata to the Os pubis), the Lamina posterior only consists of the Fascia transversalis and the Peritoneum parietale.

b Stabilising function of the M. transversus abdominis in the 'plank' position. [S700-L126]

c Contraction of the M. transversus abdominis during sit-ups. [S700-L126]

→ T 15, T 16

Clinical remarks

A rare SPIEGHEL's hernia **(Spigelian hernia)** can occur at the lateral margin of the Linea arcuata which borders the Linea semilunaris.

Surgical scars in the abdominal wall can be the starting point for **incisional hernias.**

Musculature

Muscle functions

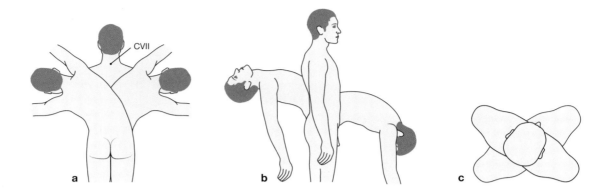

a   b   c

Fig. 2.106a–c Movement directions of the trunk. [S700-L126]
a Side-bending (lateral flexion) of the trunk. Bending to both sides up to 40° is usually normal (0°/40°). The vertebra prominens (CVII) and SI serve as reference points when determining the angle in the upright and maximal lateral flexion position. The lateral flexion of the trunk is supported by the Mm. obliquus externus abdominis, obliquus internus abdominis, quadratus lumborum, iliocostalis, psoas major, longissimus and splenius.
b Forward (flexion) and backward bending (extension) of the trunk in the vertebral joints.
The range of movements is between approximately 100° flexion and 50° extension. A straight line between the acromion of the scapula and the Crista iliaca of the femur is used to determine these angles. The forward flexion of the trunk is supported by the Mm. rectus abdominis, obliquus externus abdominis, obliquus internus abdominis and psoas major. The Mm. iliocostalis, psoas major, longissimus, splenius, spina-

lis, semispinalis, multifidus, trapezius and levatores costarum bend the spine dorsally.
c Torsion of the trunk. Bilateral anterior to posterior rotation of the trunk by approximately 40° is possible. A line connecting the acromion of the scapula on both sides serves as a reference axis. Ipsilateral rotation of the trunk is supported by Mm. obliquus internus abdominis, iliocostalis, longissimus and splenius. Rotation of the trunk to the contralateral side is achieved by the Mm. obliquus externus abdominis, semispinalis, multifidus, rotatores and levatores costarum.
The scope of movement of the individual sections of the spine is mainly limited by the vertebral joints. As for the entire spine, bending forwards (flexion) and backwards (extension) at approximately 100°/0°/50°, side-bending (lateral flexion) of 0°/40°, and torsion (rotation) of 40°/0°/40° are possible; these serve as normal reference values to assess movement restrictions.

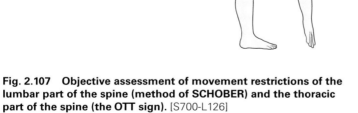

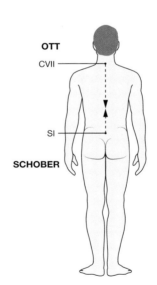

Fig. 2.107 Objective assessment of movement restrictions of the lumbar part of the spine (method of SCHOBER) and the thoracic part of the spine (the OTT sign). [S700-L126]

Clinical remarks

Method according to SCHOBER: To objectify movement restrictions of the lumbar spine, the patient is asked to stand upright and the examiner places his/her right thumb on the tip of the cranial part of the Crista sacralis mediana and the index finger of the same hand on the Proc. spinosus of a lumbar vertebra about a hand width (10 cm) above it. With maximum flexion, the distance between the two points usually increases by 5 cm (4–6 cm).

OTT sign: The same applies to the OTT sign, which measures the mobility in the area of the thoracic spine. The measuring section begins at the Proc. spinosus of the seventh cervical vertebra (Vertebra prominens) and runs for 30 cm toward the tailbone. Again, the changes in the measurement distance (normally 8 cm) are retained after flexion.

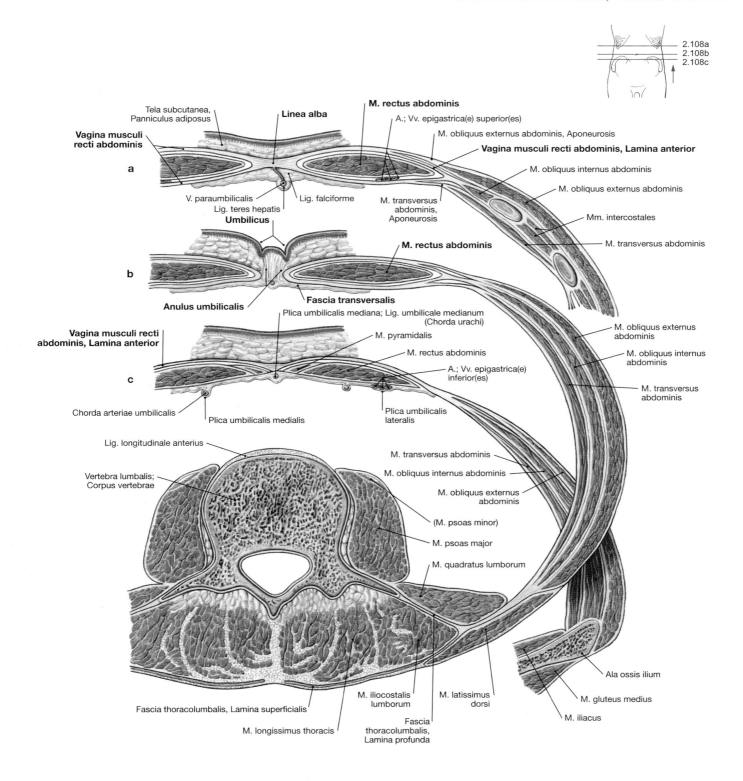

Tela subcutanea, Panniculus adiposus

Linea alba

M. rectus abdominis

A.; Vv. epigastrica(e) superior(es)

M. obliquus externus abdominis, Aponeurosis

Vagina musculi recti abdominis

Vagina musculi recti abdominis, Lamina anterior

M. obliquus internus abdominis

M. obliquus externus abdominis

a

V. paraumbilicalis

Lig. falciforme

Lig. teres hepatis

Umbilicus

M. transversus abdominis, Aponeurosis

Mm. intercostales

M. transversus abdominis

M. rectus abdominis

b

Anulus umbilicalis

Fascia transversalis

Plica umbilicalis mediana; Lig. umbilicale medianum (Chorda urachi)

M. pyramidalis

M. obliquus externus abdominis

Vagina musculi recti abdominis, Lamina anterior

M. rectus abdominis

M. obliquus internus abdominis

A.; Vv. epigastrica(e) inferior(es)

M. transversus abdominis

c

Chorda arteriae umbilicalis

Plica umbilicalis medialis

Plica umbilicalis lateralis

Lig. longitudinale anterius

M. transversus abdominis

M. obliquus internus abdominis

Vertebra lumbalis; Corpus vertebrae

M. obliquus externus abdominis

(M. psoas minor)

M. psoas major

M. quadratus lumborum

Ala ossis ilium

M. gluteus medius

M. iliacus

Fascia thoracolumbalis, Lamina superficialis

M. iliocostalis lumborum

M. latissimus dorsi

M. longissimus thoracis

Fascia thoracolumbalis, Lamina profunda

Fig. 2.108a–c   Structure of the rectus sheath, Vagina musculi recti abdominis; horizontal sections; caudal view. [S700]

The Mm. rectus abdominis and pyramidalis are stored in a fixed connective tissue sheath (Vagina musculi recti abdominis), which is formed from the aponeurosis of the oblique abdominal muscles (Mm. obliquus externus abdominis, obliquus internus abdominis and transversus abdominis as well as the Fascia transversalis and the Peritoneum parietale on the inside of the abdominal wall). All aponeuroses radiate into the median-lying Linea alba. The structure of the rectus sheath differs in the upper and lower section. The limit is the **Linea (Zona) arcuata.**

In the **upper section,** the anterior layer (Lamina anterior) of the rectus sheath is formed by the aponeurosis of the M. obliquus externus abdominis and the front portion of the aponeurosis of the M. obliquus in-

ternus abdominis; the posterior layer (Lamina posterior) consists of the posterior part of the aponeurosis of the M. obliquus internus abdominis, the aponeurosis of the M. transversus abdominis as well as the Fascia transversalis and the Peritoneum parietale **(a, b).**

In the **lower section,** all three aponeuroses run in front of the M. rectus abdominis **(c).** The posterior side of the rectus sheath is very thin here and is formed exclusively by the Fascia transversalis and the Peritoneum parietale (→ Fig. 2.105).

The navel (umbilicus) is a potential weak spot on the anterior abdominal wall, which is thinner here in the region of the umbilical pit and the Papilla umbilicalis than in other parts **(b).**

→ T 15, T 16, T 17

Abdominal wall, CT

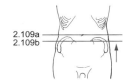

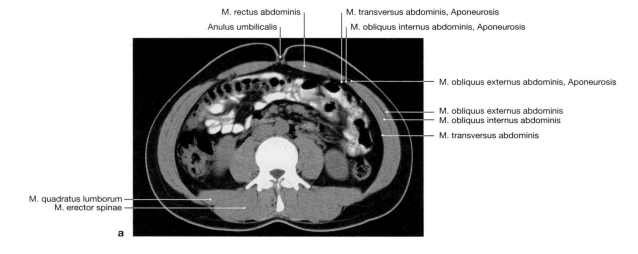

M. rectus abdominis
Anulus umbilicalis
M. transversus abdominis, Aponeurosis
M. obliquus internus abdominis, Aponeurosis
M. obliquus externus abdominis, Aponeurosis
M. obliquus externus abdominis
M. obliquus internus abdominis
M. transversus abdominis
M. quadratus lumborum
M. erector spinae

a

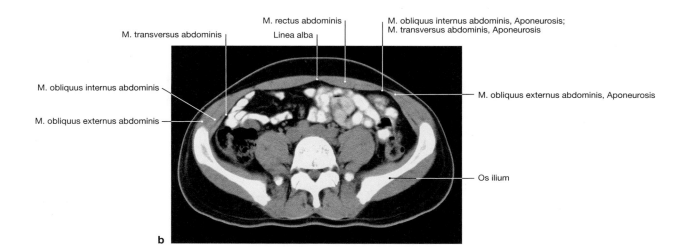

M. transversus abdominis
M. rectus abdominis
Linea alba
M. obliquus internus abdominis, Aponeurosis;
M. transversus abdominis, Aponeurosis
M. obliquus internus abdominis
M. obliquus externus abdominis, Aponeurosis
M. obliquus externus abdominis
Os ilium

b

Fig. 2.109a and b   Abdominal muscles, Mm. abdominis; computed tomography (CT) cross-sections. [S700-T893]

In the CT, the oblique and the straight abdominal muscles can be separated from each other. The M. erector spinae and the M. quadratus lumborum are also clearly visible.

Clinical remarks

Naval hernias occur in newborns as well as in adults – in the case of newborns, the naval papilla is not yet developed; in adults it occurs through the spreading of the connective tissue of the naval papilla at extreme hyperextension of the abdominal wall (pregnancy, obesity). The hernial orifice is the umbilical ring (Anulus umbilicalis).

An **omphalocele** (congenital umbilical hernia) is a birth defect resulting in the persistence of the physiological umbilical hernia during the fetal period.

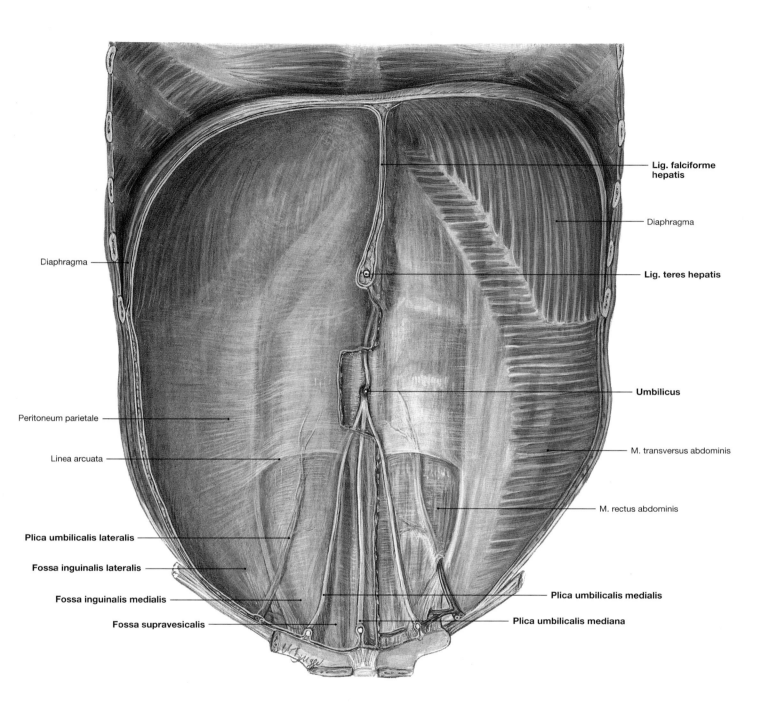

Lig. falciforme
hepatis

Diaphragma

Lig. teres hepatis

Umbilicus

M. transversus abdominis

M. rectus abdominis

Plica umbilicalis medialis

Plica umbilicalis mediana

Diaphragma

Peritoneum parietale

Linea arcuata

Plica umbilicalis lateralis

Fossa inguinalis lateralis

Fossa inguinalis medialis

Fossa supravesicalis

Fig. 2.110   Inside of the anterior abdominal wall; dorsal view. On the right side, the fascia and the peritoneum covering the diaphragm and the M. transversus abdominis have been removed. [S700]
On the inside of the abdominal wall, different folds (Plicae), pits (Fossae) and ligaments (Ligamenta) are visible. The **Lig. falciforme hepatis** (sickle-shaped band of liver) passes from the diaphragm and the liver at right angles to the side of the belly. It extends to the navel (umbilicus), as it is a developmental remnant of the mesentery of the umbilical vein in the fetus. The umbilical vein itself closes up immediately after the birth and remains as a rounded connective tissue thread **(Lig. teres hepatis)** at the edge of the Lig. falciforme hepatis. Below the umbili-

cus, the **Plica umbilicalis mediana** (containing the obliterated urachus – original urinary tract, which extends from the crown of the bladder to the navel) is visible, and lateral thereof the **Plicae umbilicales mediales** (containing the obliterated Aa. umbilicales) and **laterales** (containing the Vasa epigastrica inferiora). Cavities (Fossae supravesicales, inguinal medial and inguinal lateral) form between the folds. The **Fossa inguinalis lateralis** corresponds to the inner inguinal ring located beneath; the **Fossa inguinalis medialis** lies at the same level as the outer inguinal ring.

→ T 15, T 16, T 21

Diaphragm and posterior abdominal wall

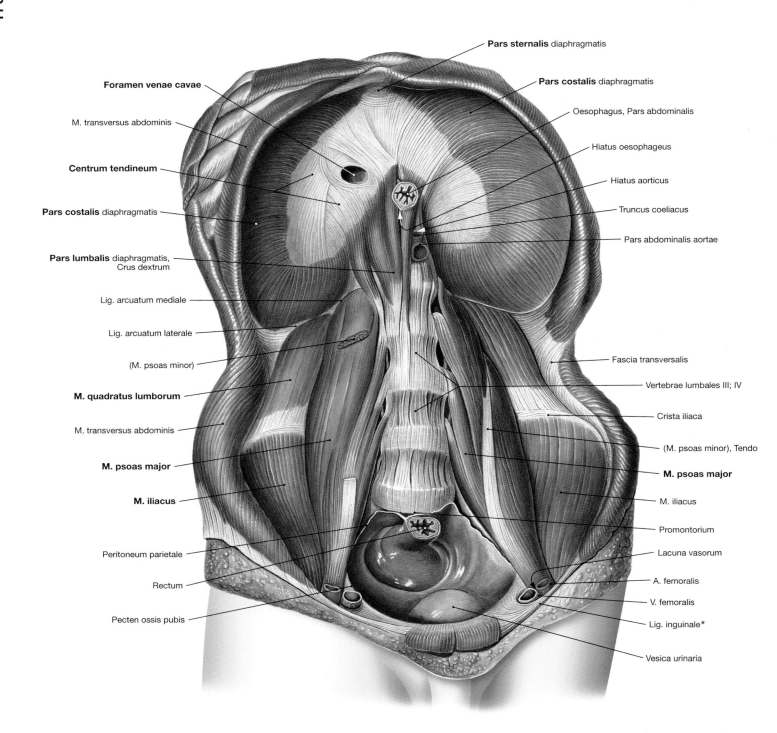

Pars sternalis diaphragmatis

Foramen venae cavae

Pars costalis diaphragmatis

M. transversus abdominis

Oesophagus, Pars abdominalis

Centrum tendineum

Hiatus oesophageus

Hiatus aorticus

Pars costalis diaphragmatis

Truncus coeliacus

Pars abdominalis aortae

Pars lumbalis diaphragmatis,
Crus dextrum

Lig. arcuatum mediale

Lig. arcuatum laterale

Fascia transversalis

(M. psoas minor)

Vertebrae lumbales III; IV

M. quadratus lumborum

Crista iliaca

M. transversus abdominis

(M. psoas minor), Tendo

M. psoas major

M. psoas major

M. iliacus

M. iliacus

Promontorium

Peritoneum parietale

Lacuna vasorum

Rectum

A. femoralis

V. femoralis

Pecten ossis pubis

Lig. inguinale*

Vesica urinaria

**Fig. 2.111   Diaphragm, Diaphragma, and abdominal muscles,
Mm. abdominis;** ventral view. [S700]
The diaphragm is composed of a central tendon plate **(Centrum tendineum)** with attached muscle groups, which have their origin at the
sternum (Pars sternalis), the ribs (Pars costalis), and the lumbar region
of the spine (Pars lumbalis).
After removal of the retroperitoneum, the paravertebral locations of the
Mm. iliopsoas (composed of a M. psoas major and M. iliacus, respectively), the M. quadratus lumborum, and, as a variant, the M. psoas
minor are visible.
Along with the **M. iliacus,** which comes from the Fossa iliaca, the **M.
psoas major** inserts at the Trochanter minor of the femur and is the

strongest flexor in the hip joint. It can move the upper body from lying
down into the sitting position and is involved in the lateral flexion of the
trunk. The **M. quadratus lumborum** originates from the Labium internum of the Crista iliaca and inserts at the XIIth rib as well as the Procc.
costales of the first to fourth lumbar vertebra. It can lower the XIIth rib
and is involved in the lateral flexion of the trunk.

* FALLOPIAN ligament or POUPART ligament

→ T 16, T 17, T 21, T 44

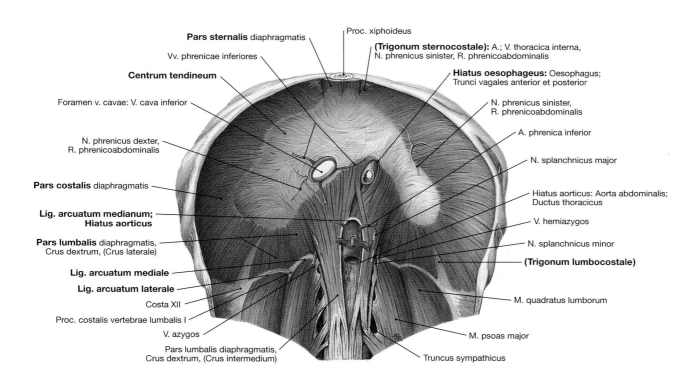

Fig. 2.112 Diaphragm, Diaphragma; caudal view. [S700-L240]
The diaphragm is divided into the Centrum tendineum, as well as into the Partes sternales, costales and lumbales. The **Trigonum sternocostale** lies between the Pars sternalis and Pars costalis, and the **Trigonum lumbocostale** (BOCHDALEK triangle) lies between the Pars cos-

talis and Pars lumbalis. The usual dictate that the Vasa thoracica interna passes through the Trigonum sternocostale, is incorrect. The vessels run ventrally in front of the Trigonum sternocostale.

→ T 21

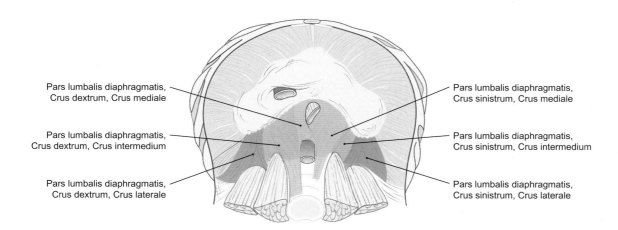

Fig. 2.113 Diaphragm, Diaphragma; caudal view. [S700-L126]
Coloured depiction of the diaphragm leg on the right side (Crus dextrum) and left side (Crus sinistrum). Each diaphragm leg is divided into Crus medial (right: yellow, left: green), Crus intermedium (light blue) and Crus lateral (red). The Crus dextrum is secured to the lumbar vertebrae bodies L1–L3 and the intervertebral discs lying in between, the Crus sinistrum to the lumbar vertebrae L1 and L2 and the intervertebral discs

in between. The Crus medial dextrum forms a loop around the oesophagus (Hiatus oesophageus). Right and left diaphragm legs are connected via the spine through a tendinous arch (Hiatus aorticus), which runs behind the aorta. The diaphragm forms the Lig. arcuatum medial (medial arcuate ligament) via the M. psoas major, and the Lig. arcuatum lateral (laterale arcuate ligament) via the M. quadratus lumborum.

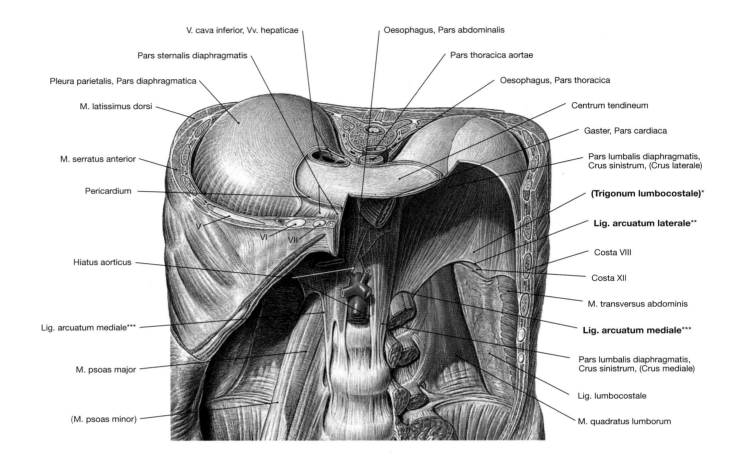

V. cava inferior, Vv. hepaticae
Oesophagus, Pars abdominalis
Pars sternalis diaphragmatis
Pars thoracica aortae
Pleura parietalis, Pars diaphragmatica
Oesophagus, Pars thoracica
M. latissimus dorsi
Centrum tendineum
Gaster, Pars cardiaca
M. serratus anterior
Pars lumbalis diaphragmatis, Crus sinistrum, (Crus laterale)
Pericardium
(Trigonum lumbocostale)*
Lig. arcuatum laterale**
Costa VIII
Hiatus aorticus
Costa XII
M. transversus abdominis
Lig. arcuatum mediale***
Lig. arcuatum mediale***
Pars lumbalis diaphragmatis, Crus sinistrum, (Crus mediale)
M. psoas major
Lig. lumbocostale
(M. psoas minor)
M. quadratus lumborum

Fig. 2.114   Diaphragm, Diaphragma, passageways and posterior abdominal wall muscles; ventral view. [S700]
The dome-shaped diaphragm runs between the thoracic and abdominal cavity (→ Fig. 2.111 and → Fig. 2.115).

*   clin.: BOCHDALEK triangle
**   lateral arcuate ligament
***   medial arcuate ligament

→ T 21

Clinical remarks

Diaphragmatic hernias are classified as congenital (Hernia diaphragmatica spuria) and acquired (Hernia diaphragmatica vera). If the shifted organs are covered by a peritoneum (hernial sac), they are called real hernias.

The **congenital** form usually presents as a breach in the diaphragm through which abdominal organs (stomach, intestine, liver, spleen) can pass into the thorax. Congenital hernias (usually the physiological weaknesses of the diaphragm in the Trigonum sterno or lumbocostale [MORGAGNI hernia] are affected) often have no hernial sac.

Acquired diaphragmatic hernias are usually sliding hernias or paraoesophageal hiatus hernias (→ Fig. 2.116). In a **hiatal hernia,** the stomach partially passes through the slit-shaped opening of the diaphragm for the passage of the oesophagus (oesophageal hiatus). An axial **sliding hernia** pulls the cardia up through the diaphragm into the thoracic cavity.

In addition, there are **mixed types.** An especially severe form is the **upside-down stomach** (thoracic stomach, where large parts of the stomach have slipped into the thoracic cavity).

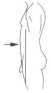

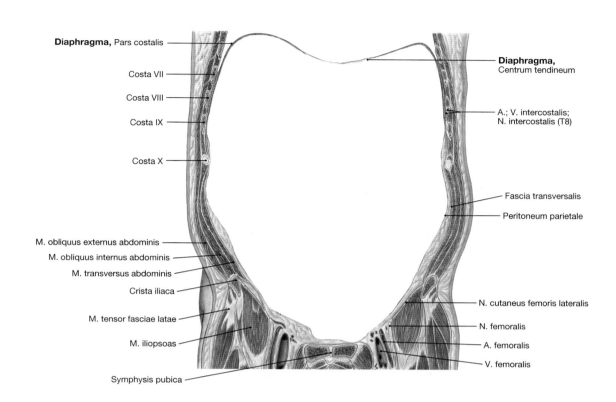

Diaphragma, Pars costalis

Costa VII

Costa VIII

Costa IX

Costa X

M. obliquus externus abdominis

M. obliquus internus abdominis

M. transversus abdominis

Crista iliaca

M. tensor fasciae latae

M. iliopsoas

Symphysis pubica

Diaphragma, Centrum tendineum

A.; V. intercostalis; N. intercostalis (T8)

Fascia transversalis

Peritoneum parietale

N. cutaneus femoris lateralis

N. femoralis

A. femoralis

V. femoralis

Fig. 2.115 Diaphragm, Diaphragma, and oblique muscles of the abdominal wall, Mm. abdominis; frontal section; ventral view. [S700-L238]
The illustration shows the dome-shaped expanse of the thin diaphragm. The Partes costales originate from the side of the IXth rib and radiate

into the Centrum tendineum. The diaphragmatic domes are positioned between the fifth and sixth intercostal spaces in resting position. The lateral abdominal wall is formed by the oblique abdominal muscles (Mm. obliquus externus abdominis, obliquus internus abdominis and transversus abdominis).

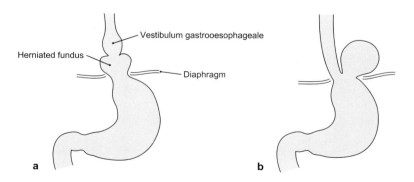

Vestibulum gastrooesophageale

Herniated fundus

Diaphragm

a

b

Fig. 2.116a and b Axial (sliding hernia) (a) and paraoesophageal hiatus hernia (b); schematic drawing. [S008-3]

Arteries of the ventral trunk wall

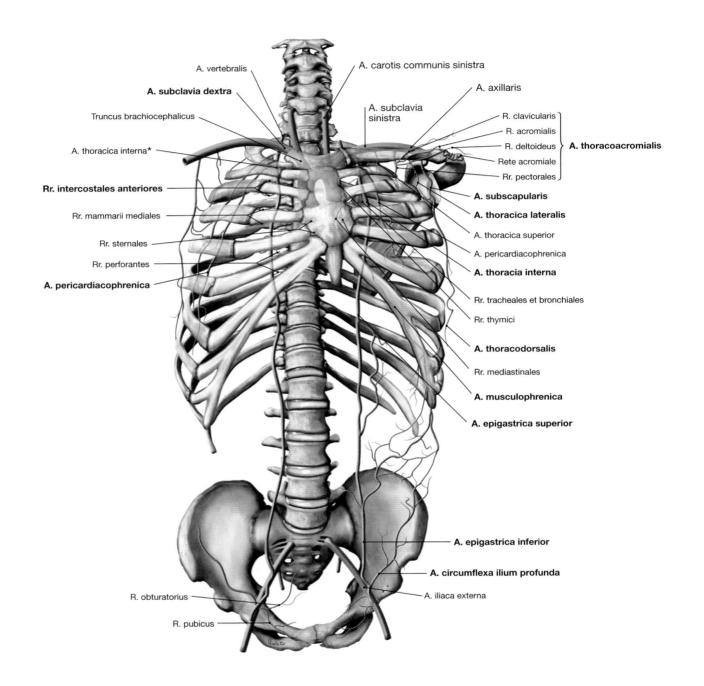

A. vertebralis

A. carotis communis sinistra

A. subclavia dextra

A. axillaris

Truncus brachiocephalicus

A. subclavia sinistra

R. clavicularis

R. acromialis

A. thoracica interna*

R. deltoideus

A. thoracoacromialis

Rete acromiale

Rr. intercostales anteriores

Rr. pectorales

Rr. mammarii mediales

A. subscapularis

A. thoracica lateralis

Rr. sternales

A. thoracica superior

Rr. perforantes

A. pericardiacophrenica

A. pericardiacophrenica

A. thoracia interna

Rr. tracheales et bronchiales

Rr. thymici

A. thoracodorsalis

Rr. mediastinales

A. musculophrenica

A. epigastrica superior

A. epigastrica inferior

A. circumflexa ilium profunda

R. obturatorius

A. iliaca externa

R. pubicus

Fig. 2.117 Arteries of the ventral wall of the trunk. [S700-L266]
The ventral wall of the trunk is supplied with blood from branches of the Aa. subclavia, axillaris, iliaca externa and femoralis. The muscles of the abdominal wall receive blood via the segmentally arranged Aa. lumbales from the Aorta abdominalis (not shown).

* clin.: A. mammaria interna

Branches of the A. thoracica interna	
• Rr. mediastinales	• Rr. perforantes
• Rr. thymici	• Rr. mammarii mediales
• Rr. bronchiales	• Rr. intercostales anteriores
• Rr. tracheales	– A. musculophrenica
• A. pericardiacophrenica	• A. epigastrica superior
• Rr. sternales	

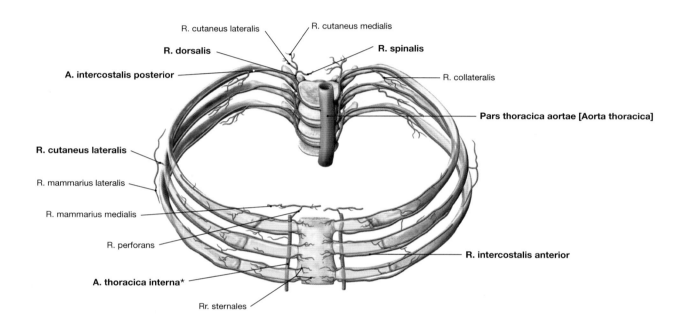

R. cutaneus lateralis
R. cutaneus medialis
R. dorsalis
R. spinalis
A. intercostalis posterior
R. collateralis
Pars thoracica aortae [Aorta thoracica]
R. cutaneus lateralis
R. mammarius lateralis
R. mammarius medialis
R. perforans
R. intercostalis anterior
A. thoracica interna*
Rr. sternales

Fig. 2.118 Arteries of the thoracic wall. [S700-L266]
The intercostal arteries form anastomoses between the A. thoracica interna and Pars thoracica aortae.

* clin.: A. mammaria interna

Branches of the Pars thoracica aortae [Aorta thoracica]

- Aa. intercostales posteriores
  - R. dorsalis
    - R. cutaneus medialis
    - R. cutaneus lateralis
  - R. spinalis
- R. collateralis
- R. cutaneus lateralis
  - Rr. mammarii lateralis

Clinical remarks

A **stenosis of the aortic isthmus,** a narrowing of the aorta in the aortic arch area, results in the formation of a vertical and a horizontal bypass circulation:
- **Vertical bypass circulation:** between the Aa. subclaviae and iliacae externae via the Aa. thoracicae internae, epigastricae superiores and epigastricae inferiores (within the rectus sheath) as well as in the area of the abdominal wall via the Aa. musculophrenicae, epigastricae inferiores and circumflexae ilium profundae

- **Horizontal bypass circulation:** between the Aa. thoracicae internae and Aorta thoracica via the Rr. intercostales anteriores and Aa. intercostales posteriores to supply the thoracic and abdominal organs. The enlargement of the intercostal arteries leads to the formation of rib notching (Clinical remarks → Fig. 2.17). A bypass circulation supports the maintenance of blood supply to parts of the trunk wall and the lower extremities (a difference in blood pressure between the upper and lower extremities is usually still measurable).

Veins of the ventral wall of the trunk

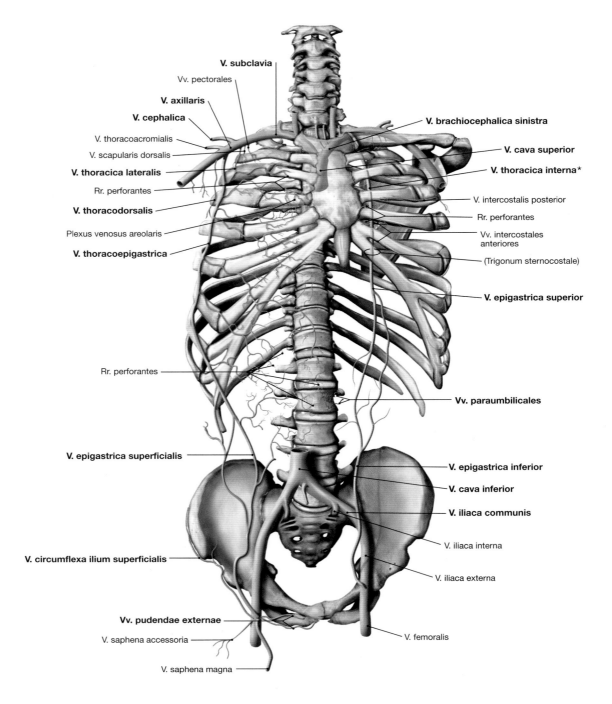

V. subclavia

Vv. pectorales

V. axillaris

V. cephalica

V. thoracoacromialis

V. scapularis dorsalis

V. thoracica lateralis

Rr. perforantes

V. thoracodorsalis

Plexus venosus areolaris

V. thoracoepigastrica

Rr. perforantes

V. epigastrica superficialis

V. circumflexa ilium superficialis

Vv. pudendae externae

V. saphena accessoria

V. saphena magna

V. brachiocephalica sinistra

V. cava superior

V. thoracica interna*

V. intercostalis posterior

Rr. perforantes

Vv. intercostales anteriores

(Trigonum sternocostale)

V. epigastrica superior

Vv. paraumbilicales

V. epigastrica inferior

V. cava inferior

V. iliaca communis

V. iliaca interna

V. iliaca externa

V. femoralis

Fig. 2.119 Veins of the anterior wall of the trunk. [S700-L266]
The veins of the anterior wall of the trunk form a superficial (right side of the body) and a deep (left side of the body) **system of anastomoses** between the Vv. cavae superior and inferior.

* clin.: V. mammaria interna

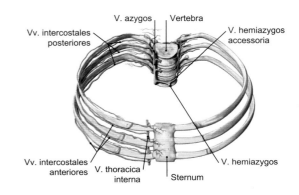

V. azygos   Vertebra

Vv. intercostales posteriores

V. hemiazygos accessoria

Vv. intercostales anteriores   V. thoracica interna

Sternum

V. hemiazygos

Fig. 2.120 Veins of the thoracic wall. [S702-L266]
The veins run alongside the arteries in the area of the thoracic wall. Ventrally the Vv. intercostales anteriores drain into the V. thoracica interna and dorsally into the Vv. azygos and hemiazygos, as well as the V. hemiazygos accessoria. They thereby form venous anastomoses between both drainage pathways.

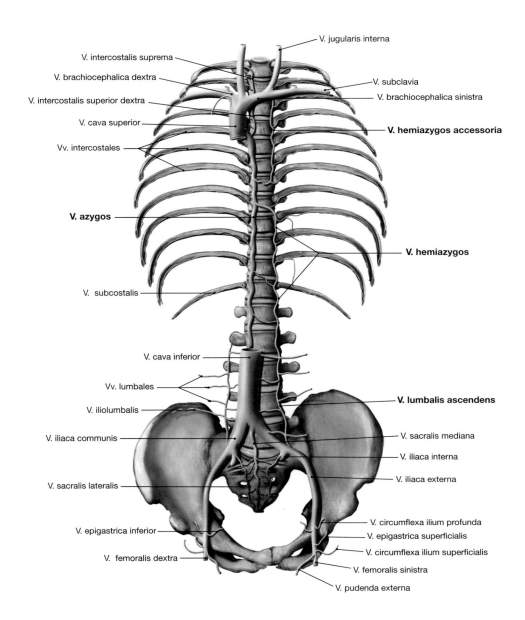

Fig. 2.121 Azygos system. [S700-L266]

The azygos system drains blood between the V. iliaca interna and V. cava superior. The V. lumbalis ascendens on the right side, which connects the V. azygos to the V. iliaca communis dextra, is covered by the V. cava inferior. In addition, there are also direct connections from the Vv. lumbales ascendentes to the V. cava inferior. In the system, the Plexus venosus sacralis and the Plexus venosi vertebrales externi and interni as well as the Vv. lumbales are activated.

Clinical remarks

The venous congestion of the V. cava superior, the V. cava inferior or the Vv. iliacae communes via either a thrombosis, a mass formation or the growth of tumours, can lead to the development of a bypass circulation between the V. cava superior and V. cava inferior **(cavocaval anastomoses)**:

* between the V. iliaca externa and V. cava superior via the V. epigastrica inferior, V. epigastrica superior, V. thoracica interna and V. brachiocephalica

* between the V. femoralis and V. cava superior via the V. circumflexa ilium superficialis/epigastrica superficialis, V. thoracoepigastrica, V. axillaris and V. brachiocephalica
* between the V. iliaca interna and V. cava superior via the Plexus venosus sacralis, Plexus venosi vertebrales externi and interni, Vv. azygos and hemiazygos
* between Vv. lumbales and V. cava superior via the Vv. lumbales ascendentes, Vv. azygos and hemiazygos. Zwischen V. iliaca externa.

Portocaval anastomoses (→ Fig. 6.101, Vol. 2).

Arteries of the thoracic wall

Trunk

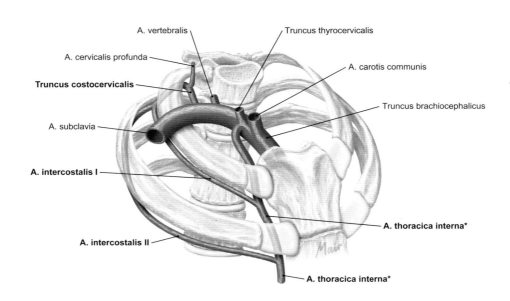

Fig. 2.122 Arteries of the thoracic wall in relation to the first and second rib. [S700-L127]

The first two posterior intercostal arteries originate from the Truncus costocervicalis which is a branch of the A. subclavia. Both intercostal arteries anastomose with their anterior counterparts from the A. thoracica interna.

* clin.: A. mammaria interna

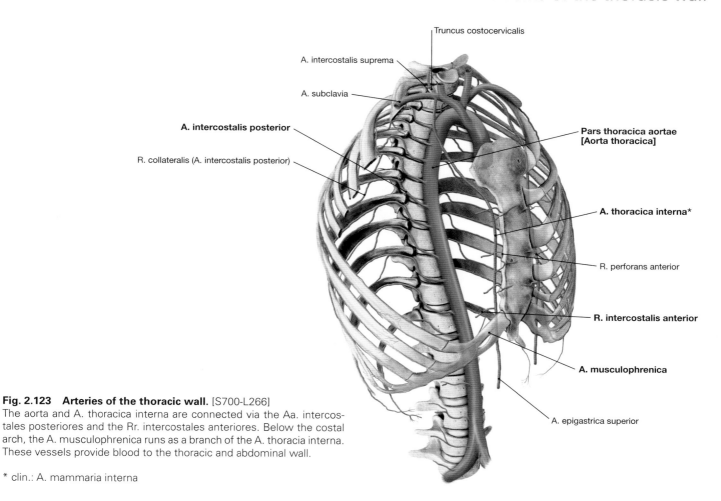

Truncus costocervicalis

A. intercostalis suprema

A. subclavia

A. intercostalis posterior

R. collateralis (A. intercostalis posterior)

Pars thoracica aortae
[Aorta thoracica]

A. thoracica interna*

R. perforans anterior

R. intercostalis anterior

A. musculophrenica

A. epigastrica superior

Fig. 2.123   Arteries of the thoracic wall. [S700-L266]
The aorta and A. thoracica interna are connected via the Aa. intercostales posteriores and the Rr. intercostales anteriores. Below the costal
arch, the A. musculophrenica runs as a branch of the A. thoracia interna.
These vessels provide blood to the thoracic and abdominal wall.

* clin.: A. mammaria interna

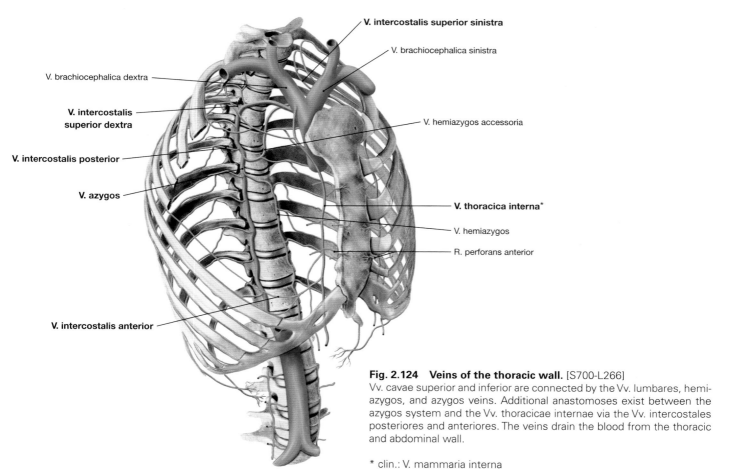

V. intercostalis superior sinistra

V. brachiocephalica sinistra

V. brachiocephalica dextra

**V. intercostalis
superior dextra**

V. hemiazygos accessoria

V. intercostalis posterior

V. azygos

V. thoracica interna*

V. hemiazygos

R. perforans anterior

V. intercostalis anterior

Fig. 2.124   Veins of the thoracic wall. [S700-L266]
Vv. cavae superior and inferior are connected by the Vv. lumbares, hemiazygos, and azygos veins. Additional anastomoses exist between the
azygos system and the Vv. thoracicae internae via the Vv. intercostales
posteriores and anteriores. The veins drain the blood from the thoracic
and abdominal wall.

* clin.: V. mammaria interna

Arteries and veins of the anterior wall of the trunk

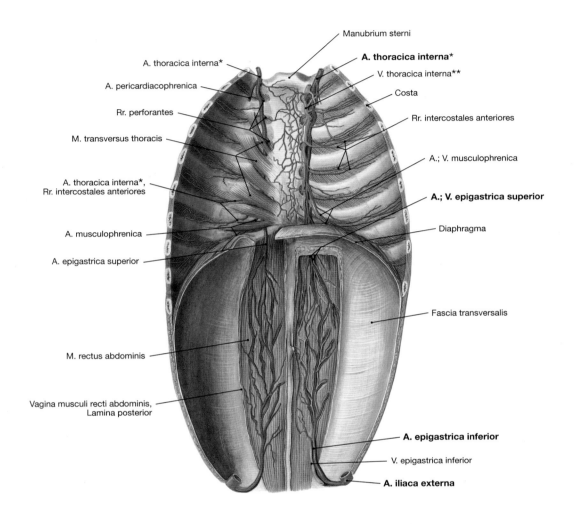

Manubrium sterni

A. thoracica interna*

A. pericardiacophrenica

Rr. perforantes

M. transversus thoracis

A. thoracica interna*,
Rr. intercostales anteriores

A. musculophrenica

A. epigastrica superior

M. rectus abdominis

Vagina musculi recti abdominis,
Lamina posterior

A. thoracica interna*

V. thoracica interna**

Costa

Rr. intercostales anteriores

A.; V. musculophrenica

A.; V. epigastrica superior

Diaphragma

Fascia transversalis

A. epigastrica inferior

V. epigastrica inferior

A. iliaca externa

Fig. 2.125 Vessels at the posterior aspect of the anterior wall of the trunk; dorsal view. [S700]

The epigastric vessels (Vasa epigastrica superiora and inferiora) run along the back of the M. transversus abdominis and are visible after removal of the rectus sheath in the upper two-thirds of the abdomen and after removal of the Fascia transversalis. The A. thoracica interna is covered on the left side of the body by the M. transversus thoracis.

Below this it passes through the Trigonum sternocostale of the diaphragm into the rectus sheath and flows into the A. epigastrica superior. The A. epigastrica inferior originates from the A. iliaca externa. Shown on the right side of the body are the associated veins.

* clin.: A. mammaria interna
** clin.: V. mammaria interna

Clinical remarks

As well as the V. saphena magna, the A. thoracica (mammaria) interna is often used for operative revascularisation of the heart in high-grade **coronary stenosis** (narrowing of the coronary arteries) as a

bypass. Bypass circulation in stenosis of the aortic isthmus are shown in Clinical remarks → Fig. 2.118; cavocaval anastomoses are shown in Clinical remarks → Fig. 2.121.

Fig. 2.126 Superficial lymphatic vessels and regional lymph nodes of the ventral wall of the trunk. [S700-L127]

The **axillary lymph nodes** (Nodi lymphoidei axillares, including the Nodi lymphoidei brachiales and pectorales) collect the lymph of the entire upper extremity, of large parts of the ventral wall of the trunk, up to the watershed area at the level of the umbilicus, as well as of the back, up to the corresponding watershed area (→ Fig. 2.127).

The **superficial inguinal lymph nodes** (Nodi lymphoidei inguinales superficiales) consist of a vertical and horizontal group. They collect the lymph of the entire lower extremity, of the ventral wall of the trunk, up to the watershed area at the level of the umbilicus, the gluteal area and the back up to the watershed area, as well as the external genitalia (including the penis), and the perineal and anal region.

In **women** the lymphatic vessels, which come from the Corpus uteri and the uterotubal junction which pass through the inguinal canal along with the Lig. teres uteri (→ Fig. 2.129), drain their lymph into the superficial inguinal lymph nodes.

In **men,** the lymph of the testis is drained into the paraaortic lymph nodes (not shown).

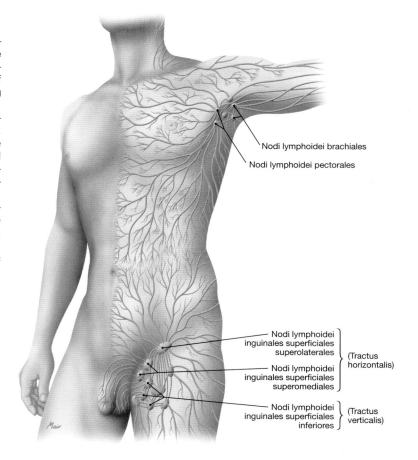

Nodi lymphoidei brachiales

Nodi lymphoidei pectorales

Nodi lymphoidei inguinales superficiales superolaterales

(Tractus horizontalis)

Nodi lymphoidei inguinales superficiales superomediales

Nodi lymphoidei inguinales superficiales inferiores

(Tractus verticalis)

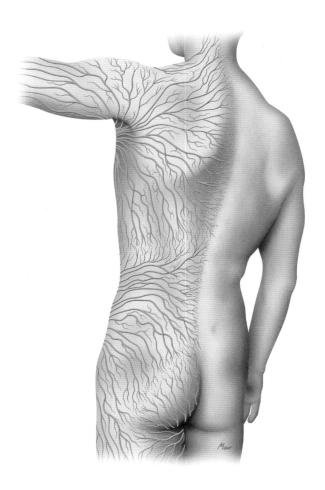

Fig. 2.127 Superficial lymphatic vessels of the posterior trunk wall. [S700-L127]

The lymph of the back area is drained above the umbilicus into the axillary lymph nodes and below thereof into the superficial inguinal lymph nodes.

Neurovascular pathways

Lymphatic vessels

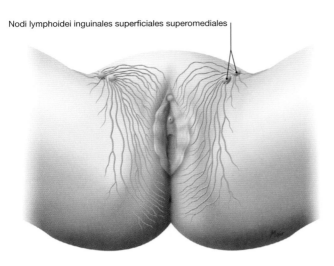

Nodi lymphoidei inguinales superficiales superomediales

Fig. 2.128 Superficial vessels and regional lymph nodes of the female external genitalia as well as of the perineal and anal region; caudal view. [S700-L127]
The lymph from the external genital, perineal and anal region is drained into the superficial inguinal lymph nodes. The first lymph station is the **Nodi lymphoidei inguinales superficiales superomediales.**

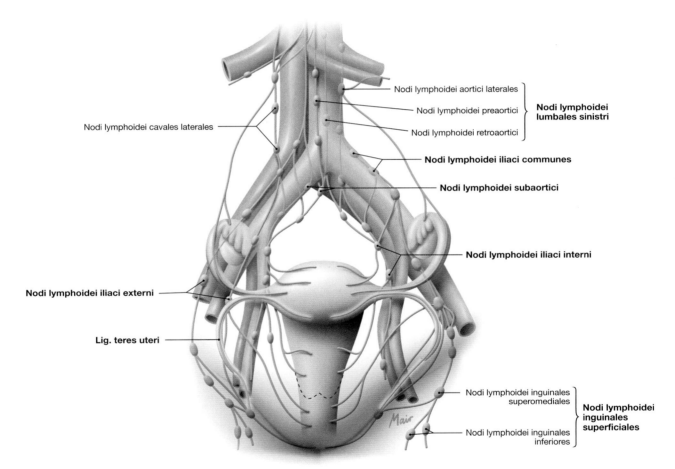

Nodi lymphoidei cavales laterales

Nodi lymphoidei aortici laterales
Nodi lymphoidei preaortici
Nodi lymphoidei retroaortici
}
**Nodi lymphoidei
lumbales sinistri**

Nodi lymphoidei iliaci communes

Nodi lymphoidei subaortici

Nodi lymphoidei iliaci interni

Nodi lymphoidei iliaci externi

Lig. teres uteri

Nodi lymphoidei inguinales superomediales
Nodi lymphoidei inguinales inferiores
}
**Nodi lymphoidei
inguinales
superficiales**

Fig. 2.129 Superficial and deep lymphatic vessels and regional lymph nodes of the vagina, uterus, uterine fallopian tube and ovary; ventral view. [S700-L127]
- The lymph of the upper two thirds of the vagina is drained into the pelvic lymph nodes, while the lower third drains into the inguinal lymph nodes.
- The lymph from the ovary, uterine FALLOPIAN tube and a part of the uterine fundus and corpus flows along the A. ovarica, which is locat-

ed in the Lig. suspensorium ovarii, to the **Nodi lymphoidei lumbales.**
- A second part of the lymph from the Fundus, Corpus and Cervix uterii is taken to the A. uterina in the **Nodi lymphoidei iliaci.**
- A third part of the lymph from the Fundus and Corpus uterii is drained along the Lig. teres uteri to the **Nodi lymphoidei inguinales superficiales** (highlighted in colour).

Clinical remarks

The inguinal lymph nodes are of clinical importance in the context of inflammation and malignancy, as an enlargement can be an initial indication of a pathological process in the catchment area. In this context, a **metastatic route** from the uterus via the lymphatic vessels at the Lig. teres uteri through the inguinal canal has to be considered for women.

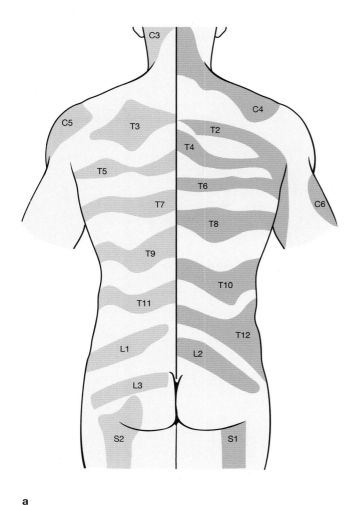

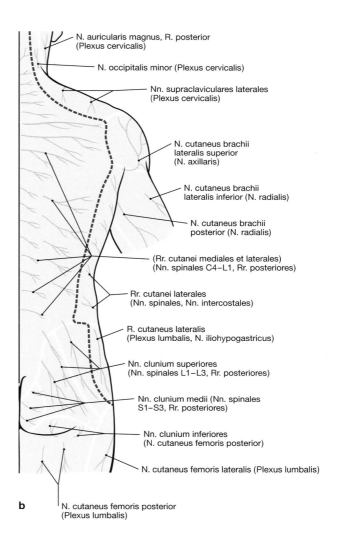

a

b

N. auricularis magnus, R. posterior
(Plexus cervicalis)

N. occipitalis minor (Plexus cervicalis)

Nn. supraclaviculares laterales
(Plexus cervicalis)

N. cutaneus brachii
lateralis superior
(N. axillaris)

N. cutaneus brachii
lateralis inferior (N. radialis)

N. cutaneus brachii
posterior (N. radialis)

(Rr. cutanei mediales et laterales)
(Nn. spinales C4–L1, Rr. posteriores)

Rr. cutanei laterales
(Nn. spinales, Nn. intercostales)

R. cutaneus lateralis
(Plexus lumbalis, N. iliohypogastricus)

Nn. clunium superiores
(Nn. spinales L1–L3, Rr. posteriores)

Nn. clunium medii (Nn. spinales
S1–S3, Rr. posteriores)

Nn. clunium inferiores
(N. cutaneus femoris posterior)

N. cutaneus femoris lateralis (Plexus lumbalis)

N. cutaneus femoris posterior
(Plexus lumbalis)

Fig. 2.130a and b   Segmental cutaneous (skin) innervation (der-matomes) and cutaneous nerves of the back; dorsal view.
[S700-L126]/[F1067-001]

a View of the dermatomes of the whole body. As many cutaneous nerves are made up of fibres from multiple spinal nerves, the dermat-omes are different to the innervation areas of the cutaneous nerves. The dermatomes are alternately presented on the left (blue) and on the right (green). For example, T7 is thus on the left-hand side in blue and T8 is on the right-hand side in green, with T9 again visible on the left-hand side in green, etc. This type of presentation is necessary to show that the dermatomes are not autonomous zones of sensitive skin innerva-tion but that they overlap to an exceptionally strong level and in varying degrees (only in the midline is the overlap very low). Regions where no colour is assigned (e.g. the area between C4, T2 and T3 around the midline), are areas where an extraordinarily large variability and a very strong interindividual overlap might occur, so that no clear assignment is possible. Presentation of the dermatomes is based on an evi-dence-based dermatome card according to LEE and co-workers (2008). In order to keep the figure clear and understandable, the dermatomes S3, S4 and S5 are not shown (they cover the area of the perineum in-cluding the anus and the external genitalia).

b Hemisectional body view of the cutaneous nerve endings. The broken red line indicates the border between the Rr. posteriores (dorsal) and Rr. anteriores (ventral) of the spinal nerves of the innervation area.

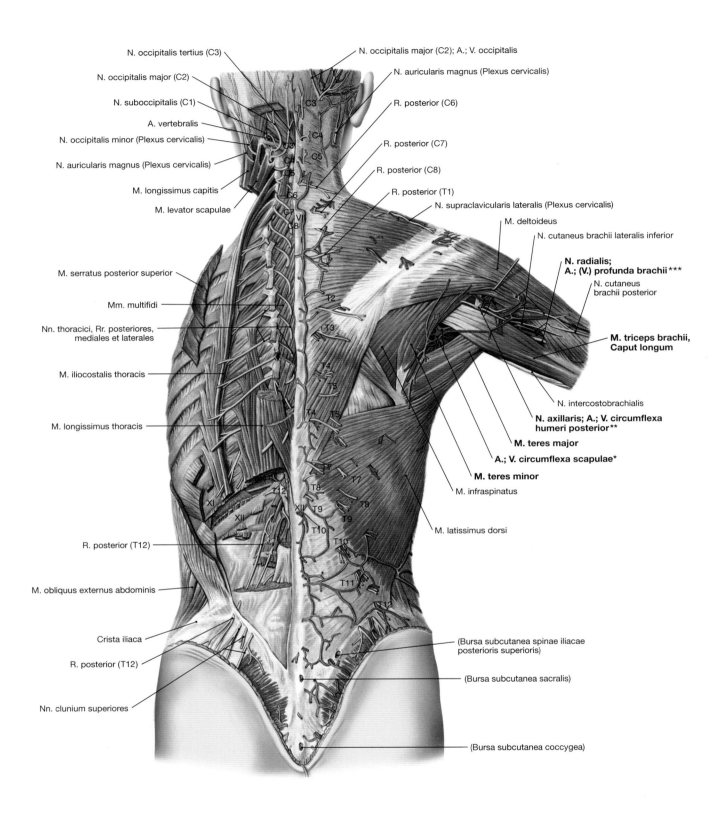

N. occipitalis tertius (C3)

N. occipitalis major (C2)

N. suboccipitalis (C1)

A. vertebralis

N. occipitalis minor (Plexus cervicalis)

N. auricularis magnus (Plexus cervicalis)

M. longissimus capitis

M. levator scapulae

M. serratus posterior superior

Mm. multifidi

Nn. thoracici, Rr. posteriores, mediales et laterales

M. iliocostalis thoracis

M. longissimus thoracis

R. posterior (T12)

M. obliquus externus abdominis

Crista iliaca

R. posterior (T12)

Nn. clunium superiores

N. occipitalis major (C2); A.; V. occipitalis

N. auricularis magnus (Plexus cervicalis)

R. posterior (C6)

R. posterior (C7)

R. posterior (C8)

R. posterior (T1)

N. supraclavicularis lateralis (Plexus cervicalis)

M. deltoideus

N. cutaneus brachii lateralis inferior

N. radialis; A.; (V.) profunda brachii *

N. cutaneus brachii posterior

M. triceps brachii, Caput longum

N. intercostobrachialis

N. axillaris; A.; V. circumflexa humeri posterior **

M. teres major

A.; V. circumflexa scapulae *

M. teres minor

M. infraspinatus

M. latissimus dorsi

(Bursa subcutanea spinae iliacae posterioris superioris)

(Bursa subcutanea sacralis)

(Bursa subcutanea coccygea)

Fig. 2.131 Vessels and nerves of the back; dorsal view; after the superficial muscles and shoulder girdle were removed on the left side. [S700]

The triangular **(medial) axillary space** is demarcated by the M. teres minor (cranial), M. teres major (caudal), and the Caput longum of the M. triceps brachii (lateral). The vessels and nerves in the triangular axillary space include the A. and V. circumflexa scapulae.

The margins of the quadrangular **(lateral) axillary space** are the M. teres minor (cranial), M. teres major (caudal), the Caput longum of the M. triceps brachii (medial), and the humerus shaft (lateral). Vessels

and nerves in the quadrangular axillary space include the A. and V. circumflexa humeri posterior and the N. axillaris.

The **triangular interval (triceps split)** is formed by the M. teres major (cranial), the Caput longum of the M. triceps brachii (medial), and the humerus shaft (lateral). The A. and V. profunda brachii and the N. radialis pass through the **triangular interval.**

*   vessels and nerves in the medial axillary space
**   vessels and nerves in the lateral axillary space
*** vessels and nerves in the triangular interval

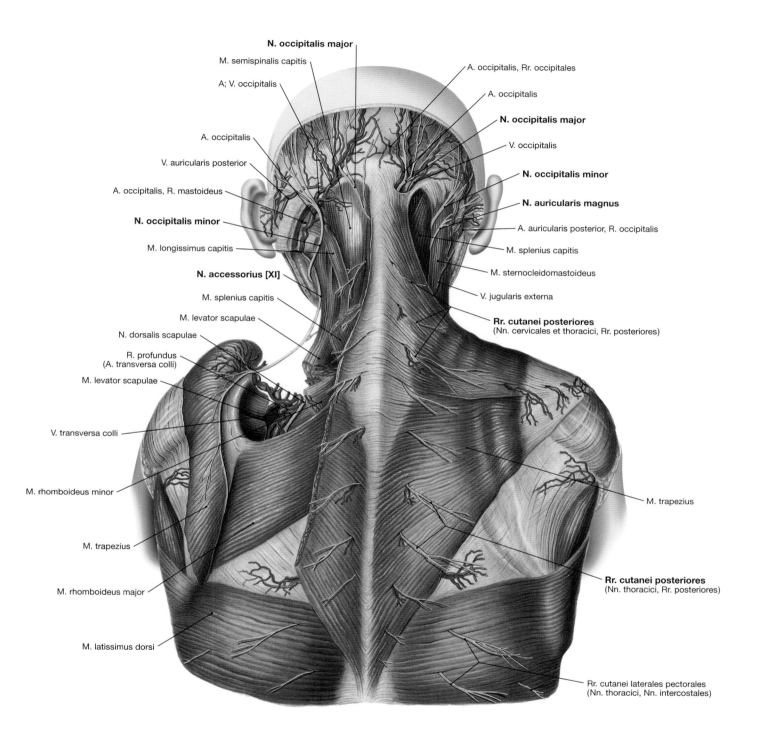

N. occipitalis major

M. semispinalis capitis

A; V. occipitalis

A. occipitalis

V. auricularis posterior

A. occipitalis, R. mastoideus

N. occipitalis minor

M. longissimus capitis

N. accessorius [XI]

M. splenius capitis

M. levator scapulae

N. dorsalis scapulae

R. profundus
(A. transversa colli)

M. levator scapulae

V. transversa colli

M. rhomboideus minor

M. trapezius

M. rhomboideus major

M. latissimus dorsi

A. occipitalis, Rr. occipitales

A. occipitalis

N. occipitalis major

V. occipitalis

N. occipitalis minor

N. auricularis magnus

A. auricularis posterior, R. occipitalis

M. splenius capitis

M. sternocleidomastoideus

V. jugularis externa

Rr. cutanei posteriores
(Nn. cervicales et thoracici, Rr. posteriores)

M. trapezius

Rr. cutanei posteriores
(Nn. thoracici, Rr. posteriores)

Rr. cutanei laterales pectorales
(Nn. thoracici, Nn. intercostales)

Fig. 2.132 Vessels and nerves of the occipital region, Regio occipitalis, neck, Regio cervicalis posterior [Regio nuchalis], and upper back area; dorsal view. [S700]
Up to the scapular line, the skin of the back receives segmental innervation from the Rr. posteriores [dorsales] of the spinal nerves (Rr. cutanei posteriores). The N. occipitalis major from C2 and the N. occipitalis

tertius from C3 (not shown) provide cutaneous innervation for the neck and occipital region (Rr. mediales of the Rr. posteriores [dorsales]). The N. occipitalis minor comes from the Plexus cervicalis (Rr. anteriores [ventrales]) via the Punctum nervosum (ERBs point). The pathway of the N. accessorius [XI] in the neck and shoulder region is also shown.

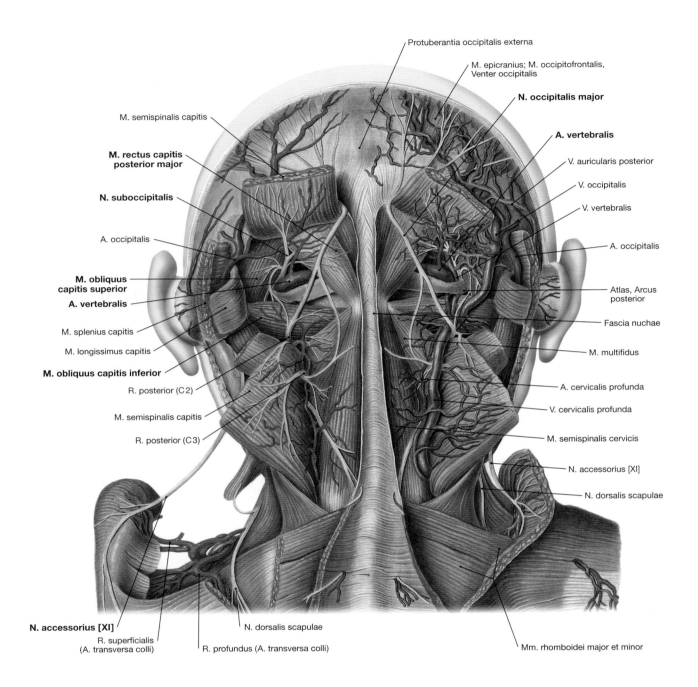

Protuberantia occipitalis externa

M. epicranius; M. occipitofrontalis, Venter occipitalis

N. occipitalis major

A. vertebralis

V. auricularis posterior

V. occipitalis

V. vertebralis

A. occipitalis

Atlas, Arcus posterior

Fascia nuchae

M. multifidus

A. cervicalis profunda

V. cervicalis profunda

M. semispinalis cervicis

N. accessorius [XI]

N. dorsalis scapulae

Mm. rhomboidei major et minor

M. semispinalis capitis

M. rectus capitis posterior major

N. suboccipitalis

A. occipitalis

M. obliquus capitis superior

A. vertebralis

M. splenius capitis

M. longissimus capitis

M. obliquus capitis inferior

R. posterior (C2)

M. semispinalis capitis

R. posterior (C3)

N. accessorius [XI]

R. superficialis (A. transversa colli)

R. profundus (A. transversa colli)

N. dorsalis scapulae

Fig. 2.133 Vessels and nerves of the occipital region, Regio occipitalis, and neck, Regio cervicalis posterior [Regio nuchalis]; dorsal view. [S700]
To demonstrate the deep neurovascular pathways on both sides, the Mm. trapezius, sternocleidomastoideus, splenius capitis, and semispinalis capitis were detached and partially removed. On both sides, the short neck muscles (Mm. recti capitis posterior minor and major as well as the Mm. obliqui capitis superior and inferior), which frame the **triangle of the vertebral artery** (Trigonum arteriae vertebralis) are visible. Besides arteries and veins, Nn. occipitalis major and suboccipitalis as well as the N. accessorius [XI] are shown.

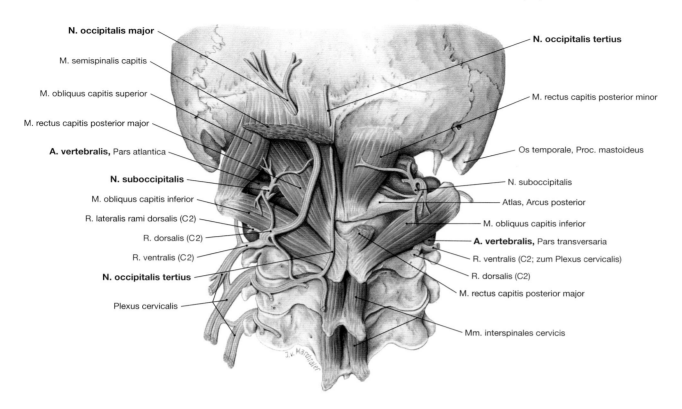

N. occipitalis major

M. semispinalis capitis

M. obliquus capitis superior

M. rectus capitis posterior major

A. vertebralis, Pars atlantica

N. suboccipitalis

M. obliquus capitis inferior

R. lateralis rami dorsalis (C2)

R. dorsalis (C2)

R. ventralis (C2)

N. occipitalis tertius

Plexus cervicalis

N. occipitalis tertius

M. rectus capitis posterior minor

Os temporale, Proc. mastoideus

N. suboccipitalis

Atlas, Arcus posterior

M. obliquus capitis inferior

A. vertebralis, Pars transversaria

R. ventralis (C2; zum Plexus cervicalis)

R. dorsalis (C2)

M. rectus capitis posterior major

Mm. interspinales cervicis

Fig. 2.134 Nerves of the neck, Regio cervicalis posterior; dorsal view. [S700]
The R. posterior from C2 continues as the **N. occipitalis major** on the occiput. The R. posterior from C3 continues cranially as the **N. occipita-**

lis tertius in the area of the Lig. nuchae. From the depths of the triangle of the vertebral artery (Trigonum arteriae vertebralis), in which the A. vertebralis lies, the R. posterior comes from C1 and innervates the short neck muscles as **N. suboccipitalis**.

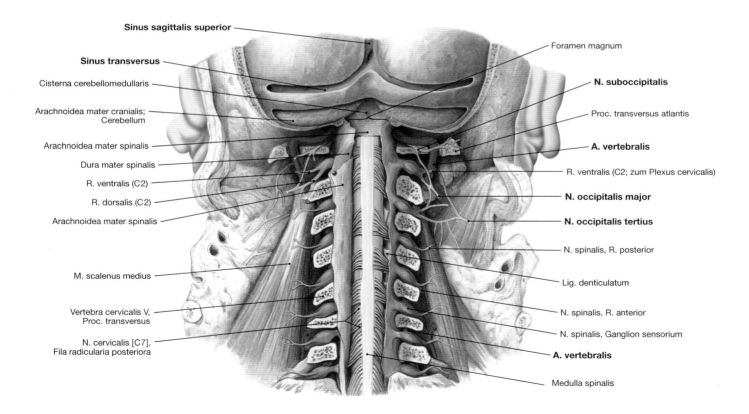

Sinus sagittalis superior

Sinus transversus

Cisterna cerebellomedullaris

Arachnoidea mater cranialis; Cerebellum

Arachnoidea mater spinalis

Dura mater spinalis

R. ventralis (C2)

R. dorsalis (C2)

Arachnoidea mater spinalis

M. scalenus medius

Vertebra cervicalis V, Proc. transversus

N. cervicalis [C7], Fila radicularia posteriora

Foramen magnum

N. suboccipitalis

Proc. transversus atlantis

A. vertebralis

R. ventralis (C2; zum Plexus cervicalis)

N. occipitalis major

N. occipitalis tertius

N. spinalis, R. posterior

Lig. denticulatum

N. spinalis, R. anterior

N. spinalis, Ganglion sensorium

A. vertebralis

Medulla spinalis

Fig. 2.135 Vessels and nerves of the deep posterior neck area, Regio cervicalis posterior, and content of the vertebral canal; dorsal view. [S700]

The vertebral canal has been opened from the dorsal side and the occipital bone removed; this provides a view of the Dura mater with the opened Sinus sagittalis superior and the Sinus transversus unobstructed. Between the cervical vertebrae, the **A. vertebralis** arises.

Trunk

Cauda equina and lumbar puncture

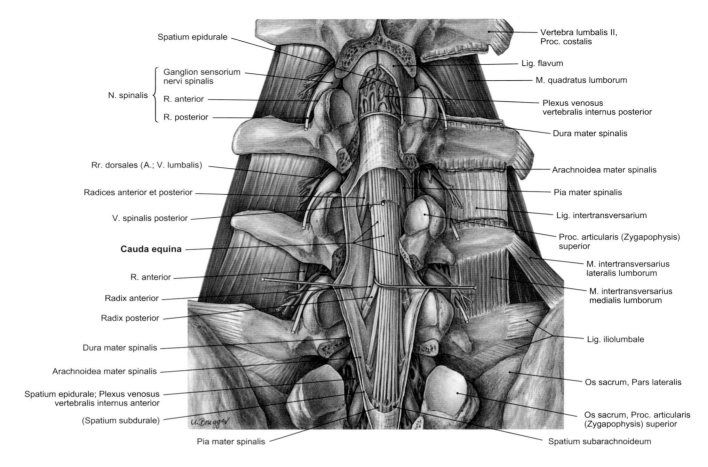

Spatium epidurale

Vertebra lumbalis II, Proc. costalis

Ganglion sensorium nervi spinalis

N. spinalis
- R. anterior
- R. posterior

Lig. flavum

M. quadratus lumborum

Plexus venosus vertebralis internus posterior

Dura mater spinalis

Rr. dorsales (A.; V. lumbalis)

Arachnoidea mater spinalis

Radices anterior et posterior

Pia mater spinalis

V. spinalis posterior

Lig. intertransversarium

Cauda equina

Proc. articularis (Zygapophysis) superior

R. anterior

M. intertransversarius lateralis lumborum

Radix anterior

M. intertransversarius medialis lumborum

Radix posterior

Dura mater spinalis

Lig. iliolumbale

Arachnoidea mater spinalis

Spatium epidurale; Plexus venosus vertebralis internus anterior

Os sacrum, Pars lateralis

(Spatium subdurale)

Os sacrum, Proc. articularis (Zygapophysis) superior

Pia mater spinalis

Spatium subarachnoideum

Fig. 2.136   Vessels and nerves of the opened vertebral canal of the lumbar spine, Regio lumbalis; dorsal view. [S700]

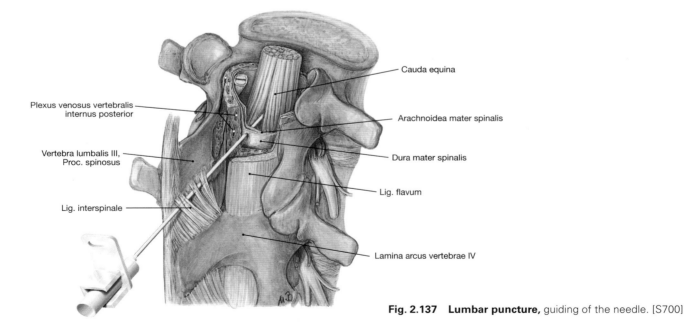

Cauda equina

Plexus venosus vertebralis internus posterior

Arachnoidea mater spinalis

Vertebra lumbalis III, Proc. spinosus

Dura mater spinalis

Lig. interspinale

Lig. flavum

Lamina arcus vertebrae IV

Fig. 2.137   Lumbar puncture, guiding of the needle. [S700]

Clinical remarks

In order to attain cerebrospinal fluid for diagnostic purposes or to apply drugs in the subarachnoid space, a **lumbar puncture** is carried out. This is conducted below the second lumbar vertebra, typically between the spinous processes of L3/L4, and L4/L5, to ensure that the spinal cord is not injured. The Cauda equina can be found at this level; here the subarachnoid space expands to its largest extent. The needle is inserted through the Ligg. supraspinale and interspinale, the epidural space, the Dura mater and the Arachnoidea until the needle enters the subarachnoid space (→ Fig. 2.137).

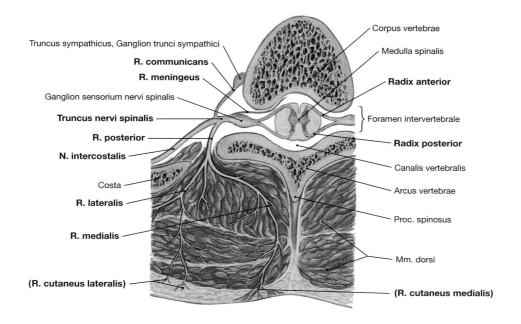

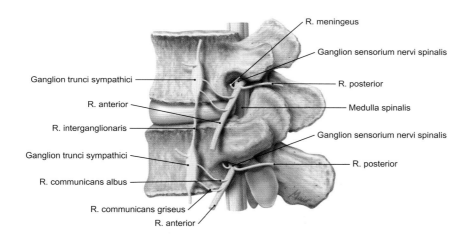

Fig. 2.138 Spinal nerve, N. spinalis, in the thoracic region; caudal view. [S700]
The root of the spinal nerve is only a few millimetres long (Truncus nervi spinalis). It is formed from the Radices anterior and posterior that merge with the Truncus nervi spinalis. The greater R. anterior (N. intercostalis in the thoracic area) and the smaller R. posterior emerge from the sympathetic trunk (Truncus sympathicus). This is divided into a medial (R. medialis) and a lateral (R. lateralis) branch that innervate the au-

tochthonous muscles (Mm. dorsi) as well as the skin of the back with their terminal ends (Rr. cutanei medialis and lateralis). The spinal nerve connects via the R. communicans with the sympathetic trunk. The R. meningeus of the spinal nerve runs downward into the vertebral canal and innervates the ligaments of the spine and the spinal cord. The N. intercostalis runs below the rib (not shown) ventrally, innervates the Mm. intercostales externi and interni and provide the Rr. cutanei lateralis and anterior for skin innervation.

Fig. 2.139 Spinal nerve, N. spinalis, in the lumbar region; lateral view from the left side. [S700-L127]

After the spinal nerve has passed through the Foramen intervertebrale it divides into the Rr. anterior, posterior, meningeus and communicans which connect with the sympathetic chain (Truncus sympathicus).

┌ Clinical remarks ─────────────────────────────────

Posterolateral disc prolapses, spondylophytes or tumours can cause the **narrowing of the Foramen intervertebrale** with compression of the spinal nerve roots and resulting nerve function loss. [S701-L126]

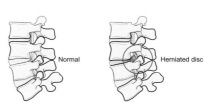

Spinal nerve

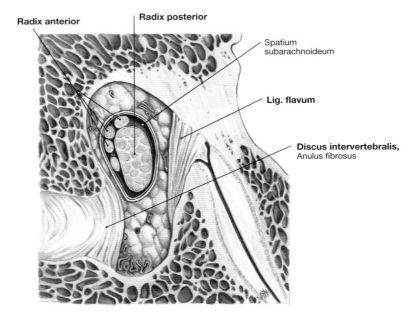

Radix anterior

Radix posterior

Spatium subarachnoideum

Lig. flavum

Discus intervertebralis, Anulus fibrosus

Fig. 2.140 Spinal nerve, N. spinalis, in the lumbar region. Sagittal section at the level of the Foramen intervertebrale; view from the left side. [B500-L240]
In the Foramen intervertebrale, the Radices anterior and posterior have not yet fused to the spinal nerve. They are still in the dural pocket and immersed in cerebrospinal fluid. Ventrally you can see the intervertebral disc (Discus intervertebralis) and dorsally the Lig. flavum, as well as the adjacent zygapophyseal joint.

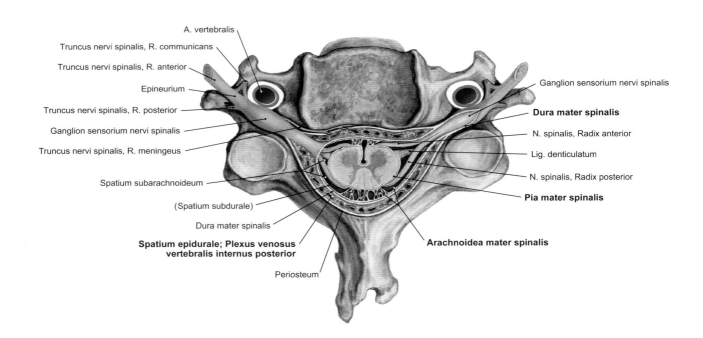

A. vertebralis

Truncus nervi spinalis, R. communicans

Truncus nervi spinalis, R. anterior

Epineurium

Truncus nervi spinalis, R. posterior

Ganglion sensorium nervi spinalis

Truncus nervi spinalis, R. meningeus

Spatium subarachnoideum

(Spatium subdurale)

Dura mater spinalis

Spatium epidurale; Plexus venosus vertebralis internus posterior

Periosteum

Ganglion sensorium nervi spinalis

Dura mater spinalis

N. spinalis, Radix anterior

Lig. denticulatum

N. spinalis, Radix posterior

Pia mater spinalis

Arachnoidea mater spinalis

Fig. 2.141 Content of the vertebral canal, Canalis vertebralis; cross-section at the level of the fifth cervical vertebra; view from cranial. [S700]
The spinal cord is surrounded by the Dura, Arachnoidea and Pia mater and immersed in cerebrospinal fluid in the subarachnoid space (Spatium subarachnoideum). In the vertebral canal, the dural sac and the exiting spinal nerve roots are surrounded and protected by adipose tissue with an embedded venous plexus (Plexus venosi vertebrales interni anterior and posterior) and with nourishing blood vessels.
See epidural anaesthesia → Fig. 12.190, Vol. 3.

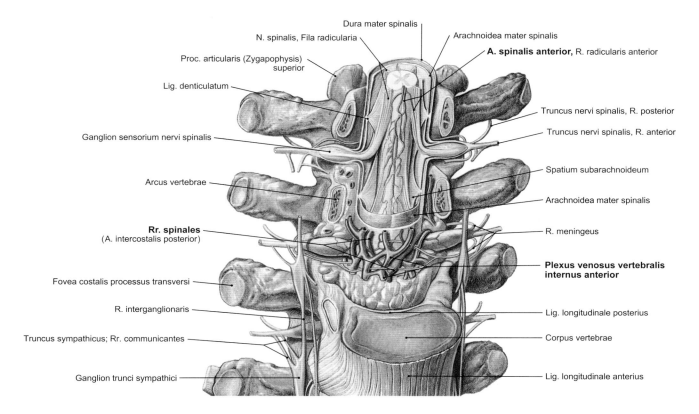

Dura mater spinalis
N. spinalis, Fila radicularia
Proc. articularis (Zygapophysis) superior
Lig. denticulatum
Ganglion sensorium nervi spinalis
Arcus vertebrae
Rr. spinales (A. intercostalis posterior)
Fovea costalis processus transversi
R. interganglionaris
Truncus sympathicus; Rr. communicantes
Ganglion trunci sympathici

Arachnoidea mater spinalis
A. spinalis anterior, R. radicularis anterior
Truncus nervi spinalis, R. posterior
Truncus nervi spinalis, R. anterior
Spatium subarachnoideum
Arachnoidea mater spinalis
R. meningeus
Plexus venosus vertebralis internus anterior
Lig. longitudinale posterius
Corpus vertebrae
Lig. longitudinale anterius

Fig. 2.142 Thoracic spine with spinal cord, Medulla spinalis, and sympathetic trunk, Truncus sympathicus; ventral view. [S700]
You can see the Spatium epidurale encapsulating the meninges in the vertebral canal, in which the Plexus venosus vertebralis internus anteri-

or, as well as the Rr. spinales of the A. intercostalis posterior are visible in its adipose tissue. The A. spinalis anterior runs along the spinal cord.

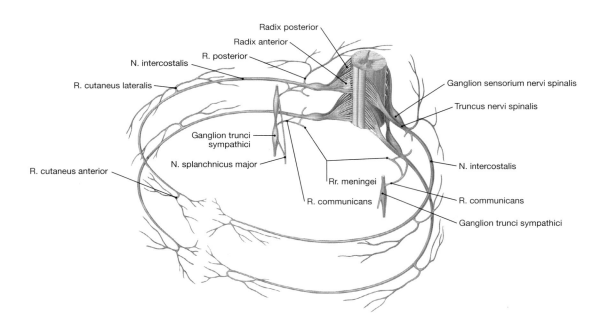

Radix posterior
Radix anterior
R. posterior
N. intercostalis
R. cutaneus lateralis
Ganglion trunci sympathici
N. splanchnicus major
R. cutaneus anterior
Rr. meningei
R. communicans

Ganglion sensorium nervi spinalis
Truncus nervi spinalis
N. intercostalis
R. communicans
Ganglion trunci sympathici

Fig. 2.143 Structure of a spinal nerve, N. spinalis, and spinal cord segment, exemplified by two thoracic nerves, Nn. thoracici; oblique superior view. [S700]
Each spinal nerve has an anterior root (Radix anterior) and a posterior root (Radix posterior). The cell bodies (perikarya) of the motor nerve fibres are located in the grey matter of the spinal cord and exit through the anterior root; the perikarya of sensory nerve fibres are located in the

dorsal root ganglion (Ganglion sensorium nervi spinalis) and enter the spinal cord via the dorsal root. Connections from the spinal cord to the Ganglion trunci sympathici (ganglion of the sympathetic trunk) are made via the Rr. communicantes. The branches of the dorsal spinal nerves are arranged segmentally; apart from the intercostal nerves II–XI, the ventral branches merge in the plexus.

Vessels and nerves of the vertebral canal

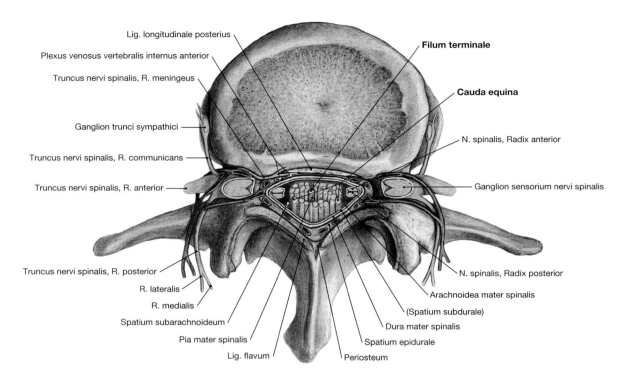

Lig. longitudinale posterius
Plexus venosus vertebralis internus anterior
Truncus nervi spinalis, R. meningeus
Ganglion trunci sympathici
Truncus nervi spinalis, R. communicans
Truncus nervi spinalis, R. anterior
Truncus nervi spinalis, R. posterior
R. lateralis
R. medialis
Spatium subarachnoideum
Pia mater spinalis
Lig. flavum

Filum terminale
Cauda equina
N. spinalis, Radix anterior
Ganglion sensorium nervi spinalis
N. spinalis, Radix posterior
Arachnoidea mater spinalis
(Spatium subdurale)
Dura mater spinalis
Spatium epidurale
Periosteum

Fig. 2.144 Content of the vertebral canal, Canalis vertebralis; cross-section at the level of the third lumbar vertebra; cranial view. [S700]
Below the first/second lumbar vertebra, the nerve roots of L2 run caudally up to and including the N. coccygeus in the dural sac as a loose bundle, to its exit points. This entire collection of nerve roots is called **Cauda equina.** Between the nerve fibre processes, the extremely thin **Filum terminale** is visible, connecting to the Conus medullaris of the spinal cord.
For lumbar puncture → Fig. 2.137.

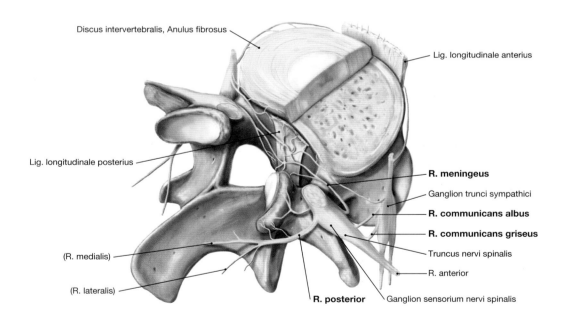

Discus intervertebralis, Anulus fibrosus
Lig. longitudinale posterius
(R. medialis)
(R. lateralis)
R. posterior

Lig. longitudinale anterius
R. meningeus
Ganglion trunci sympathici
R. communicans albus
R. communicans griseus
Truncus nervi spinalis
R. anterior
Ganglion sensorium nervi spinalis

Fig. 2.145 Nerves of the spine, Columna vertebralis; oblique view from the right. [S700-L266]
Branches of the spinal nerve are shown running to directly adjacent structures. These include the **R. meningeus** which sensorily innervates the membrane of the spinal cord, the small branches projecting from the **R. posterior** to the Capsula articularis of the zygapophyseal joints, as well as the Rr. communicantes albus and griseus connecting to the Truncus sympathicus.

Preganglionic sympathetic fibres run via the **R. communicans albus** from the lateral horn of the spinal cord to the Truncus sympathicus. Postganglionic sympathetic fibres run via the **R. communicans griseus** from the sympathetic trunk to the spinal nerve. Autonomic fibres of the sympathetic trunk innervate the spinal discs and ligaments of the spine.

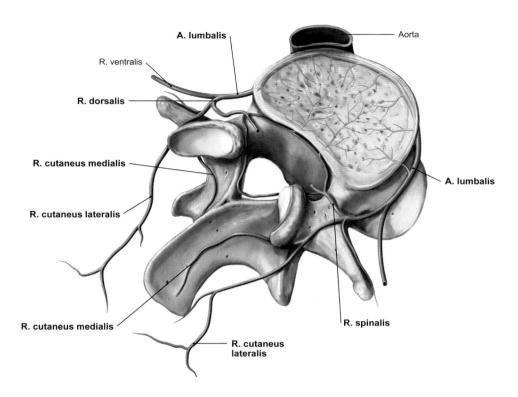

Fig. 2.146 Arteries of the vertebral canal, Canalis vertebralis, with the lumbar vertebra as an example; oblique view from the right side. [S700-L266]

In the thoracic and lumbar spine there is a strictly segmental arterial supply. Emerging as segmental branches, the paired **Aa. intercostales posteriores** from the Aorta thoracica and the paired Aa. lumbales from the Aorta abdominalis supply the adjacent vertebrae with blood. Each artery leads into a **R. dorsalis,** from which a **R. spinalis** passes through the Foramen intervertebrale of the corresponding motion segment into

the vertebral canal. The segmental spinal arteries anastomose on various levels in the vertebral canal via ascending and descending branches. The posterior artery branches reach the plates (laminae) of the vertebral arch and the spinous processes from the inside. Parallel to the eponymously named dorsal spinal nerve branches, the terminal branches of the Rr. posteriores run as **Rr. cutanei mediales** and **Rr. cutanei laterales.** They supply the posterior bony structures from the outside with blood, and the dorsal back muscles and the skin via their terminal ends.

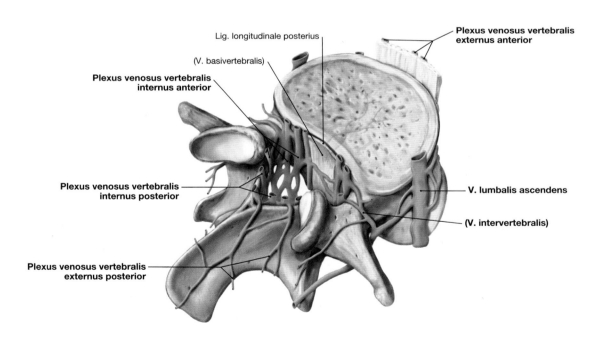

Fig. 2.147 Veins of the vertebral canal, Canalis vertebralis, oblique dorsal view from the right. [S700-L266]

The vertebral canal is filled with a dense network of veins which form the **Plexus venosi vertebrales interni anterior** and **posterior.** Located in the Spatium epidurale, this venous plexus covers the meninges with the bone marrow contained here, as well as the cauda equina. The two plexuses are connected with the **Plexus venosus vertebralis externus**

posterior via the Vv. intervertebrales. This vein drains the blood (in the area of the lumbar spine) into the paravertebral oriented Vv. lumbales ascendentes (the Vv. azygos, hemiazygos and hemiazygos accessoria run through the thoracic region). They also take blood from the disc located on the front of the vertebral body and the **Plexus venosus vertebralis externus anterior.**

Operative access to the spine

Clinical remarks

a Operative access to the cervical spine, ventrally at the level of the first tracheal ring; horizontal section. [S700-L126]
b Operative access to the cervical spine at the level of the vocal folds; horizontal section. Depending on the cause for operative in-

tervention (→ Fig. a), access to the cervical spine from the anterior, lateral or dorsal (e.g. according to FRYKHOLM) is necessary. [S700-L126]

Clinical remarks

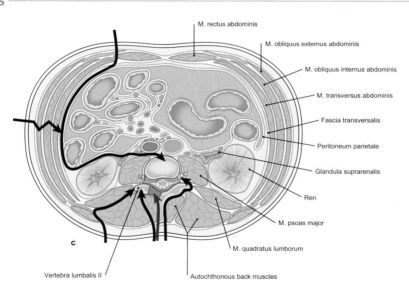

M. rectus abdominis

M. obliquus externus abdominis

M. obliquus internus abdominis

M. transversus abdominis

Fascia transversalis

Peritoneum parietale

Glandula suprarenalis

Ren

M. psoas major

M. quadratus lumborum

c

Vertebra lumbalis II

Autochthonous back muscles

c Operative access to the lumbar spine at the level of the first lumbar vortex; horizontal section. [S700-L126]

Operative access to the spine is an integral part of spine surgery for a wide variety of reasons, such as for the treatment of herniated discs, spinal canal stenosis, and for procedures in the treatment of scoliosis, vertebral fractures, tumours and metastases, birth defects or degenerative instability (e. g. vertebral slippage). The surgeon has to penetrate the soft tissue shell of the spine from the exterior.

In the case of anterior access at the level of the first **tracheal ring,** access is made at the anterior border of the M. sternocleidomastoideus. The neck viscera with the surrounding general organ fascia

is brought forward, while the carotid sheath remains at the back with its content.

Anterior, lateral, and dorsal surgical access routes are possible, dependent on the reason for surgical intervention in the **lumbar region.** In the case of an anterior and/or lateral approach, care should be taken to keep the peritoneum intact. A dorsal surgical approach is easier, with the Proc. spinosus of the lumbar vertebra serving as a reference point. The red arrow indicates the standard surgical approach (clinical 'semicircle') for medial and mediolateral access during vertebral disk prolapse surgery.

Female breast

Female breast, overview and development

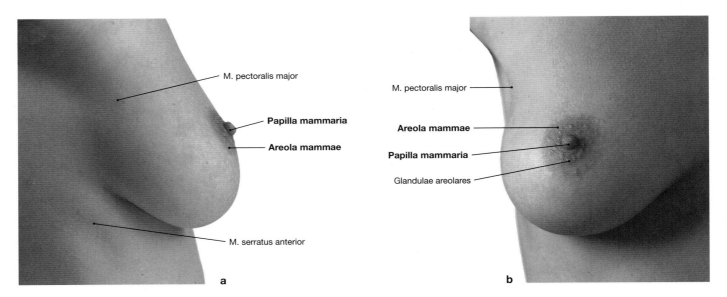

Fig. 2.148a and b   Breast, Mamma. [S700]
a Lateral view.
b Ventral view.

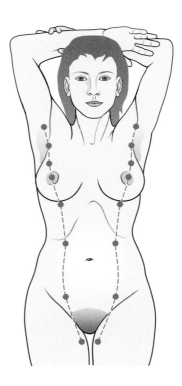

Fig. 2.149   Milk line. [S700-L126]
The mammary gland development begins in the milk line, a strip of condensed epithelium, which forms in the sixth week of development in the surface ectoderm and which extends from the armpit into the inguinal region. The milk line regresses to the area above the M. pectoralis major. Development of the breast (Mamma) takes place here.

Clinical remarks

The absence of nipples **(athelie)** or breasts **(amastia, aplasia of mammary gland)** are rare congenital anomalies that can occur unilaterally or bilaterally. The presence of supernumerary nipples or breasts are called **polythelia** or **polymastia.** This is usually hereditary and can also affect men.

The rudimentary mammary tissue usually does not develop further in men after birth. However, breast growth which continues in men (often in the context of hormonal disorders), is called **gynaecomastia.** Some female breasts are too large **(mammary hypertrophy),** causing shoulder and back pain. In such cases, breast reduction surgery is indicated.

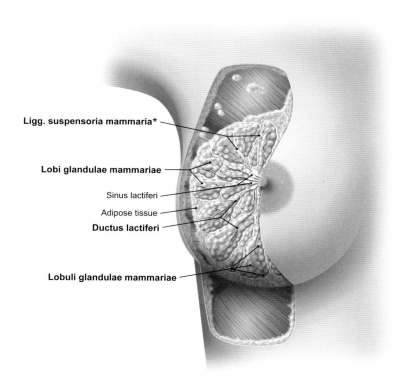

Ligg. suspensoria mammaria*

Lobi glandulae mammariae

Sinus lactiferi

Adipose tissue

Ductus lactiferi

Lobuli glandulae mammariae

Fig. 2.150 Breast, Mamma; ventral view. [S700-L127]
The breast consists of the mammary gland (Glandula mammaria) and a fibrous stroma, which contains adipose tissue. The breast has up to 20 individual lobes (lobi), each possessing a separate lactiferous duct on the nipple (Papilla mammaria). Terminal parts that are arranged in groups (lobuli) are located at the ends of the branched lactiferous ducts. During pregnancy, the glandular tissue transforms into the lactating mammary gland.

* clin.: COOPER's ligaments

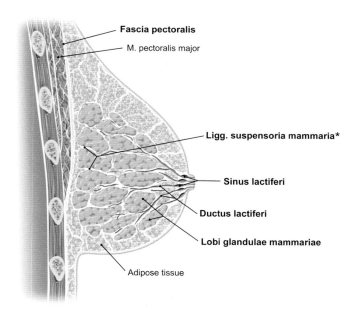

Fascia pectoralis

M. pectoralis major

Ligg. suspensoria mammaria*

Sinus lactiferi

Ductus lactiferi

Lobi glandulae mammariae

Adipose tissue

Fig. 2.151 Breast, Mamma; sagittal section. [S700-L127]
The breast is flexibly secured with strong connective tissue strands (Ligg. suspensoria mammaria, COOPER's ligaments) on the Fascia pectoralis of the M. pectoralis major.

* clin.: COOPER's ligaments

Blood supply and lymphatic drainage

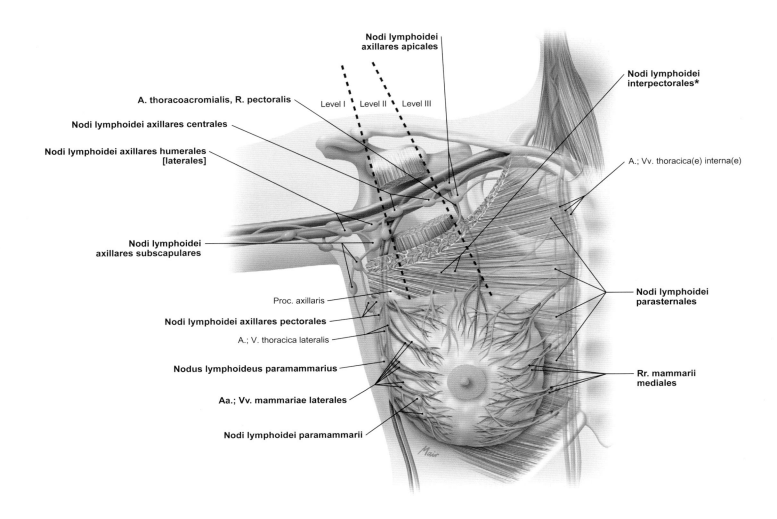

Nodi lymphoidei
axillares apicales

A. thoracoacromialis, R. pectoralis

Level I   Level II   Level III

Nodi lymphoidei axillares centrales

Nodi lymphoidei axillares humerales
[laterales]

Nodi lymphoidei
axillares subscapulares

Proc. axillaris

Nodi lymphoidei axillares pectorales

A.; V. thoracica lateralis

Nodus lymphoideus paramammarius

Aa.; Vv. mammariae laterales

Nodi lymphoidei paramammarii

Nodi lymphoidei
interpectorales*

A.; Vv. thoracica(e) interna(e)

Nodi lymphoidei
parasternales

Rr. mammarii
mediales

Fig. 2.152 Blood supply of the female mammary gland, lymphatic drainage pathways of the female breast lymphs, and location of regional lymph nodes. [S700-L127]
The lymph of almost the entire upper extremity as well as two thirds of the lymph from the mammary gland and most of the lymph from the thoracic and upper abdominal wall flows through approximately 40 axillary lymph nodes. The **Truncus subclavius** collects the lymph of the axillary lymph nodes and drains it on the right into the **Ductus lymphaticus dexter** and on the left into the **Ductus thoracicus** (not shown).

* clin.: ROTTER's lymph nodes

Clinical remarks

From a clinical, topographical and oncosurgical viewpoint, lymph nodes of the female breast are categorised into **three levels.** In doing so, the M. pectoralis minor acts as a boundary:
• Level I lies lateral of the M. pectoralis minor
• Level II lies below the M. pectoralis minor
• Level III lies medial of the M. pectoralis minor.

The parasternal lymph nodes of both sides are interconnected. The lymph is drained via level I into level II and from here into the Nodi lymphoidei axillares apicales in level III. From here, the lymph passes into the Truncus subclavius.

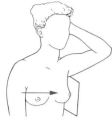

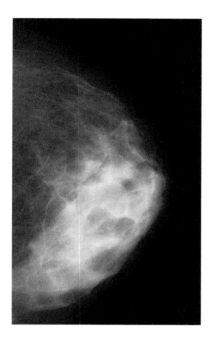

Fig. 2.153   X-ray of the breast (mammography) of a 47-year-old woman. [S700]
A mammography is an X-ray examination for the early detection of breast cancer (mammary carcinoma), the most common cancer in women.

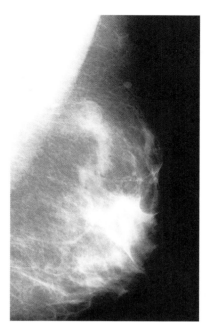

Fig. 2.154   X-ray of the breast (mammography) of a 23-year-old woman. [G198]
You can see the normal breast tissue as ill-defined white consolidations, primarily behind the nipple. In young women, the mammary tissue can be extremely tight and only contain small quantities of interspersed fat.

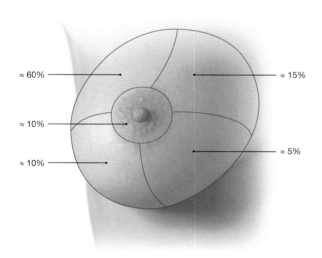

≈ 60%

≈ 15%

≈ 10%

≈ 5%

≈ 10%

Fig. 2.155   Percentage of the frequency of occurrence of breast cancer relative to the location. [S700-L127]

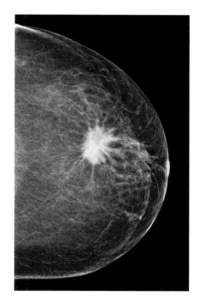

Fig. 2.156   Mammography of malignant breast cancer.
[S700-T903]

Clinical remarks

Breast cancer is responsible for 16 % of all cancer deaths in women worldwide in 2020. This means that breast cancer is the first cause of death from cancer, even before intestinal and lung cancer. In women, breast cancer is the leading cause of death between the age of 35 and 55 years. In about 60 % of all cases the upper outer quadrant of the breast is affected (→ Fig. 2.155). Breast cancer originates mostly from the epithelium of the Ductus lactiferi (ductal carci-

noma) and metastasises mainly into the axillary lymph nodes, less often into the retrosternal (parasternal) lymph nodes.
The first lymph node located in the drainage area is known as the **sentinel (guard) node**. This node is usually the first lymph node to be colonised by metastatic cells. The number of affected lymph nodes in the levels is directly related to the survival rate. Breast cancer of the medial quadrant can metastasise via the interconnected parasternal lymph nodes onto the opposite side.

Cutaneous innervation of the thoracic and abdominal wall

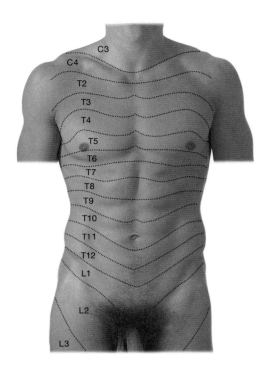

Fig. 2.157   Segmental sensory innervation of the anterior thoracic and abdominal wall (dermatomes). [S700]
Cutaneous (skin) areas which are innervated by the sensitive fibres of a single spinal nerve are called dermatomes. The nipple lies in the dermatome T4–T5; the navel in the dermatome T10.

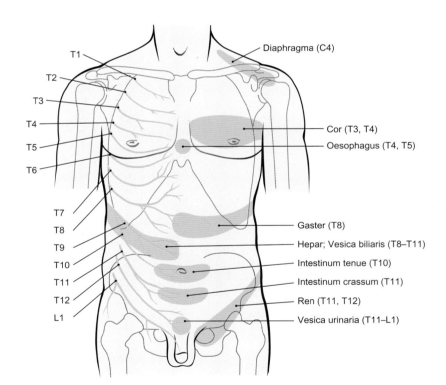

Fig. 2.158   Segmental sensory innervation of the thoracic and abdominal wall. [S700-L126]
The spinal nerves which are responsible for the innervation of the dermatomes are shown on the right side (→ Fig. 2.157).
A HEAD's zone is the name for an area in which there is a link between the somatic (= animalistic) and the autonomic nervous system via the associated spinal cord segment, due to the segmentation of the body (metamerism). Certain internal organs are assigned to this area. The HEAD's zone, which is assigned to a specific organ, can extend across several dermatomes, but usually has a point of maximal reflexivity.

Clinical remarks

Shingles **(herpes zoster)** is the most common infection of the peripheral nervous system. Herpes zoster leads to an acute neuralgia, which is limited to the dermatome of a specific sensory spinal or cranial nerve root. The cause is an infection with the varicella zoster virus, which causes chickenpox when first infected and is now re-activated. It leads to a vesicular rash (blistering), which is limited to the innervation area of a sensory root ganglion or a sensory cranial nerve.

Initially, the patient suffers from an intense, burning and localised ache, followed three to five days later by blistering. An irritation of the associated internal organ of a **HEAD's zone** (→ Fig. 2.158) can initiate a viscerocutaneous reflexive pain in a specific, mostly ipsilateral zone (zone of hyperalgesia). This phenomenon is called **referred pain**. The pain can sometimes spread to adjacent segments or to the whole of the affected body side (generalisation).

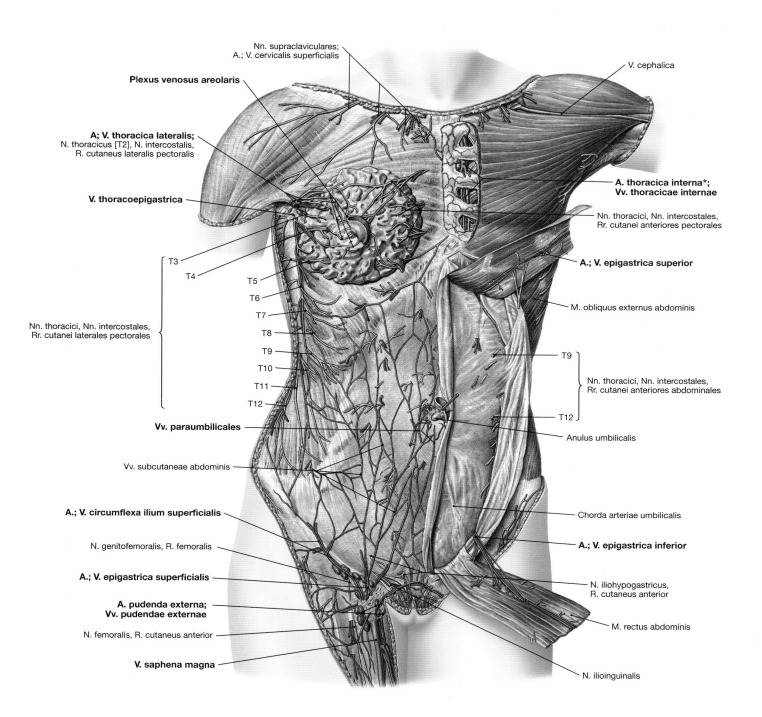

Nn. supraclaviculares;
A.; V. cervicalis superficialis

Plexus venosus areolaris

V. cephalica

A; V. thoracica lateralis;
N. thoracicus [T2], N. intercostalis,
R. cutaneus lateralis pectoralis

V. thoracoepigastrica

A. thoracica interna*;
Vv. thoracicae internae

Nn. thoracici, Nn. intercostales,
Rr. cutanei anteriores pectorales

T3
T4
T5
T6
T7

A.; V. epigastrica superior

M. obliquus externus abdominis

Nn. thoracici, Nn. intercostales,
Rr. cutanei laterales pectorales

T8
T9
T10
T11
T12

T9

Nn. thoracici, Nn. intercostales,
Rr. cutanei anteriores abdominales

T12

Vv. paraumbilicales

Anulus umbilicalis

Vv. subcutaneae abdominis

A.; V. circumflexa ilium superficialis

Chorda arteriae umbilicalis

N. genitofemoralis, R. femoralis

A.; V. epigastrica inferior

A.; V. epigastrica superficialis

N. iliohypogastricus,
R. cutaneus anterior

A. pudenda externa;
Vv. pudendae externae

M. rectus abdominis

N. femoralis, R. cutaneus anterior

V. saphena magna

N. ilioinguinalis

Fig. 2.159 Epifascial and deep vessels and nerves of the anterior
trunk wall in the female; ventral view. [S700]
On the right side of the body, the Fasciae deltoidea, pectoralis, thoracica, abdominis and lata are presented with their epifascial neurovascular
pathways and the mammary gland. The Mamma receives its blood supply from the Rr. mammarii mediales of the A. thoracic interna and via
the Rr. mammarii lateralis from the Aa. thoracica lateralis and thoracodorsalis.

On the left side of the body, the superficial fascia has been removed to
provide a clear view of the muscles. The rectus sheath is opened, the
M. rectus abdominis is cut along the middle; its parts are folded back at
the top and the bottom. On the back, you can see the Vasa epigastrica
superiora and inferiora.

* clin.: A. mammaria interna

Inner outline of the anterior abdominal wall

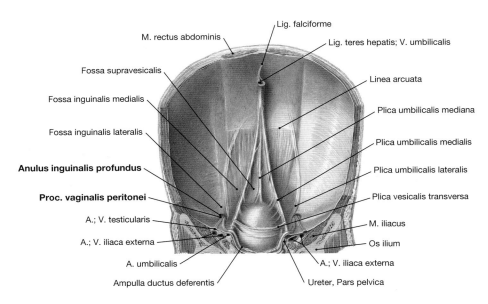

Fig. 2.160 Anterior abdominal wall of a newborn; view from inside. [S700]
In the case of a mature newborn, the descent of the testes into the scrotum (Descensus testis) is complete. At the Anulus inguinalis profundus, the Peritoneum parietale forms a shallow cavity as the Proc. vaginalis peritonei invaginates slightly into the inguinal canal.

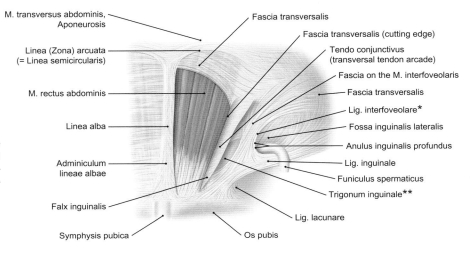

Fig. 2.161 Anterior abdominal wall; view from inside; Peritoneum parietale and Fascia transversalis are partially removed. [S700-L127]/[E633-002]
Depiction of the Trigonum inguinale (HESSELBACH's triangle) of the Lig. interfoveolare (HESSELBACH's ligament) and the Fossa inguinalis lateralis with the penetrating Funiculus spermaticus.

* clin.: HESSELBACH's ligament
** clin.: HESSELBACH's triangle

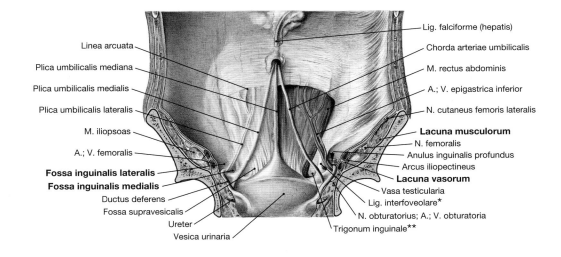

Fig. 2.162 Anterior abdominal wall; view from inside. [S700]
The Fossa inguinalis medialis, Fossa inguinalis lateralis, Lacuna vasorum and Lacuna musculorum are depicted. To view the neurovascular pathways, the Peritoneum parietale and the Fascia transversalis were removed from the right side of the body.

* clin.: HESSELBACH's ligament
** clin.: HESSELBACH's triangle

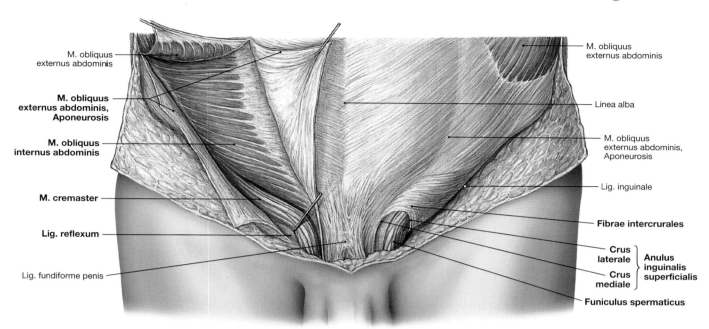

M. obliquus externus abdominis

M. obliquus externus abdominis, Aponeurosis

M. obliquus internus abdominis

M. cremaster

Lig. reflexum

Lig. fundiforme penis

M. obliquus externus abdominis

Linea alba

M. obliquus externus abdominis, Aponeurosis

Lig. inguinale

Fibrae intercrurales

Crus laterale ⎫ **Anulus**
Crus mediale ⎭ **inguinalis superficialis**

Funiculus spermaticus

Fig. 2.163 Outer inguinal ring, Anulus inguinalis superficialis; ventral view. [S700]
Boundaries of the outer inguinal ring are the **Crus medial** and **Crus lateral,** formed by the aponeurosis of the M. obliquus externus abdominis, between which the Fibrae intercrurales is spread out. The caudal margin is formed by the **Lig. reflexum** as part of the Lig. inguinale.

On the right side of the body, the aponeurosis of the M. obliquus externus abdominis is folded back and provides a view of the **M. obliquus internus abdominis.** Muscle fibres of the M. obliquus internus abdominis split off as **M. cremaster** and draw back into the scrotum along with the Funiculus spermaticus.

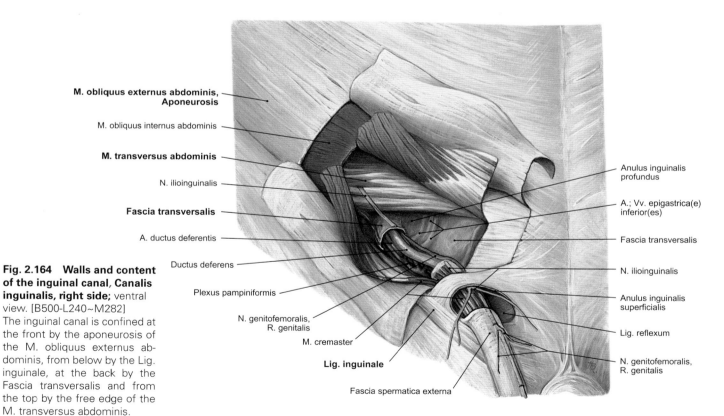

M. obliquus externus abdominis, Aponeurosis

M. obliquus internus abdominis

M. transversus abdominis

N. ilioinguinalis

Fascia transversalis

A. ductus deferentis

Ductus deferens

Plexus pampiniformis

N. genitofemoralis, R. genitalis

M. cremaster

Lig. inguinale

Fascia spermatica externa

Anulus inguinalis profundus

A.; Vv. epigastrica(e) inferior(es)

Fascia transversalis

N. ilioinguinalis

Anulus inguinalis superficialis

Lig. reflexum

N. genitofemoralis, R. genitalis

Fig. 2.164 Walls and content of the inguinal canal, Canalis inguinalis, right side; ventral view. [B500-L240~M282]
The inguinal canal is confined at the front by the aponeurosis of the M. obliquus externus abdominis, from below by the Lig. inguinale, at the back by the Fascia transversalis and from the top by the free edge of the M. transversus abdominis.

Clinical remarks

The contraction of the M. cremaster when touching the inside of the thigh is called the **cremasteric reflex,** prompting an elevation of the testis on the same side. It is a physiological extrinsic reflex. Afferent fibres run in the R. femoralis of the N. genitofemoralis, and the efferent fibres in the R. genitalis of the N. genitofemoralis.

The Anulus inguinalis profundus is the **internal hernial canal** for indirect inguinal hernias, the Fossa inguinalis medialis (HESSELBACH's triangle, → Fig. 2.162) is the internal hernial canal for direct inguinal hernias and the Septum femorale in the Lacuna vasorum is the internal hernial canal for **femoral hernias.**

Inguinal canal

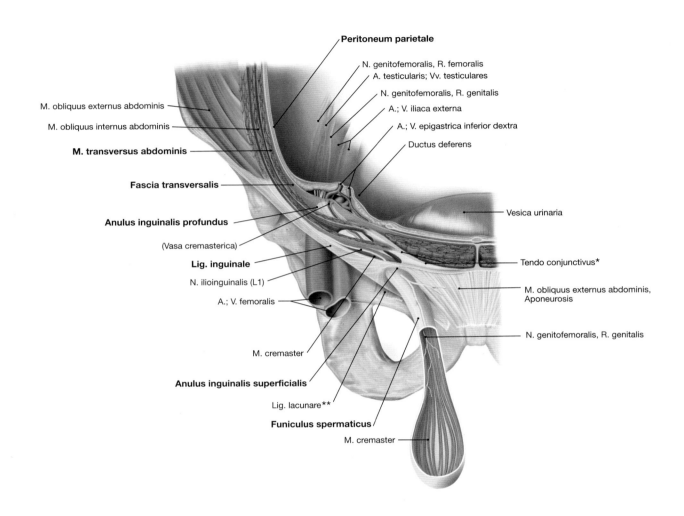

Peritoneum parietale
N. genitofemoralis, R. femoralis
A. testicularis; Vv. testiculares
N. genitofemoralis, R. genitalis
A.; V. iliaca externa
A.; V. epigastrica inferior dextra
Ductus deferens
M. obliquus externus abdominis
M. obliquus internus abdominis
M. transversus abdominis
Fascia transversalis
Anulus inguinalis profundus
(Vasa cremasterica)
Lig. inguinale
N. ilioinguinalis (L1)
A.; V. femoralis
Vesica urinaria
Tendo conjunctivus*
M. obliquus externus abdominis, Aponeurosis
N. genitofemoralis, R. genitalis
M. cremaster
Anulus inguinalis superficialis
Lig. lacunare**
Funiculus spermaticus
M. cremaster

Fig. 2.165 Inguinal canal, Canalis inguinalis, and spermatic cord, Funiculus spermaticus, right side; ventral view. [S700-L280]
The approximately 4–6 cm long inguinal canal penetrates the ventral abdominal wall above the inguinal ligament in an oblique angle from a posterior-lateral-cranial to an anterior-medial-caudal direction. The inner opening is the **Anulus inguinalis profundus,** which at the posterior is formed by the peritoneum and the Fascia transversalis, cranially by the M. transversus abdominis and caudally by the Lig. inguinale. The outer opening is the **Anulus inguinalis superficialis,** which is confined at the front by the aponeurosis of the M. obliquus externus abdominis and below by the Lig. inguinale (Lig. reflexum). The **Funiculus spermaticus** emerges from the inguinal canal. On its Fascia spermatica externa, the

N. scrotalis anterior from the N. ilioinguinalis reaches the front section of the scrotum. The **M. obliquus internus abdominis** takes the same path as the M. transversus abdominis via the Funiculus spermaticus, and provides fibres (M. cremaster) which run along the Funiculus spermaticus, enclosed in a separate fascia (Fascia cremasterica), up to the testes between the Fasciae spermaticae externa and interna. The M. cremaster plays a decisive role in the thermoregulation of the spermatogenesis.

* transversus conjoined tendon
** clin.: GIMBERNAT's ligament

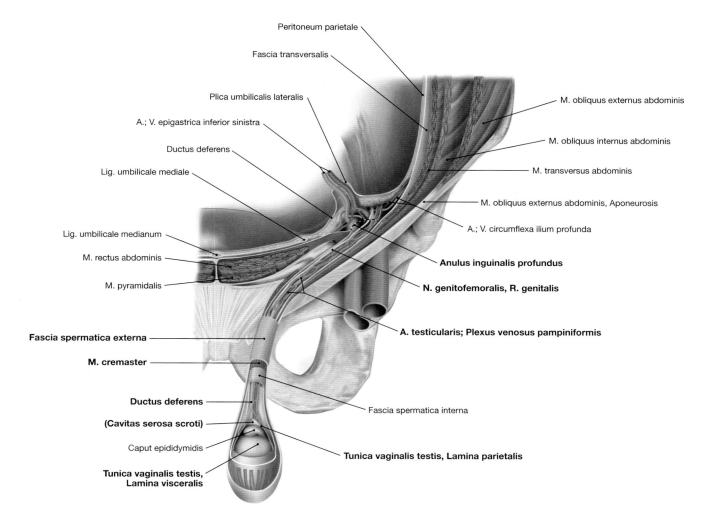

Peritoneum parietale

Fascia transversalis

Plica umbilicalis lateralis

A.; V. epigastrica inferior sinistra

Ductus deferens

Lig. umbilicale mediale

Lig. umbilicale medianum

M. rectus abdominis

M. pyramidalis

Fascia spermatica externa

M. cremaster

Ductus deferens

(Cavitas serosa scroti)

Caput epididymidis

Tunica vaginalis testis, Lamina visceralis

M. obliquus externus abdominis

M. obliquus internus abdominis

M. transversus abdominis

M. obliquus externus abdominis, Aponeurosis

A.; V. circumflexa ilium profunda

Anulus inguinalis profundus

N. genitofemoralis, R. genitalis

A. testicularis; Plexus venosus pampiniformis

Fascia spermatica interna

Tunica vaginalis testis, Lamina parietalis

Fig. 2.166 Content of the spermatic cord, Funiculus spermaticus, and testicular sheaths, left side; ventral view. [S700-L280]
Covered by the Fascia spermatica externa, M. cremaster and Fascia spermatica interna, the **spermatic cord** contains the spermatic duct (Ductus deferens), the A. ductus deferentis, the A. testicularis (a direct branch of the aorta), the Plexus pampiniformis (drains into the V. testicularis and from there on the right side into the V. cava inferior and on the left side into the V. renalis), the R. genitalis of the N. genitofemoralis and the Vestigium processus vaginalis (obliterated Proc. vaginalis testis, on the side of which the testis has descended from the abdominal cavity into the scrotum, → Fig. 2.167).

The **testis** is covered by the Laminia visceralis of the serosa (epiorchium) and is separated by the Cavum serosum scroti (a cavity) from the enveloping Lamina parietalis (periorchium). The epiorchium and periorchium are connected at the mesorchium. Externally, they are joined by the Fascia spermatica interna, fibres of the M. cremaster as well as the Fascia spermatica externa. The two testicles (testes) are embedded in the scrotum (not shown), which is padded by the membrane (Tunica dartos). The latter contains a number of myoepithelial cells, which can collectively cause the scrotum to contract and are thus involved in the thermoregulation of the spermatogenesis.

Clinical remarks

Fluid accumulation in the Cavitas serosa scroti is referred to as a **hydrocele.** Cysts within the Proc. vaginalis testis lead to swelling of the Funiculus spermaticus and are referred to as Hydrocele funiculi spermatici.
Retention cysts of the epididymis are called **spermatoceles.** Malformation of the mesorchium (attachment zone of the testis and epididymis) can lead to **testicular torsion** (common in puberty) with restriction of the venous return via the Plexus pampiniformis and

subsequent strangulation of the A. testicularis with risk of aseptic necrosis of the testes.
A back-flow of blood in the Plexus pampiniformis is called a **varicocele,** which in 80 % of all cases occurs on the left side (because the V. testicularis on the left drains into the V. renalis on the left). Causes are often obstacles in drainage, e. g. such as a renal tumour. Varicoceles can lead to infertility.

Development of the inguinal canal

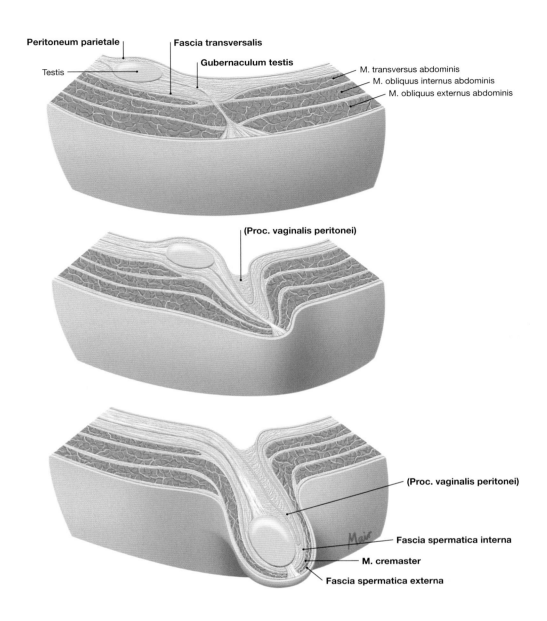

Peritoneum parietale
Fascia transversalis
Gubernaculum testis
Testis
M. transversus abdominis
M. obliquus internus abdominis
M. obliquus externus abdominis

(Proc. vaginalis peritonei)

(Proc. vaginalis peritonei)
Fascia spermatica interna
M. cremaster
Fascia spermatica externa

Fig. 2.167 Descensus testis from the seventh week (post conception) until birth. [S700-L127]
In male embryos during the fetal period, the testes located at the dorsal abdominal wall descend from the abdominal cavity into the scrotum along the lower Gubernaculum testis and below the Peritoneum parietale. The Peritoneum parietale forms a pouch in the inguinal canal (Proc. vaginalis peritonei), which extends into the scrotum and comes to lie on top of the testes. The Proc. vaginalis peritonei obliterates shortly after birth, except for a remnant that persists in close proximity to the testis (Tunica vaginalis testis).

Clinical remarks

The Descensus testis in the scrotum is a sign of fetal maturity at birth. **Disorders of the Descensus testis** occur in approx. 3 % of all newborns. The testicle can remain in the abdominal cavity or in the inguinal canal (testicular retention, cryptorchidism, ectopic testis).

Due to the high ambient temperature (spermatogenesis usually runs at 35 °C), a **testicular ectopy** as fertility problems and an increased risk of malignant degeneration may occur.

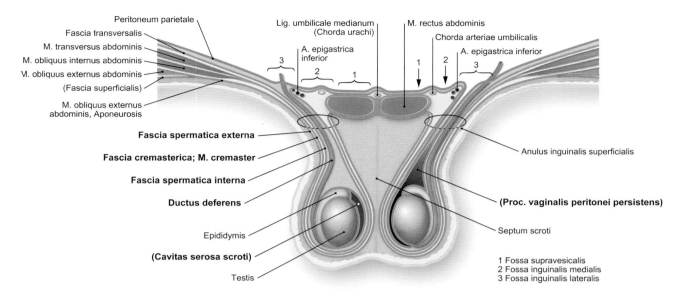

Fig. 2.168   Structure of the abdominal wall and the coverings of the spermatic cord, Funiculus spermaticus, and testes, Testis; schematic representation. For didactic reasons the inguinal canal, the spermatic cord and the scrotum are drawn on the same plane. [S700-L275]/[B500-L240]

The Descensus testis causes the testis to lie in a pouch of the abdominal wall which extends into the scrotum. Thereby the scrotum and spermatic cord have the same structure as the abdominal wall.

The fascia of the M. obliquus externus abdominis continues as the **Fascia spermatica externa** on the Funiculus spermaticus. Underneath it lies the M. cremaster (enveloped by the **Fascia crematerica**) which has separat-

ed from the M. obliquus internus abdominis. Below the M. cremaster lies the **Fascia spermatica interna,** which envelops the contents of the Funiculus spermaticus. As the next layer, the Fascia spermatica interna is a separation from the aponeurosis of the M. transversus abdominis. With the exception of a remnant in the testicular region (Tunica vaginalis testis with Lamina parietalis [periorchium] and Lamina visceralis [epiorchium]), the Proc. vaginalis is obliterated (left side of the image) and has become the **Vestigium processus vaginalis** (a fibrous cord). On the right side of the image, the Pro vaginalis testis is not closed, but persists (Proc. vaginalis peritonei persistens). There is an open connection between the abdominal cavity and Cavitas serosa scroti.

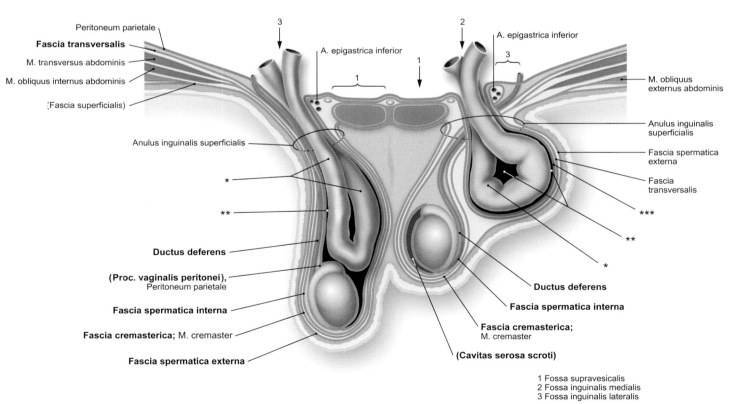

Fig. 2.169   Hernias; schematic representation. Left side of the image: lateral, indirect hernia; right side of the image: medial, direct hernia. [S700-L275]/[B500-L240]

Indirect hernias (canal hernias) enter into the inguinal canal in the Fossa inguinalis lateralis via the Anulus inguinalis profundus.

Direct inguinal hernias penetrate through the muscle-free Trigonum inguinale (HESSELBACH's triangle) into the Fossa inguinalis medialis,

which is a weak spot in the abdominal wall. Here, the posterior abdominal wall consists only of the Fascia transversalis and Peritoneum parietale (Paries dorsalis tenuis canalis inguinalis).

*   intestinal loop in the hernial sac
**   peritoneal space
*** newly formed peritoneal hernial sac

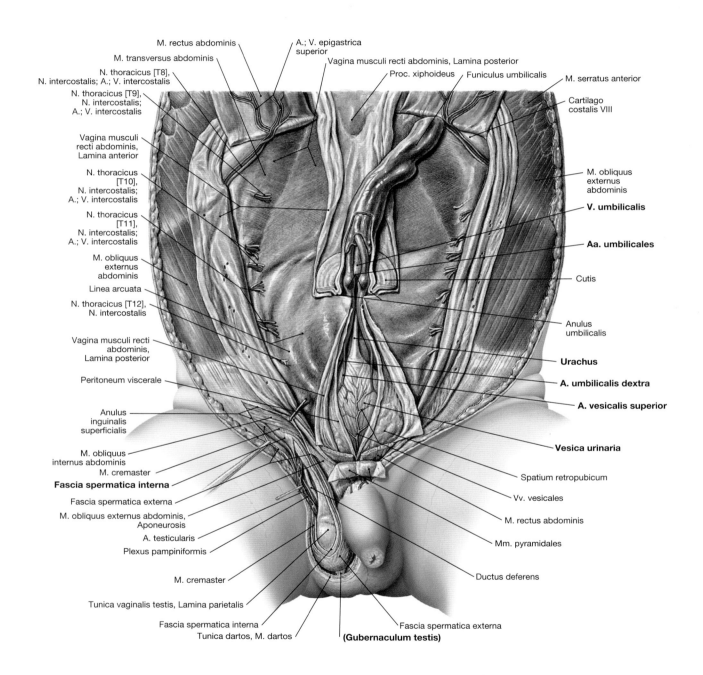

M. rectus abdominis

M. transversus abdominis

N. thoracicus [T8],
N. intercostalis; A.; V. intercostalis

N. thoracicus [T9],
N. intercostalis;
A.; V. intercostalis

Vagina musculi
recti abdominis,
Lamina anterior

N. thoracicus
[T10],
N. intercostalis;
A.; V. intercostalis

N. thoracicus
[T11],
N. intercostalis;
A.; V. intercostalis

M. obliquus
externus
abdominis

Linea arcuata

N. thoracicus [T12],
N. intercostalis

Vagina musculi recti
abdominis,
Lamina posterior

Peritoneum viscerale

Anulus
inguinalis
superficialis

M. obliquus
internus abdominis

M. cremaster

Fascia spermatica interna

Fascia spermatica externa

M. obliquus externus abdominis,
Aponeurosis

A. testicularis

Plexus pampiniformis

M. cremaster

Tunica vaginalis testis, Lamina parietalis

Fascia spermatica interna

Tunica dartos, M. dartos

A.; V. epigastrica
superior

Vagina musculi recti abdominis, Lamina posterior

Proc. xiphoideus

Funiculus umbilicalis

M. serratus anterior

Cartilago
costalis VIII

M. obliquus
externus
abdominis

V. umbilicalis

Aa. umbilicales

Cutis

Anulus
umbilicalis

Urachus

A. umbilicalis dextra

A. vesicalis superior

Vesica urinaria

Spatium retropubicum

Vv. vesicales

M. rectus abdominis

Mm. pyramidales

Ductus deferens

Fascia spermatica externa

(Gubernaculum testis)

Fig. 2.170 Anterior abdominal wall of a newborn; the Mm. recti abdominis are folded back cranially; the abdominal cavity is opened in the median plane along with the umbilical cord; on the right side the inguinal canal is prepared. [S700]

The Fascia spermatica externa is secured via remnants of the Gubernaculum testis to the base of the scrotum sac. In the area of the opened abdominal cavity up to the navel you can see the bladder with the urachus and the umbilical cord blood vessels.

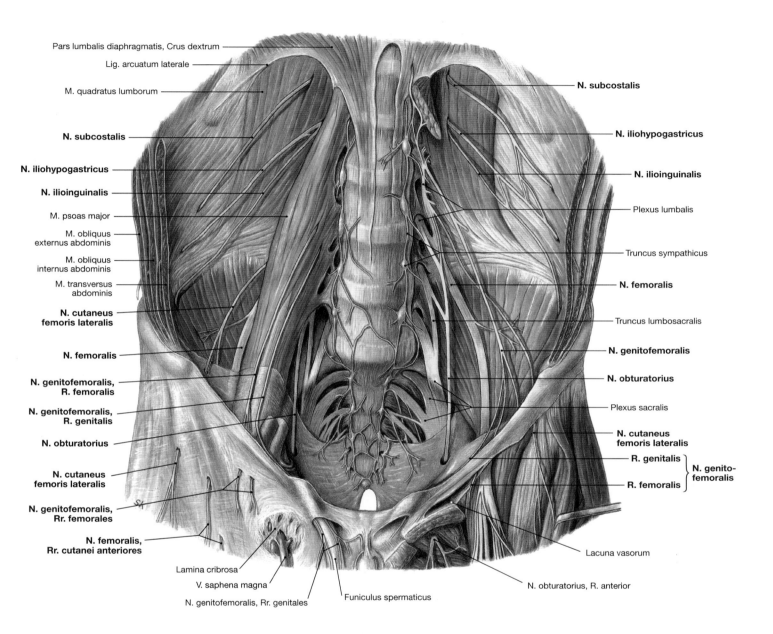

Pars lumbalis diaphragmatis, Crus dextrum

Lig. arcuatum laterale

M. quadratus lumborum

N. subcostalis

N. iliohypogastricus

N. ilioinguinalis

M. psoas major

M. obliquus externus abdominis

M. obliquus internus abdominis

M. transversus abdominis

N. cutaneus femoris lateralis

N. femoralis

N. genitofemoralis, R. femoralis

N. genitofemoralis, R. genitalis

N. obturatorius

N. cutaneus femoris lateralis

N. genitofemoralis, Rr. femorales

N. femoralis, Rr. cutanei anteriores

Lamina cribrosa

V. saphena magna

N. genitofemoralis, Rr. genitales

Funiculus spermaticus

N. subcostalis

N. iliohypogastricus

N. ilioinguinalis

Plexus lumbalis

Truncus sympathicus

N. femoralis

Truncus lumbosacralis

N. genitofemoralis

N. obturatorius

Plexus sacralis

N. cutaneus femoris lateralis

R. genitalis ⎫ N. genito-
R. femoralis ⎬ femoralis

Lacuna vasorum

N. obturatorius, R. anterior

Fig. 2.171 Posterior abdominal wall with Plexus lumbosacralis; ventral view. [S700-L238]

The Plexus lumbosacralis consists of the Plexus lumbalis (T12, L1–L3 [L4]) and the Plexus sacralis ([L4] L5, S1–S5). The Plexus lumbalis is important for the innervation of the wall of the trunk. The illustration shows the segmented exit points and the pathway of the **Rr. anteriores [ventrales] of the spinal nerves of the Plexus lumbalis,** which innervate the abdominal muscles, the inguinal region and the thigh. Cranially to caudally, these are the Nn. subcostalis (intercostalis XII), iliohypogastricus (T12, L1), ilioinguinalis (L1), genitofemoralis (L1, L2) with the R. femoralis and R. genitalis, and the N. cutaneus femoris lateralis (L2, L3). In addition, you can see the exit of the N. femoralis (L1–L4), which after crossing through the Lacuna musculorum, provides Rr. cutanei anteriores for skin innervation on the thigh, and also the N. obturatorius ([L1] L2–L4), which enters the Canalis obturatorius.

→ T 42

195

Sample exam questions

To check that you are completely familiar with the content of this chapter, sample questions from an oral anatomy exam are listed here.

Explain the structure of a vertebra:

- How do the vertebrae of the different sections of the spine differ from each other?
- What are the characteristics of the first and second cervical vertebrae?
- Which ligaments stabilise the spine and how are the cervical spine and skull connected to each other?
- Which movements can be carried out in the spine between two vertebrae and in general?
- What is meant by a motion segment?
- Which muscles are instrumental to the movements of the spine?

Explain the structure of the thoracic wall:

- Which structures must be pierced during a pleural puncture?
- What must be taken into account during a pleural puncture from an anatomical point of view?
- What is the course of the intercostal muscles and what are their functions?

Explain the structure of the abdominal wall:

- How is the rectus sheath formed?
- Where are the weak points?
- What functions do the straight and oblique abdominal muscles have?
- What passes into the abdominal wall folds?

Explain the structure of the diaphragm:

- What points of penetration do you know and what passes through them?
- Which weak spots do you know?
- What is meant by the quadratus lumborum?
- What nerves innervate the diaphragm?

Explain the blood supply in the area of the thoracic and abdominal wall:

- What arterial connections exist between the upper and lower halves of the body?

- What is meant by a vertical and horizontal bypass circulation?
- Can you name the types of cavocaval anastomoses?
- Which blood vessels run on the inside of the thoracic and abdominal wall and communicate with each other?

Explain the construction of the neck muscles and their localised structures:

- What are the short neck muscles called?
- What is meant by the vertebralis triangle?
- What are the nerves of the neck called?

Explain the structure of the epidural space:

- How is a spinal nerve structured?
- What structures are in the Foramen intervertebrale?
- To what structures do you have to pay attention in a lumbar puncture?

Specify the location and structure of the Mamma:

- What is the milk line and where does it run?
- Why is the female breast divided into quadrants?
- Name local lymph node groups in the area of the Mamma.
- From a clinical, topographical and oncosurgical viewpoint, lymph nodes of the female breast are divided into levels. Which are these and what acts as the boundary?

Explain the difference between the dermatome and the HEAD's zone:

- Can you name characteristic dermatomes on the ventral trunk wall?
- Show the HEAD's zone which is assigned to the heart. What is meant by referred pain?

Explain the structure of the inguinal canal:

- What structures run through the inguinal canal?
- How is the inguinal canal confined?
- What is the Proc. vaginalis peritonei and what happens if it does not obliterate? Explain the Descensus testis.
- What is meant by an indirect inguinal hernia, and direct?

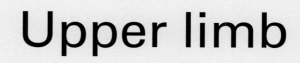

Upper limb

Surface. 200

Development. 202

Skeleton. 204

Musculature. 236

Neurovascular pathways 276

Topography 308

Cross-sectional images. 338

3

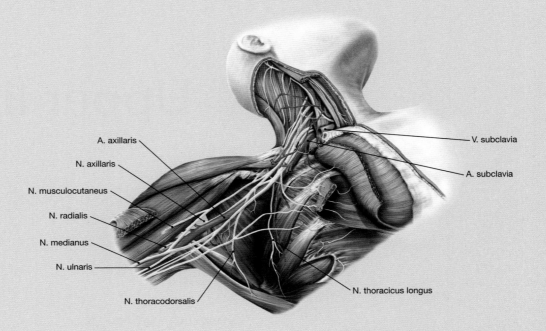

A. axillaris
N. axillaris
N. musculocutaneus
N. radialis
N. medianus
N. ulnaris
N. thoracodorsalis
V. subclavia
A. subclavia
N. thoracicus longus

Overview

The **upper limb** includes the **shoulder girdle and arm.** The shoulder girdle consists of the clavicle and the shoulder blade on each side. The arm is subdivided by joints into the upper arm, forearm and hand. The shoulder girdle and thus the whole upper limb are only anchored by the medial clavicular joint directly at the torso.

In contrast to the lower limb, which is a running and support organ, the upper limb is a **tactile and grasping organ.** In its evolutionary development, its range of motion has significantly increased. Because the wrists work together with the bones of the forearm to make a turning movement, the hand's freedom of motion increased considerably. Other features are the **differentiated mobility of the individual fin-**

gers and the **opposition** of the thumb, which enables the grasping function and is unique in its efficiency.

The muscles of the upper limb are innervated by a **nerve plexus (Plexus brachialis),** fed mainly via the spinal nerves from the spinal cord segments C5–T1. Various nerves for the shoulder and arm come from the Plexus brachialis. The blood vessels that supply the arm are the **A. and V. subclavia** and their downstream vascular branches. To a large extent the lymphatic vessels run in conjunction with the veins and are connected to the **axillary lymph nodes,** which also drain the thoracic or chest wall, including the mammary gland.

Main topics

After working through this chapter, you should be able to:

- name the basic principles of limb development and the clinically relevant variations and malformations;
- describe the bony structures of the shoulder girdle and arm as well as their joints, along with the range of motion on a skeleton;
- explain the course of the ligaments on the joints, as well as the origin, insertion (attachment) and function of all muscles of the shoulder girdle and arm, and to show these on a skeleton or dissection. With regard to the hand muscles, it is often sufficient to describe the basic principles of their course and function as well as their innervation;
- describe the arrangement of the Plexus brachialis, to show its structures on the dissection and to explain the symptoms associated with plexus lesions;
- name the functions and dysfunctions of the shoulder nerves;
- describe the pathway, function and precise symptoms associated with a lesion of the major nerves in the arm and to show these on the dissection;

- identify all arteries of the upper limb on the dissection;
- explain the vascular anastomoses of the shoulder and upper arm region;
- understand the basic principle of the venous flow in the upper limb;
- name the large epifascial veins and show them on the dissection;
- explain the principles of the lymph flow in the upper limb;
- explain the axillary lymph node stations and their clinical relevance;
- specify the neurovascular pathways, which cross the MOHRENHEIM's fossa;
- name the borders of the axillary spaces, to describe the penetrating structures and locate them on the dissection;
- explain the route of the neurovascular pathways in the cubital fossa;
- explain the construction and penetrating structures of the carpal tunnel and of the GUYON's canal.

Clinical reference

In order not to lose touch with prospective everyday clinical life with so many anatomical details, the following describes a typical case that shows why the content of this chapter is so important.

Brachial plexus lesion

Case study
Riding his motorbike, a 20-year-old man crashed into a crash barrier. He is found at the side of the road and is dazed but responsive. He is wearing motorbike clothing and does not seem to have any obvious external injuries. He is stabilised on a vacuum stretcher with a cervical collar to reduce the risk of displacing broken bones and damaging the spinal cord, and is transported to a hospital.

Result of examination
The patient is conscious, and alert and oriented. He has severe pain in different parts which relates to bruises (contusions) and abrasions of the skin. His heart rate (100/min), respiratory rate (25/min) and blood pressure (140/100 mmHg) are slightly increased.

Diagnostic procedure
Apart from contusions and skin abrasions found during the examination, the computerised tomography (CT) image shows no additional evidence of broken bones (fractures) or internal injuries. After the injuries have been bandaged, all joints are examined the next day, including measuring their movement from a neutral starting position, the neutral- zero-method. It thereby appears that the patient is unable to raise his right arm (abduct) or to flex the elbow joint (→ Fig. a). The right arm hangs down limply; the palm is turned outward towards the back, i.e. the shoulder is rotated inward. Movements of the hand and fingers are not affected. The touch sensation has been lost in a band-shaped area extending from the outside of the shoulder across the lateral forearm down to the thumb (dermatomes C5–C6). A magnetic resonance image (MRI) of the right shoulder is carried out. It shows that the spinal nerve roots of the spinal cord segments C5 and C6 have been torn away (avulsion) at their exit point from the spinal cord.

Diagnosis
Lesion of the Plexus brachialis (ERB's palsy) (→ Fig. b).

Treatment
Initially the neurosurgeons secure the torn-off (avulsed) nerve roots by suturing the surrounding connective tissue. In the setting of a scientific study, this surgical procedure is combined with the local application of a nerve growth factor (NGF) to accelerate the growth of nerve fibres. Physiotherapy is initiated in the days following the operation. After months of intense training, the patient regains limited arm movement.

Further developments
Limited functionality of the elbow joint can be restored but sensory impairment persists in the forearm and thumb.

Dissection lab
The Plexus brachialis is one of the most complex structures presenting in the dissection lab. Only after extensively studying it by using an anatomy atlas can it be dissected and explained (→ Fig. 3.102): The **Plexus brachialis** is formed by anterior branches (rami) of the spinal nerves. The nerves of the lower cervical and the upper thoracic segments (C5–T1) supply the plexus. The anterior branches of the spinal nerves combine initially to form **three trunks (trunci)** that run between the deep cervical muscles (Mm. scaleni) through the **scalene hiatus** to reach the axilla. There they form **three fascicles** surrounding the A. axillaris.

 It is advisable to study the origins of the nerves extensively in the dissection lab – otherwise it is easy to lose sight of the bigger picture!

The individual nerves then emerge from the trunci and fascicles. The cranial spinal cord segments (C5, C6) supply the proximal shoulder muscles and the corresponding skin regions via **short nerves.** The caudal segments (C8, T1) supply the forearm and hand via long nerves. The **N. musculocutaneus** activates the flexors of the elbow joint in the upper arm and forms the lateral cutaneous nerve of the forearm. The flexors in the forearm are innervated by the **N. medianus and N. ulnaris** (from the medial fascicle). The extensor muscles are controlled by the **N. radialis** (posterior fascicle).

 The Plexus brachialis is a good reference point because the nerves form an 'M'!

Back to the clinic
The symptoms show that a mixed motor and sensory lesion causes the loss of function. Considering the dysfunctions of all affected muscles and skin areas, the losses can be attributed to the spinal cord segments C5–C6. Therefore, it is likely that hitting the crash barrier caused the shoulder to be pulled downwards, leading to an avulsion of the upper nerve roots of the Plexus brachialis. Hence, the diagnosis is ERB's palsy, an upper plexus lesion.

 This is a frequent exam question as part of the anatomy of the Plexus brachialis!

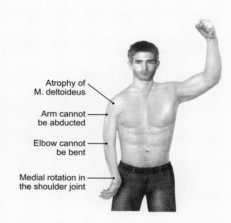

Atrophy of
M. deltoideus

Arm cannot
be abducted

Elbow cannot
be bent

Medial rotation in
the shoulder joint

Fig. a Clinical picture of an upper Plexus brachialis lesion (ERB's palsy). [S700-L238]

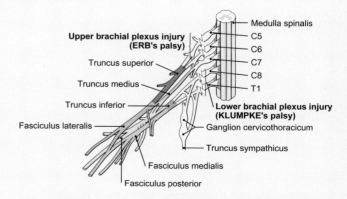

Medulla spinalis
Upper brachial plexus injury (ERB's palsy)
C5
C6
Truncus superior
C7
Truncus medius
C8
T1
Truncus inferior
Lower brachial plexus injury (KLUMPKE's palsy)
Fasciculus lateralis
Ganglion cervicothoracicum
Truncus sympathicus
Fasciculus medialis
Fasciculus posterior

Fig. b Lesions of the Plexus brachialis, types of spinal nerve lesions, right side; frontal view. [S700-L126]

Surface anatomy

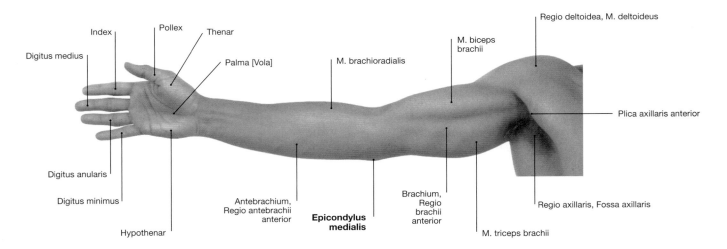

Index | Pollex | Thenar
Digitus medius
Palma [Vola]
M. brachioradialis
M. biceps brachii
Regio deltoidea, M. deltoideus

Plica axillaris anterior

Digitus anularis

Digitus minimus

Hypothenar

Antebrachium, Regio antebrachii anterior

Epicondylus medialis

Brachium, Regio brachii anterior

Regio axillaris, Fossa axillaris

M. triceps brachii

a

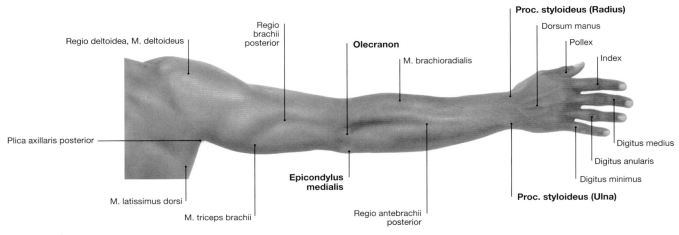

Regio deltoidea, M. deltoideus

Regio brachii posterior

Olecranon

M. brachioradialis

Proc. styloideus (Radius)

Dorsum manus

Pollex

Index

Plica axillaris posterior

Digitus medius

Digitus anularis

Digitus minimus

Epicondylus medialis

M. latissimus dorsi

M. triceps brachii

Regio antebrachii posterior

Proc. styloideus (Ulna)

b

Fig. 3.1a and b   Surface anatomy of the arm, right side. [S700]
a Ventral view.
b Dorsal view.

Clinical remarks

The surface anatomy of the arm is determined by the muscles and by some of the skeletal elements. The palpable **bony landmarks** (shown in bold in the figure) facilitate orientation during the physical examination.

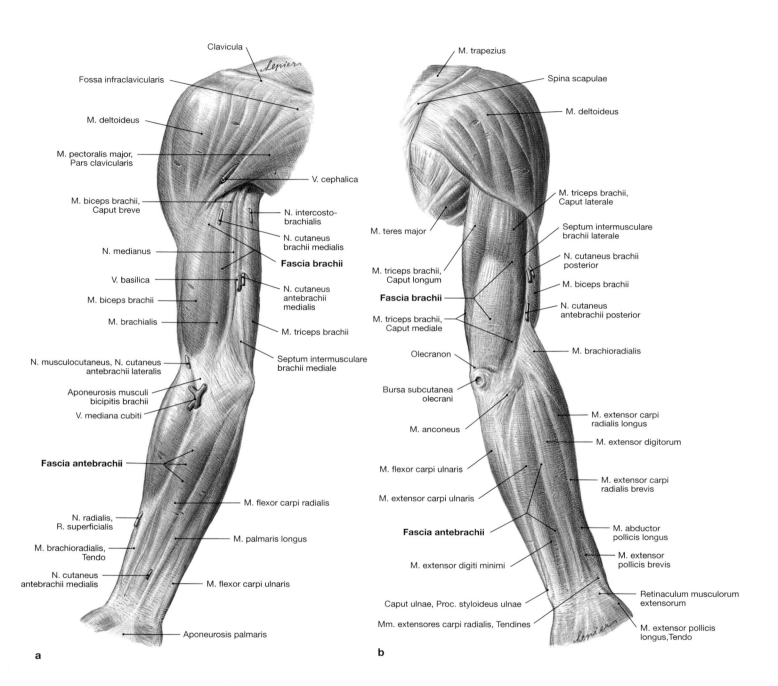

Clavicula

Fossa infraclavicularis

M. deltoideus

M. pectoralis major,
Pars clavicularis

M. biceps brachii,
Caput breve

N. medianus

V. basilica

M. biceps brachii

M. brachialis

N. musculocutaneus, N. cutaneus
antebrachii lateralis

Aponeurosis musculi
bicipitis brachii

V. mediana cubiti

Fascia antebrachii

N. radialis,
R. superficialis

M. brachioradialis,
Tendo

N. cutaneus
antebrachii medialis

V. cephalica

N. intercosto-
brachialis

N. cutaneus
brachii medialis

Fascia brachii

N. cutaneus
antebrachii
medialis

M. triceps brachii

Septum intermusculare
brachii mediale

M. flexor carpi radialis

M. palmaris longus

M. flexor carpi ulnaris

Aponeurosis palmaris

a

M. trapezius

Spina scapulae

M. deltoideus

M. triceps brachii,
Caput laterale

Septum intermusculare
brachii laterale

N. cutaneus brachii
posterior

M. biceps brachii

N. cutaneus
antebrachii posterior

M. brachioradialis

M. extensor carpi
radialis longus

M. extensor digitorum

M. extensor carpi
radialis brevis

M. abductor
pollicis longus

M. extensor
pollicis brevis

Retinaculum musculorum
extensorum

M. extensor pollicis
longus, Tendo

M. teres major

M. triceps brachii,
Caput longum

Fascia brachii

M. triceps brachii,
Caput mediale

Olecranon

Bursa subcutanea
olecrani

M. anconeus

M. flexor carpi ulnaris

M. extensor carpi ulnaris

Fascia antebrachii

M. extensor digiti minimi

Caput ulnae, Proc. styloideus ulnae

Mm. extensores carpi radialis, Tendines

b

**Fig. 3.2a and b   Fascia of the upper arm, Fascia brachii, and of the
forearm, Fascia antebrachii, right side.** [S700]
a Ventral view.
b Dorsal view.
The surface anatomy is determined primarily by the individual muscles.
They are covered with their own fasciae and form part of muscle

groups. These are covered by a shared common fascia, the fascia of the
upper arm and the forearm, which lies underneath the subcutis of the
skin. During dissection, after exposing all important subcutaneous
structures such as the cutaneous nerves and epifascial veins, the subcutaneous adipose tissue is removed completely to expose the outer
layer of fascia.

Upper limb

Development

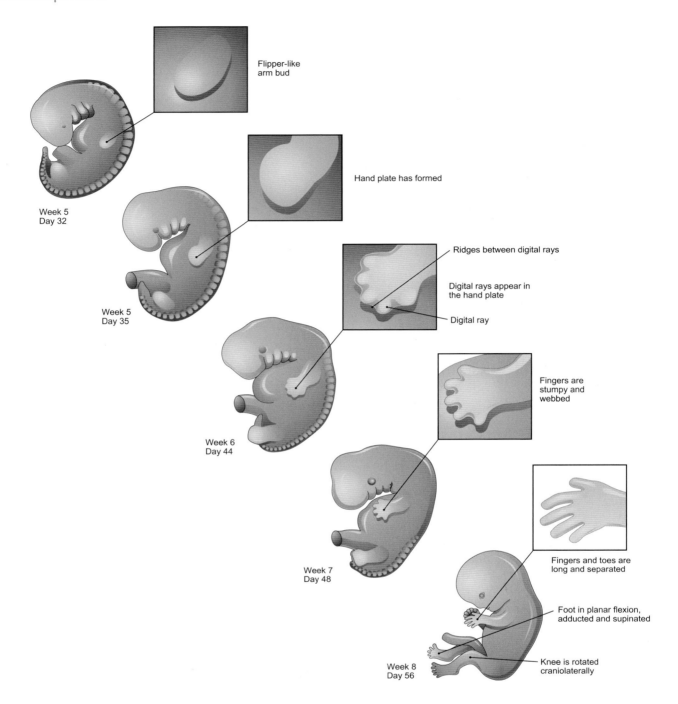

Flipper-like
arm bud

Hand plate has formed

Week 5
Day 32

Week 5
Day 35

Ridges between digital rays

Digital rays appear in
the hand plate

Digital ray

Week 6
Day 44

Fingers are
stumpy and
webbed

Fingers and toes are
long and separated

Week 7
Day 48

Foot in planar flexion,
adducted and supinated

Week 8
Day 56

Knee is rotated
craniolaterally

Fig. 3.3 Development of the limbs in week 5–8; schematic drawing. [E347-009]

The **limbs** begin to develop from **week 4.** The flipper-like **arm buds** form on day **26–27** and therefore two days earlier than the leg buds. At this time, the primordial limbs consist of a mesenchymal core of connective tissue, originating from the mesodermal somatopleura as well as a superficial ectodermal layer which later forms the epidermis of the skin (→ Fig. 3.4). The ectoderm at the distal edge of the limb buds (ectodermal marginal ridge) produces growth factors which attract precursors of muscle cells from the somites of the mesoderm in the trunk. In **week 5–6** the limb buds show signs of a **segmentation** in the primor-

dial arms and legs. From week 6 the digital rays separate from each other as a result of the programmed cell death (apoptosis) in the interpositioned tissue. By the **end of week 8** the **fingers and toes** are completely separated.

In contrast to the primordial arms, the **primordial legs in week 8** undergo a rotation, leading to a **craniolateral orientation of the knee.** This leads to the extensor muscles of the upper and lower leg lying ventrally, whereas they lie on the dorsal side on the arm. In addition, **in week 8 the foot** initially becomes **plantarflexed, adducted** and **supinated.** This foot position is generally reversed by week 11.

Clinical remarks

A **congenital clubfoot** is the most common malformation (or deformity) of the extremities. The foot is hereby fixed in plantar flexion and supination. It is therefore assumed that this deformity is caused

by the failure of the reversal of the physiological foot position of the embryo in weeks 8 to 11.

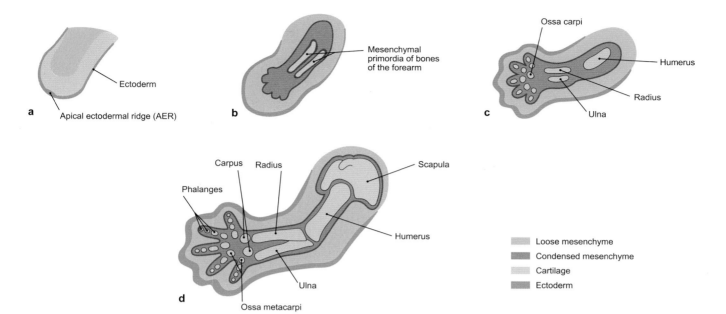

Fig. 3.4a–d Development of the cartilaginous precursors of the bones of the upper limbs in weeks 4–8; schematic longitudinal sections. [E347-009]

a In **week 4** the primordial limbs consist of a mesenchymal core of connective tissue and a layer of superficial ectoderm, that later forms the epidermis of the skin.

b The mesenchyme condenses so that – between **week 4 and week 6** on the arm and between **week 6 and week 8** on the leg – a **cartilaginous skeleton** develops as a precursor to bone. This process advances from proximal to distal.

c In this cartilaginous skeleton, nuclei or ossification centres form, which initiate the ossification and thus the conversion of the cartilaginous skeleton into bony tissue **(endochondral ossification) from week 7.**

d The ossification progresses in a specific pattern (→ Fig. 1.27).

- **Up to week 12, ossification centres (nuclei)** can be found in all bones of the upper limb, apart from the wrist. The ossification centres of the **wrist** emerge only after birth (postnatally) between the **first and eighth year of life.** An exception is the clavicle, which emerges from **week 7** without a cartilaginous precursor and thus derives directly from the mesenchyme **(desmal ossification).**
- The ossification of the lower limb is a little delayed. While the first ossification centres in the femur and leg bones emerge as early as in **week 8,** the ossification centres in the phalanges only follow between **week 9** and the **sixth month.** The tarsal bones (first to fourth year of life) and the pelvic girdle (sometimes up to the 20th year) ossify postnatally.

The **closure of the epiphyseal gaps** which signifies the completion of the longitudinal growth of the limbs, takes place at the age of **14 to 25 years,** but in most of the bones by **21 years.**

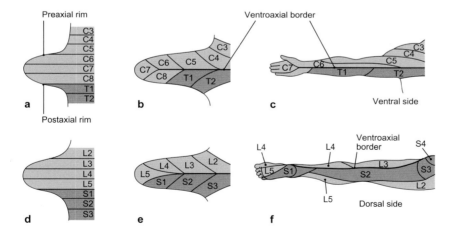

Fig. 3.5a–f Development of the dermatomes in the limb regions. [E347-009]

Sensory innervation of certain cutaneous areas is supplied by a single spinal cord segment (dermatome). In contrast to the belt-like orientation of the dermatomes on the torso, the dermatomes on the limbs in-

itially run in an almost longitudinal direction **(a, d),** following an increasingly oblique direction later in the development (→ Fig. 3.108 and → Fig. 4.145). Arms and legs show a ventroaxial border **(b, c, e, f)** with hardly any overlap of the individual areas with sensory innervation.

Clinical remarks

Looking at how the ossification **(bone age)** progresses, the future growth pattern and adult height of children can be predicted by means of X-ray examinations. In X-ray examinations to exclude broken bones (fractures), it must be taken into consideration that the

bones of children may in part still consist of ossification centres (nuclei) which have not yet been ossified or fused. Therefore the bones are not fractured.

Skeleton

Skeleton of the upper limb

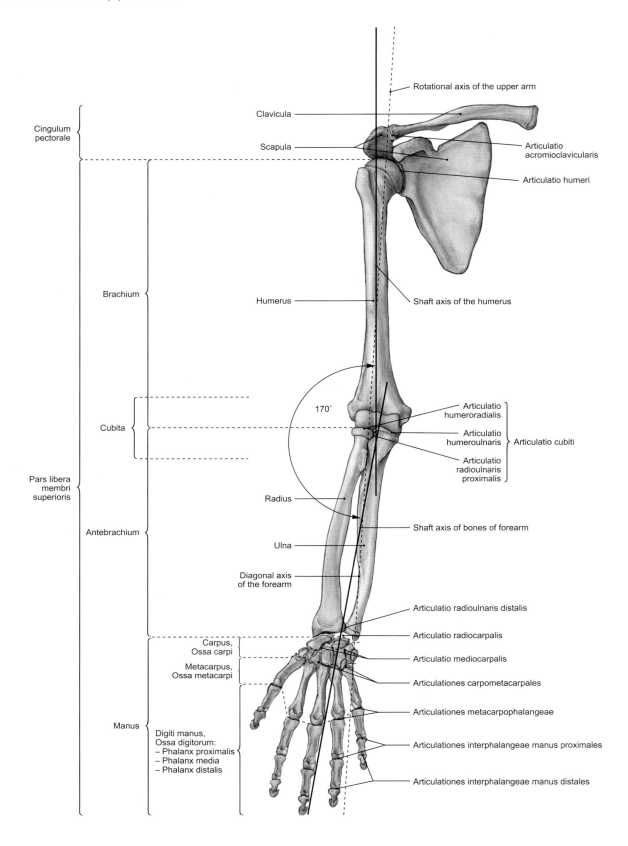

Cingulum pectorale

Brachium

Cubita

Pars libera membri superioris

Antebrachium

Manus

Rotational axis of the upper arm

Clavicula

Scapula

Articulatio acromioclavicularis

Articulatio humeri

Shaft axis of the humerus

Humerus

170°

Articulatio humeroradialis

Articulatio humeroulnaris

Articulatio cubiti

Articulatio radioulnaris proximalis

Radius

Shaft axis of bones of forearm

Ulna

Diagonal axis of the forearm

Articulatio radioulnaris distalis

Articulatio radiocarpalis

Carpus, Ossa carpi

Articulatio mediocarpalis

Metacarpus, Ossa metacarpi

Articulationes carpometacarpales

Articulationes metacarpophalangeae

Digiti manus, Ossa digitorum:
– Phalanx proximalis
– Phalanx media
– Phalanx distalis

Articulationes interphalangeae manus proximales

Articulationes interphalangeae manus distales

Fig. 3.6 Bones and joints of the upper limb, Membrum superius, right side; ventral view. [S700]
Similar to the leg, the bones of the upper arm and forearm form a **carrying angle** of 170°, open to the lateral side, which is divided in half by the transverse axis of the elbow joint. The rotational axis of the upper arm in the shoulder joint corresponds to the connecting line between the humeral head and elbow joint. It extends as the diagonal axis of the forearm from the proximal to the distal joint between the bones of the forearm (radioulnar joints). The turning or rotational movements (pronation/supination) of the forearm take place around this axis.

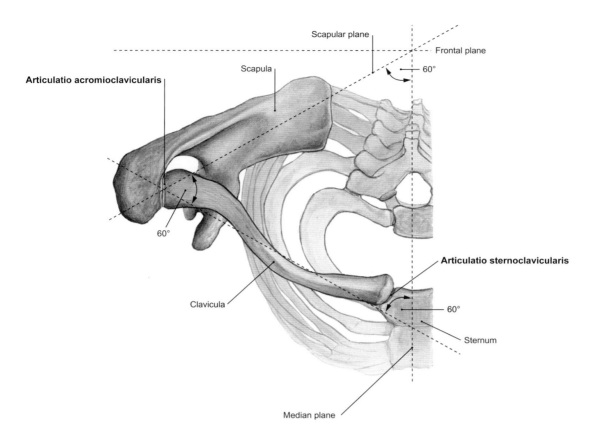

Fig. 3.7 Shoulder girdle, Cingulum pectorale, right side; cranial view. [S700]
The shoulder girdle consists of the **clavicle** (Clavicula) and the **shoulder blade** (scapula). Both bones are connected in the lateral clavicular joint (Articulatio acromioclavicularis). The clavicle articulates via the medial clavicular joint (Articulatio sternoclavicularis) with the axial skeleton.

The clavicle forms an angle of approx. 60° with both the median plane and the shoulder blade (scapular plane), respectively. The shoulder blade is positioned in the scapular plane, which again has an angle of 60° to the median plane.

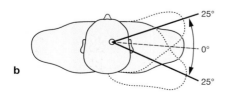

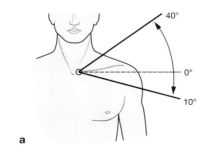

Fig. 3.8a and b   Range of movements in the shoulder girdle starting from the medial clavicular joint. [S700-L126]/[G1061]
a Elevation and depression.
b Protraction and retraction.
Both clavicular joints form functional **ball-and-socket joints,** which mostly act as a functional unit as the shoulder girdle is only connected to the axial skeleton in the medial clavicular joint. In addition to forward and backward movements (protraction and retraction), a slight lowering (depression) and a relatively substantial lifting (elevation) of the shoulder is possible. The fixed sternal end of the clavicle allows a rotation of about 45°. The range of movement of the upper limb is significantly increased by the mobility of the shoulder girdle.
Range of movements of the shoulder girdle:
- Elevation–depression: 40°–0°–10°
- Protraction–retraction: 25°–0°–25°

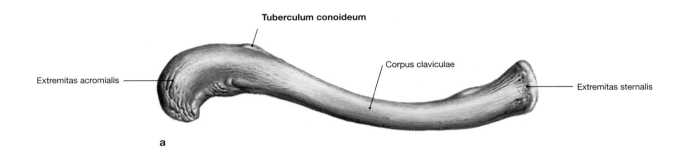

Tuberculum conoideum

Corpus claviculae

Extremitas acromialis

Extremitas sternalis

a

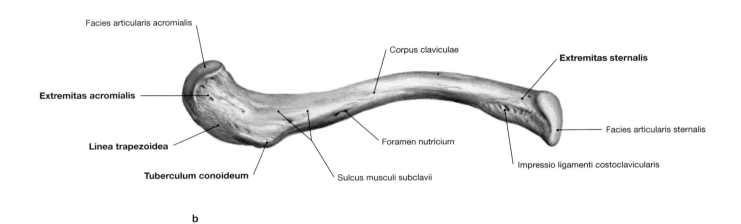

Facies articularis acromialis

Corpus claviculae

Extremitas sternalis

Extremitas acromialis

Facies articularis sternalis

Linea trapezoidea

Foramen nutricium

Tuberculum conoideum

Sulcus musculi subclavii

Impressio ligamenti costoclavicularis

b

Fig. 3.9a and b   Clavicle, Clavicula, right side. [S700]
a Cranial view. Matching an isolated clavicle to one side of the body is seldom easy. It should be noted that the Extremitas sternalis is rather clumsily designed, while the Extremitas acromialis is flat and elongated. On the skeleton, the convexity at the sternal end is directed ventrally.

b Caudal view. On the underside of the bone there are two distinctive apophyses, onto which both parts of the Lig. coracoclaviculare are attached (→ Fig. 3.21). The **Tuberculum conoideum lies medially,** the Linea trapezoidea lies laterally.

Clinical remarks

Of all the bones in the arm, the clavicle is most prone to fractures. Clavicular fractures frequently occur when falling onto an outstretched arm or directly onto the shoulder.
a The fracture is most often located in the middle third of the clavicle at the transition from the concave lateral to the convex medial part. [S701-L231]
b On physical examination, a conspicuous swelling may be visible (arrow). The arm cannot be raised and hangs loosely because the patient cannot bear the weight of the arm. [G721]
c The X-ray image of the shoulder shows the fracture. The medial bone segment of the clavicle points upward (above the arrow) where a bony fragment has formed (arrow). [G305]

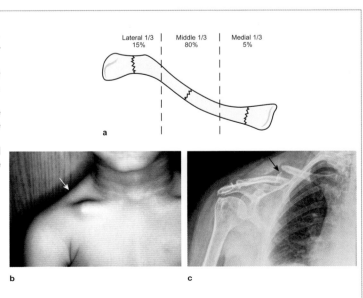

Lateral 1/3
15%

Middle 1/3
80%

Medial 1/3
5%

a

b

c

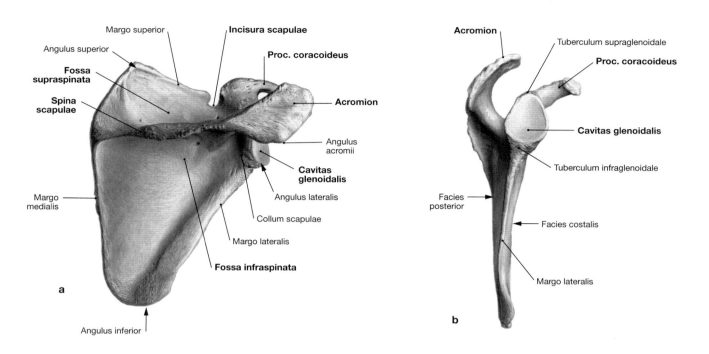

Margo superior
Angulus superior
Fossa supraspinata
Spina scapulae
Incisura scapulae
Proc. coracoideus
Acromion
Angulus acromii
Cavitas glenoidalis
Angulus lateralis
Collum scapulae
Margo lateralis
Fossa infraspinata
Margo medialis
Angulus inferior

a

Acromion
Tuberculum supraglenoidale
Proc. coracoideus
Cavitas glenoidalis
Tuberculum infraglenoidale
Facies posterior
Facies costalis
Margo lateralis

b

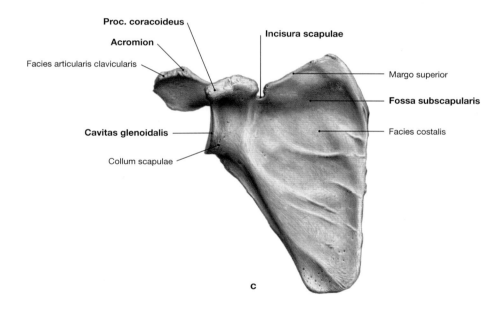

Proc. coracoideus
Acromion
Facies articularis clavicularis
Incisura scapulae
Margo superior
Fossa subscapularis
Facies costalis
Cavitas glenoidalis
Collum scapulae

c

Fig. 3.10a–c   Shoulder blade, Scapula, right side. [S700]
a Dorsal view. The shoulder blade is a flat bone with three edges and three angles. The dorsal T-shaped protrusion of the Spina scapulae serves as an important apophysis for the attachment (origin and insertion) of muscles.

b Lateral view.
c Ventral view.

Clinical remarks

The **N. suprascapularis** passes through the **Incisura scapulae,** which is bridged by the Lig. transversum scapulae superius (→ Fig. 3.21). With ossification of the ligament, a **compression** of the nerve may occur and result in a weakening of its target muscles (M. supraspinatus and M. infraspinatus), which are important for the abduction and lateral rotation of the arm.

Humerus

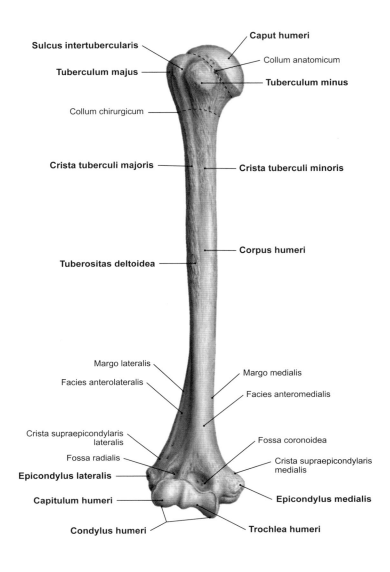

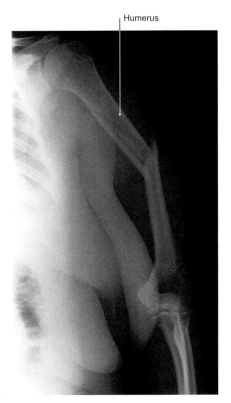

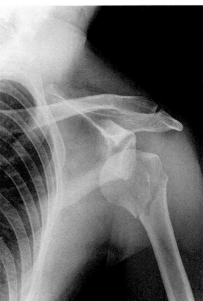

Humerus

Fig. 3.11 Bone of the upper arm, Humerus, right side; ventral view. [S700]

Along with the axis of the shaft, the head of the humerus forms an angle of 150°–180° **(collodiaphyseal angle).** In addition, the head shows a **retrotorsion** of 15°–30°, i.e. the neck of the humerus is rotated backwards in relation to the transverse axis of the distal condyles. In the proximal part of the shaft, the Tuberculum majus is located laterally and the Tuberculum minus medially.

Fig. 3.12a and b X-ray images of humeral fractures.
a Humeral shaft fracture left, which can lead to an injury of the N. radialis. [E402]
b Humeral head fracture left, at the Collum chirurgicum, can lead to an injury of the N. axillaris. [R234]

Labels on Fig. 3.11:
- Sulcus intertubercularis
- Tuberculum majus
- Collum chirurgicum
- Crista tuberculi majoris
- Tuberositas deltoidea
- Margo lateralis
- Facies anterolateralis
- Crista supraepicondylaris lateralis
- Fossa radialis
- Epicondylus lateralis
- Capitulum humeri
- Condylus humeri
- Caput humeri
- Collum anatomicum
- Tuberculum minus
- Crista tuberculi minoris
- Corpus humeri
- Margo medialis
- Facies anteromedialis
- Fossa coronoidea
- Crista supraepicondylaris medialis
- Epicondylus medialis
- Trochlea humeri

— Clinical remarks ——

Broken bones (fractures) and **dislocations** (luxations) leading to malalignments of the skeletal elements can be verified with an X-ray.

Injuries to ligaments, however, are not visible and can only be detected with ultrasound or magnetic resonance imaging (MRI).

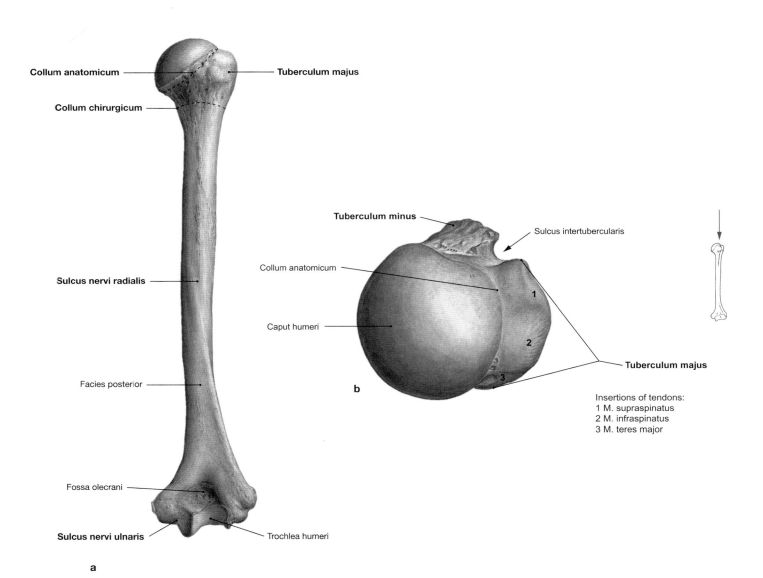

Collum anatomicum — Tuberculum majus

Collum chirurgicum

Tuberculum minus — Sulcus intertubercularis

Collum anatomicum

Sulcus nervi radialis

Caput humeri

1

2

Facies posterior

3

Tuberculum majus

b

Insertions of tendons:
1 M. supraspinatus
2 M. infraspinatus
3 M. teres major

Fossa olecrani

Sulcus nervi ulnaris — Trochlea humeri

a

Fig. 3.13a and b   Bone of the upper arm, Humerus, right side.
[S700]
a Dorsal view.
In a spiral manner, the **Sulcus nervi radialis** winds around the dorsal side of the humeral shaft which contains the N. radialis. At the posterior

side of the Epicondylus medialis, inside the **Sulcus nervi ulnaris,** lies the N. ulnaris, which can be mechanically stimulated on impact ('funny bone').
b Proximal view.

Clinical remarks

Fractures of the humerus due to a fall are relatively common. In the case of **proximal fractures,** the **supplying blood vessels** (Aa. circumflexae humeri anterior and posterior) and the N. axillaris (→ Fig. 3.116, → Fig. 3.117, → Fig. 3.118), which are looped around the humerus, may become damaged. In the case of fractures or surgical treatment of fractures in the **shaft area,** the N. radialis can be dam-

aged, resulting in clinical signs of a **radial nerve lesion** (→ Fig. 3.122). In this location, it can also be compressed (**'park bench position'**). **Distal fractures** may cause **damage to the ulnar nerve** in the Sulcus nervi ulnaris (→ Fig. 3.130). Since the nerve is extremely exposed (or vulnerable) in this area, lesions of the N. ulnaris represent one of the most common nerve lesions of the upper limb.

Skeleton

Ulna

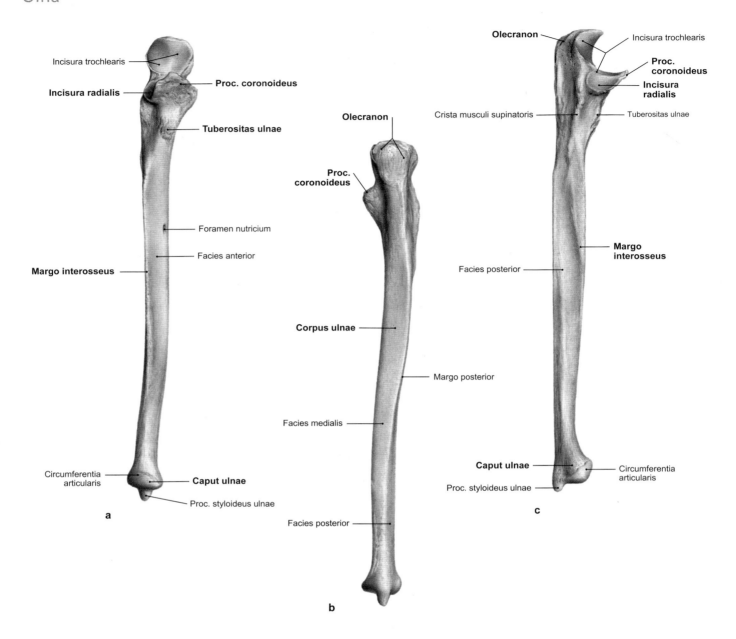

Incisura trochlearis

Incisura radialis

Proc. coronoideus

Tuberositas ulnae

Foramen nutricium

Facies anterior

Margo interosseus

Circumferentia articularis

Caput ulnae

Proc. styloideus ulnae

a

Olecranon

Proc. coronoideus

Corpus ulnae

Margo posterior

Facies medialis

Facies posterior

b

Olecranon

Incisura trochlearis

Proc. coronoideus

Incisura radialis

Crista musculi supinatoris

Tuberositas ulnae

Margo interosseus

Facies posterior

Caput ulnae

Circumferentia articularis

Proc. styloideus ulnae

c

Fig. 3.14a–c   Ulna, right side. [S700]
a Ventral view.
It is possible to match an isolated ulna to one side of the body by refer-ring to the position of the Incisura radialis, which points laterally.

b Dorsal view.
c View from the side of the radius.

Clinical remarks

When propping up on the elbows, the area of the olecranon is fre-quently used.
a This is facilitated by several **bursa** which are located under the skin and between the tendon and bone at the insertion site of the elbow extensor (M. triceps brachii). [S701-L126]
b Injuries, excessive use or infections can result in **bursitis (Bursitis olecrani).** This presents with a pronounced swelling (arrow), which is very painful to movement and touch. [G463]

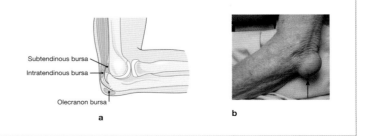

Subtendinous bursa

Intratendinous bursa

Olecranon bursa

a

b

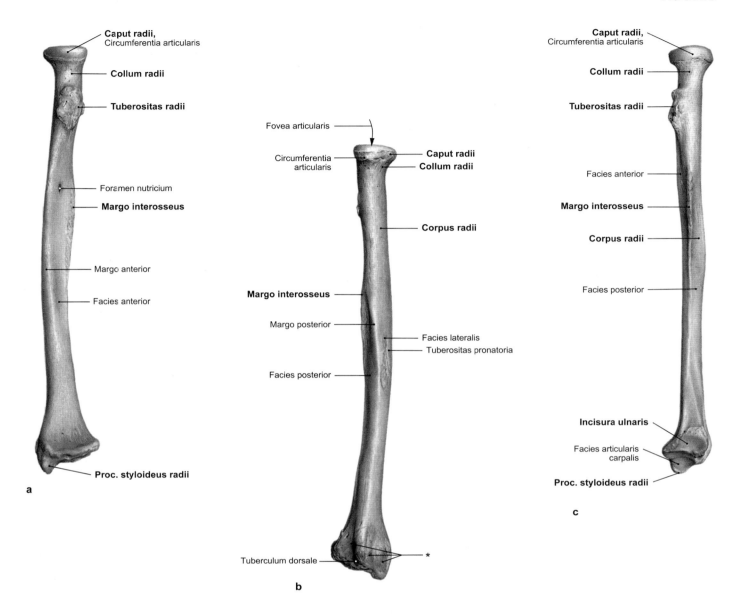

Fig. 3.15a–c   Radius, right side. [S700]
a Ventral view.
It is possible to match an isolated radius to one side of the body by referring to the position of the Proc. styloideus radii, which points laterally. In contrast, the Incisura ulnaris points in the direction of the ulna.

b Dorsal view.
c View from the side of the ulna.

* grooves and bony ridges for the insertion of extensor tendons

---

Clinical remarks

The distal **radius fracture** (COLLES' fracture) is the most common bone fracture in the human body. In most cases, it is caused by falling onto an outstretched arm. The fracture is typically within a few centimeters from the proximal wrist (carpal) joint. A lateral X-ray image shows a dislocation of the distal bone fragment, mostly with dorsal deviation (arrow). [G645]

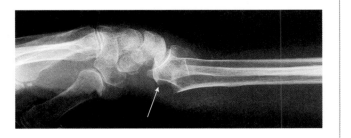

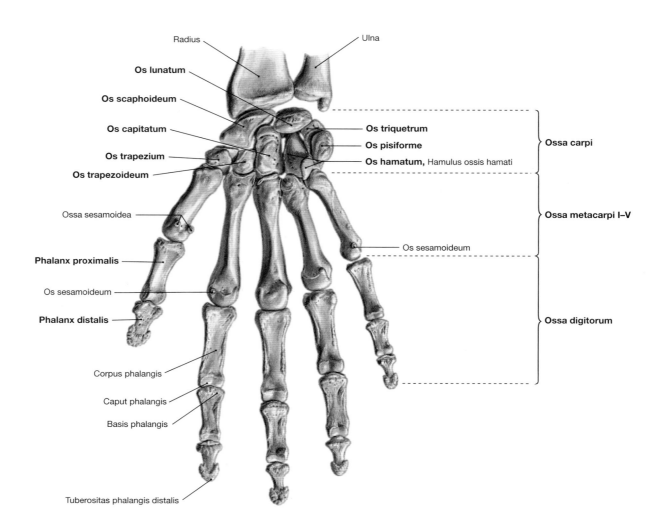

Radius

Ulna

Os lunatum

Os scaphoideum

Os capitatum

Os triquetrum

Os pisiforme

Os trapezium

Os hamatum, Hamulus ossis hamati

Os trapezoideum

Ossa sesamoidea

Os sesamoideum

Phalanx proximalis

Os sesamoideum

Phalanx distalis

Corpus phalangis

Caput phalangis

Basis phalangis

Tuberositas phalangis distalis

Ossa carpi

Ossa metacarpi I–V

Ossa digitorum

Fig. 3.16 Hand skeleton (or bones), Ossa manus, right side; palmar view. [S700]
The hand (Manus) can be divided into the wrist (Carpus, with Ossa carpi), the middle part of the hand (Metacarpus, with Ossa metacarpi) and the fingers (Digiti, with Ossa digitorum). The wrist (Carpus) consists of a proximal and a distal row. In the proximal row, aligned from the radial to the ulnar direction, are the scaphoid (Os scaphoideum), lunate (Os lunatum) and triquetral bones (Os triquetrum). The triquetral bone lies on the palmar side of the pisiform bone (Os pisiforme), which is not a carpal bone but rather a sesamoid bone (Os sesamoideum), which is embedded in the tendon of the M. flexor carpi ulnaris. The distal row

consists of the large trapezium bone (Os trapezium), the small trapezoid bone (Os trapezoideum), the capitate (Os capitatum) and the hamate bones (Os hamatum).
For many decades, there has been an amusing mnemonic for the carpal bones in anatomical literature, and it is widely used:
Some **L**overs **T**ry **P**ositions **T**hat **T**hey **C**an't **H**andle.
The digits consist of several phalanges. The bones of the wrist (or carpal bones) form the Sulcus carpi, which is the base of the carpal tunnel (→ Fig. 3.128). It is confined by the scaphoid and trapezium bones (Os scaphoideum and Os trapezium) on the radial side and by the pisiform and hamate bones (Os pisiforme and Os hamatum) on the ulnar side.

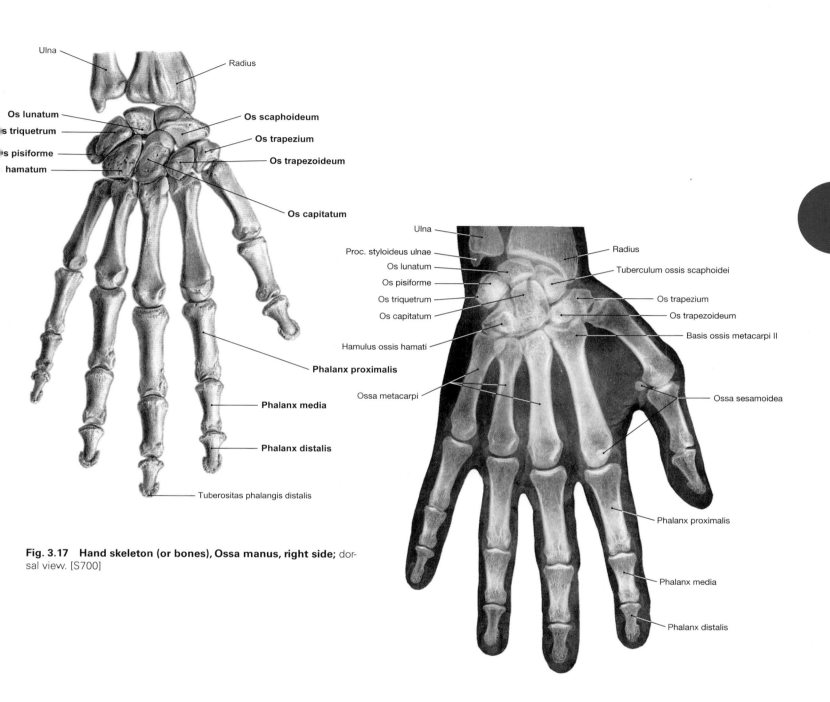

Ulna

Radius

Os lunatum

s triquetrum

s pisiforme

hamatum

Os scaphoideum

Os trapezium

Os trapezoideum

Os capitatum

Phalanx proximalis

Phalanx media

Phalanx distalis

Tuberositas phalangis distalis

Fig. 3.17 Hand skeleton (or bones), Ossa manus, right side; dorsal view. [S700]

Ulna

Proc. styloideus ulnae

Os lunatum

Os pisiforme

Os triquetrum

Os capitatum

Hamulus ossis hamati

Ossa metacarpi

Radius

Tuberculum ossis scaphoidei

Os trapezium

Os trapezoideum

Basis ossis metacarpi II

Ossa sesamoidea

Phalanx proximalis

Phalanx media

Phalanx distalis

Fig. 3.18 Hand, Manus, right side; X-ray in an anterior-posterior (AP) projection. [S700]

Clinical remarks

With **fractures** of the carpal bones, the **scaphoid** is most frequently affected. An injury to the supplying blood vessels can hereby lead to a necrosis that is visible in the X-ray image due to the decrease in bone density. Injuries can cause degenerative changes such as **oste-** **oarthritis** of the hand and finger joints which are associated with typical signs of arthritis, such as bony appositions (osteophytes) and destruction of the joint surfaces.

Skeleton

Medial clavicular joint

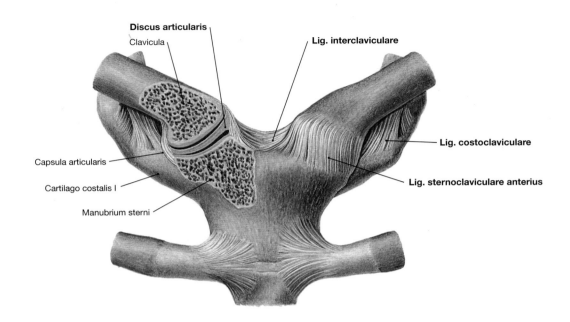

Discus articularis

Clavicula

Lig. interclaviculare

Capsula articularis

Cartilago costalis I

Manubrium sterni

Lig. costoclaviculare

Lig. sternoclaviculare anterius

Fig. 3.19 Medial clavicular joint, Articulatio sternoclavicularis; ventral view of the joint on both sides. [S700]
The medial clavicular joint is the only articulated connection between the upper limb and the axial skeleton. The slightly saddle-shaped articular surfaces – the socket of the breastbone and the head of the clavicle – are separated by a Discus articularis of fibrous cartilage, which absorbs the traction forces of lateral displacement. The joint ligaments are very stable and consist of the **Ligg. sternoclavicularia anterius** and **posterius,** which connect the two bony elements on the front and back of the joint and the **Lig. interclaviculare,** as a cranial connection between the two clavicles. From the cartilage of rib I, the **Lig. costoclaviculare** extends to the sternal end of the clavicle, and the M. subclavius to the acromial end.

Structure and function

The sternoclavicular joint is a **ball-and-socket joint** held in place by very **strong joint ligaments.** The clavicle rotates around its axis in this joint.

Overview of joints of the upper limb	
• Medial clavicular joint **(sternoclavicular joint):** ball-and-socket joint	• Proximal wrist joint **(Articulatio radiocarpalis):** condyloid joint
• Lateral clavicular joint **(Articulatio acromioclavicularis):** plane joint (acts along with the medial joint as ball-and-socket joint)	• Distal wrist joint **(Articulatio mediocarpalis):** interlocked hinge joint (along with the proximal joint, functions as condyloid joint)
• Shoulder joint **(Articulatio humeri):** ball-and-socket joint	• Wrist (or carpal) and metacarpal joints **(Articulationes intercarpales, Articulationes carpometacarpales, Articulationes intermetacarpales):** amphiarthroses, except for the carpometacarpal joint of the thumb **(Articulatio carpometacarpalis pollicis):** saddle joint

• Elbow joint **(Articulatio cubiti):** composite joint, consists of:
  – Humeroulnar joint **(Articulatio humeroulnaris):** hinge joint
  – Humeroradial joint **(Articulatio humeroradialis):** ball-and-socket joint
  – Proximal radioulnar joint **(Articulatio radioulnaris proximalis):** pivot joint
	• Metacarpophalangeal joints **(Articulationes metacarpophalangeae):** ball-and-socket joints, except for metacarpophalangeal joint of the thumb: hinge joint

• Distal radioulnar joint **(Articulatio radioulnaris distalis):** pivot joint	• Middle and distal finger joints **(Articulationes interphalangeae manus):** hinge joints

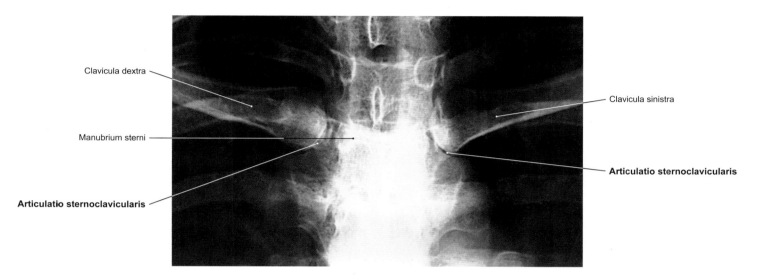

Clavicula dextra

Clavicula sinistra

Manubrium sterni

Articulatio sternoclavicularis

Articulatio sternoclavicularis

Fig. 3.20 Medial clavicular joint; ventral view, anteroposterior (AP) X-ray image. [E530]
The figure shows the right and left sternoclavicular joint. The medial bony ends of each clavicle are clearly visible. By contrast, the Manu-brium sterni is difficult to discern in the image due to overlapping verte-bral bodies.

Clinical remarks

Injuries to the medial clavicular joints are rare because of the strong ligaments; it requires a massive force to rupture those strong ligaments.

a Posterior dislocation of the sternoclavicular joint occurs as a result of direct frontal impact onto the medial clavicular part, e.g. impact against a hard object. An anterior dislocation is the result of an indi-rect force to the shoulder which causes the forceful forward move-ment of the shoulder. [S701-L126]

b The computer tomographic (CT) image of the upper thorax shows a posterior dislocatioin of the right medial sternoclavicular joint (cir-cle). The posterior dislocation is more dangerous than the medial dislocation of the clavicular bone, as several important structures behind the clavicle are at risk of being injured, including the lung, trachea, oesophagus and blood supply, such as the A./V. subclavia and the nerves of the Plexus brachialis (→ Fig. 5.135, Vol. 2). This can lead to the rupture of blood vessels and life-threatening internal bleeding. [H064-001]

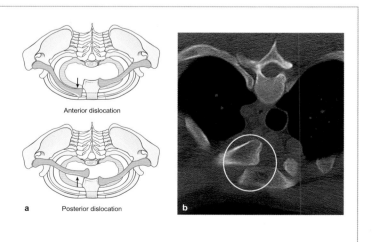

Anterior dislocation

a Posterior dislocation

b

Skeleton

Lateral clavicular joint

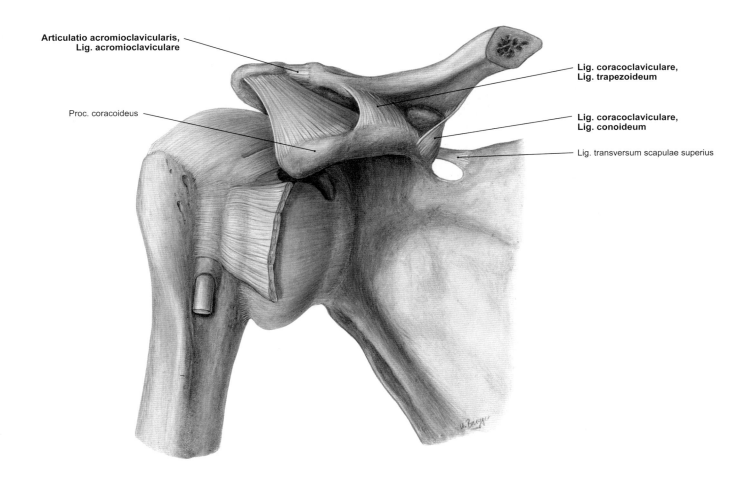

Articulatio acromioclavicularis,
Lig. acromioclaviculare

Proc. coracoideus

Lig. coracoclaviculare,
Lig. trapezoideum

Lig. coracoclaviculare,
Lig. conoideum

Lig. transversum scapulae superius

Fig. 3.21 Lateral clavicular joint, Articulatio acromioclavicularis, right side; ventral view. [S700]
The lateral clavicular joint is an articulated connection between the clavicle and the shoulder blade. There is usually a fibrocartilaginous Discus articularis between the plane joint surfaces, which only partly divides the joint cavity. The joint capsule is reinforced by the **Lig. acromioclav-**iculare. The **Lig. coracoclaviculare** is also important for the stability of the acromioclavicular joint, with two distinct ligaments which connect the Proc. coracoideus of the shoulder blade with the clavicle. The **Lig. conoideum,** which passes to the Tuberculum conoideum, lies medially. Laterally, the **Lig. trapezoideum** attaches to the Linea trapezoidea, which is located below the acromial end of the clavicle (→ Fig. 3.9b).

Clinical remarks

While the sternoclavicular joint is well protected by its stable ligaments (e.g. in the case of a fall), **injuries to the acromioclavicular or AC joint** are relatively common (→ Fig. 3.23).

Structure and function

The acromioclavicular joint is a **plane joint.** Secured by joint ligaments composed of three parts, this immobile joint connects the clavicle with the scapula and allows the shoulder girdle to rotate in the sternoclavicular joint. Functionally **both clavicular joints** therefore jointly act as a **ball-and-socket joint.** The **joint ligaments** of the acromioclavicular joint are **weak in relation** to the stress exerted by the arm actions on this joint.

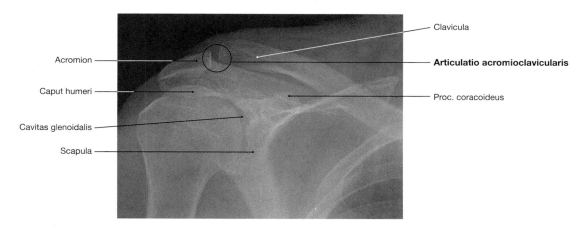

Acromion

Caput humeri

Cavitas glenoidalis

Scapula

Clavicula

Articulatio acromioclavicularis

Proc. coracoideus

Fig. 3.22 Acromioclavicular (AC) joint, right side; view from ventral, X-ray image in anteroposterior (AP) projection. [G568]
The X-ray image displays an intact AC joint. The joint appears extended because the Discus articularis is not visible on the X-ray image. The distance between the Proc. coracoideus and the clavicle is not enlarged.

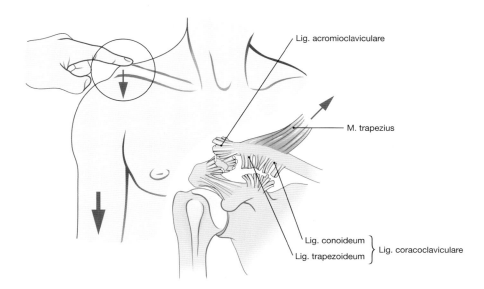

Lig. acromioclaviculare

M. trapezius

Lig. conoideum
Lig. trapezoideum } Lig. coracoclaviculare

Fig. 3.23 Injuries of the acromioclavicular joint (shoulder joint or AC joint separation). [S700-L126]/[(B500~M282-L132)/G1063]
Severe injuries to the acromioclavicular joint result in the lateral end of the clavicle pointing upwards as a result of traction from the M. trapezius muscle. This stepped formation of the lateral end of the clavicle can be pushed down with a finger (piano key sign).

Clinical remarks

In comparison to lesions to the sternoclavicular joint, **injuries to the acromioclavicular (AC) joint** are relatively more frequent. This is caused by a larger range of motion of the distal clavicular part which encircles the medial sternoclavicular joint. An AC joint injury or **AC joint separation** include the rupture of the joint ligaments. Smaller injuries include a lesion to the Lig. acromioclaviculare. With more severe injuries, this ligament is ruptured and parts of the Lig. coracoclaviculare are damaged. With severe injuries, all three ligaments are ruptured. The **classification of TOSSY** defines different levels of severity of AC injuries:

- TOSSY I: strained or partially ruptured Lig. acromioclaviculare (one ligament affected)
- TOSSY II: additional partial rupture of the Lig. coracoclaviculare (two ligaments affected)
- TOSSY III: complete rupture of the Lig. acromioclaviculare and both parts of the Lig. coracoclaviculare (all three ligaments ruptured).

The **ROCKWOOD classification** is a more relevant indicator for surgical intervention and assesses the level of horizontal instability of the AC joint. The X-ray image with AP-projection clearly shows the AC dislocation with the lateral end of the clavicle deviating upwards (arrow). As a general rule, the more the lateral end of the clavicle is dislocated, the more severe the AC lesion.
[G718]

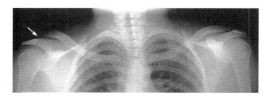

Shoulder joint

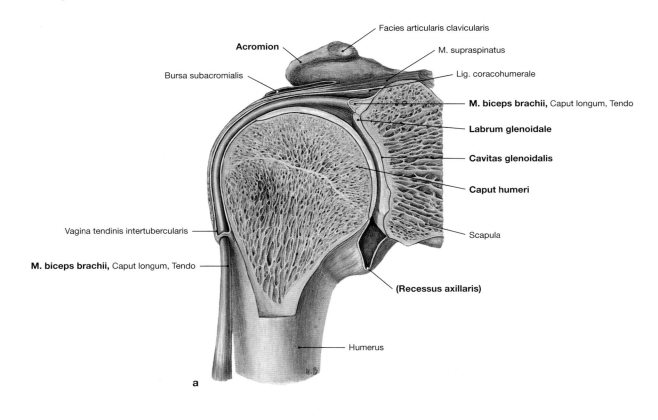

Facies articularis clavicularis

Acromion

M. supraspinatus

Bursa subacromialis

Lig. coracohumerale

M. biceps brachii, Caput longum, Tendo

Labrum glenoidale

Cavitas glenoidalis

Caput humeri

Vagina tendinis intertubercularis

M. biceps brachii, Caput longum, Tendo

Scapula

(**Recessus axillaris**)

Humerus

a

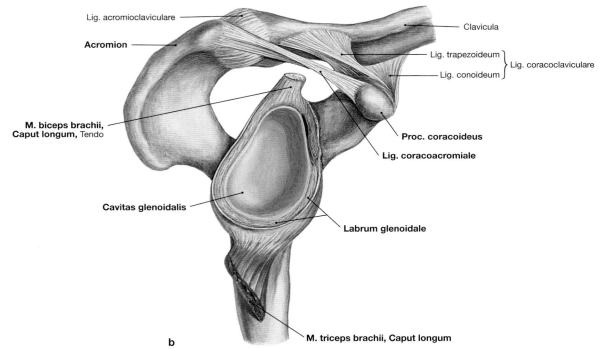

Lig. acromioclaviculare

Acromion

Clavicula

Lig. trapezoideum

Lig. conoideum

} Lig. coracoclaviculare

M. biceps brachii,
Caput longum, Tendo

Proc. coracoideus

Lig. coracoacromiale

Cavitas glenoidalis

Labrum glenoidale

M. triceps brachii, Caput longum

b

Fig. 3.24a and b   Shoulder joint, Articulatio humeri, right side.
[S700]
a Section through the scapular plane, ventral view.
b Image of the joint socket, lateral view.
The Cavitas glenoidalis of the scapula, together with the fibrocartilaginous lip (Labrum glenoidale) forms the socket of the shoulder joint, articulating with the head of the humerus. It makes for a particularly impressive ball-and-socket joint. The joint capsule (Capsula articularis) originates from the Labrum glenoidale, and on the cranial rim of the socket it also encloses the tendinous origin of the Caput longum of the M. biceps brachii. The long head of the biceps originates at the Tubercu-

lum supraglenoidale and passes through the joint capsule, while the long head of the triceps (Caput longum of the M. triceps brachii) originates at the Tuberculum infraglenoidale, outside the capsule. The joint capsule inserts at the Collum anatomicum of the humerus, so that the Tubercula majus and minus remain extra-articular. Caudally, the joint capsule has a reserve fold (Recessus axillaris). The joint capsule is reinforced on various sides by ligaments (→ Fig. 3.25) and by the radiating tendons of the rotator cuff muscles (→ Fig. 3.34 and → Fig. 3.57). The shoulder joint is covered by the acromion, the **'roof of the shoulder',** which comprises the Proc. coracoideus, the acromion as well as the **Lig. coracoacromiale,** which connects these two bony projections.

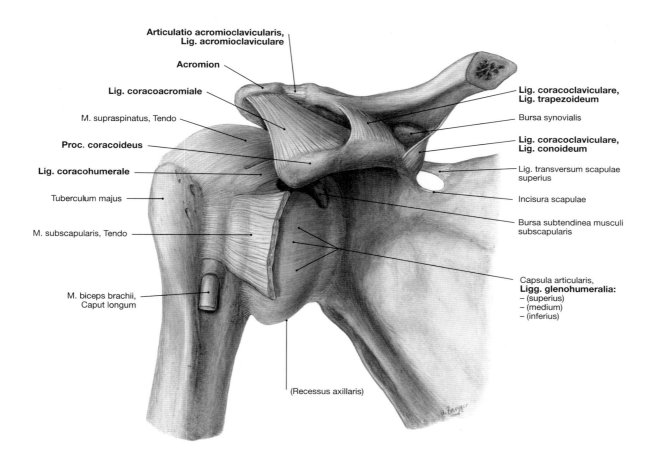

Articulatio acromioclavicularis,
Lig. acromioclaviculare

Acromion

Lig. coracoacromiale

M. supraspinatus, Tendo

Proc. coracoideus

Lig. coracohumerale

Tuberculum majus

M. subscapularis, Tendo

M. biceps brachii,
Caput longum

(Recessus axillaris)

Lig. coracoclaviculare,
Lig. trapezoideum

Bursa synovialis

Lig. coracoclaviculare,
Lig. conoideum

Lig. transversum scapulae
superius

Incisura scapulae

Bursa subtendinea musculi
subscapularis

Capsula articularis,
Ligg. glenohumeralia:
– (superius)
– (medium)
– (inferius)

Fig. 3.25 Shoulder joint, Articulatio humeri, right side; ventral view. [S700]

The joint capsule (Capsula articularis) is supported by various ligaments and by tendons of the **rotator cuff** muscles (muscle conduction). The **Lig. coracohumerale** lies cranially and extends from the Proc. coracoideus backwards into the capsule. The **Ligg. glenohumeralia** consist of various fibrous tracts and stabilise the anterior part of the capsule. Since the muscles of the rotator cuff also radiate into the capsule at the top, front and back, the bottom of the joint capsule is particularly thin

and vulnerable. The **Lig. coracoacromiale,** together with the Proc. coracoideus and the acromion, form the 'roof of the shoulder' and subsequently have no link to the joint capsule. The roof of the shoulder is an addition to the joint socket and stabilises the head of the humerus from above when pressure is exerted on the supported arm. As a 'canopy' for the joint, it also limits the abduction and anteversion of the shoulder joint, and thereby prevents the arm being raised above the horizontal plane (elevation) if the scapula is not rotated at the same time.

Structure and function

The shoulder joint is a **ball-and-socket joint** and has the **largest range of motion** of all joints of the human body. **Bones and ligaments** provide **insufficient** muscle conduction, so that joint stability is provided by the muscles of the **rotator cuff.** By projecting into the joint capsule, these muscles strengthen them directly.

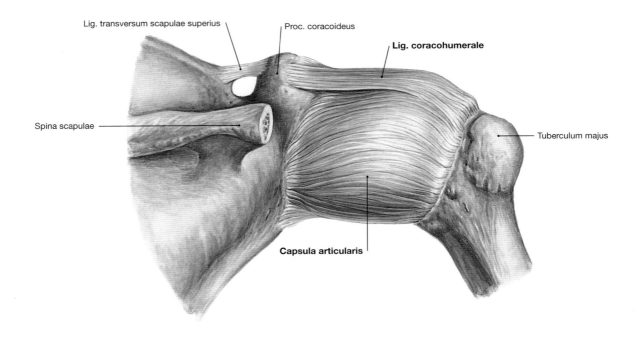

Lig. transversum scapulae superius

Proc. coracoideus

Lig. coracohumerale

Spina scapulae

Tuberculum majus

Capsula articularis

Fig. 3.26 Shoulder joint, Articulatio humeri, right side; dorsal view. [S700]

The most important muscles for movement in the shoulder joint	
Movement	**Muscle**
Anteversion	M. pectoralis major
Retroversion	M. triceps brachii
Abduction	M. deltoideus
Adduction	M. pectoralis major
External rotation	M. infraspinatus
Internal rotation	M. subscapularis

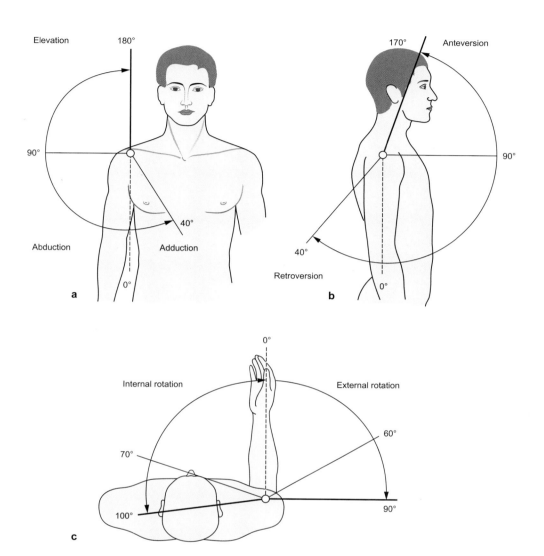

Fig. 3.27a–c   Range of motion in the shoulder joint with and without the involvement of the clavicular joints. [S700-L126]/[G1061]
a, b The shoulder joint is a **ball-and-socket joint** with three degrees of freedom of movement and has the maximum range of motion of all joints in the human body. When the movements of abduction and anteversion are exclusively performed in the shoulder joint (see thin lines), the range of motion is restricted by the roof of the shoulder. In the case of combined movements of the shoulder and the clavicular joints (see thick lines), when the shoulder blade is rotated, the range of motion is significantly increased. Then even the abduction of the arm above the horizontal plane **(elevation)** is possible. The rotation of the scapula, enabled by the M. serratus anterior and the M. trapezius, already starts at the beginning of the abduction movement.

c In order to be able to examine the rotation of the shoulder joint, the position of the forearm has to be at a right-angle to the elbow joint, like a pointer. If the arm is extended, this is usually combined with an additional turning movement of the forearm.
Range of motion in the shoulder joint alone:
* Abduction–adduction: 90°–0°–40°
* Anteversion–retroversion: 90°–0°–40°
* External rotation–internal rotation: 60°–0°–70°
Range of motion in the shoulder joint with clavicular joints:
* Abduction–adduction: 180°–0°–40°
* Anteversion–retroversion: 170°–0°–40°
* External rotation–internal rotation: 90°–0°–100°

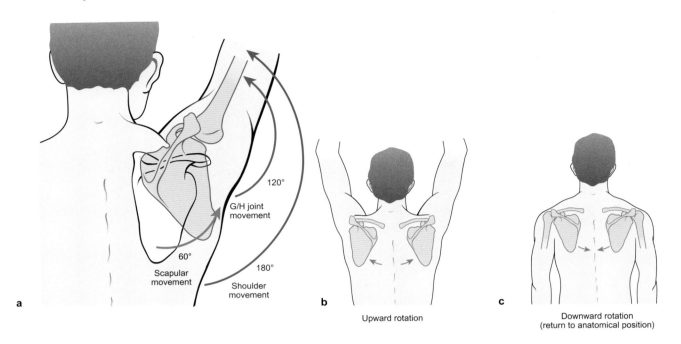

Fig. 3.28a–c Combined movements of scapula and humerus.
[S701-L126]
The elevation of the arm is facilitated by the combined movement of the scapula and humerus.

a With elevation, the movement of the scapula and humerus in relation to each other is 1:2. At a complete abduction of 180° of the shoulder girdle, the AC joint and humerus (glenohumeral joint, G/H joint) contribute 60° and 120° to this movement, respectively.

b, c Guided by the muscles of the shoulder girdle, the gliding motion of the scapula on the thoracic wall rotates the socket of the shoulder joint upward or downward. The combined movement of the scapula and humerus is called a **scapulohumeral motion**.

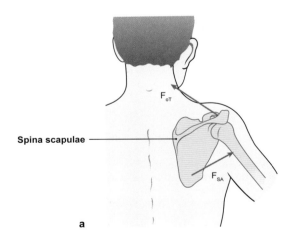

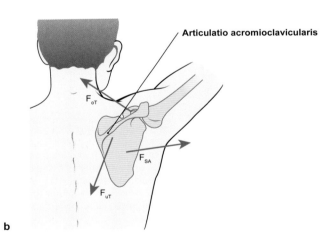

Fig. 3.29a and b Effects of muscle groups around the scapula on the combined movements of the scapula and humerus.
[S701-L126]
The muscle groups, into which the scapula is embedded, jointly engage during arm elevation.

a With an arm abduction of less than 100°, the Fossa glenoidalis joint socket rotates while the medial part of the Spina scapulae serves as an axis and is held in place. The Pars descendens of the M. trapezius (F_{oT}) opposes the action of the M. deltoideus, which provides the majority of muscle force for the abduction of the arm. The M. serratus anterior (F_{SA}) pulls the Angulus inferior of the scapula laterally forward.

b Elevation of the arm above 100° results in the rotation of the scapula in the acromioclavicular joint. This is possible because the Pars ascendens of the M. trapezius (F_{uT}) abuts the M. serratus anterior (F_{SA}). This combined contraction secures the scapula against the trunk. The Pars descendens of the M. trapezius (F_{oT}) then facilitates the rotation of the scapula with the joint socket pointing upward.

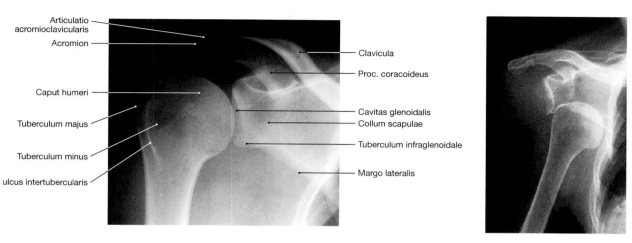

Articulatio acromioclavicularis

Acromion

Caput humeri

Tuberculum majus

Tuberculum minus

Sulcus intertubercularis

Clavicula

Proc. coracoideus

Cavitas glenoidalis
Collum scapulae

Tuberculum infraglenoidale

Margo lateralis

Fig. 3.30 Shoulder joint, Articulatio humeri, right side; X-ray image in an anterior-posterior (AP) projection. [S700-T902]

Fig. 3.31 Dislocation of the right shoulder joint; X-ray image of the right shoulder in anteroposterior (AP) projection; ventral view. [R234]
The X-ray image shows a dislocated right shoulder joint. The humerus head is dislocated caudally beneath the Proc. Coracoideus (Luxatio subcoracoidea).

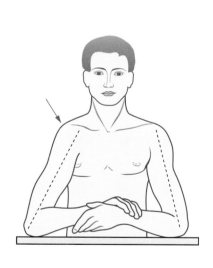

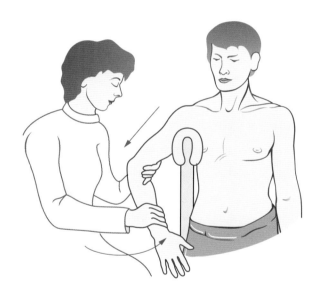

Fig. 3.32 Clinical findings associated with a dislocation of the right shoulder joint. [S700-L126]/[B500]
Physical examination reveals a different shape to the right shoulder (arrow) which appears to have slumped because the M. deltoideus and humerus head are displaced caudally. The arm on the right side seems to be longer.

Fig. 3.33 Repositioning of the shoulder dislocation. [S700-L126]/[R234]
Using the ARLT method, the injured arm is laid over the back of a padded chair. The physician pulls the arm which is flexed at a right angle towards the humerus until the head of the humerus pops back into the socket.

Clinical remarks

Dislocation of the shoulder is the most frequent dislocation of the human body. The shoulder is prone to dislocation due to a weak bony and ligamentous support system. The Luxatio subcoracoidea is the most frequent type (90 %), where the humerus head repositions itself below the Proc. coracoideus.

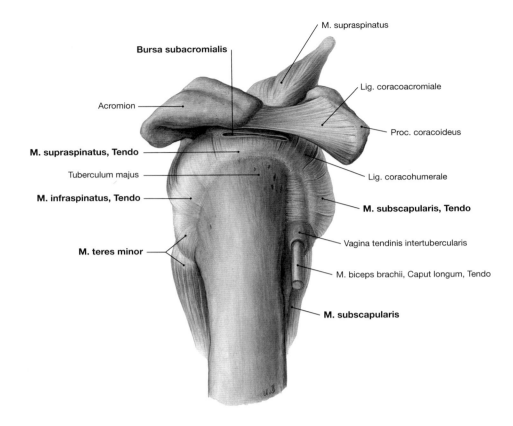

Fig. 3.34 **Shoulder joint, Articulatio humeri, right side;** lateral
view. [S700]
The tendons of various muscles radiate into the joint capsule and stabilise it. These muscles are defined as **rotator cuff: the M. subscapularis
lies at the front,** the **M. supraspinatus** at the top, and the **M. infraspinatus** and **M. teres minor** radiate from the posterior into the capsule.
The capsule is only weak on the bottom.
In the area of the shoulder joint, there are various small bursae, some
of which link partially with the joint capsule and form side extensions of

the joint. The **Bursa subcoracoidea** below the Proc. coracoideus usually communicates with the **Bursa subtendinea musculi subscapularis,**
located below the tendinous attachment point of the muscle
(→ Fig. 3.25), which is often connected with the joint cavity (→ Fig. 3.56).
The **Bursa subacromialis,** on the other hand, lies on the tendon of the
M. supraspinatus and is mostly linked to the **Bursa subdeltoidea.**
These two bursae together form the so-called **'subacromial space'**
and allow a low-friction movement of the humeral head and of the tendons of the rotator cuff under the acromion.

Clinical remarks

Scapulohumeral movements are frequently affected because the
bony and ligamentous support in the shoulder joint is weak. **Lesions
of the rotator cuff** can occur as a result. The tendon of the M. supraspinatus is particularly prone to injury since it can be jammed in
below the acromion during arm abduction.
a Degenerative changes to the supraspinatus tendon can frequently
be diagnosed in an X-ray (AP) projection image (white arrow). [G217]

b Abductions of the arm between 60° and 120° can be painful if the
tendon of the M. supraspinatus is trapped under the acromion **(impingement syndrome).** Additionally, **calcifications** of degenerative
lesions in the subacromial space can cause pain and limit the range
of motion in the shoulder joint. [S701-L126]

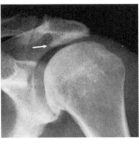

a

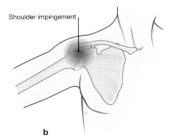

b

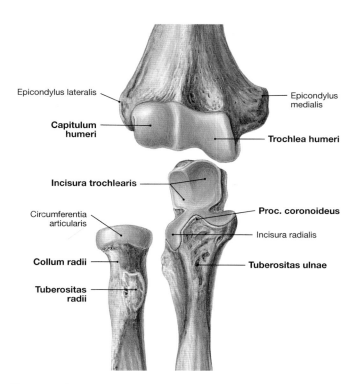

Fig. 3.35 **Bony parts of the elbow joint, Articulatio cubiti;** ventral view. The cartilage-covered joint surfaces are shown in blue. [S700]

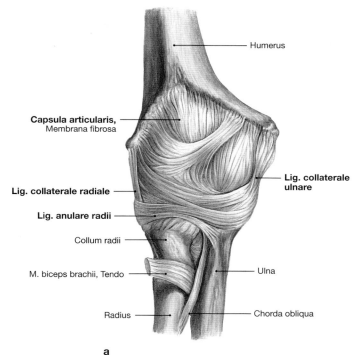

a

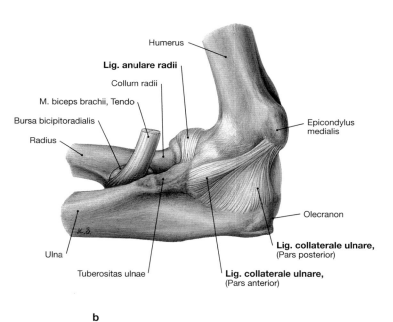

b

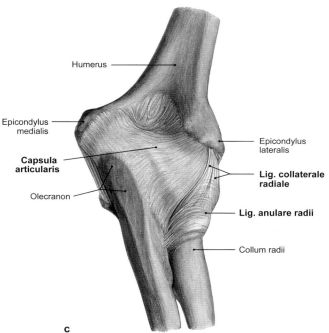

c

Fig. 3.36a–c **Elbow joint, Articulatio cubiti, right side.** [S700]
a Ventral view.
b Medial view.
c Dorsal view.
The elbow joint is a composite joint (Articulatio composita), in which the humerus, the radius and the ulna articulate in three partial joints.

- **Articulatio humeroulnaris:** hinge joint with the Trochlea humeri as the joint head and the Incisura trochlearis of the ulna as the joint socket
- **Articulatio humeroradialis:** ball-and-socket joint with the Capitulum humeri as the ball and the Fovea articularis of the radius as the socket
- **Articulatio radioulnaris proximalis:** pivot joint with the Circumferentia articularis of the Caput radii as the ball and the Incisura radialis of the ulna as the socket.

The joint capsule (Capsula articularis) encloses the cartilaginous joint surfaces of all three bones. The capsule is reinforced by strong ligaments. Two **collateral ligaments** stabilise the elbow joint medially and laterally. Medially, the **Lig. collaterale ulnare** connects the Epicondylus medialis of the humerus to the Proc. coronoideus (Pars anterior) and olecranon (Pars posterior) of the ulna. The **Lig. collaterale radiale** originates from the bottom of the Epicondylus lateralis and radiates into the **annular ligament (Lig. anulare radii),** which is attached at the anterior and posterior sides of the Incisura radialis of the ulna. Due to the this ligament looping around the head of the radius, it allows the radius to engage in rotational movements around its axis.

Elbow joint

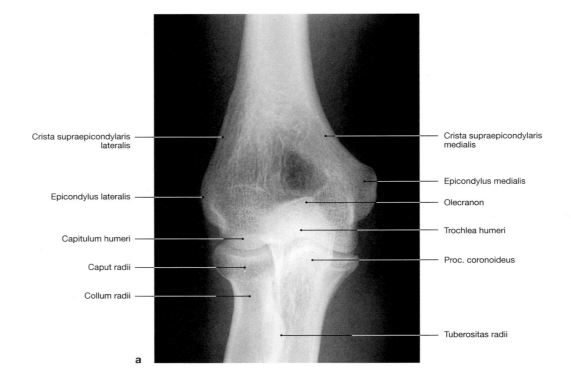

Crista supraepicondylaris lateralis

Epicondylus lateralis

Capitulum humeri

Caput radii

Collum radii

Crista supraepicondylaris medialis

Epicondylus medialis

Olecranon

Trochlea humeri

Proc. coronoideus

Tuberositas radii

a

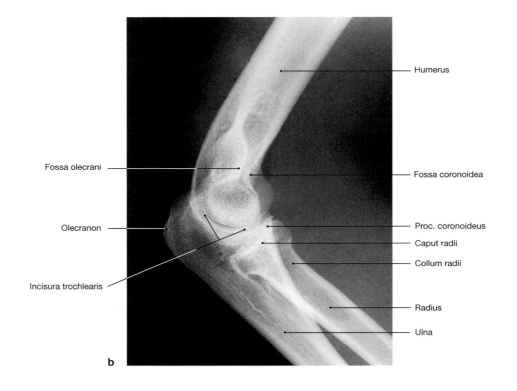

Fossa olecrani

Olecranon

Incisura trochlearis

Humerus

Fossa coronoidea

Proc. coronoideus

Caput radii

Collum radii

Radius

Ulna

b

Fig. 3.37a and b Elbow joint, Articulatio cubiti, right side.
[S700-T902]
a X-ray in anterior-posterior (AP) projection.
b X-ray in lateral projection.

Clinical remarks

In the extended position of the elbow joint, both epicondyles of the humerus are in line with the olecranon (→ Fig. 3.37a). Fractures or dislocations may result in deviations from the normal position (→ Fig. 3.40).

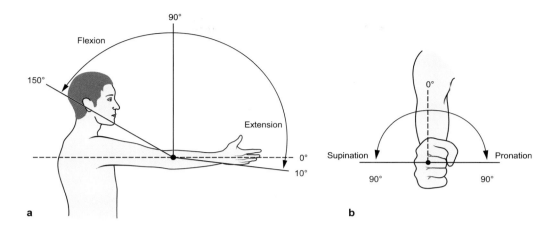

a

b

Fig. 3.38a and b Range of motion in the elbow joint, Articulatio cubiti. [S700-L126]/[G1061]
The elbow joint enables hinge movements between the humerus and the ulna and between the humerus and the radius, as well as rotational movements between the humerus and the radius, and the radius and the ulna. Together, the partial joints therefore behave like a **pivot-hinge joint** (trochoginglymus). The bony parts of the humeroulnar joint provide strong guidance during movements.
a Flexion and extension. Flexion is limited in the upper arm flexors by soft tissue and extension is restricted by the bone characteristics of the olecranon. The transverse axis of movement in the hinge joint is positioned in the centre of the Trochlea humeri.

b The turning movement of the elbow also involves the distal radioulnar joint (→ Fig. 3.43). The rotational movement is secured by the Lig. anulare radii **(ligament conduction)**. Although the articular surfaces of the humeroradial joint resemble those of a ball-and-socket joint, abduction and adduction are not possible, because the radius is tied to the ulna by the ring ligament and can therefore only follow the hinge movements of the humeroulnar joint.
Range of motion in the elbow joint:
- Extension–flexion: 10°–0°–150°
- Supination–pronation: 90°–0°–90°

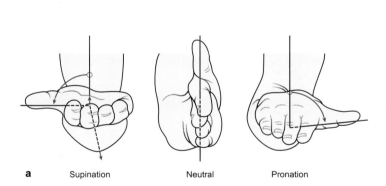

a   Supination   Neutral   Pronation

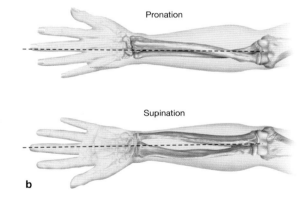

b

Fig. 3.39a and b Rotational movements in the elbow joint, Articulatio cubiti.
With rotational movements in the elbow joint, the radius moves around the ulna in a circular movement, known as **supination** and **pronation**.
a In the neutral position (neutral-zero method) with the thumb pointing upwards, rotational movement can lead to **supination** (palm pointing upward) or **pronation** (palm pointing downward) of the forearm. [S701-L126]

b In the supinated forearm, the radius and ulna are parallel to each other, whereas during pronation they cross over each other. The elbow joint is therefore supinated in the neutral position so that positional terms such as medial and lateral are unambiguous. [S701-L127]
Hint for dissection: During the dissection and study of the arm, it is easier to place the arm in a supinated position. It can be particularly confusing with the cadaver in a prone position to identify the muscles and neurovascular bundles in a pronated arm.

The most important muscles for movement of the elbow, Articulatio cubiti		
Movement		**Muscles**
Flexion		M. biceps brachii
Extension		M. triceps brachii
Supination		M. biceps brachii (with flexed elbow) M. supinator (with extended elbow)
Pronation		M. pronator teres

Upper limb

Elbow joint

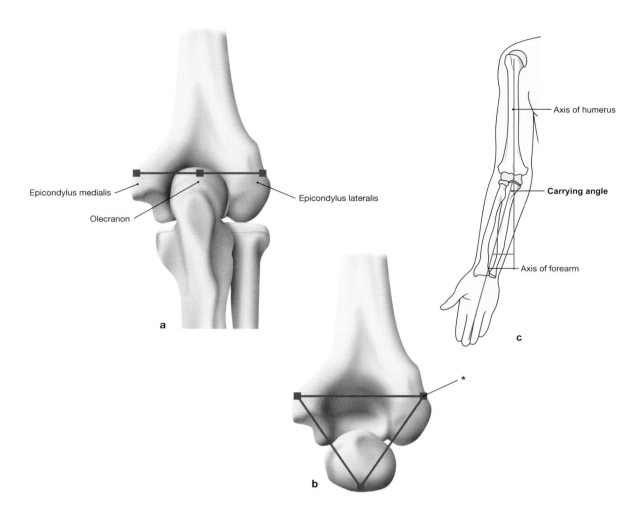

Epicondylus medialis

Olecranon

Epicondylus lateralis

a

b

*

Axis of humerus

Carrying angle

Axis of forearm

c

Fig. 3.40a–c HUETER triangle.
a The tips of the epicondyles of the humerus and the olecranon are aligned in the extended elbow joint. [S700-L127]
b In a flexed position, the tips of the epicondyles of the humerus and the olecranon form an equilateral triangle (HUETER triangle). Bone fractures and dislocations result in a deviation from this triangular formation and is an important reference point in diagnostic imaging. [S700-L127]

c When the supinated arms are placed close to the body they deviate 5°–10° from the longitudinal axis and point outward. This is called the **carrying angle.** This prevents the arms from hitting the pelvis during walking or sports activities while allowing them to swing freely. Fractures or dislocations of the elbow can alter this angle and can be helpful for diagnostic purposes. [S701-L231]
* clin.: HUETER triangle

Clinical remarks

Dislocations of the elbow joint occur during severe traumata. A fall from a great height or a crash with a motorbike or car can cause a dorsal dislocation and involves the displacement of the proximal ends of the forearm bones posterior to the olecranon. All the bones involved may be fractured. Dislocations of the elbow joint cause severe pain, swelling of the joint and deviation from the carrying angle and the HUETER triangle. Additionally, the N. ulnaris runs through the dorsal part of the joint and can be damaged. Complex injuries with fractures and dislocation require surgical repositioning and stabilisation and frequently result in permanent defects, such as instability and a reduced range of motion in the elbow joint.
Ventral dislocation of the elbow joint. [E813]

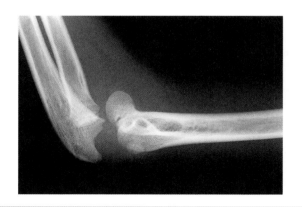

Structure and function

The elbow joint is a composite joint which is secured by very **stable ligaments.** Because the head of the radius is secured in a ligamen-

tous loop, it loses some of its freedom to abduct/adduct. The elbow joint therefore **functions as a swivel and a hinge joint**.

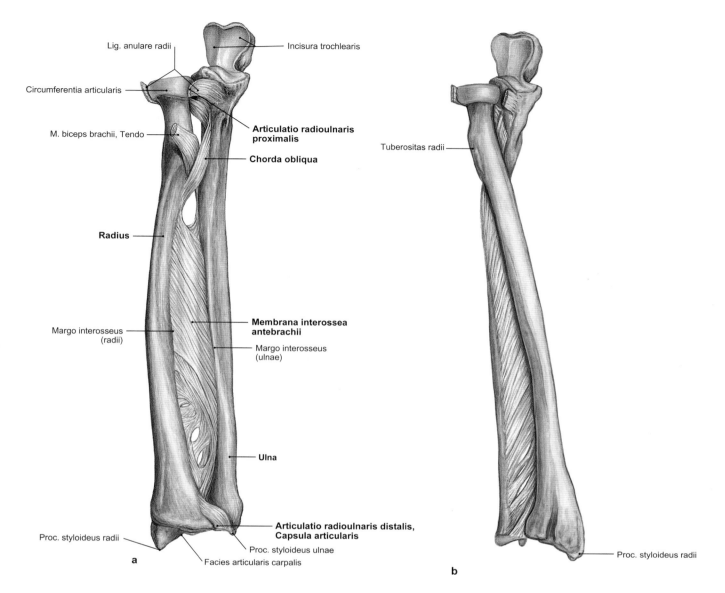

Fig. 3.41a and b   Joints of the bones of the forearm, right side; ventral view. [S700]
a View of supinated position.
b View of pronated position.
The bones of the forearm are connected by the tough Membrana interossea antebrachii, the fibres of which run predominantly in a proximal to distal direction from the radius to the ulna. Proximally it is supplemented by the Chorda obliqua that runs in the opposite direction. The figures illustrate how the radius is twisted around the ulna. In the supinated position of the forearm, both bones are parallel to each other, but cross over each other in the pronated position.

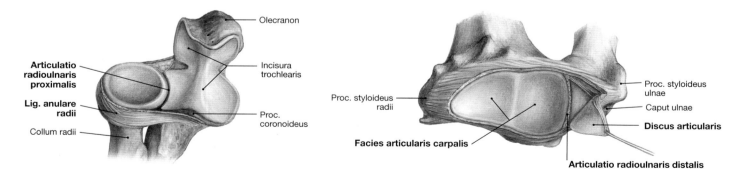

Fig. 3.42   Proximal radioulnar joint, Articulatio radioulnaris proximalis, right side; proximal view from ventral. [S700]
The proximal radioulnar joint is a **pivot joint** and part of the elbow joint. The common axis of movement for both the proximal and the distal radioulnar joints is the oblique axis of the forearm, which connects the Caput radii and the Caput ulnae.

Fig. 3.43   Distal radioulnar joint, Articulatio radioulnaris distalis, right side; dorsal view from distal. [S700]
The distal radioulnar joint is also a **pivot joint** and lies adjacent to the proximal wrist. It is formed by the Caput ulnae and the Incisura ulnaris of the radius. The surface of the proximal wrist joint consists of the Facies articularis carpalis of the radius and the Discus articularis, which separates the Articulatio radioulnaris distalis from the proximal wrist joint.

Carpal and metacarpal joints

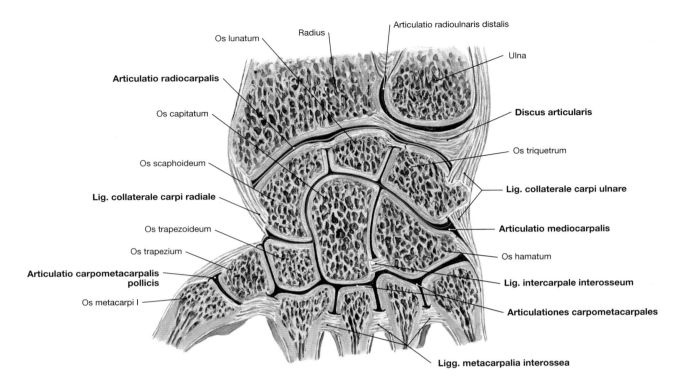

Os lunatum
Radius
Articulatio radioulnaris distalis
Ulna
Articulatio radiocarpalis
Os capitatum
Os scaphoideum
Discus articularis
Os triquetrum
Lig. collaterale carpi radiale
Lig. collaterale carpi ulnare
Os trapezoideum
Articulatio mediocarpalis
Os trapezium
Os hamatum
Articulatio carpometacarpalis pollicis
Lig. intercarpale interosseum
Os metacarpi I
Articulationes carpometacarpales
Ligg. metacarpalia interossea

Fig. 3.44 Carpal (wrist) and metacarpal joints, Articulationes carpi, right side; palmar view; surface section parallel to the back of the hand. [S700]

These include, in addition to the smaller articulated bones of the carpal and metacarpal bones, the two wrist joints.

- The **proximal wrist joint (Articulatio radiocarpalis)** connects the forearm bones (socket) with the proximal row of the carpal bones (head) and is a condyloid (ellipsoid) joint. The ulna is separated from the Os triquetrum by the Discus articularis (→ Fig. 3.43).
- In the **distal wrist joint (Articulatio mediocarpalis),** the proximal and distal rows of the carpal bones articulate in a wavy line with

each other. According to the morphology of the joint surfaces it is an interlocking hinge joint, which along with the proximal joint functions as a condyloid joint.

- The **Articulationes carpometacarpales II to V** between the carpal and metacarpal bones and the **Articulationes intermetacarpales** between the bases of the metacarpal bones are usually tight amphiarthroses which allow relatively little movement. In contrast, the **carpometacarpal joint of the thumb** (Articulatio carpometacarpalis pollicis) is very flexible and enables flexion and extension as well as abduction and adduction.

Clinical remarks

Fractures of the carpal and metacarpal bones are frequent.

a Scaphoid (navicular) fracture: This is the most frequent carpal fracture (Os scaphoideum, arrow). Falling onto the outstretched arm can injure both the scaphoid bone as well as the artery branches leading from the A. radialis. This can result in necrosis of the bone which is evident from the decreased bone density. Additionally, scaphoid injuries can result in degenerative changes, including osteoarthritis of the wrist joints. [G719]

b Boxer fracture: Fracture of the distal end of the fifth metacarpal bone. This type of fracture can occur when hitting something hard or a hard part of the human body with great force, such as a punch to the chin in boxing, and the little finger or ring finger is fractured. [E513-002]

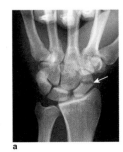

a

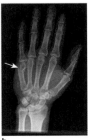

b

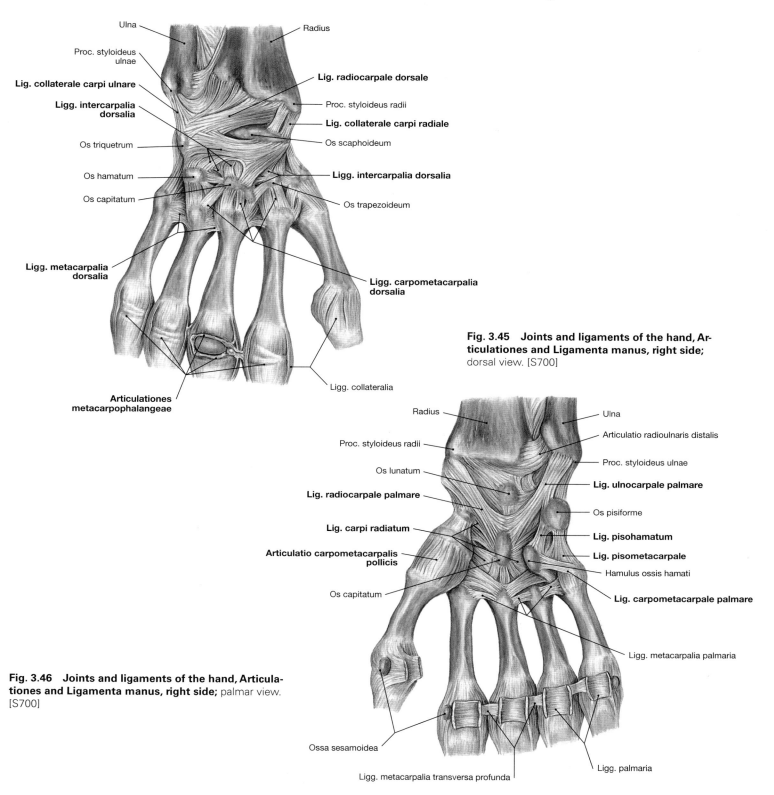

Ulna

Radius

Proc. styloideus ulnae

Lig. collaterale carpi ulnare

Ligg. intercarpalia dorsalia

Os triquetrum

Os hamatum

Os capitatum

Ligg. metacarpalia dorsalia

Articulationes metacarpophalangeae

Lig. radiocarpale dorsale

Proc. styloideus radii

Lig. collaterale carpi radiale

Os scaphoideum

Ligg. intercarpalia dorsalia

Os trapezoideum

Ligg. carpometacarpalia dorsalia

Ligg. collateralia

Fig. 3.45   Joints and ligaments of the hand, Articulationes and Ligamenta manus, right side; dorsal view. [S700]

Radius

Ulna

Articulatio radioulnaris distalis

Proc. styloideus radii

Proc. styloideus ulnae

Os lunatum

Lig. ulnocarpale palmare

Lig. radiocarpale palmare

Os pisiforme

Lig. carpi radiatum

Lig. pisohamatum

Articulatio carpometacarpalis pollicis

Lig. pisometacarpale

Hamulus ossis hamati

Os capitatum

Lig. carpometacarpale palmare

Ligg. metacarpalia palmaria

Fig. 3.46   Joints and ligaments of the hand, Articulationes and Ligamenta manus, right side; palmar view. [S700]

Ossa sesamoidea

Ligg. palmaria

Ligg. metacarpalia transversa profunda

Ligaments of the carpal and metacarpal bones

- Ligg. radiocarpalia palmare and dorsale and Lig. ulnocarpale palmare
- Ligg. collateralia carpi radiale and ulnare: originating from the Procc. styloidei
- Ligg. intercarpalia palmaria, dorsalia and interossea
- Lig. carpi radiatum: star-shaped (radiating) ligament originating at the Os capitatum
- Lig. pisohamatum: continuation of the tendon of the M. flexor carpi ulnaris to the Os hamatum
- Lig. pisometacarpale: continuation of the tendon of the M. flexor carpi ulnaris to the Ossa metacarpi IV and V
- Ligg. carpometacarpalia palmaria and dorsalia
- Ligg. metacarpalia palmaria, dorsalia and interossea

Movements of wrist and finger joints

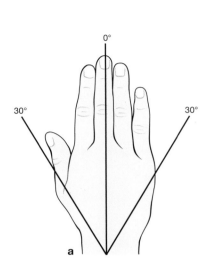

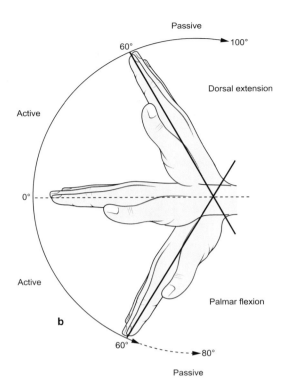

Fig. 3.47a and b   Range of motion of the wrist joints.
a The proximal and distal wrist joints function as **condyloid (ellipsoid) joints** and are both involved in the movements of the hand. Therefore, combined movement axes can be indicated, both running through the Os capitatum. The **ulnar and radial abduction movements** occur mainly in the **proximal wrist joint** with a combined dorsal-palmar axis running through the centre of the Os capitatum. [S700-L126]/[G1061]
b The **p**almar flexion is predominantly mediated by the **p**roximal wrist joint, while the **d**orsal extension predominantly takes place in the **d**istal wrist joint (ppdd – mnemonic!). The transverse axis of these movements also runs through the centre of the Os capitatum. As most of the other carpal and metacarpal joints are amphiarthroses, their ranges of motion

are negligible. In contrast, the **carpometacarpal joint of the thumb** is very flexible and facilitates flexion and extension as well as abduction and adduction. These movements can be combined for circumduction and opposition of the thumb, which is important for grasping objects. [S700-L126]/[G1062]
Range of motion in the wrist joints:
- Ulnar abduction–radial abduction: 30°– 0°– 30°
- Dorsal extension–palmar flexion: 60°– 0°– 60°
Range of motion of the carpometacarpal joint of the thumb:
- Extension–flexion: 30°– 0°– 40°
- Abduction–adduction: 10°– 0°– 40°

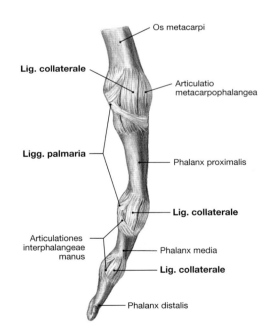

Fig. 3.48   Finger joints, Articulationes digiti, right side; lateral view, sagittal section. [S700]
This includes the metacarpophalangeal, proximal and distal interphalangeal joints of the hand.
The **metacarpophalangeal joints** (Articulationes metacarpophalangeae) are **ball-and-socket joints** between the heads of the metacarpal bones and the bases of the proximal phalanges. The metacarpophalangeal joint of the thumb, however, is a hinge joint.
The **proximal and distal interphalangeal joints** (Articulationes interphalangeae manus proximales and distales) between the heads and bases of the individual phalanges are **hinge joints.**

Fig. 3.49   Ligaments of the finger joints, Articulationes digiti, right side; lateral view. [S700]
- **Ligg. collateralia:** medial and lateral
- **Lig. palmare:** ventral
- **Lig. metacarpale transversum profundum:** connects the palmar ligaments to the metacarpophalangeal joints.

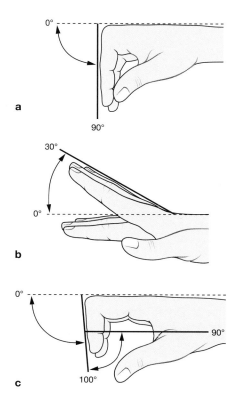

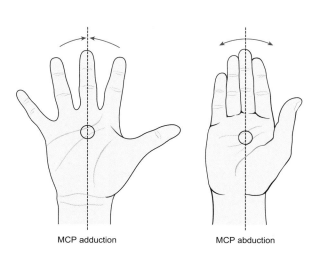

MCP adduction   MCP abduction

Fig. 3.50   Movements of the metacarpophalangeal (MCP) joints. [S701-L126]

The metacarpophalangeal joints are **ball-and-socket joints** which allow flexion, extension, adduction and abduction movements. Adduction and abduction always relate to the middle finger of the hand, as it is located in the midline of the wrist joint.

Range of motion in the metacarpophalangeal joints:
- Dorsal extension–palmar flexion: 30°– 0°– 90°
- Ulnar abduction–radial abduction: (20–40)°– 0°– (20–40)°

Fig. 3.51a–c   Range of motion of the finger joints. [S700-L126]/ [G1061]

The metacarpophalangeal joints allow flexion and extension as well as radial and ulnar abduction movements. Rotation of the fingers is only possible if fingers are extended passively. The saddle joint of the thumb allows only hinge movements. This also applies to all proximal and distal interphalangeal joints, which can only bend or flex from the normal position.

Range of motion in the proximal interphalangeal joints:
- Dorsal extension–palmar flexion: 0°– 0°–100°

Range of motion in the distal interphalangeal joints:
- Dorsal extension–palmar flexion: 0°– 0°– 90°

Clinical remarks

Clinically the following **terms and abbreviations** are often used for the finger joints:
- **MCP** (= **m**eta**c**arpo**p**halangeal joint)
- **PIP** (= **p**roximal **i**nter**p**halangeal joint)
- **DIP** (= **d**istal **i**nter**p**halangeal joint)

Skeleton

Movements of wrist and finger joints

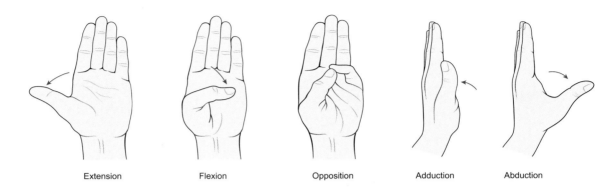

| Extension | Flexion | Opposition | Adduction | Abduction |

Fig. 3.52 Range of motion of the thumb. [S701-L126]
The key joint enabling the gripping movement of the hand is the **carpometacarpal joint (CMC)** of the thumb. This joint is a saddle joint between the Os trapezium and the base of the Os metacarpi I (→ Fig. 3.44). As expected from a joint with two degrees of freedom in movement, the saddle joint facilitates flexion/extension and adduction/abduction. These movements can also be combined to enable the thumb to oppose the other fingers and the palm. Objects can hereby be grasped purposefully.

Range of motion of the CMC of the thumb:
- Extension–flexion: 30°– 0°– 40°
- Abduction–adduction: 10°– 0°– 40°

The metacarpophalangeal joint (MCP) and the proximal interphalangeal joint (PIP) are hinge joints which only support flexion and extension movements.

Range of motion of the MCP of the thumb:
- Extension–flexion: 0°– 0°– 50°

Range of motion of the PIP of the thumb:
- Extension–flexion: 0°– 0°– 80°

Clinical remarks

Injuries to the small joints of the hands and fingers are frequent and result in painful swellings of the aflicted joints.
a The lateral X-ray image shows a dislocated proximal interphalangeal joint of the ring finger (arrow). [E339-01]
b Injuries to the ligaments or overextension of the joints can result in small fractures at the insertion site of ligaments or muscles which are called **avulsion fractures** (arrow). [E380]

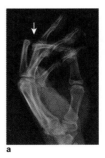
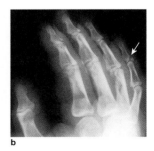

Structure and function

The **proximal wrist joint** (ellipsoidal or condyloid synovial joint) and the **distal wrist joint** (interlocked hinge joint) show distinct differences in their joint surfaces but work as **one functional unit.** The joint ligaments are complex and create relative stability.
The **carpometacarpal saddle joint of the thumb** is critically important for the gripping motion, whereas the other joints are largely in-
flexible amphiarthroses. The proximal metacarpophalangeal ball-and-socket joints are much more flexible than the hinge joint of the thumb, which is functionally more akin to the interphalangeal joints of the fingers and thumb. The joints of the fingers are stabilised by tight ligaments.

Muscles for the movement of the wrist (carpal) joints

Movement		Muscles
Palmar flexion		M. palmaris longus, M. flexor carpi radialis, M. flexor carpi ulnaris, M. flexor digitorum superficialis, M. flexor digitorum profundus
Dorsal extension		M. extensor digitorum, M. extensor digiti minimi, M. extensor carpi ulnaris, M. abductor pollicis longus, M. extensor pollicis brevis, M. extensor pollicis longus, M. extensor indicis, M. extensor carpi radialis longus, M. extensor carpi radialis brevis
Ulnar abduction		M. flexor carpi ulnaris, M. extensor carpi ulnaris
Radial abduction		M. flexor carpi radialis, M. extensor carpi radialis longus, M. extensor carpi radialis brevis

Most important flexors and extensors of the phalangeal joints

Movement	MCP	PIP	DIP
Flexion of fingers	Mm. interossei palmares, Mm. interossei dorsales	M. flexor digitorum superficialis	M. flexor digitorum profundus
Extension of fingers	M. extensor digitorum	M. extensor digitorum	Mm. lumbricales
Flexion of thumb	M. flexor pollicis longus	M. flexor pollicis longus	-
Extension of thumb	M. extensor pollicis brevis	M. extensor pollicis longus	-

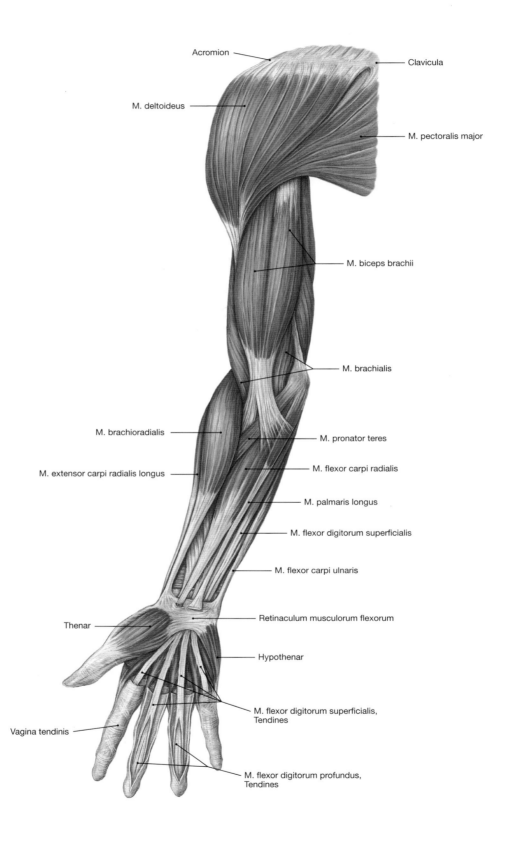

Acromion

Clavicula

M. deltoideus

M. pectoralis major

M. biceps brachii

M. brachialis

M. brachioradialis

M. pronator teres

M. extensor carpi radialis longus

M. flexor carpi radialis

M. palmaris longus

M. flexor digitorum superficialis

M. flexor carpi ulnaris

Retinaculum musculorum flexorum

Thenar

Hypothenar

M. flexor digitorum superficialis,
Tendines

Vagina tendinis

M. flexor digitorum profundus,
Tendines

Fig. 3.53   Ventral muscles of the shoulder and arm, right side;
ventral view. [S700]

→ T 26–T 40

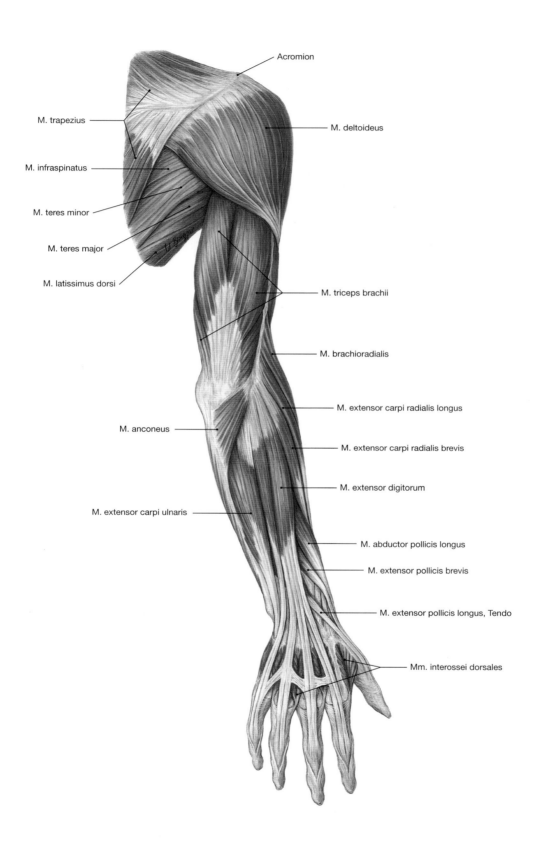

Acromion

M. trapezius

M. deltoideus

M. infraspinatus

M. teres minor

M. teres major

M. latissimus dorsi

M. triceps brachii

M. brachioradialis

M. extensor carpi radialis longus

M. anconeus

M. extensor carpi radialis brevis

M. extensor digitorum

M. extensor carpi ulnaris

M. abductor pollicis longus

M. extensor pollicis brevis

M. extensor pollicis longus, Tendo

Mm. interossei dorsales

Fig. 3.54   Dorsal muscles of the shoulder and arm, right side; dorsal view. [S700]

Arm muscles

[S700]

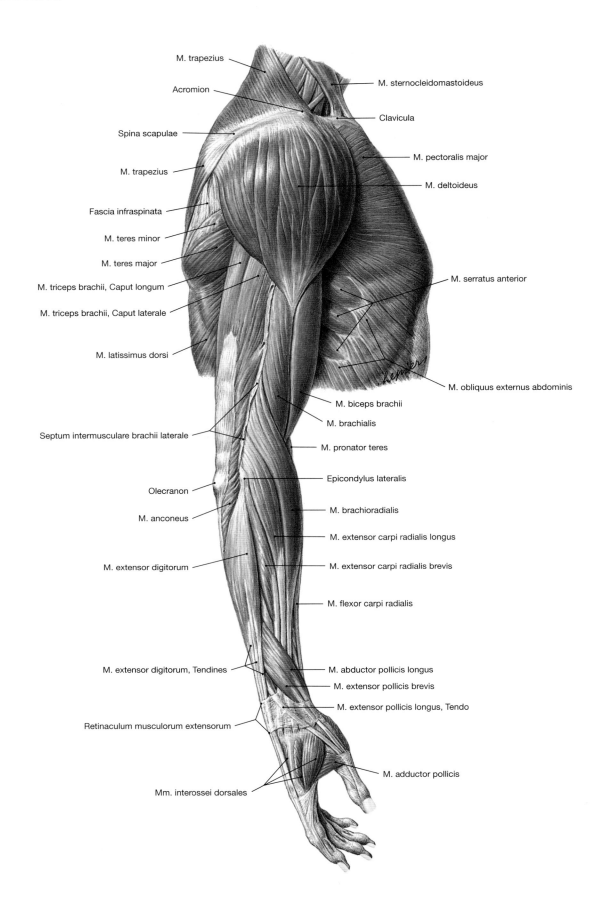

M. trapezius

Acromion

Spina scapulae

M. trapezius

Fascia infraspinata

M. teres minor

M. teres major

M. triceps brachii, Caput longum

M. triceps brachii, Caput laterale

M. latissimus dorsi

Septum intermusculare brachii laterale

Olecranon

M. anconeus

M. extensor digitorum

M. extensor digitorum, Tendines

Retinaculum musculorum extensorum

Mm. interossei dorsales

M. sternocleidomastoideus

Clavicula

M. pectoralis major

M. deltoideus

M. serratus anterior

M. obliquus externus abdominis

M. biceps brachii

M. brachialis

M. pronator teres

Epicondylus lateralis

M. brachioradialis

M. extensor carpi radialis longus

M. extensor carpi radialis brevis

M. flexor carpi radialis

M. abductor pollicis longus

M. extensor pollicis brevis

M. extensor pollicis longus, Tendo

M. adductor pollicis

Fig. 3.55 Muscles of the arm and chest, right side; lateral view.

→ T 26–T 40

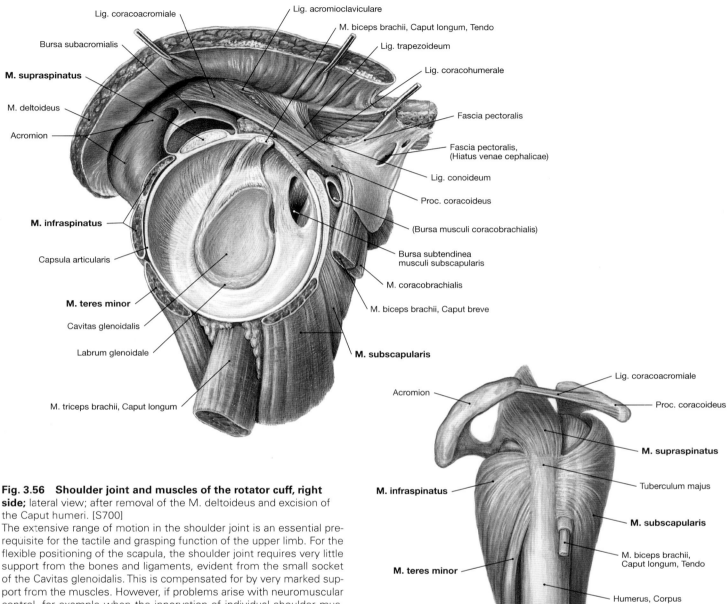

Lig. coracoacromiale
Lig. acromioclaviculare
M. biceps brachii, Caput longum, Tendo
Bursa subacromialis
Lig. trapezoideum
M. supraspinatus
Lig. coracohumerale
M. deltoideus
Acromion
Fascia pectoralis
Fascia pectoralis, (Hiatus venae cephalicae)
Lig. conoideum
M. infraspinatus
Proc. coracoideus
(Bursa musculi coracobrachialis)
Capsula articularis
Bursa subtendinea musculi subscapularis
M. coracobrachialis
M. teres minor
M. biceps brachii, Caput breve
Cavitas glenoidalis
Labrum glenoidale
M. subscapularis
M. triceps brachii, Caput longum

Acromion
Lig. coracoacromiale
Proc. coracoideus
M. supraspinatus
M. infraspinatus
Tuberculum majus
M. subscapularis
M. biceps brachii, Caput longum, Tendo
M. teres minor
Humerus, Corpus

Fig. 3.56 Shoulder joint and muscles of the rotator cuff, right side; lateral view; after removal of the M. deltoideus and excision of the Caput humeri. [S700]

The extensive range of motion in the shoulder joint is an essential pre-requisite for the tactile and grasping function of the upper limb. For the flexible positioning of the scapula, the shoulder joint requires very little support from the bones and ligaments, evident from the small socket of the Cavitas glenoidalis. This is compensated for by very marked support from the muscles. However, if problems arise with neuromuscular control, for example when the innervation of individual shoulder muscles is disrupted as a result of lesions or disorders of the nerves, or if the muscular equilibrium of these muscles is disturbed, a stable articular connection at the end points of movement can no longer be guaranteed. Dislocations occur when shearing forces act in tangential directions on the Cavitas glenoidalis, particularly in the case of a fall.

The tendons of those muscles directly adjacent to the shoulder joint radiate into the joint capsule and form a tight rotator cuff around the head of the humerus. The **M. subscapularis** (anterior), the **M. supraspinatus** (superior), the **M. infraspinatus** (posterosuperior) and the **M. teres minor** (posteroinferior) are all involved. Apart from the M. subscapularis, which inserts at the Tuberculum minus, all other muscles of the rotator cuff have their insertions at the Tuberculum majus and the Crista tuberculi majoris. The M. deltoideus is not part of this muscle group, as it does not radiate into the joint capsule, but passes over the joint.

Fig. 3.57 Muscles of the rotator cuff; lateral view. [S700]

The following muscles of the rotator cuff radiate into and insert at the joint capsule and stabilise the following: **M. subscapularis** (anterior), the **M. supraspinatus** (superior), the **M. infraspinatus** (posterosuperior), and the **M. teres minor** (posteroinferior). The inferior part of the joint capsule lacks any reinforcement and is thus prone to dislocations of the shoulder. With the exception of the M. subscapularis inserting at the Tuberculum minus, all other rotator cuff muscles insert at the Tuberculum majus.

→ T 28, T 30

Clinical remarks

In addition to their role in various movements (kinematics), the muscles of the rotator cuff are very important in maintaining the correct position of the humeral head in the articular cavity (statics). Imbalanced equilibrium of muscle forces, particularly a relative weakness of the adducting (lower) portions of the muscles, may cause an **elevation of the humeral head**.

Musculature

Muscles of the shoulder girdle

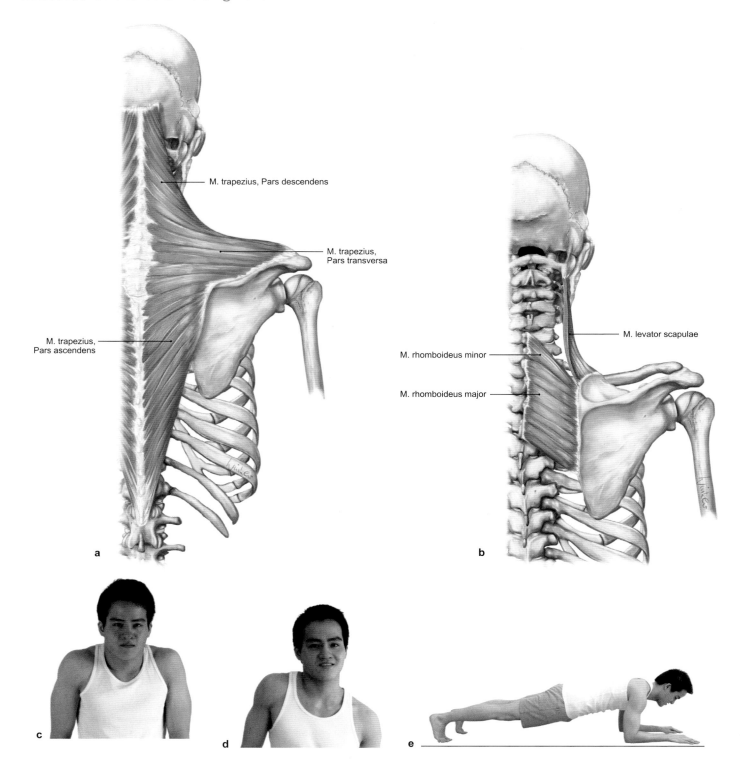

Fig. 3.58a–e   Muscles of the shoulder girdle.
In the shoulder area, there are two muscle groups. The **muscles of the shoulder girdle** insert at the scapula or clavicle, and primarily move the shoulder girdle and only indirectly move the arm. The **shoulder musculature,** on the other hand, insert at the humerus and move it directly. According to their location, these muscles are divided into a dorsal and a ventral subgroup. The **dorsal** muscles of the shoulder girdle include the **M. trapezius, M. levator scapulae and Mm. rhomboidei.**
The scapula is secured to the torso mainly by the M. levator scapulae and Mm. rhomboidei and supported by the M. trapezius. These muscles secure the scapula and therewith the arm and connect them to the spine. Hence they are named spinoscapular muscles.
a M. trapezius. [S700-L266]

b M. levator scapulae and Mm. rhomboidei. [S700-L266]
c The M. trapezius and Mm. rhomboidei are used to lift the scapulae upwards and bring both closer together, as when shrugging. [S701-L271]
d Unilateral lifting of the shoulder is achieved by contraction of the M. levator scapulae on that side. [S701-L271]
e The spinoscapular muscles oppose the traction forces and fix the scapula medially to the torso when carrying heavy loads, or during plank and pull-up exercises or weight-lifting. [S701-L271]
Note: The dorsal muscles of the shoulder girdle are also presented as superficial muscles of the back when shown with the torso (→ Fig. 2.82, → Fig. 2.83).

→ T 29

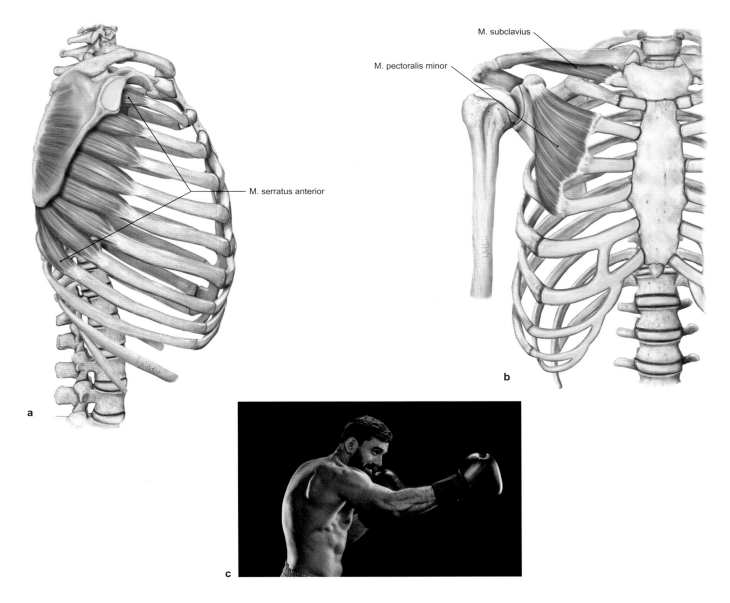

M. subclavius

M. pectoralis minor

M. serratus anterior

a

b

c

Fig. 3.59a–c Ventral muscles of the shoulder girdle.
M. serratus anterior, M. pectoralis minor and **M. subclavius** are **ventral** muscles of the shoulder girdle.

a M. serratus anterior. The main function of the **M. serratus anterior** and also of the M. trapezius is the rotation of the scapula, which is necessary for raising the arm above the horizontal plane (elevation). The scapula and the humerus work together for coordinated movements called scapulohumeral movements (→ Fig. 3.27). As the M. serratus anterior crosses below the scapula before inserting at the medial margin, it stabilises the medial edge of the scapula on the trunk and, for example when doing press-ups, prevents it being lifted up from the trunk. Thereby it is possible to lift the entire body up when lying down. [S700-L266]

b M. pectoralis minor and M. subclavius. The **M. pectoralis minor** lowers the scapula or, similar to the M. serratus anterior, acts as an auxiliary respiratory muscle by raising the ribs when the arms are propped up. Because the M. pectoralis minor inserts ventrally at the

Proc. coracoideus of the scapula, it prevents the scapula from slipping off dorsally when carrying something heavy. Along with the spinoscapular muscles on the back of the trunk (→ Fig. 3.58), the M. pectoralis minor as well as the M. serratus anterior secure the scapula to the torso.

The **M. subclavius** actively stabilises the sternoclavicular joint. [S700-L266]

c When throwing a punch, e.g. during boxing, the M. serratus anterior supports this movement by pulling forward the entire shoulder girdle at the torso. [J787]

Note for dissection: Exarticulation of the medial end of the clavicle from the sternoclavicular joint requires severing the joint ligaments as well as the M. subclavius.

Note: The ventral muscles are also depicted on the ventral abdominal wall → Fig. 2.103, → Fig. 2.104, → Fig. 2.105.

→ T 26

Clinical remarks

The ventral muscles of the shoulder girdle stabilise the trunk. Of clinical relevance is only the paralysis of the **M. serratus anterior** because the affected arm can no longer be elevated. When propping up on the arm, the medial margin of the scapula lifts off the torso,

which is a diagnostic sign called **Scapula alata.** Usually the cause is a lesion of the N. thoracicus longus which can be trapped under the scapula when carrying heavy loads (backpack palsy).

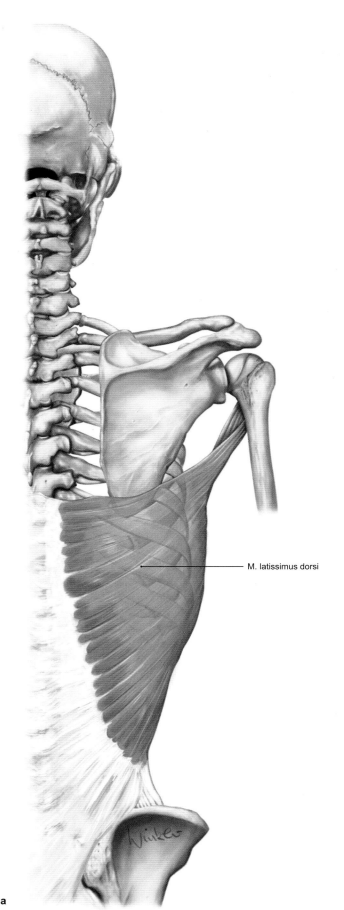

M. latissimus dorsi

a

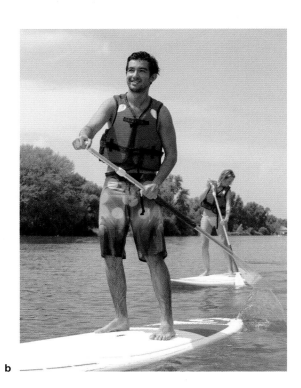

b

Fig. 3.60a and b   Muscles of the shoulder: M. latissimus dorsi.
In contrast to the muscles of the shoulder girdle, shoulder muscles act directly on the shoulder joint.

a The **M. latissimus dorsi** is a broad **dorsal** shoulder muscle capable of initiating a powerful retroversion movement from an anteverted position (trajectory movement) and can induce a slight adduction and internal rotation in the shoulder joint. [S700-L266]

b In a neutral position, the relatively weak lever of the M. latissimus dorsi means it is not essential for any shoulder movements. However, for many sports exercises this muscle plays an important role when doing something like pull-ups on a bar or sled-pulling. The same muscle supports the reaching forward movement and backward push of the arms during paddling. [J787]

The M. latissimus dorsi can also serve as an auxiliary respiratory muscle during expiration by compressing the thorax ('cough muscle').

→ T 30

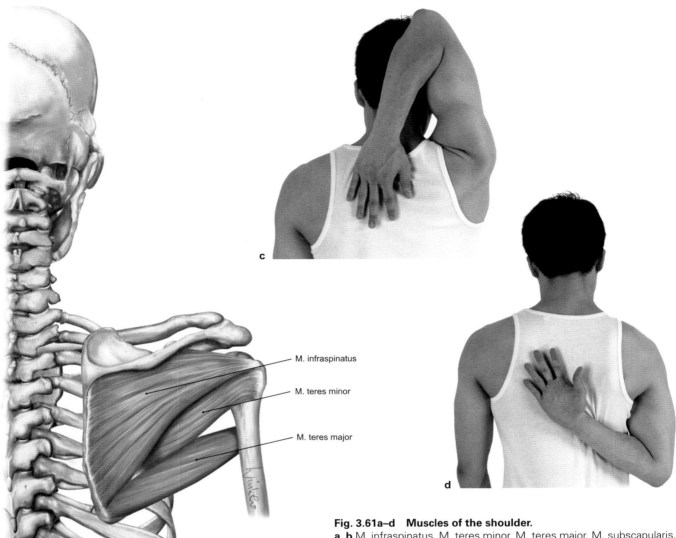

M. infraspinatus

M. teres minor

M. teres major

a

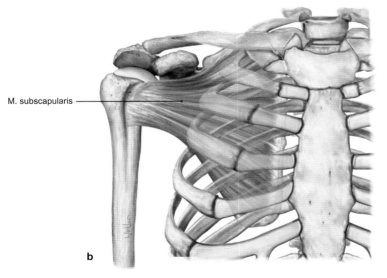

M. subscapularis

b

c

d

Fig. 3.61a–d   Muscles of the shoulder.
a, b M. infraspinatus, M. teres minor, M. teres major, M. subscapularis.
The **dorsal** shoulder muscles include the **M. latissimus dorsi, M. in-fraspinatus, M. teres minor, M. teres major** and **M. subscapularis.**
The two most important muscles of this group for movements in the
shoulder joint are the M. infraspinatus and the M. subscapularis. Both
muscles are part of the rotator cuff and stabilise the shoulder joint by
inserting their tendons into the joint capsule (→ Fig. 3.56, → Fig. 3.57).
[S700-L266]
c The **M. infraspinatus** enables a strong external rotation of the arm.
This is the most important muscle for external rotation in the shoulder
and its functional impairment leads to noticeable restrictions in shoulder movement. The **M. teres minor** supports the external rotational
movement. Both muscles are used when moving the hand from a position above the head down the back, as when scratching one's back.
Although the M. teres minor is not essential for any movement of the
shoulder, it stabilises the shoulder joint as part of the rotator cuff. This
stabilising role becomes important when injuries to the rotator cuff occur (→ Fig. 3.57), which most frequently involve the tendon of the
M. supraspinatus. [S701-L271]
Shoulder movements against a resistance, as in some sports activities,
activate the **M. teres major.** This muscle is otherwise not that relevant
for movements from a neutral position. The M. teres major supports the
M. latissimus dorsi during retroversion and adduction of the shoulder.
[S701-L271]
d Of this group of muscles, the **M. subscapularis** is uniquely located at
the anterior side of the scapula and is the antagonist for the M. infraspinatus. The M. subscapularis is the most important internal rotator in the
shoulder joint and is necessary for crossing the arms behind the back
or to scratch one's back. Patients readily notice the impairment of this
muscle because many everyday movements are negatively affected.
[S701-L271]

→ T 30

Musculature

Muscles of the shoulder

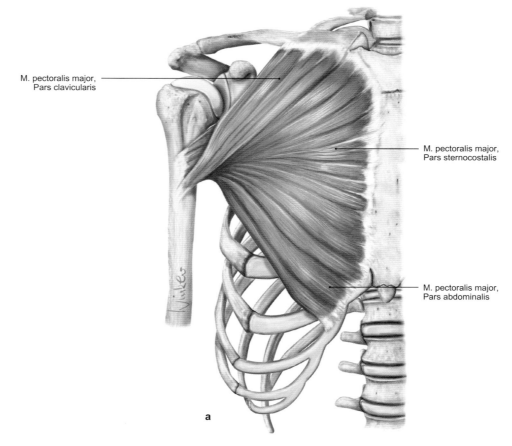

M. pectoralis major,
Pars clavicularis

M. pectoralis major,
Pars sternocostalis

M. pectoralis major,
Pars abdominalis

a

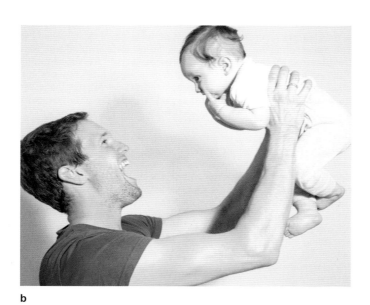

b

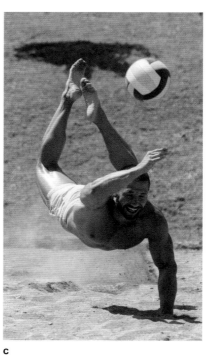

c

Fig. 3.62a–c Muscles of the shoulder: M. pectoralis major.
a The **M. pectoralis major** is the only shoulder muscle located **ventrally.** It is the strongest muscle for anteversion and adduction in the shoulder joint. Without this muscle, it is not possible to cross the arms in
front of the torso. [S700-L266]
b The M. pectoralis major is required when lifting up an object in front
of the body, pulling down a weight in front of the body, or when doing
pull-ups on a bar. [R476-K383]

c The M. pectoralis major is also used to provide support or to brace
oneself when jumping or falling to the ground. In an anteversion position of the arm, both the M. latissimus dorsi and the M. pectoralis major
can facilitate a strong retroversion movement (lifting movement). [J787]

→ T 27

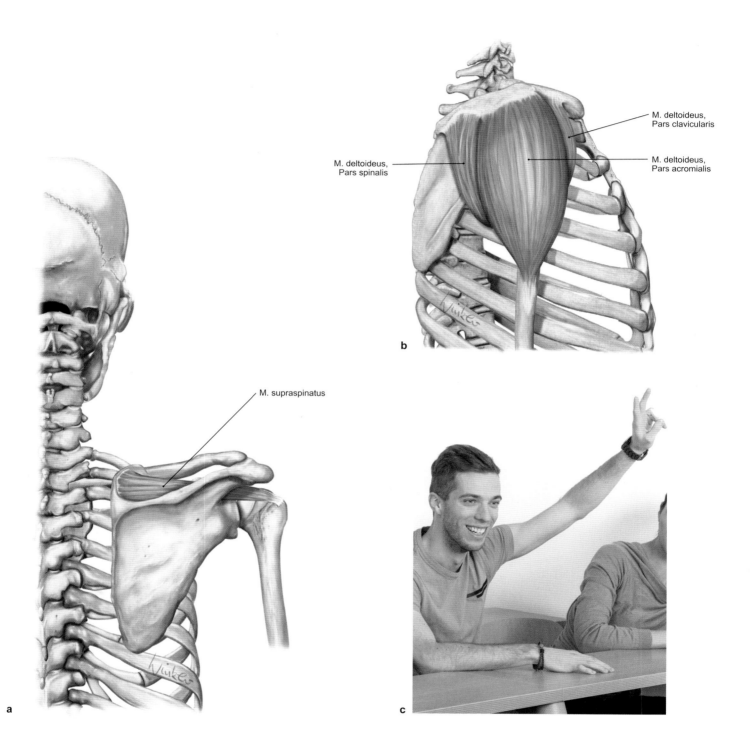

M. deltoideus,
Pars clavicularis

M. deltoideus,
Pars acromialis

M. deltoideus,
Pars spinalis

M. supraspinatus

Fig. 3.63a–c   Muscles of the shoulder.
The **lateral** shoulder muscles include the **M. supraspinatus** and the **M. deltoideus.**
a M. supraspinatus. The M. supraspinatus supports the M. deltoideus during abduction and initiates this arm movement (starter function). The M. supraspinatus is part of the rotator cuff and stabilises the shoulder joint by inserting its tendon into the joint capsule (→ Fig. 3.56, → Fig. 3.57). [S700-L266]

b M. deltoideus. The M. deltoideus is the most important abductor muscle in the shoulder joint but its functionally distinct parts can support all other movements of the shoulder as well. [S700-L266]
c The M. deltoideus is the most important abductor shoulder muscle to elevate the arm. [J787]

→ T 28

Muscles of the shoulder

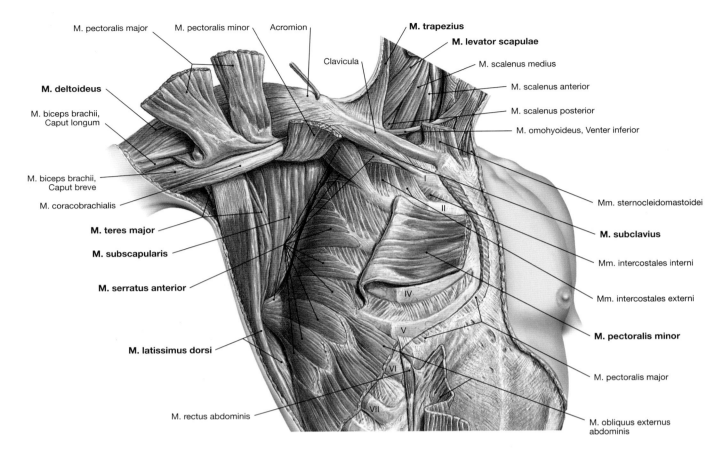

M. pectoralis major — M. pectoralis minor — Acromion — **M. trapezius**

M. levator scapulae

M. deltoideus

Clavicula

M. scalenus medius

M. scalenus anterior

M. biceps brachii, Caput longum

M. scalenus posterior

M. omohyoideus, Venter inferior

M. biceps brachii, Caput breve

M. coracobrachialis

M. teres major

M. subscapularis

M. serratus anterior

Mm. sternocleidomastoidei

M. subclavius

Mm. intercostales interni

Mm. intercostales externi

M. pectoralis minor

M. latissimus dorsi

M. pectoralis major

M. rectus abdominis

M. obliquus externus abdominis

Fig. 3.64 Muscles of the shoulder girdle and shoulder, right side; ventral view; roman numerals denote the corresponding ribs. [S700] The anterior group (M. serratus anterior, M. pectoralis minor and M. subclavius) of muscles of the shoulder girdle are most visible here, whereas of the dorsal muscles, only the M. levator scapulae and a part of the M. trapezius are shown. The M. pectoralis minor has been unfolded so that the origins of the M. serratus anterior on ribs I to 9 can be seen. The abduction position of the arm gives a clear view of the M. subscapularis which broadly covers the ventral area of the scapula.

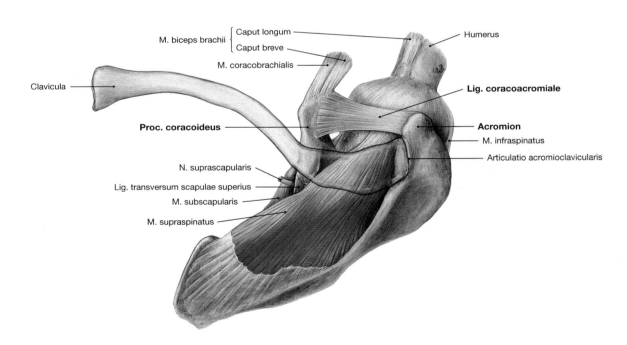

M. biceps brachii — Caput longum — Humerus

Caput breve

M. coracobrachialis

Clavicula

Lig. coracoacromiale

Proc. coracoideus

Acromion

M. infraspinatus

Articulatio acromioclavicularis

N. suprascapularis

Lig. transversum scapulae superius

M. subscapularis

M. supraspinatus

Fig. 3.65 Position of the M. supraspinatus in relation to the roof of the shoulder. [S700]
The 'roof of the shoulder' consists of the acromion and the Proc. coracoideus which are connected by the Lig. coracoacromiale. The attaching tendon of the M. supraspinatus crosses underneath the roof of the shoulder before it radiates into the joint capsule. It is therefore understandable why this tendon can be compressed when the arm is abducted and therefore often exhibits painful degenerative changes (impingement syndrome, → Fig. 3.34).

→ T 28, T 30, T 31

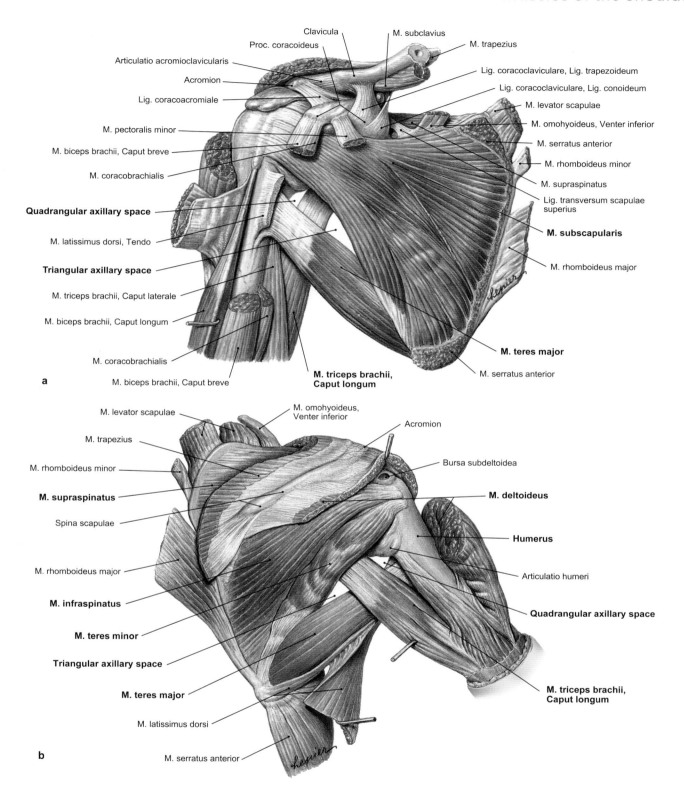

Clavicula
M. subclavius
M. trapezius
Proc. coracoideus
Articulatio acromioclavicularis
Lig. coracoclaviculare, Lig. trapezoideum
Acromion
Lig. coracoclaviculare, Lig. conoideum
Lig. coracoacromiale
M. levator scapulae
M. pectoralis minor
M. omohyoideus, Venter inferior
M. biceps brachii, Caput breve
M. serratus anterior
M. coracobrachialis
M. rhomboideus minor
M. supraspinatus
Quadrangular axillary space
Lig. transversum scapulae superius
M. latissimus dorsi, Tendo
M. subscapularis
Triangular axillary space
M. rhomboideus major
M. triceps brachii, Caput laterale
M. biceps brachii, Caput longum
M. coracobrachialis
M. teres major
M. serratus anterior
a
M. biceps brachii, Caput breve
M. triceps brachii, Caput longum

M. levator scapulae
M. omohyoideus, Venter inferior
Acromion
M. trapezius
M. rhomboideus minor
Bursa subdeltoidea
M. supraspinatus
M. deltoideus
Spina scapulae
M. rhomboideus major
Humerus
M. infraspinatus
Articulatio humeri
M. teres minor
Quadrangular axillary space
Triangular axillary space
M. teres major
M. triceps brachii, Caput longum
M. latissimus dorsi
b
M. serratus anterior

Fig. 3.66a and b   Muscles of the shoulder girdle and shoulder, right side. [S700]
a Ventral view.
b Dorsal view.
Most of the muscles of the shoulder girdle have been removed to expose the shoulder muscles, so that only the muscle origins remain. In the ventral view it is particularly easy to recognise the M. subscapularis and its entire course. The course of the M. teres major is also easily recognisable. From its origin at the Angulus inferior of the scapula, it crosses underneath the humerus before inserting on the Crista tuberculi minoris. The M. supraspinatus lies below the M. trapezius and runs (not shown here) underneath the roof of the shoulder to the upper part of the Tuberculum majus.

The M. infraspinatus and M. teres minor insert below this point. The dissection specimens show both axillary spaces, which lie between the M. teres major and M. teres minor and are laterally bordered by the humerus: the two muscles diverge in a V-shape from their origins at the scapula and leave a gap between them, which is divided by the long head of the M. triceps brachii into the **triangular medial axillary space** (Spatium axillare mediale) and into the **quadrangular lateral axillary space** (Spatium axillare laterale). The A. and V. circumflexa scapulae pass through the medial axillary space on their way to the rear side of the shoulder blade. Together with the A. and V. circumflexa humeri posterior, the N. axillaris passes through the lateral axillary space (→ Fig. 3.165, → Fig. 3.167).

→ T 27, T 28, T 30, T 32

Muscles of the upper arm

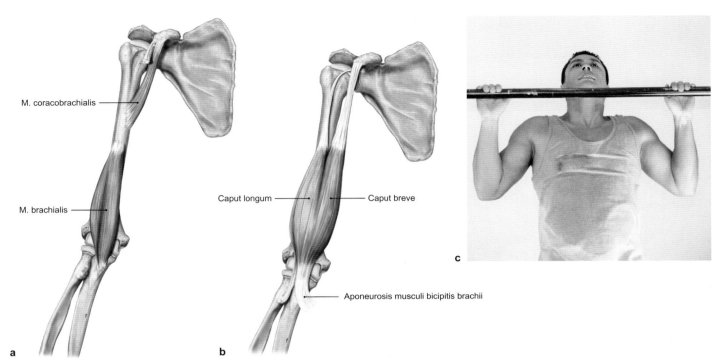

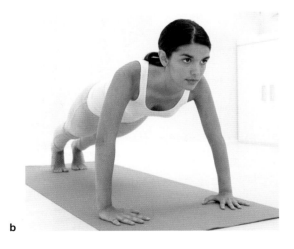

c

M. coracobrachialis

M. brachialis

Caput longum — Caput breve

Aponeurosis musculi bicipitis brachii

a   **b**

Fig. 3.67a–c   Ventral muscles of the upper arm, right side; ventral view.
a M. coracobrachialis and M. brachialis. The **M. coracobrachialis** is situated on the anterior side of the upper arm, originates on the Proc. coracoideus and inserts medially on the humerus. In contrast to the other two ventral muscles, the muscle acts only on the shoulder joint and is involved in its adduction, internal rotation and anteversion. Originating from the distal anterior surface of the humerus, the **M. brachialis** runs to the joint capsule and the Tuberositas ulnae. On the elbow joint alone it acts as a strong flexor and is referred to as *Brachialgewalt* in German (brute force). [S700-L266]
b M. biceps brachii. Contrary to the M. coracobrachialis and M. brachialis, the M. biceps brachii is a double-jointed muscle which facilitates

movements in the shoulder and elbow joints. The M. biceps brachii with its Caput breve originates from the Proc. coracoideus and therefore has the same functions as the M. coracobrachialis in the shoulder joint. The Caput longum originates at the Tuberculum supraglenoidale of the scapula and has an abducting function. However, its action on the elbow joint is significant. As it inserts at the Tuberositas radii, the M. biceps brachii is the **most important flexor in the elbow joint** and in particular the strongest supinator of the forearm in a flexed position. [S700-L266]
c All three flexor muscles of the upper arm act jointly when the shoulder and elbow joints are flexed together, such as when doing a pull-up. [J787]

→ T 31

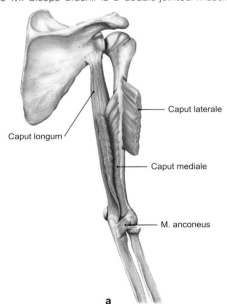

Caput laterale

Caput longum

Caput mediale

M. anconeus

a

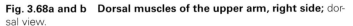

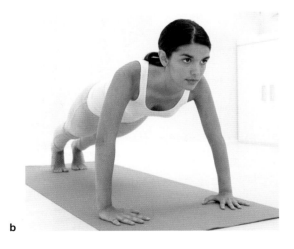

b

Fig. 3.68a and b   Dorsal muscles of the upper arm, right side; dorsal view.
a M. triceps brachii and M. anconeus. The **M. triceps brachii** is located on the back of the upper arm and originates from the Tuberculum infraglenoidale with its Caput longum, while its Caput laterale and Caput mediale originate widely from the back of the humerus. In addition to its minor involvement in the adduction and retroversion of the shoulder joint, it is the most import extensor of the elbow joint due to its great size, course, and insertion on the olecranon. The M. anconeus

also inserts at the lateral olecranon. This muscle has split off from the M. triceps brachii and represents an isolated fourth muscle head, creating a similar scenario as with the M. quadriceps femoris on the upper leg. [S700-L266]
b The M. triceps brachii is the most important extensor of the elbow joint and enables pushing up from the arms when lying down. This movement is slightly supported by the M. anconeus. [J787]

→ T 32

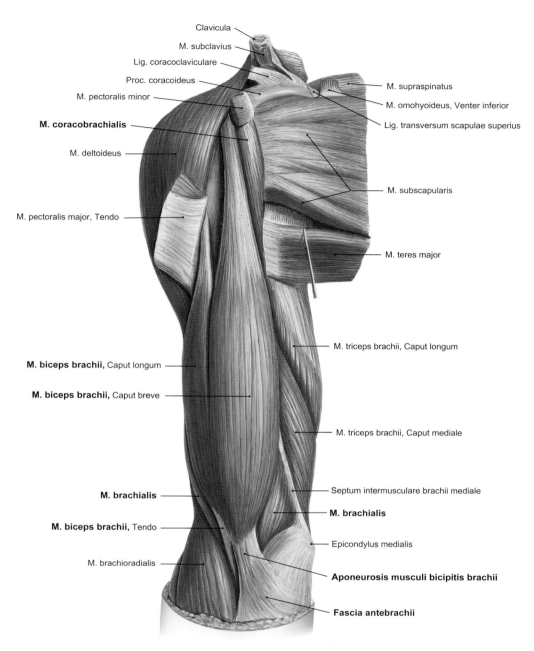

Clavicula

M. subclavius

Lig. coracoclaviculare

Proc. coracoideus

M. pectoralis minor

M. coracobrachialis

M. deltoideus

M. pectoralis major, Tendo

M. supraspinatus

M. omohyoideus, Venter inferior

Lig. transversum scapulae superius

M. subscapularis

M. teres major

M. triceps brachii, Caput longum

M. biceps brachii, Caput longum

M. biceps brachii, Caput breve

M. triceps brachii, Caput mediale

M. brachialis

M. biceps brachii, Tendo

M. brachioradialis

Septum intermusculare brachii mediale

M. brachialis

Epicondylus medialis

Aponeurosis musculi bicipitis brachii

Fascia antebrachii

Fig. 3.69   Ventral muscles of the upper arm, right side; ventral view. [S700]
The M. coracobrachialis lies medially of the M. biceps brachii. The M. biceps brachii originates at the Proc. coracoideus with its Caput breve and at the Tuberculum supraglenoidale with its Caput longum. In addition to its main insertion on the Tuberositas radii, the M. biceps brachii also ex-

tends into the forearm fascia (Fascia antebrachii) with its Aponeurosis musculi bicipitis brachii. The M. brachialis is located underneath the M. biceps brachii, so that only a part of its muscle belly can be recognised on both sides of the inserting tendon of the M. biceps brachii.

→ T 31

Clinical remarks

Degenerative changes in the shoulder joint can lead to a **rupture of the biceps tendon.**
a This usually means the tendon of the Caput longum tears. This tendon runs freely through the joint cavity close to the Tuberculum supraglenoidale of the scapula. [S701-L126]
b This rupture occurs most frequently in elderly people and presents as a muscular bulge when flexing it ('Popeye deformity'). Functional impairment is small because the short biceps tendon remains intact. [F276-005]

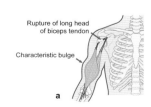

Rupture of long head of biceps tendon

Characteristic bulge

a

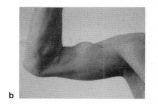

b

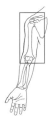

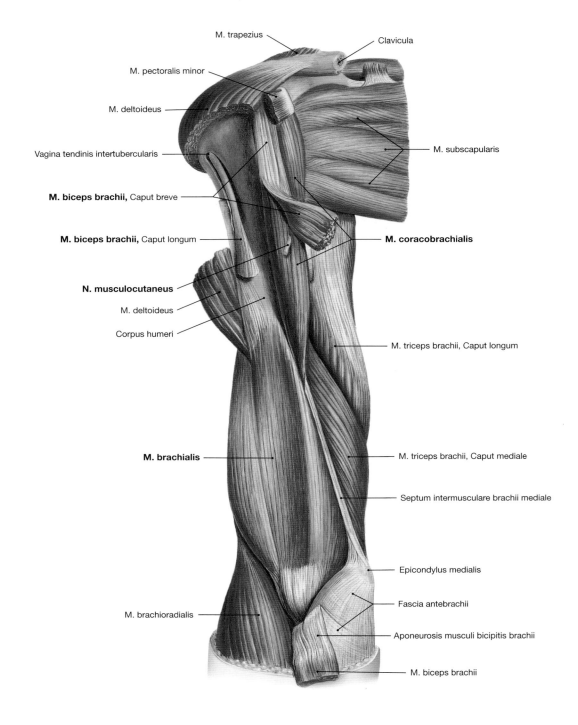

M. trapezius

Clavicula

M. pectoralis minor

M. deltoideus

M. subscapularis

Vagina tendinis intertubercularis

M. biceps brachii, Caput breve

M. biceps brachii, Caput longum

M. coracobrachialis

N. musculocutaneus

M. deltoideus

Corpus humeri

M. triceps brachii, Caput longum

M. brachialis

M. triceps brachii, Caput mediale

Septum intermusculare brachii mediale

Epicondylus medialis

Fascia antebrachii

M. brachioradialis

Aponeurosis musculi bicipitis brachii

M. biceps brachii

Fig. 3.70 Ventral muscles of the upper arm, right side; ventral view; after removal of the M. biceps brachii. [S700]
The M. biceps brachii was removed to reveal the underlying M. brachialis. The M. coracobrachialis can be easily identified, because it is usually pierced by the N. musculocutaneus which innervates the three muscles on the ventral side of the upper arm (M. coracobrachialis, M. biceps brachii, M. brachialis).

→ T 31

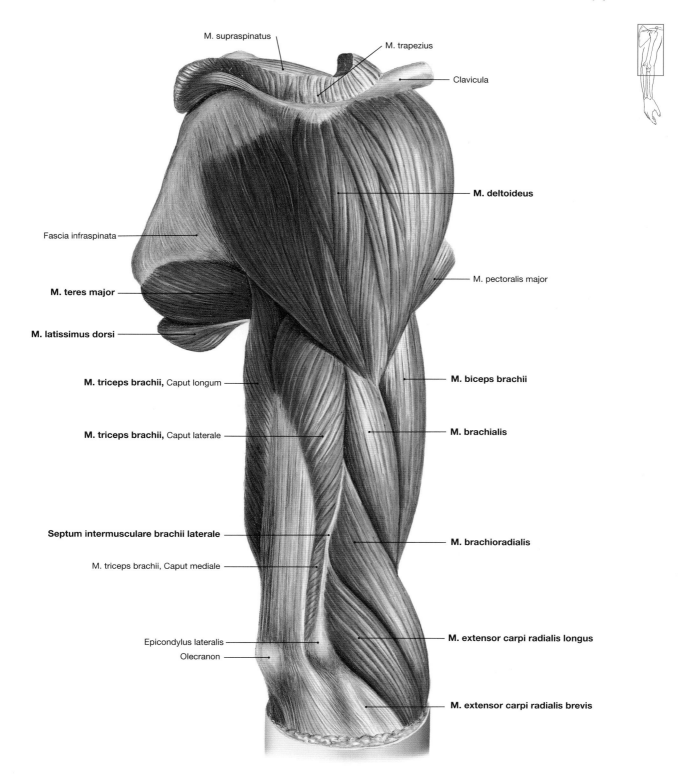

M. supraspinatus

M. trapezius

Clavicula

M. deltoideus

Fascia infraspinata

M. pectoralis major

M. teres major

M. latissimus dorsi

M. triceps brachii, Caput longum

M. biceps brachii

M. triceps brachii, Caput laterale

M. brachialis

Septum intermusculare brachii laterale

M. brachioradialis

M. triceps brachii, Caput mediale

Epicondylus lateralis

Olecranon

M. extensor carpi radialis longus

M. extensor carpi radialis brevis

Fig. 3.71 Dorsal muscles of the shoulder and upper arm as well as ventral muscles of the upper arm, right side; dorsolateral view. [S700]

The M. triceps brachii almost completely covers the posterior aspect of the upper arm. Only the Caput longum and the Caput laterale, which both cover the Caput mediale, are visible here. All three muscle bellies insert on the olecranon. Separated by the Septum intermusculare brachii laterale, the flexor muscles (M. brachialis, M. biceps brachii) attach on the ventral side. The radial extensor muscles of the forearm also have their origins on the lateral aspect of the distal upper arm. From proximally to distally, these include the M. brachioradialis, M. extensor carpi radialis longus and M. extensor carpi radialis brevis. In addition to the M. deltoideus, other shoulder muscles, such as the M. teres major, the M. latissimus dorsi and the M. supraspinatus are visible here.

→ T 29, T 30, T 32

Muscles of the upper arm

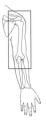

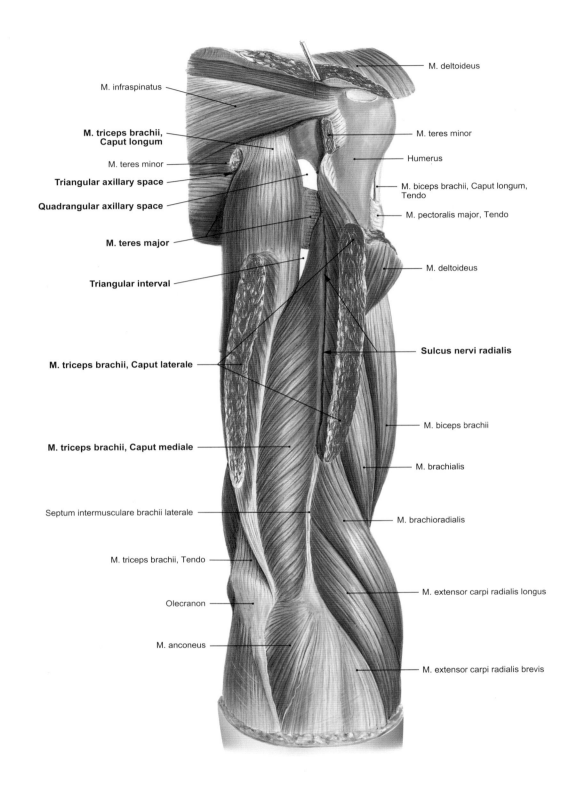

M. infraspinatus

M. deltoideus

M. triceps brachii, Caput longum

M. teres minor

M. teres minor

Humerus

Triangular axillary space

Quadrangular axillary space

M. biceps brachii, Caput longum, Tendo

M. pectoralis major, Tendo

M. teres major

M. deltoideus

Triangular interval

Sulcus nervi radialis

M. triceps brachii, Caput laterale

M. biceps brachii

M. triceps brachii, Caput mediale

M. brachialis

Septum intermusculare brachii laterale

M. brachioradialis

M. triceps brachii, Tendo

M. extensor carpi radialis longus

Olecranon

M. anconeus

M. extensor carpi radialis brevis

Fig. 3.72 Dorsal muscles of the shoulder and upper arm, right side; dorsal lateral view; after splitting the Caput laterale of the M. triceps brachii. [S700]

The Caput longum of the M. triceps brachii originates from the Tuberculum infraglenoidale of the scapula. The Caput laterale originates proximally and laterally of the Sulcus nervi radialis. After splitting the Caput laterale, the Caput mediale is visible, which originates distally and medially of the Sulcus nervi radialis on the humerus. In addition, both **axil-** lary spaces, which are separated by the Caput longum, are visible between the M. teres minor and M. teres major (→ Fig. 3.64). Passing through the so-called **triangular interval,** which lies distally of the M. teres major, the N. radialis reaches the dorsal side of the upper arm. It is bordered medially by the Caput longum and laterally by the Caput laterale of the M. triceps brachii.

→ T 30, T 32

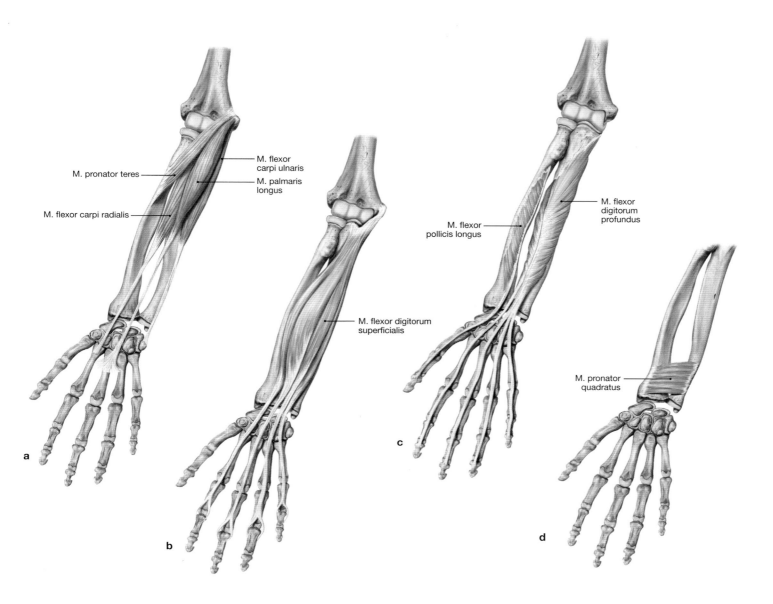

M. pronator teres

M. flexor carpi ulnaris

M. palmaris longus

M. flexor carpi radialis

M. flexor digitorum superficialis

M. flexor pollicis longus

M. flexor digitorum profundus

M. pronator quadratus

a

b

c

d

Fig. 3.73a–d   Ventral muscles of the forearm, right side; ventral view. [S700-L266]

The flexors of the forearm lie on the ventral side and are subdivided into a superficial and a deep group by the radial and ulnar neurovascular pathways. Within these two groups the muscles lie in two layers on top of each other, so that **four different layers** can be distinguished:

• superficial layer
• middle layer
• deep layer
• deepest layer.

a Superficial layer. From radial to ulnar, the superficial layer consists of the M. pronator teres, M. flexor carpi radialis, M. palmaris longus and M. flexor carpi ulnaris. These muscles have their common origin at the Epicondylus medialis of the humerus and are **flexors in the elbow joint** and, apart from the M. pronator teres, they are also flexors of the **wrists.** The **M. pronator teres** crosses the diagonal axis of the forearm and is therefore the **most important pronator,** together with the M. pronator quadratus which lies in the deepest layer. The M. palmaris longus, which may be absent unilaterally or bilaterally in up to 20 % of the cases, tenses the palmar aponeurosis in addition to flexing the wrist. When acting together with its antagonist on the extensor side,

the M. flexor carpi ulnaris induces the ulnar abduction, whereas the M. flexor carpi radialis supports the radial abduction.

b Middle layer. The **M. flexor digitorum superficialis** constitutes the middle layer. It consists of four parts and its tendons extend to the palmar sides of the middle phalanges of the second to fifth fingers. Therefore, in addition to the elbow joints and wrists it also flexes the **proximal interphalangeal** and to a somewhat lesser extent the **metacarpophalangeal joints of the fingers.**

c Deep layer. The deep layer comprises the **M. flexor pollicis longus** on the radial side and the M. flexor digitorum profundus on the **ulnar side.** Both these muscles originate from the anterior aspect of the forearm and therefore do not act on the elbow joint. As they continue up to the palmar sides of the distal phalanges, they flex the wrist and, in addition to the **distal interphalangeal joints of the fingers and the thumb,** they also flex the **metacarpophalangeal and the proximal interphalangeal joints** to a lesser extent.

d Deepest layer. Below the long flexor tendons, the **M. pronator quadratus connects** the front sides of the ulna and the radius.

→ T 33, T 34

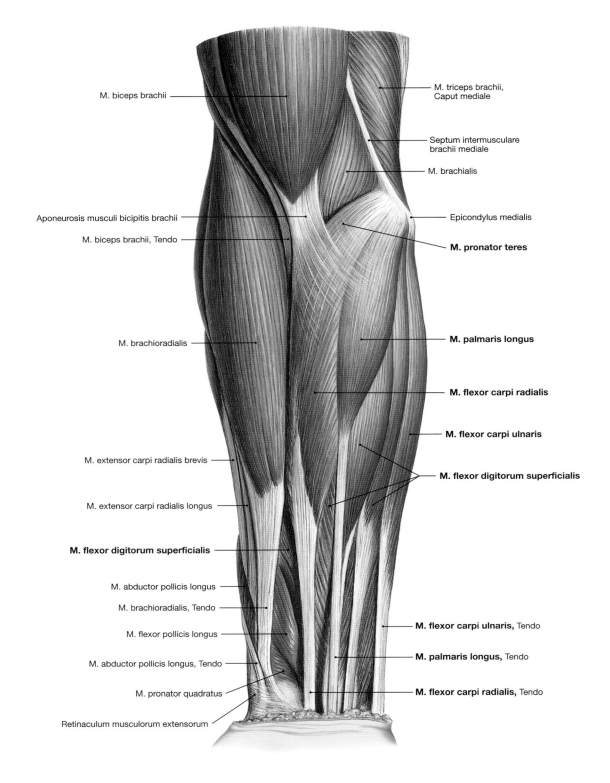

M. biceps brachii

M. triceps brachii, Caput mediale

Septum intermusculare brachii mediale

M. brachialis

Aponeurosis musculi bicipitis brachii

Epicondylus medialis

M. biceps brachii, Tendo

M. pronator teres

M. brachioradialis

M. palmaris longus

M. flexor carpi radialis

M. flexor carpi ulnaris

M. extensor carpi radialis brevis

M. flexor digitorum superficialis

M. extensor carpi radialis longus

M. flexor digitorum superficialis

M. abductor pollicis longus

M. brachioradialis, Tendo

M. flexor carpi ulnaris, Tendo

M. flexor pollicis longus

M. palmaris longus, Tendo

M. abductor pollicis longus, Tendo

M. pronator quadratus

M. flexor carpi radialis, Tendo

Retinaculum musculorum extensorum

Fig. 3.74   Superficial layer of the ventral muscles of the forearm, right side; ventral view. [S700]
From radial to ulnar, the superficial flexor muscles of the forearm consist of the M. pronator teres, M. flexor carpi radialis, M. palmaris longus and M. flexor carpi ulnaris. Parts of the M. flexor digitorum superficialis, which form the middle layer, are visible between the M. palmaris lon-

gus and M. flexor carpi ulnaris as well as between the inserting tendons of these muscles. Radial to the superficial flexor muscles lies the radial muscle group of the forearm, which belongs to the extensor muscles because of their innervation and their effect on the wrists.

→ T 33

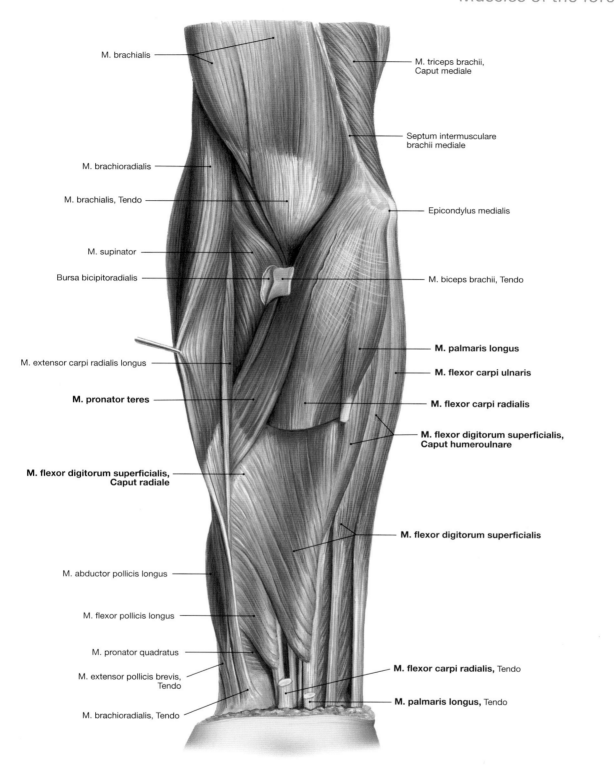

M. brachialis

M. triceps brachii,
Caput mediale

Septum intermusculare
brachii mediale

M. brachioradialis

M. brachialis, Tendo

Epicondylus medialis

M. supinator

Bursa bicipitoradialis

M. biceps brachii, Tendo

M. extensor carpi radialis longus

M. palmaris longus

M. flexor carpi ulnaris

M. pronator teres

M. flexor carpi radialis

**M. flexor digitorum superficialis,
Caput humeroulnare**

**M. flexor digitorum superficialis,
Caput radiale**

M. flexor digitorum superficialis

M. abductor pollicis longus

M. flexor pollicis longus

M. pronator quadratus

M. extensor pollicis brevis,
Tendo

M. flexor carpi radialis, Tendo

M. palmaris longus, Tendo

M. brachioradialis, Tendo

**Fig. 3.75   Middle layer of the ventral muscles of the forearm,
right side;** ventral view; after partial removal of the M. flexor carpi radialis and M. palmaris longus. [S700]
The full extent of the M. pronator teres is visible after removal of the
Aponeurosis musculi bicipitis brachii and folding back of the M. brachioradialis. Below the superficial layer of the flexor muscles lies the middle
layer of the ventral muscles of the forearm, which consists of the four
muscle bellies of the M. flexor digitorum superficialis. The entire width
of this muscle only becomes visible when the M. flexor carpi radialis
and the M. palmaris longus are pulled apart or have been cut away, as

shown here. The Caput humeroulnare of the M. flexor digitorum superficialis originates from the Epicondylus medialis of the humerus and
from the Proc. coronoideus of the ulna. Its Caput radiale originates at
the anterior aspect of the radius.
On closer examination, it is clear that the bellies of the M. flexor digitorum are not on the same plane. Only the muscular parts for the third
and fourth fingers are visible here, as they cover the muscle bellies re-
lating to the second and fifth fingers.

→ T 33

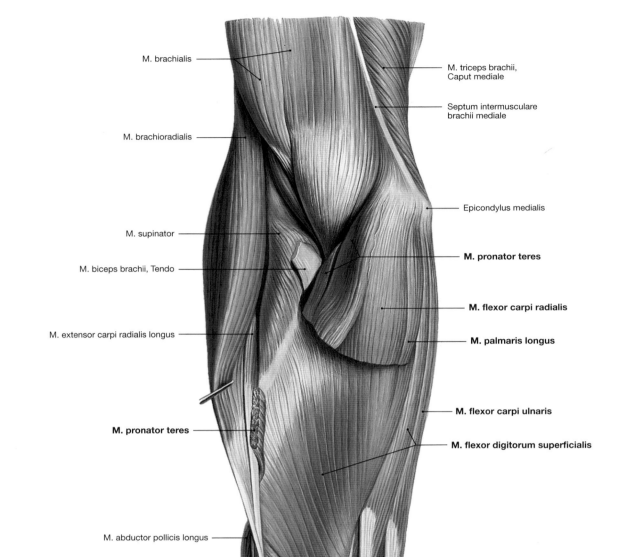

M. brachialis

M. triceps brachii, Caput mediale

Septum intermusculare brachii mediale

M. brachioradialis

Epicondylus medialis

M. supinator

M. pronator teres

M. biceps brachii, Tendo

M. flexor carpi radialis

M. extensor carpi radialis longus

M. palmaris longus

M. flexor carpi ulnaris

M. pronator teres

M. flexor digitorum superficialis

M. abductor pollicis longus

M. flexor pollicis longus

M. pronator quadratus

M. abductor pollicis longus, Tendo

M. flexor carpi radialis, Tendo

M. brachioradialis, Tendo

M. palmaris longus, Tendo

Fig. 3.76 Middle layer of the ventral muscles of the forearm, right side; ventral view; after extensive removal of the M. flexor carpi radialis, M. palmaris longus and M. pronator teres. [S700]
In contrast to → Fig. 3.75, the M. pronator teres was additionally split here to expose the origins of the M. flexor digitorum superficialis. The

Caput humeroulnare originates from the Epicondylus medialis of the humerus and from the Proc. coronoideus of the ulna. The Caput radiale originates from the anterior aspect of the radius.

→ T 33

─ **Clinical remarks** ─────────────────────────

After a stroke or lesions of the central nervous system, an **abnormal muscular hypertonicity** can occur in the form of **spasticity** or even without any major injury in the form of **dystonia.** Spasticity often affects entire muscle groups. Sometimes dystonia manifests selectively in individual flexor muscles, e.g. with writer's cramp, or some-

times only in a single muscle belly, e.g. of the M. flexor digitorum superficialis. To enable a targeted treatment, e.g. the inhibition of signal transmission to the motor end plates by injection of the botulinum toxin, a very precise understanding of the function and topography of the muscles is necessary.

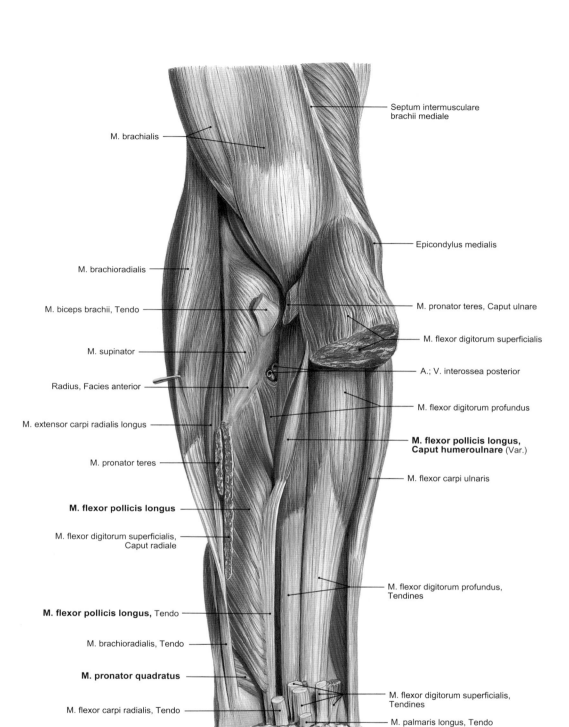

M. brachialis

Septum intermusculare
brachii mediale

Epicondylus medialis

M. brachioradialis

M. biceps brachii, Tendo

M. pronator teres, Caput ulnare

M. flexor digitorum superficialis

M. supinator

A.; V. interossea posterior

Radius, Facies anterior

M. flexor digitorum profundus

M. extensor carpi radialis longus

**M. flexor pollicis longus,
Caput humeroulnare** (Var.)

M. pronator teres

M. flexor carpi ulnaris

M. flexor pollicis longus

M. flexor digitorum superficialis,
Caput radiale

M. flexor digitorum profundus,
Tendines

M. flexor pollicis longus, Tendo

M. brachioradialis, Tendo

M. pronator quadratus

M. flexor carpi radialis, Tendo

M. flexor digitorum superficialis,
Tendines

M. palmaris longus, Tendo

Fig. 3.77 Deep and deepest layer of the ventral muscles of the forearm, right side; ventral view; after removal of the superficial flexor muscles. [S700]
When all superficial muscles have been pulled apart or removed, the deep flexor muscles become visible as shown here. The M. flexor digitorum profundus originates from the anterior aspect of the ulna and from the Membrana interossea antebrachii. The M. flexor pollicis longus

originates from the anterior aspect of the radius and in up to 40 % of all cases with an additional Caput humeroulnare from the Epicondylus medialis and the Proc. coronoideus. The M. pronator quadratus is situated below the flexor tendons on the distal forearm where it passes along the anterior aspect of both the bones from the ulna to the radius.

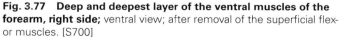

→ T 34

Muscles of the forearm

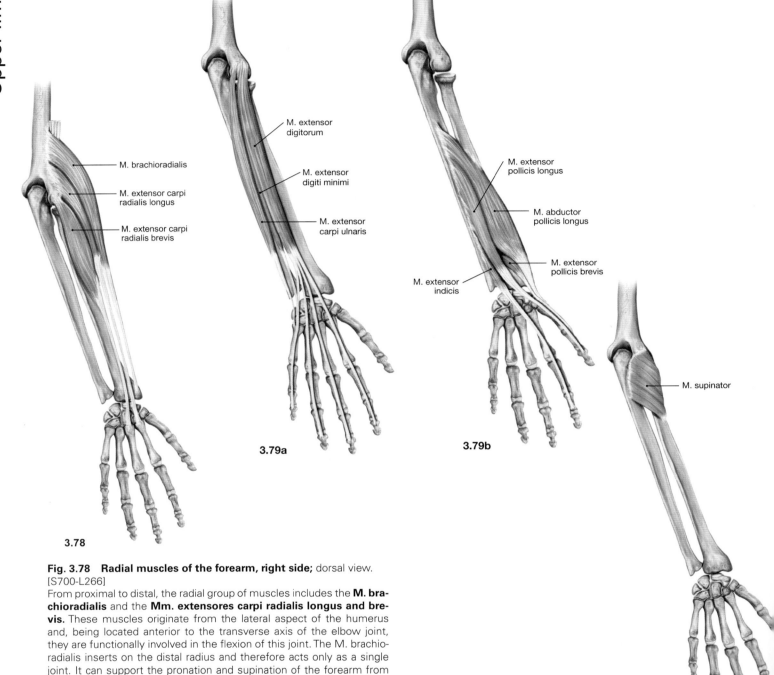

M. brachioradialis

M. extensor carpi radialis longus

M. extensor carpi radialis brevis

3.78

M. extensor digitorum

M. extensor digiti minimi

M. extensor carpi ulnaris

3.79a

M. extensor pollicis longus

M. abductor pollicis longus

M. extensor pollicis brevis

M. extensor indicis

3.79b

M. supinator

3.79c

Fig. 3.78   Radial muscles of the forearm, right side; dorsal view. [S700-L266]
From proximal to distal, the radial group of muscles includes the **M. brachioradialis** and the **Mm. extensores carpi radialis longus and brevis.** These muscles originate from the lateral aspect of the humerus and, being located anterior to the transverse axis of the elbow joint, they are functionally involved in the flexion of this joint. The M. brachioradialis inserts on the distal radius and therefore acts only as a single joint. It can support the pronation and supination of the forearm from the respectively opposing positions. The Mm. extensores carpi radialis longus and brevis are extensors of the wrists and facilitate the radial abduction.

→ T 35

Fig. 3.79a–c   Dorsal muscles of the forearm, right side; dorsal view. [S700-L266]
a Superficial layer. The superficial extensors all originate at the **Epicondylus lateralis.** Excessive stress on the point of origin of these tendons can cause very unpleasant pain ('tennis elbow'). From radial to ulnar, this muscle group includes the **M. extensor digitorum,** the **M. extensor digiti minimi,** and the **M. extensor carpi ulnaris.** The M. extensor digitorum and M. extensor digiti minimi radiate into the dorsal aponeuroses of the second to fifth digits. Therefore, these muscles extend into the wrists as well as into the metacarpophalangeal and proximal interphalangeal joints of the fingers. As the middle tract of the dorsal aponeurosis ends on the middle phalanges, the muscles are not involved in extending the distal interphalangeal joints.

b Deep layer. Distally from radial to ulnar, the deep layer consists of the **M. abductor pollicis longus, M. extensor pollicis brevis, M. extensor pollicis longus** and **M. extensor indicis.** The M. abductor pollicis longus abducts the thumb in the saddle joint, whereas the Mm. extensores pollicis brevis and longus extend the carpometacarpal and distal interphalangeal joints. The M. extensor indicis extends the index finger in the carpometacarpal and proximal interphalangeal joints.
c Deep layer. Proximally, the deep layer of the wrist extensor muscles includes the **M. supinator** which winds around the radius. It is the strongest supinator when the elbow joint is extended.

→ T 36, T 37

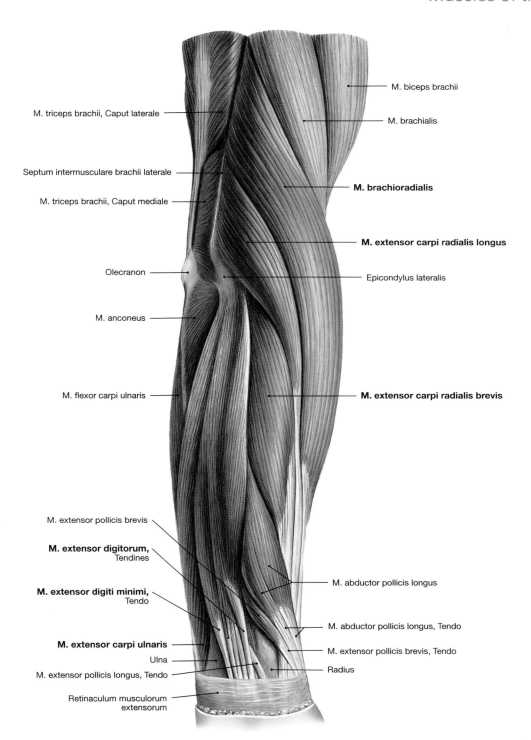

M. biceps brachii

M. triceps brachii, Caput laterale

M. brachialis

Septum intermusculare brachii laterale

M. brachioradialis

M. triceps brachii, Caput mediale

M. extensor carpi radialis longus

Olecranon

Epicondylus lateralis

M. anconeus

M. flexor carpi ulnaris

M. extensor carpi radialis brevis

M. extensor pollicis brevis

M. extensor digitorum,
Tendines

M. abductor pollicis longus

M. extensor digiti minimi,
Tendo

M. abductor pollicis longus, Tendo

M. extensor carpi ulnaris

M. extensor pollicis brevis, Tendo

Ulna

M. extensor pollicis longus, Tendo

Radius

Retinaculum musculorum
extensorum

**Fig. 3.80 Superficial layer of the dorsal muscles of the forearm
and of the distal part of the upper arm, right side;** lateral view.
[S700]
The muscles of the radial muscle group are particularly visible in the
lateral view. From proximal to distal there are the M. brachioradialis and
the Mm. extensores carpi radialis longus and brevis. The superficial extensor muscles (M. extensor digitorum, M. extensor digiti minimi and

M. extensor carpi ulnaris) follow in the ulnar direction. Between these
muscle groups, the distal parts of the deep extensor muscles are visible distally (thus, they are not completely covered by the superficial
extensors). On the distal upper arm, the fascia on the M. anconeus has
been removed. This muscle belongs to the extensor muscles of the
upper arm.

→ T 31, T 32, T 36

Muscles of the forearm

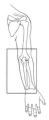

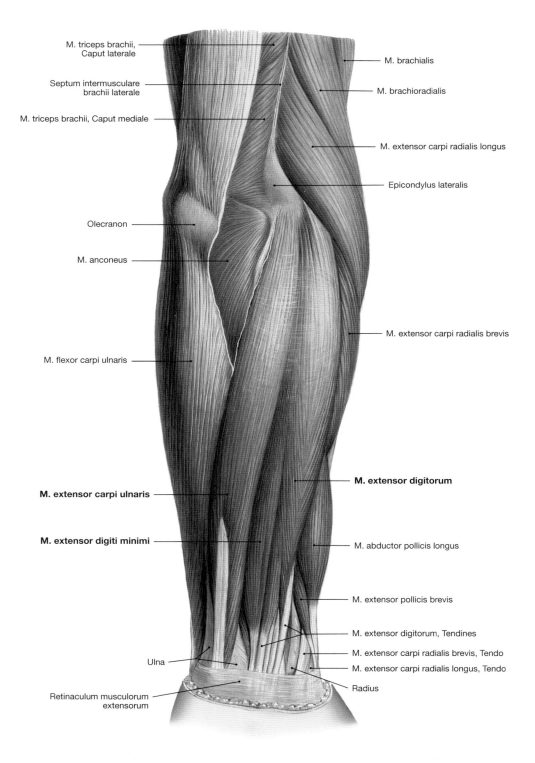

M. triceps brachii, Caput laterale

Septum intermusculare brachii laterale

M. triceps brachii, Caput mediale

Olecranon

M. anconeus

M. flexor carpi ulnaris

M. extensor carpi ulnaris

M. extensor digiti minimi

Ulna

Retinaculum musculorum extensorum

M. brachialis

M. brachioradialis

M. extensor carpi radialis longus

Epicondylus lateralis

M. extensor carpi radialis brevis

M. extensor digitorum

M. abductor pollicis longus

M. extensor pollicis brevis

M. extensor digitorum, Tendines

M. extensor carpi radialis brevis, Tendo

M. extensor carpi radialis longus, Tendo

Radius

Fig. 3.81 Superficial layer of the dorsal muscles of the forearm and of the distal part of the upper arm, right side; dorsal view. [S700]

The superficial extensor muscles of the forearm are visible here. From radial to ulnar, this muscle group includes the M. extensor digitorum, M. extensor digiti minimi and M. extensor carpi ulnaris. The M. extensor carpi ulnaris joins the M. flexor carpi ulnaris of the superficial flexor group in the ulnar direction.

→ T 36

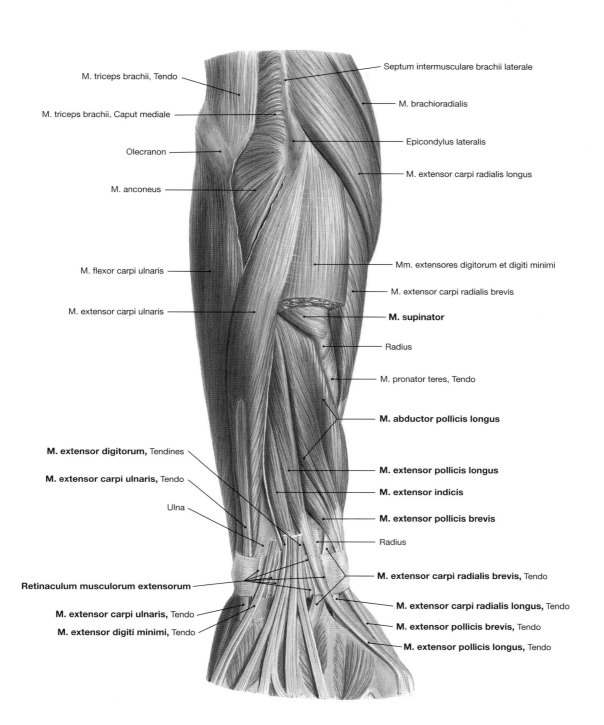

M. triceps brachii, Tendo

M. triceps brachii, Caput mediale

Olecranon

M. anconeus

M. flexor carpi ulnaris

M. extensor carpi ulnaris

Septum intermusculare brachii laterale

M. brachioradialis

Epicondylus lateralis

M. extensor carpi radialis longus

Mm. extensores digitorum et digiti minimi

M. extensor carpi radialis brevis

M. supinator

Radius

M. pronator teres, Tendo

M. abductor pollicis longus

M. extensor digitorum, Tendines

M. extensor carpi ulnaris, Tendo

Ulna

M. extensor pollicis longus

M. extensor indicis

M. extensor pollicis brevis

Radius

M. extensor carpi radialis brevis, Tendo

Retinaculum musculorum extensorum

M. extensor carpi ulnaris, Tendo

M. extensor digiti minimi, Tendo

M. extensor carpi radialis longus, Tendo

M. extensor pollicis brevis, Tendo

M. extensor pollicis longus, Tendo

Fig. 3.82   Deep layer of the dorsal muscles of the forearm, right side; dorsal view; after partial removal of the Mm. extensores digitorum and digiti minimi. [S700]

After removal of the superficial extensors of the forearm, the proximal parts of the deep extensor muscles beneath become visible. The deep layer consists proximally of the M. supinator; it is followed from radial to ulnar by the M. abductor pollicis longus, M. extensor pollicis brevis, M. extensor pollicis longus and M. extensor indicis.

The Retinaculum musculorum extensorum forms **six tendon compartments,** through which the tendons of the extensor muscles pass to the dorsal side of the hand. In this dissection, the third, fourth and fifth tendon compartments have been opened.

Tendon compartments on the back of the hand are, from radial to ulnar:
*   First compartment: M. abductor pollicis longus and M. extensor pollicis brevis
*   Second compartment: Mm. extensores carpi radialis longus and brevis
*   Third compartment: M. extensor pollicis longus
*   Fourth compartment: M. extensor digitorum and M. extensor indicis
*   Fifth compartment: M. extensor digiti minimi
*   Sixth compartment: M. extensor carpi ulnaris.

→ T 37

Muscles of the forearm

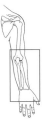

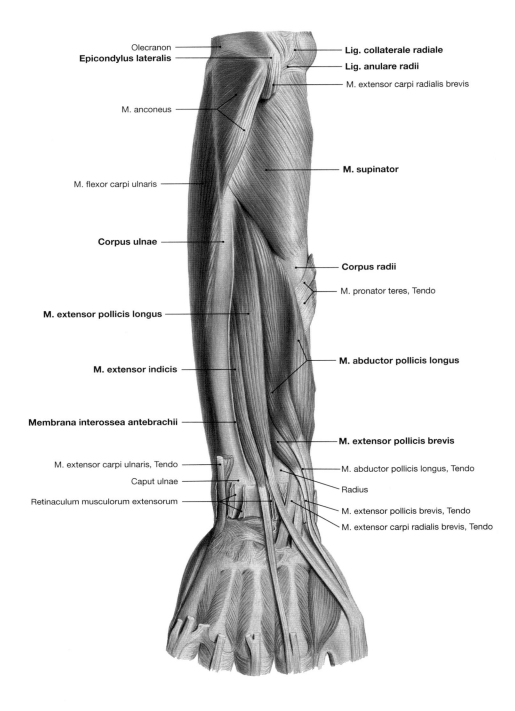

Olecranon
Epicondylus lateralis
M. anconeus
M. flexor carpi ulnaris
Corpus ulnae
M. extensor pollicis longus
M. extensor indicis
Membrana interossea antebrachii
M. extensor carpi ulnaris, Tendo
Caput ulnae
Retinaculum musculorum extensorum

Lig. collaterale radiale
Lig. anulare radii
M. extensor carpi radialis brevis
M. supinator
Corpus radii
M. pronator teres, Tendo
M. abductor pollicis longus
M. extensor pollicis brevis
M. abductor pollicis longus, Tendo
Radius
M. extensor pollicis brevis, Tendo
M. extensor carpi radialis brevis, Tendo

Fig. 3.83   Deep layer of the dorsal muscles of the forearm, right side; dorsal view; after complete removal of the superficial extensor muscles. [S700]

The superficial extensor muscles have been completely removed to show the origins of the deep extensor muscles. The M. supinator originates from the Epicondylus lateralis of the humerus, the radial ligaments (Lig. collaterale radiale and Lig. anulare radii) as well as the Crista m. supinatoris of the ulna. With its insertion, it encompasses the radius above and below the Tuberositas radii. The two muscles on the radial side (M. abductor pollicis longus, M. extensor pollicis brevis) have

tendons passing through the first tendon compartment, and originate from the dorsal sides of the radius and the ulna as well as from the Membrana interossea antebrachii. In contrast, the two muscles on the ulnar side (M. extensor pollicis longus and M. extensor indicis) originate exclusively from the ulna and the Membrana interossea. Their tendons pass through the third and fourth compartments. In this dissection, all six compartments underneath the Retinaculum musculorum extensorum have been opened.

→ T 37

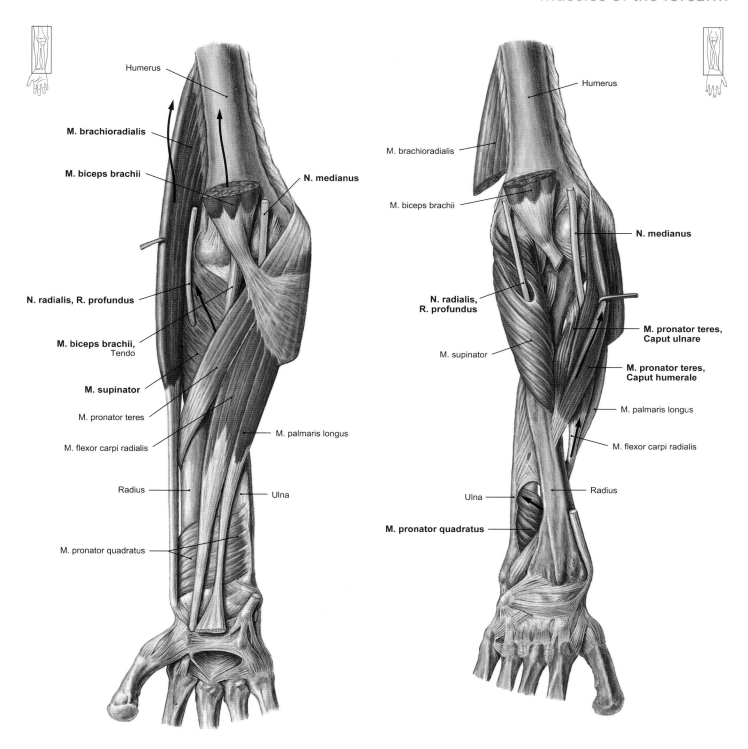

Humerus

M. brachioradialis

M. biceps brachii

N. medianus

N. radialis, R. profundus

M. biceps brachii,
Tendo

M. supinator

M. pronator teres

M. flexor carpi radialis

M. palmaris longus

Radius

Ulna

M. pronator quadratus

Humerus

M. brachioradialis

M. biceps brachii

N. medianus

**N. radialis,
R. profundus**

M. supinator

**M. pronator teres,
Caput ulnare**

**M. pronator teres,
Caput humerale**

M. palmaris longus

M. flexor carpi radialis

Radius

Ulna

M. pronator quadratus

Fig. 3.84 Forearm, antebrachium, supinated position, right side; ventral and palmar view. The arrows indicate the direction of traction of the most important supinator muscles. [S700]

As a general rule, all muscles involved in pronation or supination cross the **diagonal axis of the forearm** (→ Fig. 3.6), which corresponds to the rotational axis of this movement. In addition, it can be noted that all relevant supinator and pronator muscles have **insertions on the radius.** The **most important supinator muscles** are the **M. biceps brachii** (in particular with the arm flexed), **M. supinator** (with extended arm), and **M. brachioradialis** (from a pronated position).

The M. supinator is pierced by the R. profundus of the N. radialis. Compression or entrapment of the N. radialis can develop here, which among other things can cause a paralysis of the deep extensor muscles (→ Fig. 3.122).

Fig. 3.85 Forearm, antebrachium, pronated position, right side; ventral view in the elbow region and dorsal view in the hand region, respectively. The arrows indicate the direction of traction of the **most important pronator muscles,** which are the **M. pronator teres, M. pronator quadratus** and **M. brachioradialis** (from a supinated position). The M. flexor carpi radialis and M. palmaris longus have a weak pronation effect. [S700]

The N. medianus passes between the two heads of the M. pronator teres, and can rarely also be compressed in this location (→ Fig. 3.126).

→ T 31, T 34, T 35, T 37

Musculature

Tendons of the back of the hand

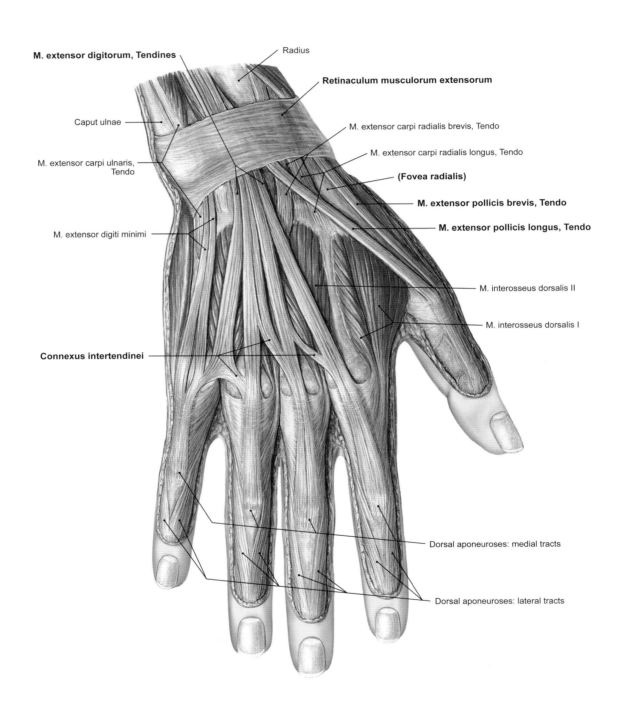

M. extensor digitorum, Tendines

Radius

Retinaculum musculorum extensorum

Caput ulnae

M. extensor carpi radialis brevis, Tendo

M. extensor carpi radialis longus, Tendo

M. extensor carpi ulnaris, Tendo

(Fovea radialis)

M. extensor pollicis brevis, Tendo

M. extensor pollicis longus, Tendo

M. extensor digiti minimi

M. interosseus dorsalis II

M. interosseus dorsalis I

Connexus intertendinei

Dorsal aponeuroses: medial tracts

Dorsal aponeuroses: lateral tracts

Fig. 3.86 Tendons of the back of the hand, Dorsum manus, right side; dorsal view. [S700]
The inserting tendons of the extensor muscles pass beneath the Retinaculum musculorum extensorum to the dorsal side of the thumb and to the dorsal aponeuroses of the fingers. The tendons of the M. extensor digitorum are connected by bridges (Connexus intertendinei), which slightly restrict a selective extension of individual fingers. The back of the hand does not have its own muscles. The Mm. interossei dorsales, which are visible below the extensor tendons, are included in the muscles of the palm. A shallow depression, bordered by the tendons of the M. extensor pollicis brevis and the M. extensor pollicis longus, is called the Fovea radialis (**snuffbox** or tabatière).

→ T 36

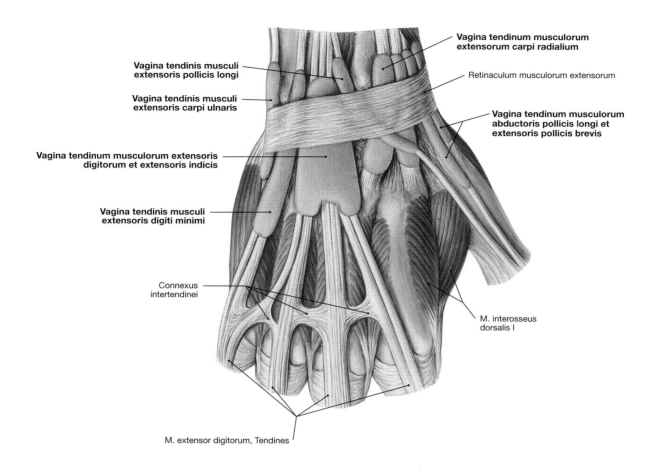

Vagina tendinum musculorum extensorum carpi radialium

Vagina tendinis musculi extensoris pollicis longi

Retinaculum musculorum extensorum

Vagina tendinis musculi extensoris carpi ulnaris

Vagina tendinum musculorum abductoris pollicis longi et extensoris pollicis brevis

Vagina tendinum musculorum extensoris digitorum et extensoris indicis

Vagina tendinis musculi extensoris digiti minimi

Connexus intertendinei

M. interosseus dorsalis I

M. extensor digitorum, Tendines

Fig. 3.87 Dorsal carpal tendon sheaths, Vaginae tendinum, of the back of the hand, right side; dorsal view. [S700]
The tendons of the extensor muscles pass through six compartments or tunnels beneath the Retinaculum musculorum extensorum (→ Fig. 3.83). The individual muscles have for the most part their own **tendon sheaths,** which facilitate gliding of the tendons between the retinaculum and the bones of the hand. The tendons of the M. extensor digitorum and M. extensor indicis thus share a common tendon sheath.

Structure and function

The **snuffbox** (or tabatière, or Foveola radialis) is a triangular depression between the tendons of the M. extensor pollicis longus and brevis (→ Fig. 3.86). This depression is called the snuffbox because it was used in the past to hold snuff (ground tobacco) before inhaling it via the nose. The **Os scaphoideum** and the **Os trapezium** are palpable at the bottom of this depression. Running through the snuffbox are the (→ Fig. 3.155, → Fig. 3.180):
• A. radialis
• R. superficialis of the N. radialis
• V. cephalica antebrachia.

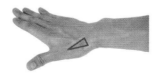

[S701-L271]

Clinical remarks

Tenderness in the **snuffbox** is frequently a sign of a **fractured Os scaphoideum** as a result of a fall onto the wrist joint. This scaphoid fracture is often overlooked with an accompanying fracture of the distal radius as the latter is more symptomatic.

Musculature

Superficial layer of the hand muscles

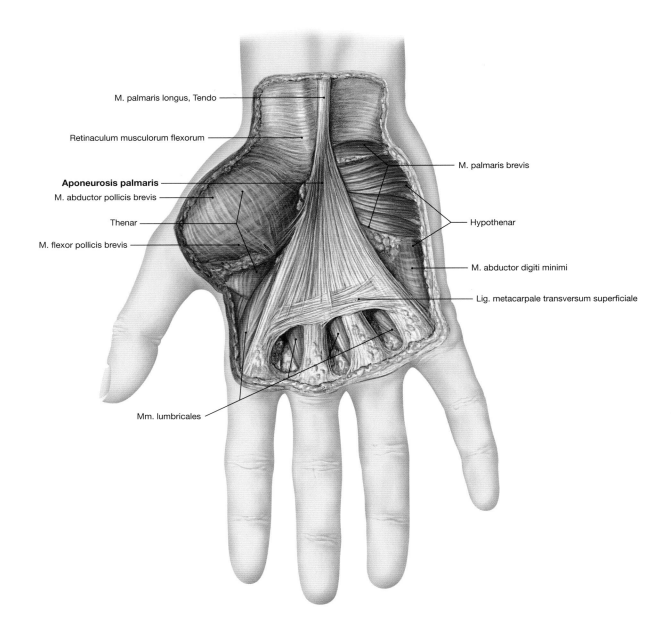

M. palmaris longus, Tendo

Retinaculum musculorum flexorum

Aponeurosis palmaris

M. abductor pollicis brevis

Thenar

M. flexor pollicis brevis

Mm. lumbricales

M. palmaris brevis

Hypothenar

M. abductor digiti minimi

Lig. metacarpale transversum superficiale

Fig. 3.88   Superficial muscle layer of the palm of the hand, Palma manus, right side; palmar view. [S700]

The muscles of the palm of the hand consist of **three groups.** The two marginal fingers (thumb and little finger) each have their own muscle group on their side of the palm. The muscles of the thumb form the thenar eminence (thenar) and the muscles of the little finger form the hypothenar eminence (hypothenar). The muscles of the palm lie in-between. These three muscle groups form **three overlying layers.** During dissection attention must be paid to the neurovascular structures running between the individual layers (→ Fig. 3.176, → Fig. 3.177, → Fig. 3.178). The **palmar aponeurosis** (Aponeurosis palmaris) lies

very close to the surface of the palm. It consists of longitudinal fibres and in particular, proximal to the metacarpophalangeal joint, of strongly developed transverse fibres **(Lig. metacarpale transversum superficiale).** Proximally the palmar aponeurosis is attached to the Retinaculum musculorum flexorum and is tensed by the M. palmaris longus. Distally it is attached to the tendon sheaths of the flexor muscles and the ligaments of the metacarpophalangeal joints of the fingers.

On the thenar eminence, the M. abductor pollicis brevis and the M. flexor pollicis brevis lie from radial to ulnar. The M. palmaris brevis and M. abductor digiti minimi lie superficially on the hypothenar eminence.

→ T 33, T 38–T40

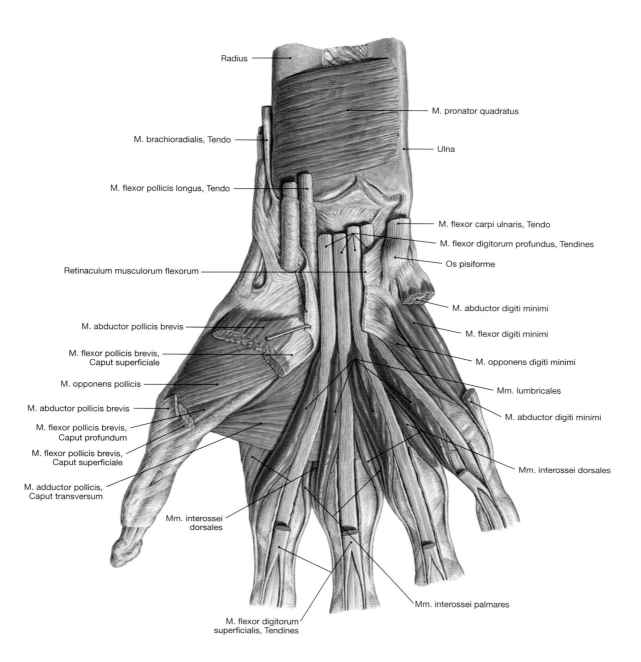

Radius

M. pronator quadratus

M. brachioradialis, Tendo

Ulna

M. flexor pollicis longus, Tendo

M. flexor carpi ulnaris, Tendo

M. flexor digitorum profundus, Tendines

Os pisiforme

Retinaculum musculorum flexorum

M. abductor digiti minimi

M. abductor pollicis brevis

M. flexor digiti minimi

M. flexor pollicis brevis, Caput superficiale

M. opponens digiti minimi

M. opponens pollicis

Mm. lumbricales

M. abductor pollicis brevis

M. abductor digiti minimi

M. flexor pollicis brevis, Caput profundum

M. flexor pollicis brevis, Caput superficiale

Mm. interossei dorsales

M. adductor pollicis, Caput transversum

Mm. interossei dorsales

Mm. interossei palmares

M. flexor digitorum superficialis, Tendines

Fig. 3.89 Middle layer of muscles in the palm of hand, Palma manus, right side; palmar view; after removal of the palmar aponeurosis and the superficial muscles. [S700]
The three muscle groups in the palm of the hand (Palma manus) form three overlying layers. After removal of the superficial muscles, the muscles of the middle layer can be defined. These comprise the M. opponens pollicis and M. adductor pollicis on the thenar eminence, and the M. flexor digiti minimi and M. opponens digiti minimi on the hypothenar eminence, both of which are located radial to the superficial M. abductor digiti minimi. In the palm, the tendons of the M. flexor

digitorum superficialis run to the middle phalanges and the tendons of the M. flexor digitorum profundus to the distal phalanges of the fingers. The tendons of the deep flexor muscle pierce the superficial flexor tendons (removed in this illustration). The tendons of the M. flexor digitorum profundus are the origin of the four Mm. lumbricales which also belong to the middle layer of muscles (for the function of the Mm. lumbricales → Fig. 3.96). The tendon of the M. flexor pollicis longus runs to the distal phalanx of the thumb.

→ T 34, T38–T 40

Tendon sheaths of the palm of the hand

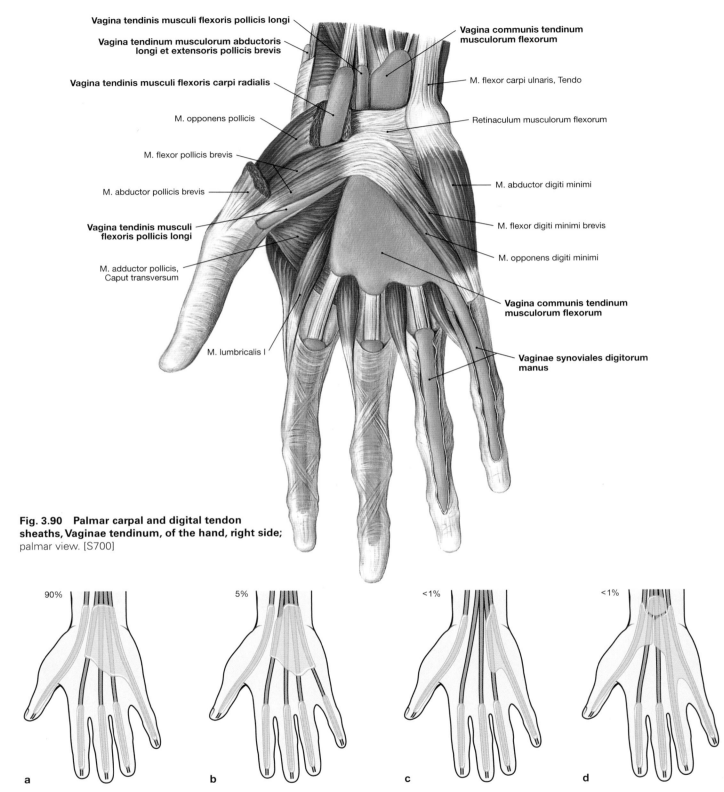

Vagina tendinis musculi flexoris pollicis longi

Vagina tendinum musculorum abductoris longi et extensoris pollicis brevis

Vagina tendinis musculi flexoris carpi radialis

M. opponens pollicis

M. flexor pollicis brevis

M. abductor pollicis brevis

Vagina tendinis musculi flexoris pollicis longi

M. adductor pollicis, Caput transversum

M. lumbricalis I

Vagina communis tendinum musculorum flexorum

M. flexor carpi ulnaris, Tendo

Retinaculum musculorum flexorum

M. abductor digiti minimi

M. flexor digiti minimi brevis

M. opponens digiti minimi

Vagina communis tendinum musculorum flexorum

Vaginae synoviales digitorum manus

Fig. 3.90 Palmar carpal and digital tendon sheaths, Vaginae tendinum, of the hand, right side; palmar view. [S700]

90%   5%   <1%   <1%

a   b   c   d

Fig. 3.91a–d   Variants of the palmar tendon sheaths. [S700-L126] In contrast to the dorsal side there are usually only two tendon sheaths for the flexor tendons of the fingers. The **radial** tendon sheath surrounds the tendon of the M. flexor pollicis longus and extends to its distal phalanx. The **ulnar** tendon sheath encloses all the tendons of the Mm. flexores digitorum superficialis and profundus at the wrists and extends to the distal phalanx only on the little finger. The other fingers have their own tendon sheaths in the area of the phalanges.

Clinical remarks

The arrangement of the tendon sheaths is of clinical importance as **bacterial infections** can quickly spread into the sheaths (phlegmon). Inflammation may spread to the ulnar tendon sheath and to the little finger (V-phlegmon) and, in the case of insufficient antibiotic therapy, may lead to stiffening of the entire hand.

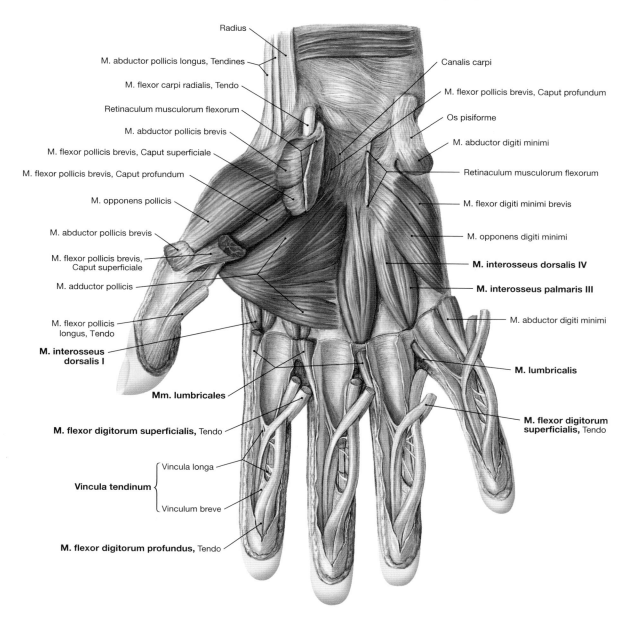

Radius

M. abductor pollicis longus, Tendines

M. flexor carpi radialis, Tendo

Retinaculum musculorum flexorum

M. abductor pollicis brevis

M. flexor pollicis brevis, Caput superficiale

M. flexor pollicis brevis, Caput profundum

M. opponens pollicis

M. abductor pollicis brevis

M. flexor pollicis brevis, Caput superficiale

M. adductor pollicis

M. flexor pollicis longus, Tendo

M. interosseus dorsalis I

Mm. lumbricales

M. flexor digitorum superficialis, Tendo

Vincula tendinum { Vincula longa
Vinculum breve

M. flexor digitorum profundus, Tendo

Canalis carpi

M. flexor pollicis brevis, Caput profundum

Os pisiforme

M. abductor digiti minimi

Retinaculum musculorum flexorum

M. flexor digiti minimi brevis

M. opponens digiti minimi

M. interosseus dorsalis IV

M. interosseus palmaris III

M. abductor digiti minimi

M. lumbricalis

M. flexor digitorum superficialis, Tendo

Fig. 3.92 Deep muscle layer of the palm of the hand, Palma manus, right side; palmar view; after removal of the tendons of the long flexor muscles of the fingers. [S700]
The three muscle groups of the palm form three overlying layers. After removal of the long flexor tendons, the muscles of the deep layer become visible. The Mm. interossei comprise three **Mm. interossei palmares** and four **Mm. interossei dorsales,** all of which flex the metacarpophalangeal joints (for the course and function of the Mm. interossei (→ Fig. 3.93, → Fig. 3.94 and → Fig. 3.95). Since the palmar and dorsal muscles partly originate from different metacarpal bones, muscles of both groups are visible in the palmar view. However, the Mm. interossei

dorsales lie in fact, as their name suggests, further dorsal between the Ossa metacarpi, so that only the dorsal muscles are apparent when looking at the back of the hand (→ Fig. 3.86).
The inserting tendons of the **Mm. interossei** run palmar to the transverse axis of the metacarpophalangeal joints. Therefore, the Mm. interossei are the **main flexors of the metacarpophalangeal joints.**
The illustration shows how the tendons of the deep flexor muscles pierce through the superficial flexor tendons. The tendons are attached to the phalanges by small ligaments (Vincula tendinum).

→ T 38, T 39

Clinical remarks

Knowledge of the function and course of the flexor muscles of the fingers is important when **examining cuts.** If it is not possible to flex the distal interphalangeal joints, the M. flexor digitorum profundus is

affected. If, however, the flexion in the proximal interphalangeal joints is restricted while the distal joints can still be bent, this indicates an isolated injury of the M. flexor digitorum superficialis.

Deep layer of the hand muscles

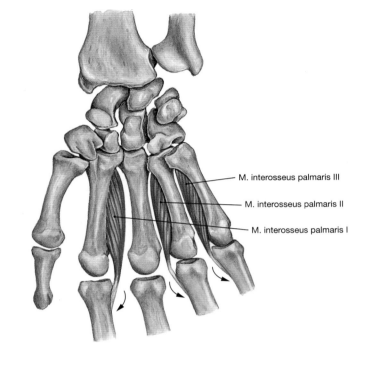

Fig. 3.93 **Mm. interossei palmares, right side;** palmar view. [S700]
The three Mm. interossei palmares originate from the ulnar aspect of
the Os metacarpi II and from the radial aspect of the Ossa metacarpi IV
and V. They insert on the same (ipsilateral) side of the corresponding
proximal phalanx of the fingers, and their inserting tendons additionally
radiate into the lateral tracts of the dorsal aponeuroses (arrows). They
therefore **flex** the **metacarpophalangeal joints** of the fingers and
somewhat **extend** the **proximal and distal interphalangeal joints.**

→ T 39

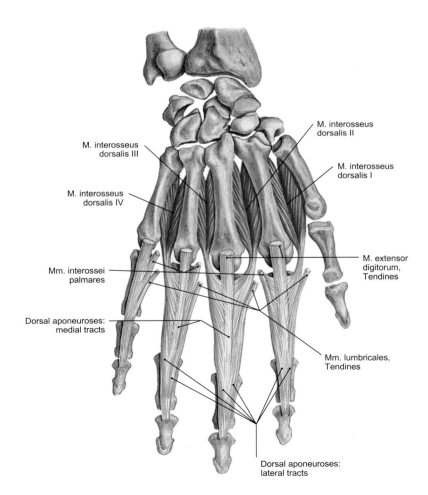

Fig. 3.94 **Mm. interossei dorsales, right side;** dorsal
view. [S700]
The four Mm. interossei dorsales originate with two
heads from opposing surfaces of the metacarpals I–V.
They begin on both sides of the proximal phalanx of the
middle finger, on the ulnar side of the ring finger, and on
the radial side of the index finger. With a small part of
their inserting tendons, they also radiate into the lateral
tracts of the dorsal aponeuroses of the fingers. Just like
the palmar interosseous muscles, they **flex** the **metacarpophalangeal joints** of the fingers and **extend** the
proximal and distal interphalangeal joints.

→ T 39

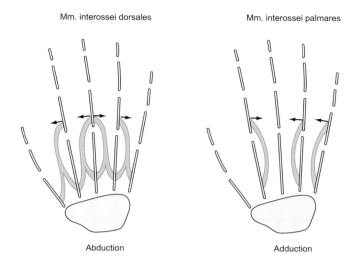

Mm. interossei dorsales   Mm. interossei palmares

Abduction   Adduction

Fig. 3.95 Schematic drawing of the position of the Mm. interossei, illustrating their effect on abduction and adduction of the fingers. [S700-L126]/[C185]
According to their course which is shown on → Fig. 3.93 and → Fig. 3.94, the **Mm. interossei dorsales** can spread the fingers **(abduction)** and can move the middle finger medially and laterally. **The Mm. interossei palmares** on the other hand bring the fingers together **(adduction).**

Their effect on the flexion and extension of the finger joints is clear from the course of their tendons in relation to the transverse axis of the finger joints and is explained on→ Fig. 3.97, → Fig. 3.98 and → Fig. 3.99.

→ T 39

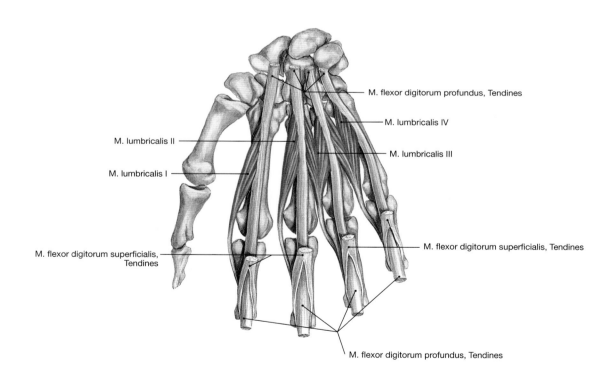

M. flexor digitorum profundus, Tendines

M. lumbricalis IV

M. lumbricalis II

M. lumbricalis III

M. lumbricalis I

M. flexor digitorum superficialis, Tendines

M. flexor digitorum superficialis, Tendines

M. flexor digitorum profundus, Tendines

Fig. 3.96 Mm. lumbricales, right side; palmar view. [S700]
The two radial Mm. lumbricales originate with one head, but both the two ulnar lumbricales originate with two heads from the tendons of the M. flexor digitorum profundus. All muscles insert on the radial side of the proximal phalanges of fingers II–V and their tendons radiate into the

lateral tracts of the dorsal aponeuroses of the fingers. Therefore, they **flex** the **metacarpophalangeal joints of the fingers** a little and **extend** the **proximal and distal interphalangeal joints.**

→ T 39

Deep layer of the hand muscles

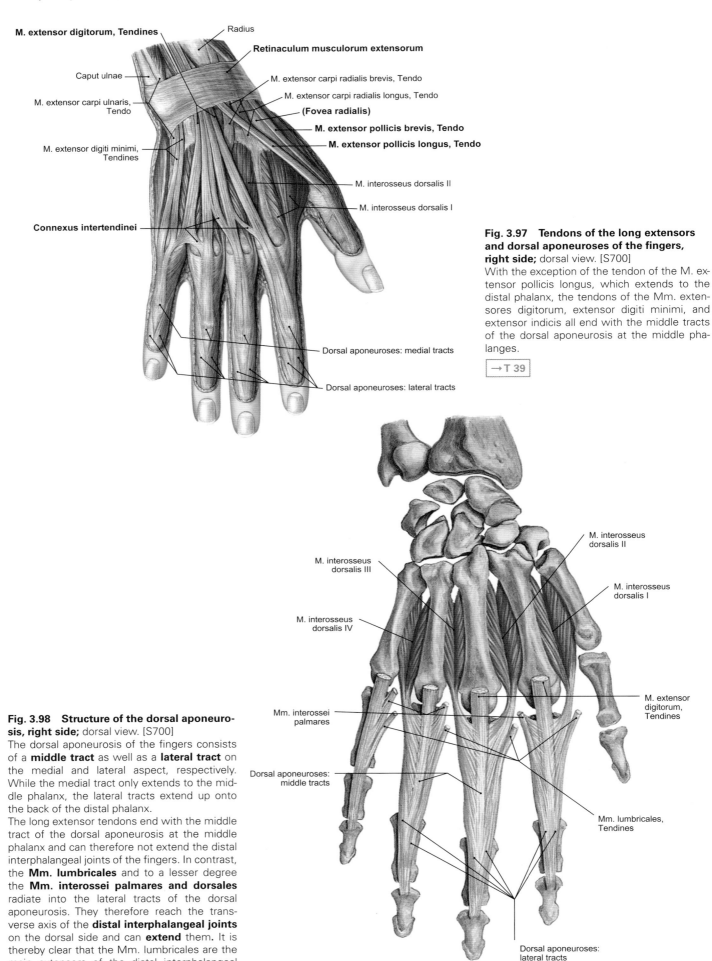

M. extensor digitorum, Tendines

Radius

Caput ulnae

Retinaculum musculorum extensorum

M. extensor carpi ulnaris, Tendo

M. extensor carpi radialis brevis, Tendo

M. extensor carpi radialis longus, Tendo

(Fovea radialis)

M. extensor digiti minimi, Tendines

M. extensor pollicis brevis, Tendo

M. extensor pollicis longus, Tendo

M. interosseus dorsalis II

M. interosseus dorsalis I

Connexus intertendinei

Dorsal aponeuroses: medial tracts

Dorsal aponeuroses: lateral tracts

Fig. 3.97   Tendons of the long extensors and dorsal aponeuroses of the fingers, right side; dorsal view. [S700]
With the exception of the tendon of the M. extensor pollicis longus, which extends to the distal phalanx, the tendons of the Mm. extensores digitorum, extensor digiti minimi, and extensor indicis all end with the middle tracts of the dorsal aponeurosis at the middle phalanges.

→ T 39

M. interosseus dorsalis II

M. interosseus dorsalis III

M. interosseus dorsalis I

M. interosseus dorsalis IV

M. extensor digitorum, Tendines

Mm. interossei palmares

Dorsal aponeuroses: middle tracts

Mm. lumbricales, Tendines

Fig. 3.98   Structure of the dorsal aponeurosis, right side; dorsal view. [S700]
The dorsal aponeurosis of the fingers consists of a **middle tract** as well as a **lateral tract** on the medial and lateral aspect, respectively. While the medial tract only extends to the middle phalanx, the lateral tracts extend up onto the back of the distal phalanx.
The long extensor tendons end with the middle tract of the dorsal aponeurosis at the middle phalanx and can therefore not extend the distal interphalangeal joints of the fingers. In contrast, the **Mm. lumbricales** and to a lesser degree the **Mm. interossei palmares and dorsales** radiate into the lateral tracts of the dorsal aponeurosis. They therefore reach the transverse axis of the **distal interphalangeal joints** on the dorsal side and can **extend** them. It is thereby clear that the Mm. lumbricales are the main extensors of the distal interphalangeal joints.

Dorsal aponeuroses: lateral tracts

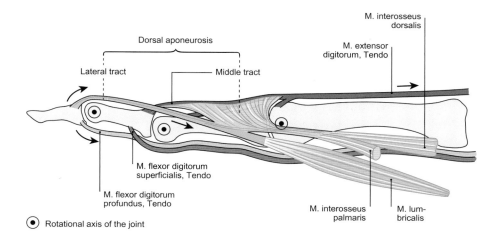

Rotational axis of the joint

Fig. 3.99 Action of the flexor and extensor muscles with the middle finger as an example; lateral view. [S700-L126]/[G1064]
The function of the tendons of the forearm and hand muscles is determined by their course in relation to the axes of the finger joints and by their insertion at the middle or distal interphalangeal joints of the fingers. The tendons of the **long flexor muscles of the fingers** (Mm. flexores digitorum superficialis and profundus) run palmar to the transverse axis of the finger joints, whereas the tendons of the **extensor muscles of the forearm** (M. extensor digitorum, M. extensor digiti minimi, M. extensor indicis) run dorsally. The M. flexor digitorum superficialis as well as the finger extensors have their insertions on the middle phalanges, so that these muscles cannot act on the distal interphalangeal joints. In contrast, the M. flexor digitorum profundus inserts on the palmar aspect of the distal phalanges so that it acts as the main flexor of the distal interphalangeal joints.

The course of the **Mm. interossei** and **Mm. lumbricales** is more complicated: both muscle groups run palmar to the transverse axis of the metacarpophalangeal joints and therefore act very effectively. On the middle phalanges however they change to the dorsal side, and radiate

with different parts into the middle and lateral tracts of the dorsal aponeurosis. As the Mm. lumbricales contribute specifically to the lateral tracts of the dorsal aponeurosis, it is understandable why they are the main extensors of the distal phalanges.

Flexor muscles of the finger joints:
Each joint has a predominant flexor muscle. In the distal interphalangeal joint, the M. flexor digitorum profundus is the only muscle that flexes.
* **Metacarpophalangeal (MCP) joints:** Mm. interossei palmares and dorsales, to a lesser extent also the Mm. lumbricales
* **Proximal interphalangeal (PIP) joints:** M. flexor digitorum superficialis (also flexes the metacarpophalangeal joint)
* **Distal interphalangeal (DIP) joints:** M. flexor digitorum profundus (also flexes the middle interphalangeal and metacarpophalangeal joints).

Extensor muscles of the finger joints:
* **MCP and PIP joints:** M. extensor digitorum, M. extensor digiti minimi, M. extensor indicis
* **DIP joints of the fingers:** Mm. lumbricales, to a lesser extent also Mm. interossei palmares and dorsales.

Most important flexor and extensor muscles of the finger and the thumb			
Function	**MCP**	**PIP**	**DIP**
Flexion of finger	Mm. interossei palmares, Mm. interossei dorsales	M. flexor digitorum superficialis	M. flexor digitorum profundus
Extension of finger	M. extensor digitorum	M. extensor digitorum	Mm. lumbricales
Flexion of thumb	M. flexor pollicis longus	M. flexor pollicis longus	-
Extension of thumb	M. extensor pollicis brevis	M. extensor pollicis longus	-

Musculature

Flexor mechanism of the fingers

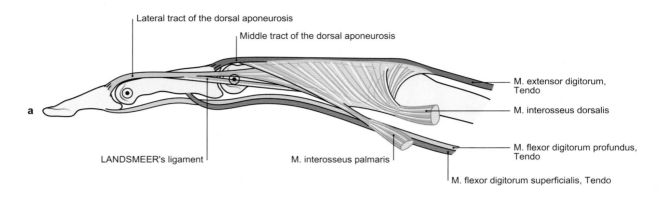

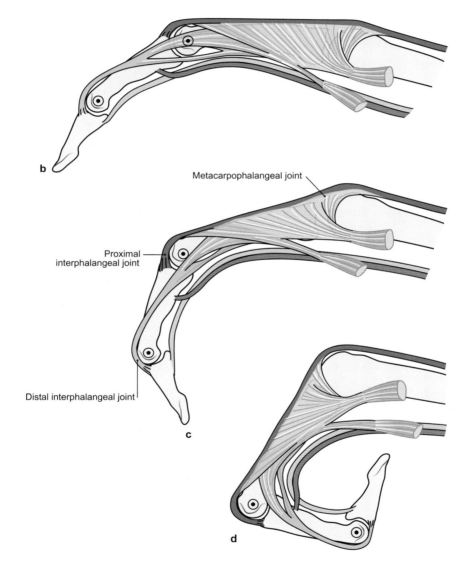

Lateral tract of the dorsal aponeurosis

Middle tract of the dorsal aponeurosis

M. extensor digitorum, Tendo

M. interosseus dorsalis

M. flexor digitorum profundus, Tendo

M. flexor digitorum superficialis, Tendo

LANDSMEER's ligament

M. interosseus palmaris

a

b

Metacarpophalangeal joint

Proximal interphalangeal joint

Distal interphalangeal joint

c

d

Fig. 3.100a–d Flexor mechanism of the fingers; lateral view. [S700-L126]/[(B500-L132)/(G1064/G1065)]

During flexion of the fingers, the long flexor muscles act together with the short palmar muscles. This results in the following sequence:

a Flexion in the distal interphalangeal (DIP) joint. Flexion is initiated by the **M. flexor digitorum profundus.**

b Flexion in the proximal interphalangeal (PIP) joint. Flexion of the distal joint **puts stress** on the **fibre tracts** between the proximal phalanx and the dorsal aponeurosis, thereby initiating the flexion of the PIP joint.

c Flexion in the proximal interphalangeal (PIP) joint. The flexion in the PIP joint is actively supported by the **M. flexor digitorum superficialis.** Flexing the PIP joint applies tension on the tendons of the Mm. interossei and Mm. lumbricales because they run dorsal to the transverse axis of the PIP joint.

d Flexion in the metacarpophalangeal joint (MCP): Contraction of the **Mm. interossei and Mm. lumbricales** results in flexion of the MCP joint because their tendons run palmar to the transverse axis.

In this way, there is a progressive flexion from the distal to the proximal joints!

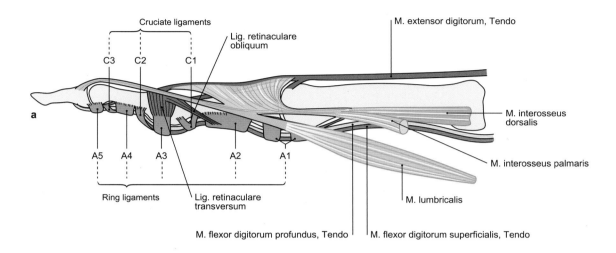

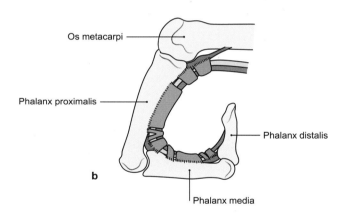

Fig. 3.101a and b Structure and function of the flexor and extensor tendons of the fingers; lateral view. [S700-L126]/[(B500-M282)/G1064]
a Extended finger.
b Bent finger.
The outer fibrous layer **(Vagina fibrosa)** of the tendon sheaths is attached to the phalanges and/or the joint capsules of the fingers with annular and cross-shaped fibres **(Pars anularis and Pars cruciformis),**

which in clinical terms are also known as **annular and cruciate ligaments** and are abbreviated as A1–A5 and C1–C3. This ensures that the ends of the tendons are firmly attached to the bones and cannot lift with flexion.

Clinical remarks

Ruptures of the so-called annular and cruciate ligaments of the tendon sheaths are especially common in climbing sports because these structures are put under tremendous pressure.

Plexus brachialis

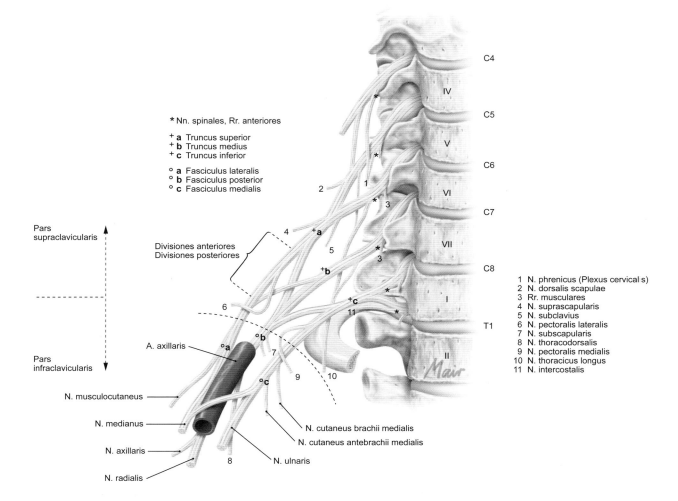

* Nn. spinales, Rr. anteriores

+ **a** Truncus superior
+ **b** Truncus medius
+ **c** Truncus inferior

° **a** Fasciculus lateralis
° **b** Fasciculus posterior
° **c** Fasciculus medialis

Pars supraclavicularis

Divisiones anteriores
Divisiones posteriores

Pars infraclavicularis

A. axillaris

N. musculocutaneus

N. medianus

N. axillaris

N. radialis

N. cutaneus brachii medialis
N. cutaneus antebrachii medialis

N. ulnaris

C4
C5
C6
C7
C8
T1

1 N. phrenicus (Plexus cervicalis)
2 N. dorsalis scapulae
3 Rr. musculares
4 N. suprascapularis
5 N. subclavius
6 N. pectoralis lateralis
7 N. subscapularis
8 N. thoracodorsalis
9 N. pectoralis medialis
10 N. thoracicus longus
11 N. intercostalis

Fig. 3.102 Brachial plexus, Plexus brachialis (C5–T1): segmentation of nerves, right side; ventral view. [S700-L127]
The upper limb is innervated by the **Plexus brachialis.** The brachial plexus is formed by the Rr. anteriores of the spinal nerves of the lower cervical and upper thoracic spinal cord segments **(C5–T1).** The Plexus brachialis is the body's most complex network of nerves and it is necessary to get to know its principles of construction before studying the individual nerves or familiarising oneself on a cadaver.
The ventral roots of the spinal nerves first form three **trunci** (superior, middle and inferior) staged one above the other. Each trunk splits into an anterior and posterior part (**divisions**) of which the nerve fibres mix anew to form **fasciculi** arranged around the A. axillaris. Projecting from these fasciculi are the long nerves for the arm. Nerves for the shoulder however branch off directly from the trunci.
The Rr. anteriores of the spinal nerves C5-T1 first merge to form three layered **trunci** which then regroup into **fasciculi** at the level of the clavicle. The individual fasciculi are named according to their relative position to the A. axillaris. The **Truncus superior** contains nerve fibres from the spinal segments **C5–C6,** the **Truncus medius** from **C7,** and the **Truncus inferior** from **C8–T1.** The dorsal divisions (Divisiones posteriores) of all three trunks form the **Fasciculus posterior** (with nerve fibres from **C5–T1**). The ventral divisions (Divisiones anteriores) of the Truncus superior and the Truncus medius supply the **Fasciculus lateralis** (lateral of the A. axillaris, nerve fibres from **C5–C7**), and the anterior part of the Truncus inferior continues as the **Fasciculus medialis** (medial of the A. axillaris, nerve fibres from **C8–T1**). Visualising this structure of the Plexus brachialis gives us a better understanding of the individual nerves, with only a few exceptions.
Topographically the Plexus brachialis can be divided into two parts. The **supraclavicular part** (Pars supraclavicularis) includes the trunci and the

nerves originating from these trunks or from the Rr. anteriores of the spinal nerves (C5–T1). The **infraclavicular part** (Pars infraclavicularis) consists of the fasciculi. The nerves of the arm (→ Fig. 3.119) originate from the infraclavicular part, while the supraclavicular part is responsible for the innervation of the shoulder.

Pars supraclavicularis:
* Muscle branches to the Mm. scaleni and M. longus colli (C5–C8)
* N. dorsalis scapulae (C3–C5)
* N. thoracicus longus (C5–C7)
* N. suprascapularis (C4–C6)
* N. subclavius (C5–C6).

Pars infraclavicularis:
Fasciculus posterior (C5–T1):
* N. axillaris (C5–C6)
* N. radialis (C5–T1)
* Nn. subscapulares (C5–C7)
* N. thoracodorsalis (C6–C8).

Fasciculus lateralis (C5–C7):
* N. musculocutaneus (C5–C7)
* N. medianus, Radix lateralis (C6–C7)
* N. pectoralis lateralis (C5–C7).

Fasciculus medialis (C8–T1):
* N. medianus, Radix medialis (C8–T1)
* N. ulnaris (C8–T1)
* N. cutaneus brachii medialis (C8–T1)
* N. cutaneus antebrachii medialis (C8–T1)
* N. pectoralis medialis (C8–T1).

→ T 24, T 25

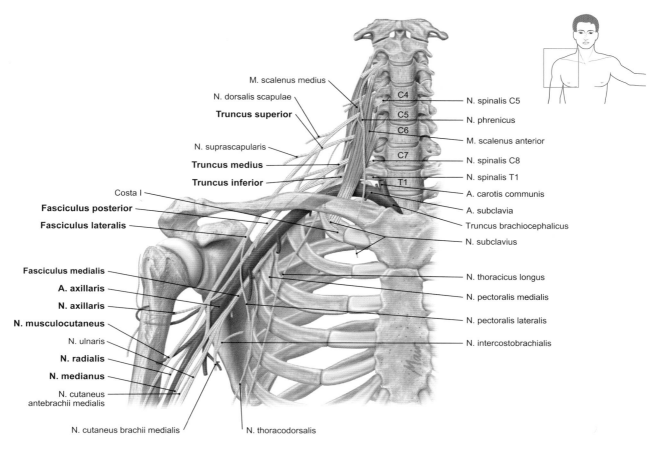

Fig. 3.103 Organisation and location of the Plexus brachialis with its nerves; right side; ventral view. [S701-L127]
The figure shows the exact pathway of the nerves of the Plexus brachialis. The trunci and A. subclavia run through the **anterior scalene fissure** (hiatus) between the M. scalenus anterior and medius. The trunci lie above the clavicle, are split into the divisions to the rear of the clavicle, and form fasciculi below the clavicle.

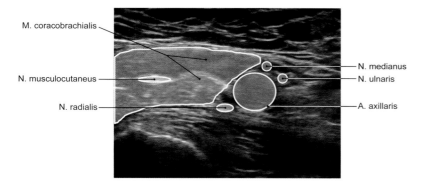

Fig. 3.104 Ultrasound image of the Plexus brachialis with plexus anaesthesia, right side. [S700-T863]
This ultrasound image shows the nerves which emerge on the arm from the three fascicles of the Plexus brachialis. The **N. medianus** and the **N. ulnaris** originate from the medial fascicle and can be defined medially around the **A. axillaris.** The **N. radialis** which continues the pathway of the posterior fascicle, passes dorsally below the artery and is therefore visible over a longer section. Laterally, the **N. musculocutaneus** can be recognised after it enters the M. coracobrachialis.

Clinical remarks

As general anaesthesia is subjected to various risks, there is an increasing tendency to perform interventions using **regional anaesthesia,** in which local anaesthetics are applied to individual nerves or plexuses. When injecting these substances, it is important to show the relevant nerves and surrounding structures, such as blood vessels, using ultrasound. For this purpose, a detailed knowledge of topographical anatomy is needed, as shown here with the Plexus brachialis as an example.

Location of the different parts of the Plexus brachialis	
Part	**Anatomical landmark**
Spinal nerves (Rr. anteriores)	Proc. transversi of cervical vertebrae
Trunci	Scalene fissure (hiatus)
Divisions	Clavicle
Fascicles	A. axillaris
Nerves	Humerus

Neurovascular pathways

Plexus brachialis

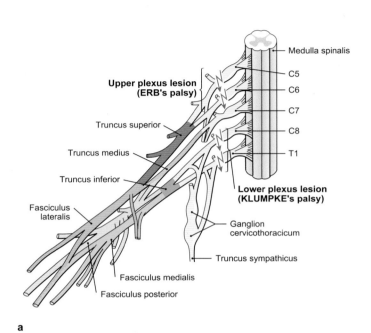

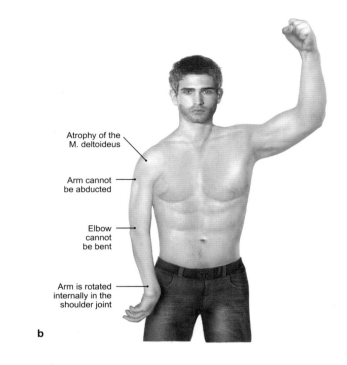

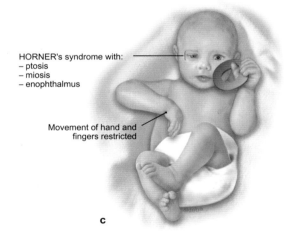

Fig. 3.105a–c Lesions of the Plexus brachialis; view from ventral.
a Upper and lower plexus lesion. Lesions of the Plexus brachialis are caused by an avulsion of the spinal nerve roots, which supply the trunci of the Plexus brachialis. [S702-L126]
b Clinical symptoms of the upper plexus lesion (ERB's palsy), right side. The shoulder is positioned close to the trunk (adduced) and rotat-

ed inward, the arm cannot bend at the elbow joint. Function of the hand is not impaired. [S702-L238]
c Clinical symptoms of the lower plexus lesion (KLUMPKE's palsy), right side. Shoulder and elbow functions are unaffected, hand and finger movements are restricted. A HORNER's syndrome is frequently associated with KLUMPKE's palsy. [S702-L238]

Clinical remarks

Severe injuries of the shoulder and arm (motorcycle accidents, abnormal position at birth, improper surgical positioning) can lead to lesions of the Plexus brachialis. Depending on the affected truncus, a distinction is made between:
- **Upper plexus paralysis (ERB, nerve roots of C5–C6 for the Truncus superior)**
Pathomechanism: increased distance between neck and shoulder. Typical signs are a paresis (paralysis) of the abductors and lateral rotators of the shoulder and upper arm flexors, as well as the M. supinator. This results in adduction and internal rotation of the shoulder with an extended elbow joint and normal hand function.

- **Lower plexus paralysis (KLUMPKE, nerve roots of C8–T1 for the Truncus inferior)**
Pathomechanism: increased distance between torso and shoulder. In this case there is a paresis of the long flexor muscles of the fingers and the short muscles of the hand, with normal function of the shoulder and elbow joints. This is frequently associated with **HORNER's syndrome** (miosis, ptosis, enophthalmus), since the preganglionic neurons of the cervical sympathetic chain also leave the spinal segments C8–T1 via the anterior roots.

The Truncus medius (C7) may be involved in both the upper and lower lesions, which is indicated by the paralysis of the M. triceps brachii and of the extensor muscles of the fingers.
In the case of a **complete lesion,** the mobility of the entire arm, including the hand, is impaired.

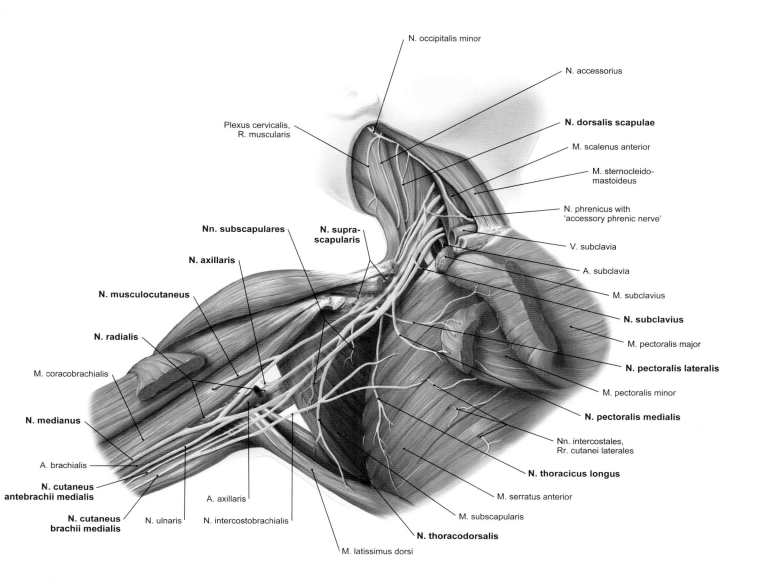

N. occipitalis minor

N. accessorius

N. dorsalis scapulae

M. scalenus anterior

M. sternocleido-mastoideus

N. phrenicus with 'accessory phrenic nerve'

V. subclavia

A. subclavia

M. subclavius

N. subclavius

M. pectoralis major

N. pectoralis lateralis

M. pectoralis minor

N. pectoralis medialis

Nn. intercostales, Rr. cutanei laterales

N. thoracicus longus

M. serratus anterior

M. subscapularis

N. thoracodorsalis

M. latissimus dorsi

Plexus cervicalis, R. muscularis

Nn. subscapulares

N. supra-scapularis

N. axillaris

N. musculocutaneus

N. radialis

M. coracobrachialis

N. medianus

A. brachialis

N. cutaneus antebrachii medialis

N. cutaneus brachii medialis

N. ulnaris

A. axillaris

N. intercostobrachialis

Fig. 3.106   Nerves of the Plexus brachialis, right side; ventral view after cutting through the Mm. pectorales major and minor near their insertion. [S700-L266]

The nerves of the **supraclavicular part** (Pars supraclavicularis) of the Plexus brachialis originate from the trunci or partly from the Rr. anteriores of the spinal nerves, and provide the innervation of the shoulder muscles. The **N. dorsalis scapulae** has the furthest cranial origin, and penetrates the M. scalenus medius. In a ventral view it is only visible if the head can be greatly extended backwards and sideways, as shown here. Further caudally, the **N. thoracicus longus** also passes through the M. scalenus medius. A specific feature of its pathway is that it runs below the Plexus brachialis to the chest wall, where it descends down the M. serratus anterior, which it innervates. The **N. suprascapularis** emerges characteristically from the Truncus superior and turns dorsally, where it passes through the Incisura scapulae below the Lig. transversum scapulae superius to the dorsal side of the scapula. The **N. subclavius** is usually inconspicuous and difficult to depict. It innervates the M. subclavius and sometimes sends off a branch to the N. phrenicus ('accessory phrenic nerve').

The nerves of the **infraclavicular part** (Pars infraclavicularis) originate directly from the fascicles. The nerves of the arm as well as of the shoulder derive from the infraclavicular part.

The **Fasciculus posterior (C5–T1)** sends small nerves medially, including the two **Nn. subscapulares** and the **N. thoracodorsalis.** The **N. axillaris** branches off and runs through the lateral axillary space, whereas the **N. radialis** continues its pathway through the triangular interval to the dorsal side of the upper arm. From the **Fasciculus lateralis (C5–C7),** the **N. pectoralis lateralis** initially branches off to the pectoral muscles, before the **N. musculocutaneus** passes laterally, where it usually penetrates the M. coracobrachialis. The remaining nerve fibres form the lateral part of the **N. medianus** (Radix lateralis). The medial part (Radix medialis) of the N. medianus comes from the **Fasciculus medialis (C8–T1),** after it has provided the **N. pectoralis medialis,** as well as the **N. ulnaris** and the sensory **Nn. cutanei brachii and antebrachii mediales.** Branches of the intercostal nerves often accompany the nerve to the upper arm as the Nn. intercostobrachiales.

→ T 24

Cutaneous innervation of the upper limb

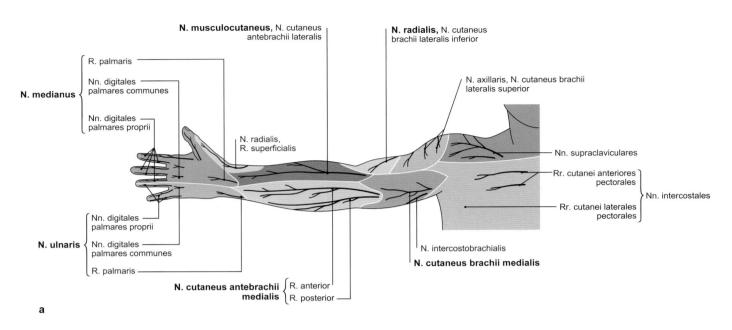

N. musculocutaneus, N. cutaneus antebrachii lateralis

N. radialis, N. cutaneus brachii lateralis inferior

N. medianus
- R. palmaris
- Nn. digitales palmares communes
- Nn. digitales palmares proprii

N. radialis, R. superficialis

N. axillaris, N. cutaneus brachii lateralis superior

Nn. supraclaviculares

Rr. cutanei anteriores pectorales

Nn. intercostales

Rr. cutanei laterales pectorales

N. ulnaris
- Nn. digitales palmares proprii
- Nn. digitales palmares communes
- R. palmaris

N. intercostobrachialis

N. cutaneus brachii medialis

N. cutaneus antebrachii medialis
- R. anterior
- R. posterior

a

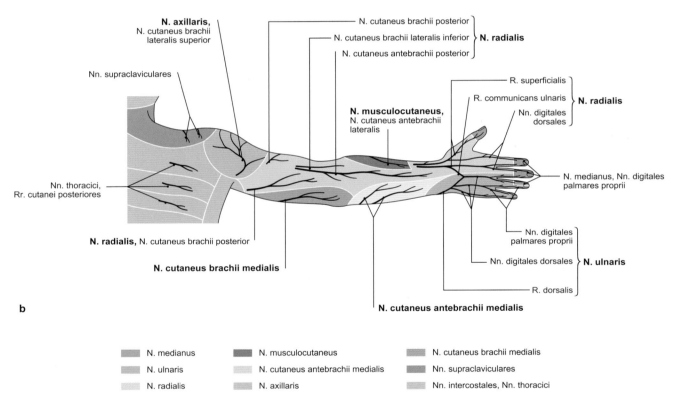

N. axillaris, N. cutaneus brachii lateralis superior

N. cutaneus brachii posterior

N. cutaneus brachii lateralis inferior

N. cutaneus antebrachii posterior

N. radialis

Nn. supraclaviculares

R. superficialis

R. communicans ulnaris

N. radialis

Nn. digitales dorsales

N. musculocutaneus, N. cutaneus antebrachii lateralis

N. medianus, Nn. digitales palmares proprii

Nn. thoracici, Rr. cutanei posteriores

Nn. digitales palmares proprii

N. ulnaris

N. radialis, N. cutaneus brachii posterior

Nn. digitales dorsales

N. cutaneus brachii medialis

R. dorsalis

N. cutaneus antebrachii medialis

b

N. medianus	N. musculocutaneus	N. cutaneus brachii medialis
N. ulnaris	N. cutaneus antebrachii medialis	Nn. supraclaviculares
N. radialis	N. axillaris	Nn. intercostales, Nn. thoracici

Fig. 3.107a and b   Cutaneous nerves of the upper limb, right side.
[S700-L127]
a Ventral view.
b Dorsal view.
All nerves of the infraclavicular part of the **Plexus brachialis** participate in the sensory innervation of the **shoulder** and **arm.** The lateral aspect of the shoulder is innervated by the N. axillaris. The lateral and dorsal sides of the upper arm, and the dorsal sides of the forearm and the ra-dial 2½ fingers are innervated by the N. radialis. The N. musculocutaneus supplies the lateral aspect of the forearm. The N. cutaneus brachii medialis and the N. cutaneus antebrachii medialis innervate the medial aspect of the arm. The N. medianus (palmar side of the radial 3½ fingers) and the N. ulnaris (palmar side of the ulnar 1½ fingers and dorsal side of the ulnar 2½ fingers) supply the hand.

→ T 24

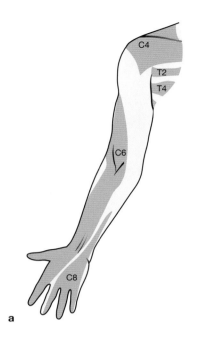

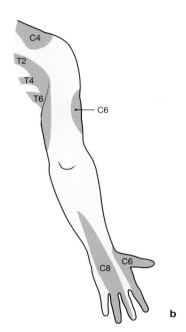

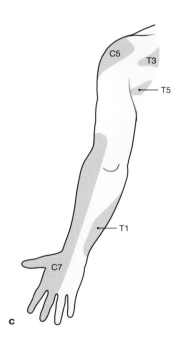

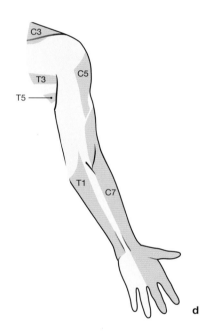

Fig. 3.108a–d Segmental innervation of the skin (dermatomes) of the upper limb, right side. [S700-L126]/[F1067-001]
a, b Ventral view.
c, d Dorsal view.
Certain areas of the skin are sensorily innervated by a single spinal cord segment. These cutaneous areas are referred to as **dermatomes.** Because the cutaneous nerves of the arm contain sensory nerve fibres from several spinal cord segments, the dermatomes are not exactly congruent with the areas supplied by the cutaneous nerves (→ Fig. 3.107). In contrast to the torso, where the dermatomes are ar-

ranged in a belt-like pattern, their distribution on the arm is largely **along the longitudinal axis** (see Development → Fig. 3.5).
For clarity, the dermatomes are depicted for the right (green) and left (blue) side of the body, respectively. This shows that the dermatomes partially overlap. This is particularly true for the thumb and index finger, which are both innervated by C6 and C7. In contrast, the middle finger is not supplied by C6 but instead by C7 and partially C8. Dermatome C8 extends to the ring finger and little finger.

→ T 25

Clinical remarks

Demarcating the borders of dermatomes are of great importance in the diagnosis of **herniated discs** and of narrowing **(stenosis) of the vertebral canal** or of the spinal nerve foramina (openings): an injury to segment **C6** causes restricted sensation in the radial forearm and

thumb; with compression to **C7,** this is most noticeable in the **middle finger.** The **little finger** is mostly affected with lesions to segment **C8.** Sensitivity to the ulnar side of the forearm is reduced when **T1** is affected.

Upper limb

Shoulder nerves from the Pars supraclavicularis of the Plexus brachialis

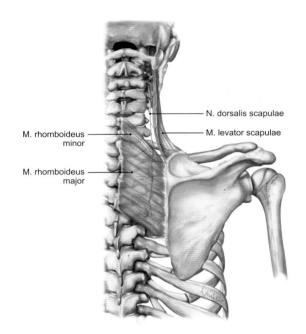

M. rhomboideus minor

M. rhomboideus major

N. dorsalis scapulae

M. levator scapulae

Fig. 3.109   N. dorsalis scapulae (C3–C5), right side; dorsal view. [S700-L266]
The shoulder nerves originate from the Pars supraclavicularis (→ Fig. 3.109, → Fig. 3.110 and → Fig. 3.111) as well as from the Pars infraclavicularis (→ Fig. 3.113, → Fig. 3.114 and → Fig. 3.115) of the Plexus brachialis.
The **N. dorsalis scapulae** innervates the Mm. rhomboidei and the M. levator scapulae, both of which secure the scapula to the torso and pull it in a medial and upward direction. The nerve leaves the Plexus brachialis at the furthest cranial point, penetrates into the M. scalenus medius and draws the lower edge of the M. levator scapulae (indicator muscle!) dorsally.
Shoulder nerves derived from the Pars supraclavicularis:
* N. dorsalis scapulae (C3–C5)
* N. thoracicus longus (C5–C7)
* N. suprascapularis (C4–C6)
* N. subclavius (C5–C6).

→ T 24

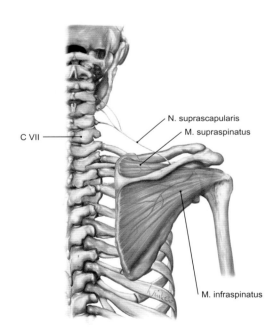

C VII

N. suprascapularis

M. supraspinatus

M. infraspinatus

Fig. 3.110   N. suprascapularis (C4–C6), right side; dorsal view. [S700-L266]
The **N. suprascapularis** innervates the **M. supraspinatus** (supports abduction) and the **M. infraspinatus** (most important external rotator of the shoulder!). The N. suprascapularis originates from the Truncus superior and runs dorsally above the clavicle. It passes below the **Lig. transversum scapulae superius** through the Incisura scapulae, and on the dorsal side of the scapula into the Fossa supraspinata, and then turns laterally around the Spina scapulae into the Fossa infraspinata. At the base of the Spina scapulae, it is sometimes covered by fibres of connective tissue which are referred to as **Lig. transversum scapulae inferius.**

→ T 24

Clinical remarks

Lesions of the shoulder nerves of the Pars supraclavicularis:
* **N. dorsalis scapulae:** the scapula is displaced laterally and slightly lifts off the thorax. An isolated lesion is rare due to the protected location.

* **N. suprascapularis:** impaired external rotation (M. infraspinatus is the most important muscle) and, to a lesser degree, impaired abduction of the shoulder (M. supraspinatus). In addition to injuries in the lateral neck region, nerve entrapments in the Incisura scapulae are also possible.

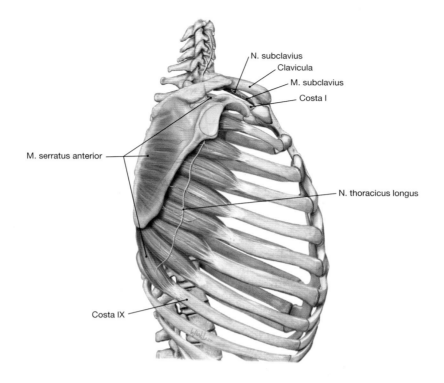

Fig. 3.111   N. thoracicus longus (C5–C7) and N. subclavius (C5–C6), right side; lateral view. [S700-L266]

The **N. thoracicus longus** penetrates the M. scalenus medius and then passes below the Plexus brachialis and the clavicle to the lateral side of the thorax, where it descends on the **M. serratus anterior** and innervates it. The M. serratus anterior contributes substantially to the rotation of the scapula. The muscle is necessary for the elevation of the arm in order to ensure that the abduction movement of the head of the humerus is not restricted by the roof of the shoulder.

The **N. subclavius** innervates the **M. subclavius,** which actively stabilises the sternoclavicular joint. The N. subclavius abuts the M. subclavius and occasionally provides a branch to the N. phrenicus ('accessory phrenic nerve').

→ T 24

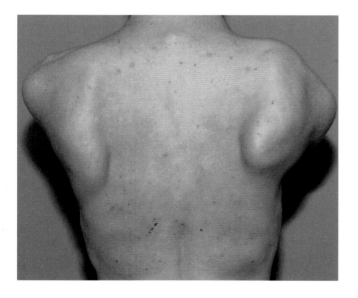

Fig. 3.112   Scapula alata caused by lesions of the N. thoracicus longus, on both sides; dorsal view. [R261]

The protruding medial margin of the scapula indicates a lesion of the N. thoracicus longus and is referred to as **Scapula alata.** Despite the adverse effect of the elevation, this symptom may not be perceived by the patient, but can be used diagnostically. The protrusion of the medial margin of the scapula is most noticeable when the patient leans against the floor or a wall, as shown here, and the M. serratus anterior is unable to keep the shoulder blade secured to the torso.

Clinical remarks

Lesions of the shoulder nerves of the Pars supraclavicularis:
- **N. thoracicus longus:** elevation impossible! The medial margin of the scapula protrudes wing-like from the torso (**Scapula alata**). This lesion is frequently caused by carrying heavy loads on the back ('backpack palsy') whereby the nerve can become entrapped under the clavicle. Incision wounds to the chest wall can also lead to a lesion of the nerve.
- An isolated lesion of the N. subclavius is very rare and has no clear clinical symptoms.

Shoulder nerves from the Pars infraclavicularis of the Plexus brachialis

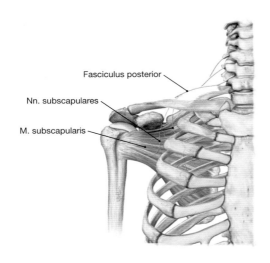

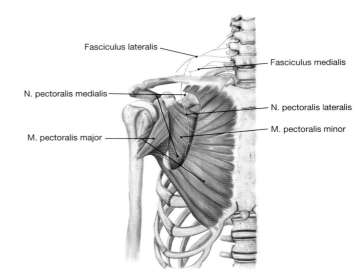

Fig. 3.113 Nn. subscapulares (C5–C7), right side; ventral view. [S700-L266]

The shoulder nerves originate from the Pars supraclavicularis (→ Fig. 3.109, → Fig. 3.110 and → Fig. 3.111) as well as the Pars infraclavicularis (→ Fig. 3.113, → Fig. 3.114 and → Fig. 3.115) of the Plexus brachialis.

There are usually two **Nn. subscapulares** which innervate the **M. subscapularis** (the most important internal rotator of the shoulder joint!). Since the Nn. subscapulares descend directly from the posterior fascicle to the front of the scapula, they are very well protected.

Shoulder nerves of the Pars infraclavicularis:

* Nn. subscapulares (C5–C7) from the Fasciculus posterior
* N. thoracodorsalis (C6–C8) from the Fasciculus posterior
* N. pectoralis lateralis (C5–C7) from the Fasciculus lateralis
* N. pectoralis medialis (C8–T1) from the Fasciculus medialis
* N. axillaris (C5–C6) from the Fasciculus posterior.

→ T 24

Fig. 3.114 Nn. pectorales lateralis (C5–C7) and medialis (C8–T1), right side; ventral view. [S700-L266]

These nerves are named according to their origin from the respective fascicles, not from their position (generally, the **N. pectoralis medialis** is located laterally and the **N. pectoralis lateralis** medially!). Both nerves innervate the **Mm. pectorales major and minor.** The M. pectoralis major is the most important muscle for the adduction and anteversion of the shoulder joint.

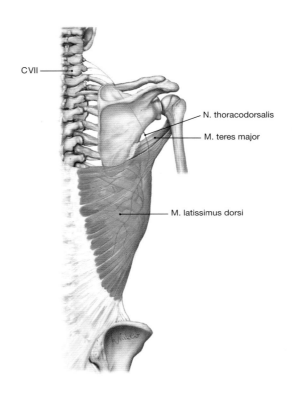

Fig. 3.115 N. thoracodorsalis (C6–C8), right side; dorsal view. [S700-L266]

The **N. thoracodorsalis** accompanies the eponomously named artery and vein to the medial side of the M. latissimus dorsi, and sends a branch to the M. teres major.

→ T 24

Clinical remarks

Lesions of shoulder nerves from the Pars infraclavicularis: in general, isolated injuries of individual infraclavicular shoulder nerves are rare due to their protected location.

* **Nn. subscapulares:** weak medial rotation of the humerus; lesions may be caused by a proximal humeral fracture.
* **Nn. pectorales:** impairment of adduction and anteversion. As a clinical and diagnostic sign, the arms cannot be crossed **in front of** the torso. The anterior axillary fold is sunken.

* **N. thoracodorsalis:** impaired adduction of the retroverted arm. The arms cannot be crossed **behind** the back, as this would require retroversion, adduction and internal rotation. The posterior axillary fold is sunken. Considering the size of the M. latissimus dorsi, these are mostly minor symptoms with movements made from the neutral position, because this muscle is, just like the M. teres major, not essential for movements of the shoulder joint! But the impairment may become obvious with gymnastics or other sports.

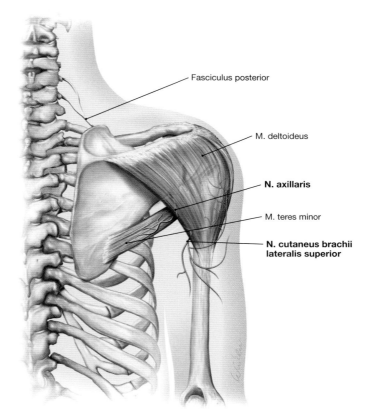

Fasciculus posterior

M. deltoideus

N. axillaris

M. teres minor

N. cutaneus brachii
lateralis superior

**Fig. 3.116 Pathway and supply area of the N. axillaris (C5–C6),
right side;** dorsal view. [S700-L266]
The **N. axillaris** originates from the Fasciculus posterior, traverses the
lateral axillary space along with the A. circumflexa humeri posterior
and runs around the surgical neck (Collum chirurgicum) of the humerus
to reach the dorsal side of the arm. Here it innervates the **M. deltoideus** (the most important abductor in the shoulder joint!) and the **M. teres
minor.** Its sensory terminal branch (N. cutaneus brachii lateralis superi-
or [purple]) emerges posteriorly at the lower margin of the M. deltoideus and innervates the lateral aspect of the shoulder.

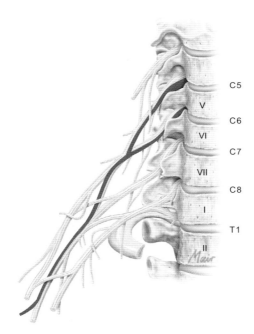

C5

V

C6

VI

C7

VII

C8

I

T1

II

Fig. 3.117 Segmentation of the N. axillaris, right side; ventral
view. [S700-L127]

→ T 24

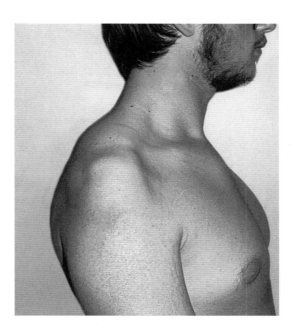

**Fig. 3.118 Lesion of the N. axillaris: paralysis and atrophy of the
M. deltoideus.** [S700-T917]

Clinical remarks

Lesion of the N. axillaris: it can be injured in proximal humeral fractures and shoulder dislocations. The **abduction of the arm is se-
verely impaired** and a **complete sensory loss affects the lateral**
side of the shoulder. In the case of a long-lasting nerve lesion, the
full roundness of the shoulder is lost due to muscle atrophy
(→ Fig. 3.118).

Arm nerves of the Plexus brachialis

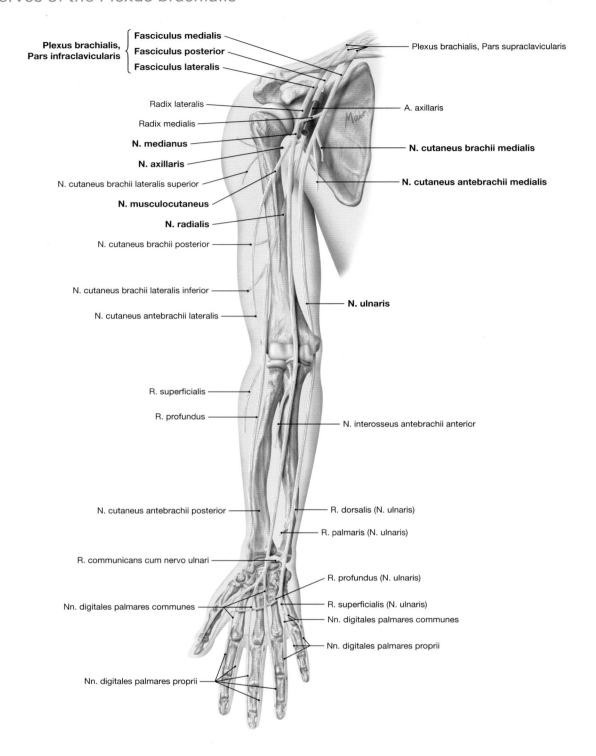

Plexus brachialis, Pars infraclavicularis
- **Fasciculus medialis**
- **Fasciculus posterior**
- **Fasciculus lateralis**

Plexus brachialis, Pars supraclavicularis

Radix lateralis

A. axillaris

Radix medialis

N. medianus

N. axillaris

N. cutaneus brachii medialis

N. cutaneus brachii lateralis superior

N. cutaneus antebrachii medialis

N. musculocutaneus

N. radialis

N. cutaneus brachii posterior

N. cutaneus brachii lateralis inferior

N. ulnaris

N. cutaneus antebrachii lateralis

R. superficialis

R. profundus

N. interosseus antebrachii anterior

N. cutaneus antebrachii posterior

R. dorsalis (N. ulnaris)

R. palmaris (N. ulnaris)

R. communicans cum nervo ulnari

R. profundus (N. ulnaris)

Nn. digitales palmares communes

R. superficialis (N. ulnaris)

Nn. digitales palmares communes

Nn. digitales palmares proprii

Nn. digitales palmares proprii

Fig. 3.119 Brachial plexus, Plexus brachialis (C5–T1): nerves of the arm, right side; ventral view. [S700-L127]

The nerves of the arm, as well as some shoulder nerves (→ Fig. 3.113, → Fig. 3.114, → Fig. 3.115 and → Fig. 3.116) originate from the infraclavicular part of the Plexus brachialis. The N. radialis continues the pathway of the Fasciculus posterior. The N. musculocutaneus and the lateral root (Radix lateralis) of the N. medianus originate from the Fasciculus lateralis. The Fasciculus medialis is divided into the medial root (Radix medialis) of the N. medianus and into the N. ulnaris, as well as into the sensory nerves on the medial side of the upper arm (N. cutaneus brachii medialis) and of the forearm (N. cutaneus antebrachii medialis).

Arm nerves of the Pars infraclavicularis:
Fasciculus posterior (C5–T1):
- N. radialis (C5–T1).

Fasciculus lateralis (C5–C7):
- N. musculocutaneus (C5–C7)
- N. medianus, Radix lateralis (C6–C7).

Fasciculus medialis (C8–T1):
- N. medianus, Radix medialis (C8–T1)
- N. ulnaris (C8–T1)
- N. cutaneus brachii medialis (C8–T1)
- N. cutaneus antebrachii medialis (C8–T1).

→ T 24

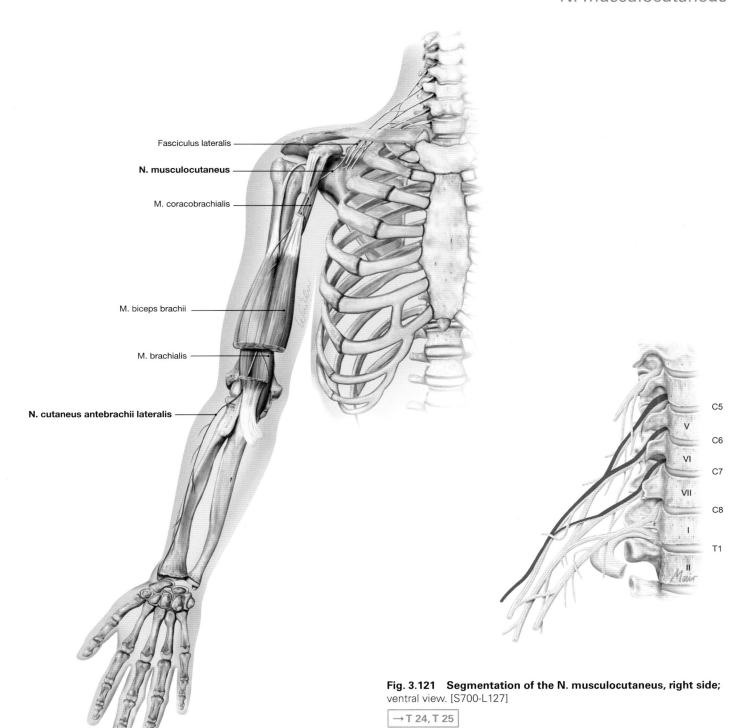

Fasciculus lateralis

N. musculocutaneus

M. coracobrachialis

M. biceps brachii

M. brachialis

N. cutaneus antebrachii lateralis

C5
V
C6
VI
C7
VII
C8
I
T1
II

Fig. 3.121   Segmentation of the N. musculocutaneus, right side; ventral view. [S700-L127]

→ T 24, T 25

Fig. 3.120   Pathway and supply area of the N. musculocutaneus (C5–C7), right side; ventral view. [S700-L266]
The **N. musculocutaneus** originates from the Fasciculus lateralis. It usually pierces the **M. coracobrachialis,** runs distally between the M. biceps brachii and M. brachialis, where its sensory terminal branch (N. cutaneus antebrachii lateralis [purple]) emerges between these two muscles and reaches the cubital fossa laterally. It supplies the three

ventral muscles of the upper arm **(M. coracobrachialis, M. biceps brachii, M. brachialis)** with motor fibres and the radial forearm with sensory fibres.
Since the N. musculocutaneus penetrates the M. coracobrachialis, this nerve helps with orientation when dissecting the Plexus brachialis (indicator nerve!) (→ Fig. 3.161 and → Fig. 3.162).

Clinical remarks

Lesion of the N. musculocutaneus: this nerve is at risk with shoulder dislocations. If it is damaged, the **flexion of the elbow joint is significantly reduced,** but is maintained to a certain degree by the radial group of the extensors (innervated by the N. radialis) and the superficial flexor muscles of the forearm (innervated by the N. medi-

anus) which also promote flexion in the elbow joint. The supination of the flexed arm and the biceps reflex are weakened due to the paralysis of the M. biceps brachii. The **sensory deficit on the radial forearm** can be mitigated, because the innervation areas of the medial and the dorsal sensory nerves often overlap.

N. radialis

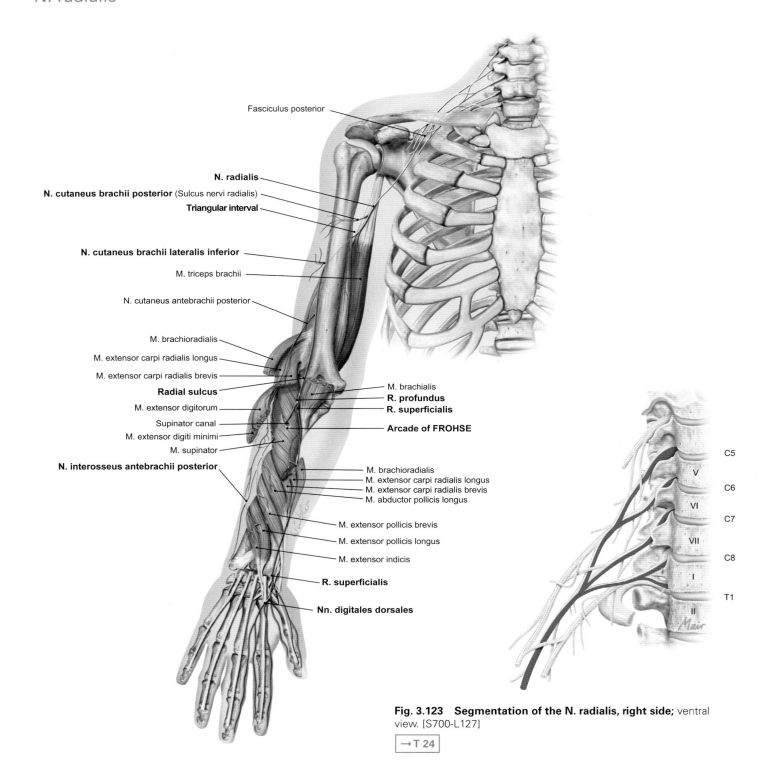

Fasciculus posterior

N. radialis

N. cutaneus brachii posterior (Sulcus nervi radialis)

Triangular interval

N. cutaneus brachii lateralis inferior

M. triceps brachii

N. cutaneus antebrachii posterior

M. brachioradialis

M. extensor carpi radialis longus

M. extensor carpi radialis brevis

Radial sulcus

M. extensor digitorum

Supinator canal

M. extensor digiti minimi

M. supinator

N. interosseus antebrachii posterior

M. brachialis

R. profundus

R. superficialis

Arcade of FROHSE

M. brachioradialis
M. extensor carpi radialis longus
M. extensor carpi radialis brevis
M. abductor pollicis longus

M. extensor pollicis brevis

M. extensor pollicis longus

M. extensor indicis

R. superficialis

Nn. digitales dorsales

C5

V

C6

VI

C7

VII

C8

I

T1

II

Fig. 3.123 Segmentation of the N. radialis, right side; ventral view. [S700-L127]

→ T 24

Fig. 3.122 Pathway and innervation area of the N. radialis (C5–T1), right side; ventral view (the dorsal side is visible here due to the pronated position of the forearm). The sensory cutaneous branches are highlighted in purple. [S700-L266]

The N. radialis originates from the Fasciculus posterior and passes through the **triangular interval** (→ Fig. 3.72) between the Caput longum and Caput laterale of the M. triceps brachii to reach the dorsal side of the humerus, winding around it in the Sulcus nervi radialis. Before entering the sulcus, it provides motor branches to the **M. triceps brachii** and the sensory branch to the back of the upper arm. The sensory branch to the back of the forearm, however, leaves from the Sulcus nervi radialis. Then the N. radialis enters between the M. brachioradialis and M. brachialis from laterally **(in the radial sulcus)** into the cubital fossa, where it divides into a R. superficialis and a R. profundus. Prior to its division, it sends muscle branches to the **M. brachioradialis** and the **Mm. extensores carpi radialis longus and brevis.**

The **R. superficialis** initially runs with the A. radialis below the M. brachioradialis; then, however, it changes distally to the dorsal side of the hand, to supply the first interdigital space (Spatium interosseum) between the thumb and index finger (autonomous area!) and the back of the radial 2½ fingers with sensory nerve fibres.

In contrast, the **R. profundus** penetrates the **M. supinator (supinator canal)** below the cubital fossa, and **also innervates the muscle,** and then turns to the dorsal side of the forearm, where it provides muscle branches to **all extensors of the forearm.** At the entrance of the supinator canal, the muscle fascia forms a crescent-shaped reinforcement **(arcade of FROHSE).** The terminal sensory branch is the N. interosseus antebrachii posterior, which supplies the wrists dorsally.

Autonomous area of sensory innervation: first interdigital space between thumb and index finger.

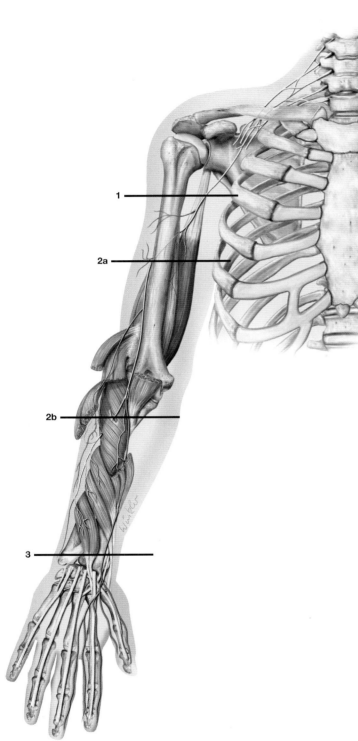

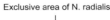
Exclusive area of N. radialis

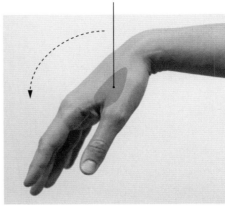

Fig. 3.125 **Proximal lesion of the radial nerve: wrist drop** with sensory disturbances in the first interdigital space. [S700]

→ T 24

Clinical remarks

With **lesions of the N. radialis,** a distinction is made between three different lesions:

* **Proximal lesion** in the area of the **axilla:** in the past often caused by crutches, but today more often due to incorrect positioning during surgery. A **dysfunction of the M. triceps brachii** with reduced elbow extension and triceps reflex, as well as a sensory loss on the back of the upper arm only occur in the case of proximal lesions (additional to the symptoms caused by lesions in the area of the humeral shaft), because these nerve fibres branch off early, before entering the Sulcus nervi radialis (→ Fig. 3.124, 1).
* **Intermediate lesion** near the **humeral shaft or the cubital fossa:** possible causes are a shaft fracture or nerve compression **(park bench position)** or squeezing against the humerus. Nerve lesions in the cubital area can be caused by dislocations or high fractures of the radius, as well as by compression in the arcade of FROHSE or in the supinator canal **(supinator syndrome).** Lesions in the area of the **humeral shaft** (→ Fig. 3.124, 2a) result in a **wrist drop** (→ Fig. 3.125) due to the dysfunction of all forearm extensors, including the radial group, as well as an impairment of the finger and thumb extension and supination with an extended arm. In addition, a sensory deficit occurs on the dorsal side of the forearm, in the first interdigital space (autonomous area), and on the dorsal side of the radial 2½ fingers. If it is only the **R. profundus** that is entrapped while passing through the M. supinator (→ Fig. 3.124, 2b), there are no sensory deficits and the effect on the innervation of the wrist is negligible. A wrist drop does **not** occur if only the finger extensors are impaired, whereas the Mm. extensores carpi radiales are sufficient for stabilisation of the wrist as part of the otherwise intact radial muscle group. Due to active insufficiency of the flexors, which cannot be compensated for by the extension of the wrists, a **strong fist closure** is not achievable.
* **Distal lesion of the R. superficialis** in the **wrist area** (→ Fig. 3.124, 3), due to a distal radius fracture (the most common fracture in humans): the sensory deficit is confined to the first interdigital space and to the back of the radial 2½ fingers.

Fig. 3.124 **Lesion sites of the radial nerve (C5–T1); right side;** dorsal view (marked with bars). The sensory cutaneous branches are highlighted in purple. [S700-L266]
Sensory autonomous area: first interdigital space
Common lesion sites (marked with bars):
1 Proximal lesion in the **axillary region**
2 Intermediate lesion near the **humeral shaft (a)** or **cubital fossa (b)**
3 Distal lesion in the **wrist area**

N. medianus

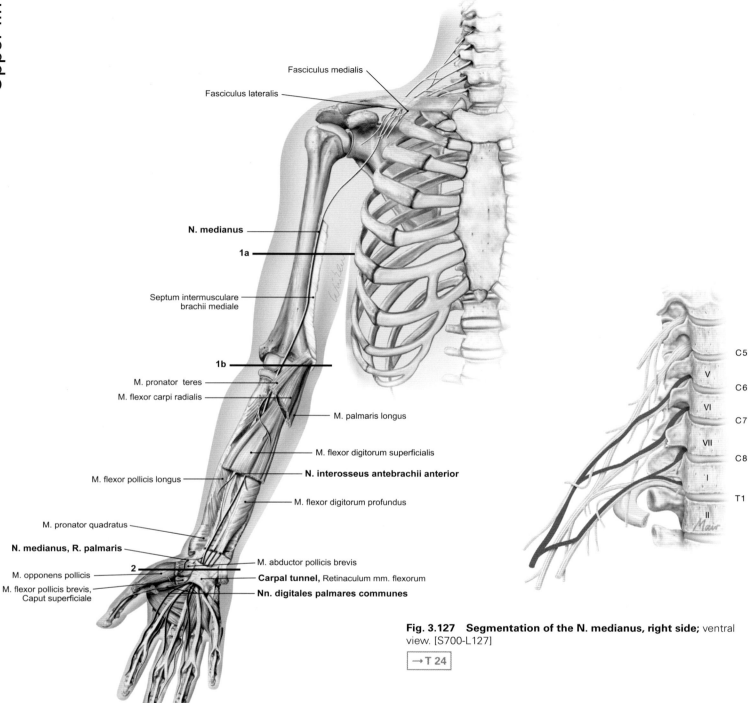

Fig. 3.127   **Segmentation of the N. medianus, right side;** ventral view. [S700-L127]

→ T 24

Fig. 3.126   Pathway, supply area and lesion sites of the N. medianus (C6–T1), right side; ventral view. The sensory cutaneous branches are highlighted in purple. [S700-L266]

The N. medianus consists of a lateral and a medial root that emerge from the respective fascicles. Firstly, it runs along the medial upper arm in the Sulcus bicipitalis medialis without providing any branches. The nerve then enters medially into the cubital fossa and passes **between the two heads of the M. pronator teres** into the intermuscular layer between the superficial and deep flexors of the forearm. Here it innervates **all flexor muscles of the forearm,** apart from the M. flexor carpi ulnaris and the ulnar head of the M. flexor digitorum profundus, of which the deep muscles are supplied by the N. interosseus antebrachii anterior. In addition, this nerve provides sensory innervation to the palmar side of the wrist. The N. medianus passes between the tendons of the finger flexors through **the carpal tunnel** (Canalis carpi) and enters into the palm, where it divides into three Nn. digitales palmares communes. These nerves provide muscular branches to the **thumb muscles** (apart from the M. adductor pollicis and the Caput profundum of the M. flexor pollicis brevis) and to the two radial **Mm. lumbricales.** They then divide into the sensory terminal branches, which supply the palmar side of the radial 3½ fingers, and also the dorsal side of the distal phalanges.

Sensory autonomous area: distal phalanges of the index and middle fingers

Common lesion sites (marked with bars):

1 Proximal lesion in the area of the **Sulcus bicipitalis medialis (a)** or **in the cubital fossa (b)**

2 Distal lesion in the **wrist** area and in the **carpal tunnel.**

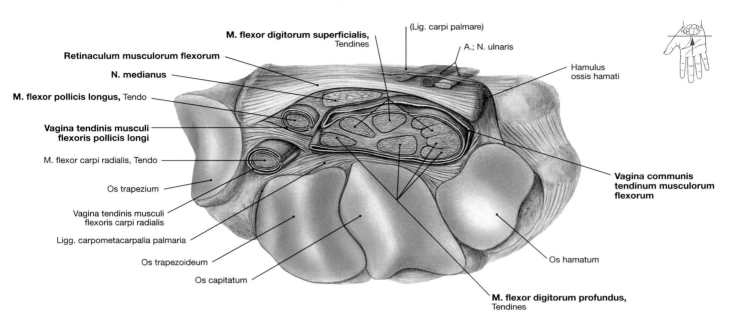

M. flexor digitorum superficialis, Tendines

(Lig. carpi palmare)

A.; N. ulnaris

Retinaculum musculorum flexorum

N. medianus

M. flexor pollicis longus, Tendo

Vagina tendinis musculi flexoris pollicis longi

M. flexor carpi radialis, Tendo

Os trapezium

Vagina tendinis musculi flexoris carpi radialis

Ligg. carpometacarpalia palmaria

Os trapezoideum

Os capitatum

Hamulus ossis hamati

Vagina communis tendinum musculorum flexorum

Os hamatum

M. flexor digitorum profundus, Tendines

Fig. 3.128   Carpal tunnel, Canalis carpi, right side; distal view; cross-section at the level of the carpometacarpal joints. [S700] Together with the carpal bones, the Retinaculum musculorum flexorum forms the carpal tunnel through which the N. medianus and the tendons of the long finger flexor muscles run (→ Fig. 3.177). Inflammation (tendinitis) or swelling in the area of the carpal tunnel can lead to a compression of the N. medianus. Functional deficits caused by compression of the N. medianus in the carpal tunnel are referred to as **carpal tunnel syndrome**.

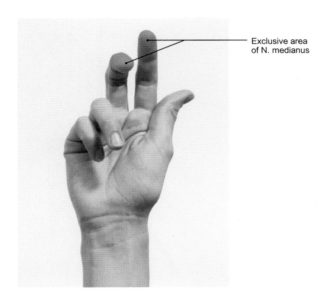

Exclusive area of N. medianus

Fig. 3.129   Proximal lesion of the N. medianus: 'benediction sign' with sensory deficits in the distal phalanges of the index and middle fingers. [S700]

Clinical remarks

Lesions of the N. medianus:
A distinction is made between proximal and distal lesions:
- **Proximal lesion** in the Sulcus bicipitalis medialis (→ Fig. 3.126, 1a; e.g. in the case of incision wounds) or in the cubital region (→ Fig. 3.126, 1b): in the cubital fossa, the N. medianus can become entrapped or compressed due to distal humerus fractures, incorrect taking of blood or intravenous injection, or when emerging between the heads of the M. pronator teres (pronator teres syndrome). Only a proximal nerve lesion causes the **'benediction sign'**, in which the thumb, index and middle fingers can no longer be bent in the proximal and distal interphalangeal joints (→ Fig. 3.129). The reason is a lack of innervation to the superficial as well as the radial part of the deep finger flexor muscles. All other symptoms are similar to those of the distal lesion.
- **Distal lesions** in the **wrist area** (e.g. when cutting the arteries with suicidal intention) or compression of the N. medianus in the carpal tunnel (**carpal tunnel syndrome,** the most common nerve injury of the upper limb; → Fig. 3.126, 2): these do not result in the 'benediction sign', because the motor branches to the finger flexor muscles branch off early at the forearm! However, the result can be an **'ape hand'**, since the atrophy of the thenar eminence leads to a constant adduction position of the thumb due to the predominant activity of the M. adductor pollicis (innervated by the N. ulnaris). The **opposition test** (SCHAEFFER's test) is **negative,** due to dysfunction of the M. opponens pollicis, and as a result the distal phalanges of the thumb and little finger cannot touch each other. The **'bottle sign'** signifies that the abduction of the thumb is insufficient (dysfunction of the M. abductor pollicis brevis), and an object can therefore not be grasped fully. **Sensory deficiencies** afflict the palmar side of the radial 3½ fingers. There is typically pain at night that radiates proximally.

N. ulnaris

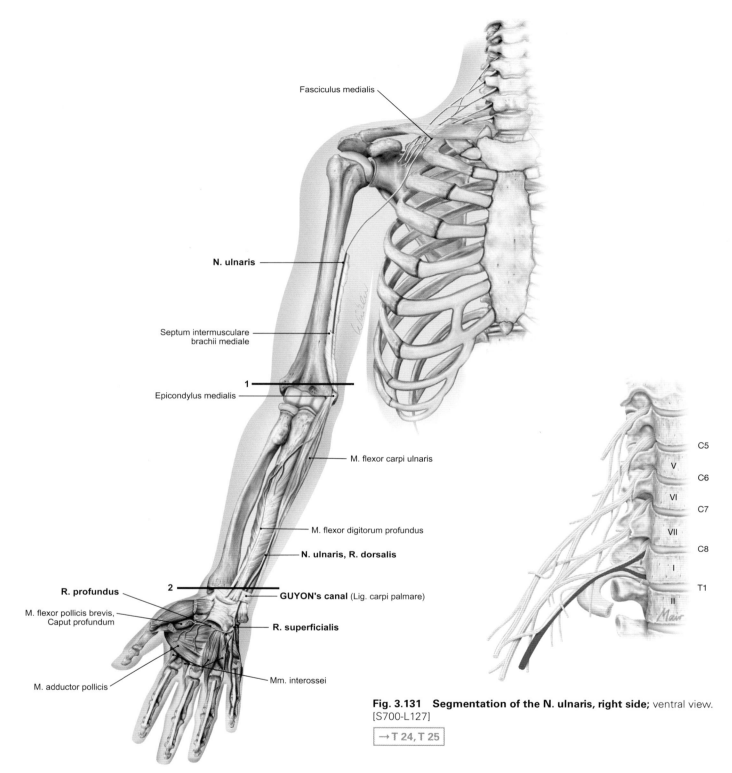

Fasciculus medialis

N. ulnaris

Septum intermusculare
brachii mediale

1

Epicondylus medialis

M. flexor carpi ulnaris

M. flexor digitorum profundus

N. ulnaris, R. dorsalis

R. profundus

2

GUYON's canal (Lig. carpi palmare)

M. flexor pollicis brevis,
Caput profundum

R. superficialis

M. adductor pollicis

Mm. interossei

C5
V
C6
VI
C7
VII
C8
I
T1
II

Fig. 3.131   Segmentation of the N. ulnaris, right side; ventral view.
[S700-L127]

→ T 24, T 25

**Fig. 3.130   Pathway, supply area and lesion sites of the N. ulnaris
(C8–T1), right side;** ventral view. The sensory cutaneous branches are
highlighted in purple. [S700-L266]
The N. ulnaris originates from the Fasciculus medialis and runs in the
Sulcus bicipitalis medialis along the medial upper arm, then it penetrates the Septum intermusculare brachii mediale and passes onto the
dorsal side of the Epicondylus medialis, where it is in direct contact
with the bone in the **Sulcus nervi ulnaris ('funny bone')**. It provides no
branches to the upper arm. In the forearm, the N. ulnaris passes along
with the A. ulnaris below the M. flexor carpi ulnaris to the wrist, where
it enters through the GUYON's canal into the palm. Its R. dorsalis continues to the dorsal side of the hand and supplies the ulnar 2½ fingers
with sensory innervation. In the forearm, the N. ulnaris provides motor
innervation to the **M. flexor carpi ulnaris** and to the **ulnar part of the**

M. flexor digitorum profundus. Branching off in the palm of the hand,
the R. profundus follows the deep palmar arterial arch to innervate the
hypothenar muscles, as well as all the **Mm. interossei,** the two ulnar
Mm. lumbricales, the **M. adductor pollicis** and the deep head of the
M. flexor pollicis brevis. The R. superficialis provides motor innervation only to the **M. palmaris brevis** and continues in the sensory R.
digitalis palmaris communis, which divides into terminal branches for
the innervation of the palmar surfaces of the ulnar 1½ fingers (and dorsally of the distal phalanges).
Sensory autonomous area: distal phalanx of the little finger
Common lesion sites (marked with bars):
1 Proximal lesion in the area of the Epicondylus medialis (cubital tunnel syndrome)
2 Distal lesion in the GUYON's canal (ulnar canal).

Upper limb

3

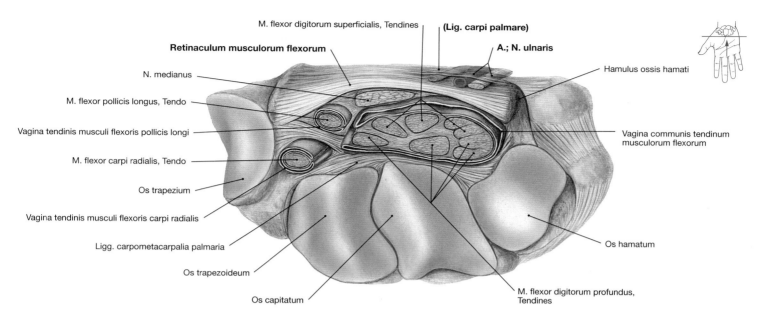

Fig. 3.132 **GUYON's canal, right side;** distal view; cross-section at the level of the carpometacarpal joints. [S700]

The GUYON's canal is formed by the Retinaculum musculorum flexorum and its superficial fibres (Lig. carpi palmare). The N. ulnaris, to-

gether with the A. and V. ulnaris, runs through the GUYON's canal (→ Fig. 3.177). Swellings or chronic pressure may cause a compression of the N. ulnaris **(GUYON's canal syndrome)**.

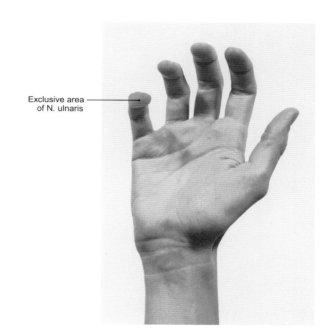

Fig. 3.133 **Proximal and distal lesions of the N. ulnaris: 'claw hand'** with sensory deficit in the distal phalanx of the little finger. [S700]

Clinical remarks

Lesions of the N. ulnaris: a distinction is made between proximal and distal lesions which cannot, however, be clearly separated:

- **Proximal lesion** in the Sulcus nervi ulnaris **(cubital tunnel syndrome)**, usually due to chronic compression and made worse when leaning on the arm: this is the second most common nerve lesion of the upper limb.
- **Distal lesion** in the **GUYON's canal,** mostly due to chronic compression.

The clinical symptoms of proximal and distal lesions are similar. In both cases, the result is a **'claw hand'**, since the (clearly visible) atrophy of the Mm. interossei and of the two ulnar Mm. lumbricales impedes flexion in the metacarpopharyngeal joints in particular, and

extension in the distal interphalangeal joints. The **opposition test** is **negative,** due to dysfunction of the M. opponens digiti minimi, which means the distal phalanges of the thumb and little finger cannot touch each other. The **FROMENT's sign** (holding a sheet of paper between the thumb and index finger) indicates that insufficient adduction of the thumb is compensated for by the bending of its distal phalanx (the M. flexor pollicis longus is innervated by the N. medianus). **Sensory deficits** occur in the palmar side of the ulnar 1½ fingers. If a compression injury occurs in the palm of the hand (hypothenar hammer syndrome), only the R. profundus is affected and sensory symptoms can be missing.

Arteries of the arm

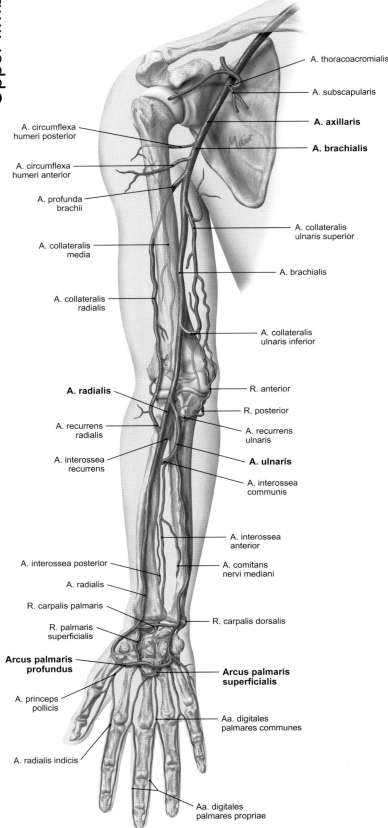

A. thoracoacromialis

A. subscapularis

A. axillaris

A. brachialis

A. circumflexa
humeri posterior

A. circumflexa
humeri anterior

A. profunda
brachii

A. collateralis
media

A. collateralis
radialis

A. collateralis
ulnaris superior

A. brachialis

A. collateralis
ulnaris inferior

A. radialis

R. anterior

R. posterior

A. recurrens
radialis

A. recurrens
ulnaris

A. interossea
recurrens

A. ulnaris

A. interossea
communis

A. interossea
anterior

A. interossea posterior

A. comitans
nervi mediani

A. radialis

R. carpalis palmaris

R. carpalis dorsalis

R. palmaris
superficialis

**Arcus palmaris
profundus**

**Arcus palmaris
superficialis**

A. princeps
pollicis

Aa. digitales
palmares communes

A. radialis indicis

Aa. digitales
palmares propriae

Arteries of the upper limb

Branches of the A. subclavia:
- A. vertebralis (→ Chapter 8)
- A. thoracica interna (→ Chapter 2)
- Truncus thyrocervicalis
  - A. thyroidea inferior
  - A. cervicalis ascendens
  - A. transversa cervicis/colli
  - A. suprascapularis
- Truncus costocervicalis
  - A. intercostalis suprema
  - A. profunda cervicis

Branches of the A. axillaris:
- A. thoracica superior (inconstant)
- A. thoracoacromialis
- A. thoracica lateralis
- A. subscapularis
  - A. circumflexa scapulae
  - A. thoracodorsalis
- A. circumflexa humeri anterior
- A. circumflexa humeri posterior

Branches of the A. brachialis:
- A. profunda brachii
  - A. collateralis media
  - A. collateralis radialis
- A. collateralis ulnaris superior
- A. collateralis ulnaris inferior

Branches of the A. radialis:
- A. recurrens radialis
- R. carpalis palmaris
- R. carpalis dorsalis → Rete carpale dorsale → Aa. metacarpales dorsales → Aa. digitales dorsales
- R. palmaris superficialis → Arcus palmaris superficialis
- A. princeps pollicis
- A. radialis indicis
- Arcus palmaris profundus → Aa. metacarpales palmares

Branches of the A. ulnaris:
- A. recurrens ulnaris
- A. interossea communis
  - A. interossea anterior
    - A. comitans nervi mediani
  - A. interossea posterior with A. interossea recurrens
- R. carpalis dorsalis
- R. carpalis palmaris
- R. palmaris profundus → Arcus palmaris profundus
- Arcus palmaris superficialis → Aa. digitales palmares

Fig. 3.134 Arteries of the upper limb, right side; ventral view. [S700-L127]

The **A. axillaris** is the continuation of the A. subclavia and extends from rib I to the lower margin of the M. pectoralis major. It is located between the three fascicles of the Plexus brachialis and the two roots of the N. medianus. In the upper arm it continues in the **A. brachialis,** which passes together with the N. medianus through the Sulcus bicipitalis medialis, and enters medially into the cubital fossa. There it divides into the A. radialis and the A. ulnaris. The **A. radialis** follows the radius between the superficial and deep flexor muscles up to the wrist, where it runs through the Fovea radialis (snuffbox) in the dorsal direction, and then passes back into the palm between the heads of the M. interosseus dorsalis I. It is the main tributary of the deep palmar arch (**Arcus palmaris profundus**). The **A. ulnaris** provides the A. interossea communis, passes along with the N. ulnaris below the M. flexor carpi ulnaris to the wrist and further along through the GUYON's canal into the palm, where it continues into the superficial palmar arch (**Arcus palmaris superficialis**).

Clinical remarks

In a complete physical examination, the **pulse** of the A. radialis and A. ulnaris is palpated on the radial and ulnar sides of the proximal wrist, respectively, to exclude any occlusion of the blood vessels by **arteriosclerosis** or blood clots (**emboli**).

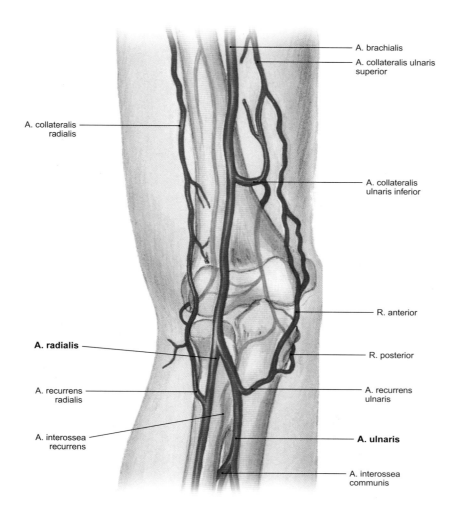

A. brachialis
A. collateralis ulnaris superior
A. collateralis radialis
A. collateralis ulnaris inferior
A. radialis
R. anterior
R. posterior
A. recurrens radialis
A. recurrens ulnaris
A. interossea recurrens
A. ulnaris
A. interossea communis

Fig. 3.135 Collateral circulation of the elbow region, Rete articulare cubiti, right side; ventral view, section of the cubital fossa. [S700] In the cubital and elbow region, a collateral or bypass circulation for the main trunk of the A. brachialis is formed by anastomoses of the **four collateral arteries** (A. collateralis media and A. collateralis radialis from the A. profunda brachii, A. collateralis ulnaris superior and A. collateralis ulnaris inferior from the A. brachialis) with the **three recurrent arteries** (A. recurrens radialis, A. recurrens ulnaris and A. interossea recurrens from the eponymously-named blood vessels).

Structure and function

Rete articulare cubiti
The **collateral arteries** (A. collateralis media, A. collateralis radialis, A. collateralis ulnaris superior, A. collateralis ulnaris inferior) and the **recurrent arteries** (A. recurrens radialis, A. recurrens ulnaris, A. interossea recurrens) form a collateral circulation in the elbow region (Rete articulare cubiti).

Clinical remarks

In the event of acute injuries, the collateral and recurrent arteries of the Rete articulare cubiti allow for a tourniquet to be applied to the **A. brachialis in the cubital fossa,** without endangering the blood supply of the forearm.

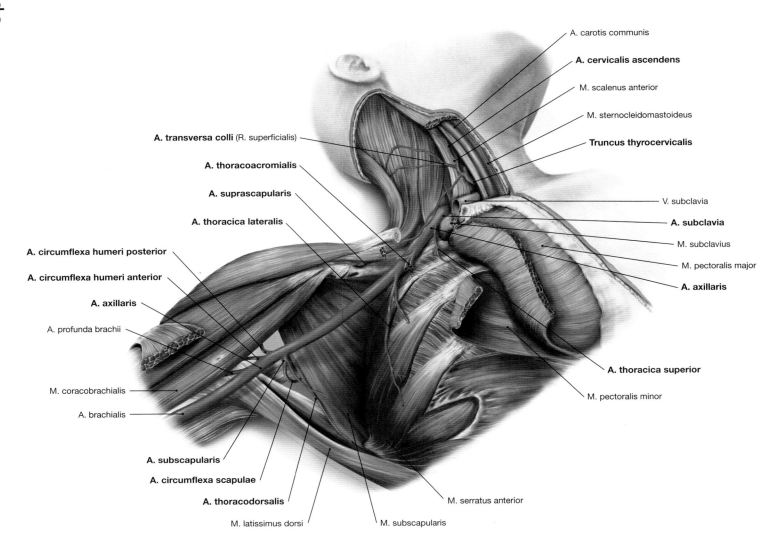

A. carotis communis

A. cervicalis ascendens

M. scalenus anterior

M. sternocleidomastoideus

Truncus thyrocervicalis

V. subclavia

A. subclavia

M. subclavius

M. pectoralis major

A. axillaris

A. transversa colli (R. superficialis)

A. thoracoacromialis

A. suprascapularis

A. thoracica lateralis

A. circumflexa humeri posterior

A. circumflexa humeri anterior

A. axillaris

A. profunda brachii

M. coracobrachialis

A. brachialis

A. thoracica superior

M. pectoralis minor

A. subscapularis

A. circumflexa scapulae

A. thoracodorsalis

M. serratus anterior

M. latissimus dorsi

M. subscapularis

Fig. 3.136 Arteries of the shoulder, right side; ventral view after severing the Mm. pectorales major and minor near their insertion. [S700-L266]

This illustration shows the arteries of the shoulder which partly derive from the A. subclavia (→ Fig. 3.139) and mainly from the A. axillaris (→ Fig. 3.140). The A. suprascapularis and the A. transversa cervicis/colli originate from the Truncus thyrocervicalis of the A. subclavia. The **A. suprascapularis** runs dorsally behind the clavicle where it crosses the Lig. transversum scapulae superius to the dorsal side of the scapula. As shown here, it is often only the superficial branch of the **A. transversa cervicalis/colli** (R. superficialis) which originates from the Truncus thyrocervicalis and passes into the lateral cervical region to reach the inferior side of the M. trapezius. The deep branch (R. profundus) is in this case the last vessel branching directly off the A. subclavia and

passing deep in through the fascicles of the Plexus brachialis (not visible here).

The first branch of the A. axillaris is the **A. thoracica superior,** which runs off onto the upper chest wall. Then the **A. thoracoacromialis** branches off in a ventral-cranial direction, and immediately divides into its terminal branches (→ Fig. 3.138) before the **A. thoracica lateralis** descends along the lateral margin of the M. pectoralis minor. The next branch is the **A. subscapularis,** which as a strong, often short arterial trunk runs caudally and soon divides into the A. circumflexa scapulae and the A. thoracodorsalis. The A. circumflexa scapulae passes through the medial axillary space to the dorsal side of the scapula. The **Aa. circumflexae humeri anterior and posterior** then originate and loop around the neck of the humerus, whereby the artery to the dorsal side of the upper arm enters through the lateral axillary space.

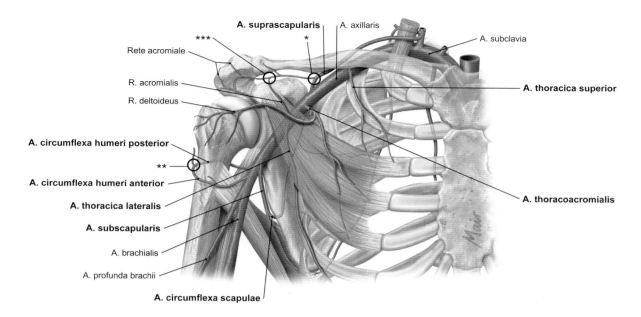

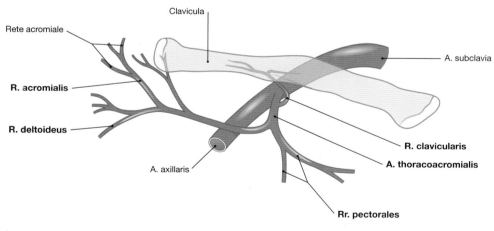

Fig. 3.137 Anastomoses between the A. subclavia and A. axillaris, right side; ventral view. [S700-L127]

The A. axillaris is divided into three sections relative to the pathway of the M. pectoralis minor. Thereby section 1 lies proximally and medially to the muscle, section 2 lies dorsally, and section 3 distally, and thereby laterally, to the M. pectoralis minor.

Scapular anastomoses:

- The **A. circumflexa scapulae** from the A. subscapularis (from the A. axillaris) passes through the medial axillary space to the dorsal side, where it anastomoses in the Fossa infraspinata with the **A. suprascapularis** (from the circulatory area of the A. subclavia) (*).

- The **A. circumflexa scapulae** can anastomose with the **A. dorsalis scapulae** (branch of the A. transversa cervicis/colli from the circulatory area of the A. subclavia) in the Fossa infraspinata via a branch at the medial margin of the scapula. This connection (if present) is mostly poorly developed.

- The **R. acromialis of the A. thoracoacromialis** (from the A. axillaris) can also anastomose with the **A. suprascapularis** (***).

Upper arm anastomoses:

- The **A. circumflexa humeri anterior** anastomoses (**) with the **A. circumflexa humeri posterior,** which passes through the lateral axillary space.

Fig. 3.138 Branches of the A. thoracoacromialis. [S700-L126]

The **A. thoracoacromialis** is a major branch of the A. axillaris and is divided into four terminal branches:

- Rr. pectorales to the Mm. pectorales
- R. clavicularis to the M. subclavius
- R. deltoideus to the M. deltoideus
- R. acromialis to the Rete acromiale.

Clinical remarks

The **scapular anastomoses** between the A. suprascapularis and A. dorsalis scapulae from the circulatory area of the A. subclavia with the A. circumflexa scapulae from the A. axillaris are important for collateral circulation of the blood supply to the arm, e.g. if the vessel is obstructed when the Truncus thyrocervicalis and the A. subscapularis branch off, or if a tourniquet must be applied in the case of a vascular injury. The arteries in the shoulder area can be visualised by angiography. The Proc. coracoideus serves as an anatomical landmark.

[H063-001]

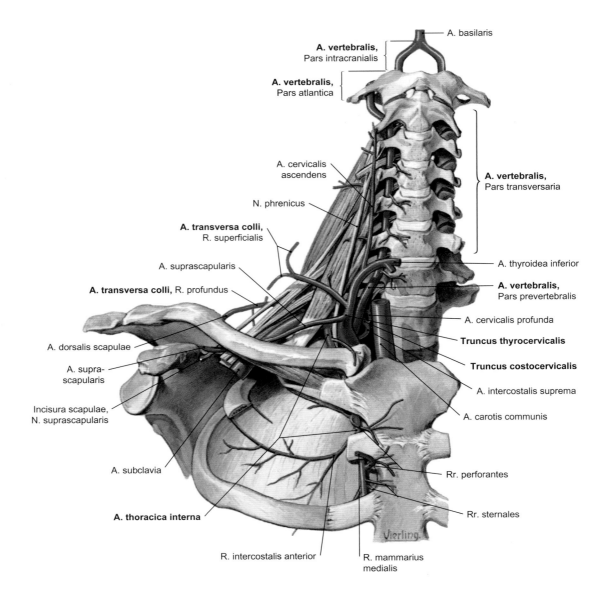
A. subclavia

A. basilaris

A. vertebralis,
Pars intracranialis

A. vertebralis,
Pars atlantica

A. cervicalis
ascendens

A. vertebralis,
Pars transversaria

N. phrenicus

A. transversa colli,
R. superficialis

A. suprascapularis

A. thyroidea inferior

A. transversa colli, R. profundus

A. vertebralis,
Pars prevertebralis

A. dorsalis scapulae

A. cervicalis profunda

Truncus thyrocervicalis

A. supra-
scapularis

Truncus costocervicalis

Incisura scapulae,
N. suprascapularis

A. intercostalis suprema

A. carotis communis

A. subclavia

Rr. perforantes

A. thoracica interna

Rr. sternales

R. intercostalis anterior

R. mammarius
medialis

Vierling.

Fig. 3.139   Branches of the A. subclavia, right side; ventral view after removal of the superficial neck muscles, as well as all shoulder/shoulder girdle and thoracic muscles. [G1066-O1109]

In addition to the arm, the branches of the **A. subclavia** supply the neck area and its organs, as well as parts of the ventral thoracic or chest wall and parts of the brain. Together with the Plexus brachialis, the artery passes through the scalene hiatus, and usually has four branches, of which the A. suprascapularis and the A. transversa cervicis/colli contribute to the blood supply of the upper extremity.

- **A. vertebralis:** descending medially of the M. scalenus anterior in the cranial direction, it supplies neck muscles and the cervical spine, spinal cord, brainstem, inner ear, cerebellum and posterior parts of the cerebrum.
- **A. thoracica interna:** running caudally, it descends about 1 cm laterally to the sternal edge and supplies the mediastinum and diaphragm as well as the anterior thoracic wall.
- **Truncus thyrocervicalis:** this generally strong vascular trunk runs in a cranial direction and divides into four branches:
  - **A. thyoidea inferior:** the strongest branch of the Truncus thyrocervicalis supplies the thyroid gland, hypopharynx, oesophagus, larynx and trachea.
  - **A. cervicalis ascendens:** thin vessel on the M. scalenus anterior.

- **A. transversa cervicis** (= A. transversa colli): runs in a lateral direction and splits into two branches:
  - R. superficialis: crosses the Plexus brachialis and continues to the bottom of the M. trapezius.
  - R. profundus: crosses over the fascicles of the Plexus brachialis and abuts the **A. dorsalis scapulae** along the Margo medialis of the scapula. It sometimes anastomoses on the dorsal side of the scapula with the A. suprascapularis, and the A. circumflexa scapulae (→ Fig. 3.137).
- **A. suprascapularis:** passes behind the clavicle and abuts the N. suprascapularis. In contrast to this nerve, it follows the Lig. transversum scapulae superius into the Fossa supraspinata and runs below the Lig. transversum scapulae inferius into the Fossa infraspinata to supply the muscles there. The A. suprascapularis usually anastomoses with the A. circumflexa scapulae and via thin branches with the A. dorsalis scapulae (**scapular anastomoses).**
- **Truncus costocervicalis:** this short vascular trunk runs caudally and divides into two branches:
  - A. intercostalis suprema: supplies the upper two intercostal spaces.
  - A. profunda cervicis: for prevertebral neck muscles.

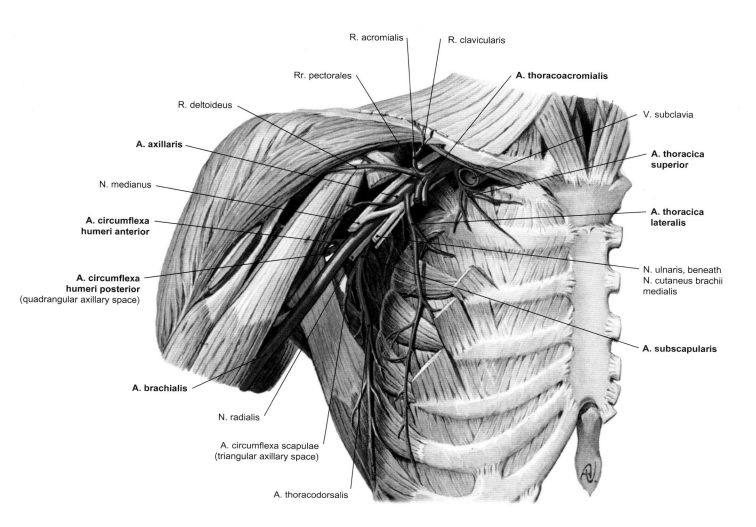

R. acromialis

R. clavicularis

Rr. pectorales

A. thoracoacromialis

R. deltoideus

V. subclavia

A. axillaris

**A. thoracica
superior**

N. medianus

**A. circumflexa
humeri anterior**

**A. thoracica
lateralis**

**A. circumflexa
humeri posterior**
(quadrangular axillary space)

N. ulnaris, beneath
N. cutaneus brachii
medialis

A. subscapularis

A. brachialis

N. radialis

A. circumflexa scapulae
(triangular axillary space)

A. thoracodorsalis

Fig. 3.140 Branches of the A. axillaris, right side; ventral view after removal of the Mm. pectorales major and minor. [G1066-O1109]
The branches of the **A. axillaris** supply the shoulder and parts of the anterior thoracic wall. Usually there are six branches associated with the three sections of the A. axillaris (→ Fig. 3.137):
First segment (medial of the M. pectoralis minor):
* **A. thoracica superior:** this inconstant thin vessel supplies the muscles of the upper thoracic wall.
Second segment (dorsal of the M. pectoralis minor):
* **A. thoracoacromialis:** the short vessel originates in the Trigonum clavipectorale, runs in a ventral-cranial direction and divides into four terminal branches (→ Fig. 3.138).
* **A. thoracica lateralis:** it descends laterally along the M. pectoralis minor in a caudal direction and provides Rr. mammarii laterales to supply the breast gland.
Third segment (lateral of M. pectoralis minor):
* **A. subscapularis:** the short, strong vessel descends caudally and divides into several branches:

– The **A. circumflexa scapulae** passes through the **medial axillary space** on the back of the scapula into the Fossa infraspinata and anastomoses with branches of the A. suprascapularis and often via thin branches with the A. dorsalis scapulae **(scapular anastomoses).**
– The **A. thoracodorsalis** continues the pathway of the A. subscapularis and accompanies the N. thoracodorsalis to the M. latissimus dorsi.
* **A. circumflexa humeri anterior:** it passes as a thin vessel around the front of the proximal humeral shaft.
* **A. circumflexa humeri posterior:** this artery can also branch off prior to the A. circumflexa scapulae, or can originate directly from the M. subscapularis, passing through the **lateral axillary space** and anastomosing with the A. circumflexa humeri anterior **(upper arm anastomoses).**

3

Upper limb

A. brachialis

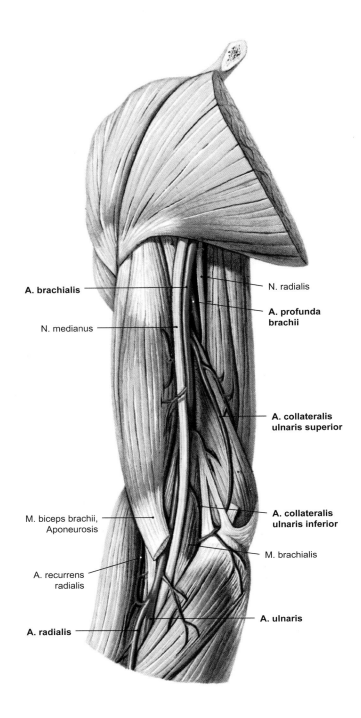

A. brachialis

N. medianus

N. radialis

A. profunda brachii

A. collateralis ulnaris superior

M. biceps brachii, Aponeurosis

A. collateralis ulnaris inferior

M. brachialis

A. recurrens radialis

A. ulnaris

A. radialis

Fig. 3.141 Branches of the A. brachialis, right side; medial-ventral view. [G1066-O1109]

The **A. brachialis** runs along the inside of the arm (Sulcus bicipitalis medialis) in the neurovascular bundle of the upper arm to the cubital fossa, where it divides into the **A. radialis** and **A. ulnaris.** The A. brachialis supplies the humerus, the elbow joint and the muscles of the upper arm. It provides three large vascular branches:

- **A. profunda brachii:** it passes with the N. radialis through the **triangular interval** and is divided into:

- **A. collateralis media:** passes to the dorsal vascular plexus on the elbow joint (Rete articulare cubiti → Fig. 3.135), and
- **A. collateralis radialis:** continues its pathway along the Sulcus nervi radialis to the Rete articulare cubiti.
- **A. collateralis ulnaris superior:** it runs with the N. ulnaris to the Rete articulare cubiti.
- **A. collateralis ulnaris inferior:** it originates just above the cubital fossa and runs to the Rete articulare cubiti.

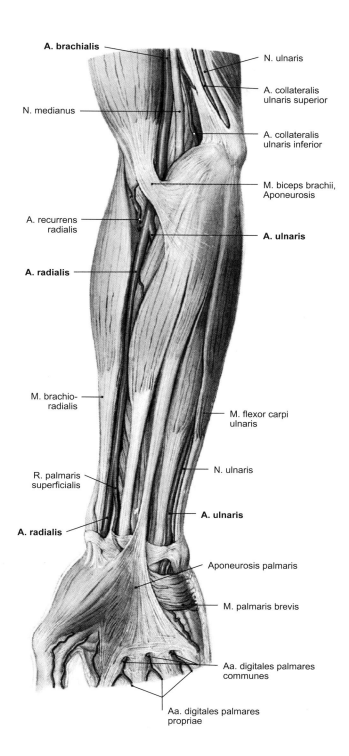

Fig. 3.142 **A. radialis and A. ulnaris, right side;** medial-ventral view. [B500]

On the radial side of the N. medianus, the **A. brachialis** enters the cubital fossa, where it provides the **A. ulnaris** dorsally of the M. pronator teres, while the **A. radialis** continues its pathway beneath the M. brachioradialis to the proximal wrist. It passes through the **Fovea radialis (snuffbox)** dorsally, and then returns to the palm of the hand between the heads of the M. interosseus dorsalis I. There it is the main tributary of the deep palmar arch **(Arcus palmaris profundus, → Fig. 3.144).**

Branches of the A. radialis:

- **A. recurrens radialis:** it passes beneath the M. brachioradialis to the Rete articulare cubiti.

- **Rr. carpales palmaris and dorsalis:** these branches supply the carpus of the hand. The dorsal branch forms the Rete carpale dorsale, providing the **Aa. metacarpales dorsales** which together with the **Aa. digitales dorsales** supply the back of the hand and fingers (→ Fig. 3.179).

- **R. palmaris superficialis:** it forms the superficial palmar arch (Arcus palmaris superficialis) together with the A. ulnaris.

- **A. princeps pollicis:** it supplies the palmar surface of the thumb (→ Fig. 3.144).

- **A. radialis indicis:** it runs along the radial side of the index finger.

- **Arcus palmaris profundus:** (→ Fig. 3.144).

Neurovascular pathways

A. radialis and A. ulnaris

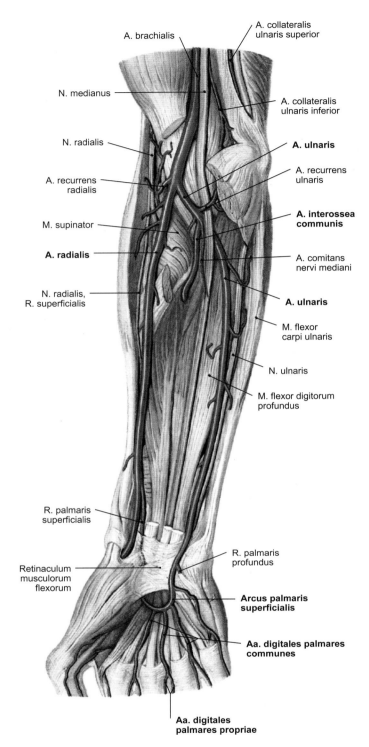

A. brachialis

A. collateralis
ulnaris superior

N. medianus

A. collateralis
ulnaris inferior

N. radialis

A. ulnaris

A. recurrens
radialis

A. recurrens
ulnaris

M. supinator

**A. interossea
communis**

A. radialis

A. comitans
nervi mediani

N. radialis,
R. superficialis

A. ulnaris

M. flexor
carpi ulnaris

N. ulnaris

M. flexor digitorum
profundus

R. palmaris
superficialis

R. palmaris
profundus

Retinaculum
musculorum
flexorum

**Arcus palmaris
superficialis**

**Aa. digitales palmares
communes**

Aa. digitales
palmares propriae

Fig. 3.143   A. radialis and A. ulnaris, right side; medial-ventral view after removal of the superficial flexor muscles of the forearm and of the palmar nerves of the hand. [B500]
The **A. ulnaris** branches off the A. brachialis dorsal to the M. pronator teres, provides the A. interossea communis and then runs along with the N. ulnaris beneath the M. flexor carpi ulnaris to the proximal wrist. It passes with the nerve through the **GUYON's canal** and is the main tributary of the superficial palmar arch **(Arcus palmaris superficialis).**
Branches of the A. ulnaris:

- **A. recurrens ulnaris:** it runs beneath the M. pronator teres to the Rete articulare cubiti.
- **A. interossea communis:** it is a short, strong blood vessel and is divided into the
  - **A. interossea anterior:** it runs on the Membrana interossea antebrachii and penetrates it on the way to the Rete carpale dorsale.

- **A. comitans nervi mediani:** this usually thin vessel accompanies the N. medianus.
- **A. interossea posterior:** it passes through the Membrana interossea antebrachii to the Rete carpale dorsale. Below the M. anconeus it provides the **A. interossea recurrens** which leads to the Rete articulare cubiti.
- **R. carpalis dorsalis:** branch leading to the Rete carpale dorsale.
- **R. palmaris profundus:** it leads to the Arcus palmaris profundus.
- **Arcus palmaris superficialis:** The superficial palmar arch lies under the palmar aponeurosis on the tendons of the long flexor muscles, is supplied mainly by the A. ulnaris, and anastomoses with the R. palmaris superficialis of the A. radialis, which closes the arch. The **Aa. digitales palmares communes,** which divide into the **Aa. digitales palmares propriae,** originate from the superficial palmar arch. These vessels represent the finger arteries.

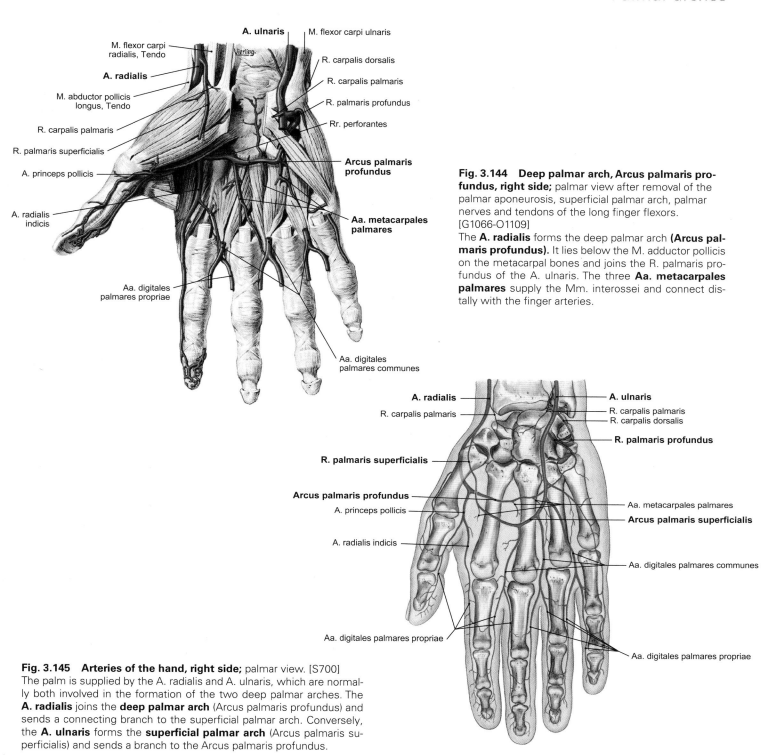

M. flexor carpi radialis, Tendo
A. ulnaris
M. flexor carpi ulnaris
A. radialis
R. carpalis dorsalis
M. abductor pollicis longus, Tendo
R. carpalis palmaris
R. carpalis palmaris
R. palmaris profundus
R. palmaris superficialis
Rr. perforantes
A. princeps pollicis
Arcus palmaris profundus
A. radialis indicis
Aa. metacarpales palmares
Aa. digitales palmares propriae
Aa. digitales palmares communes

Fig. 3.144 Deep palmar arch, Arcus palmaris profundus, right side; palmar view after removal of the palmar aponeurosis, superficial palmar arch, palmar nerves and tendons of the long finger flexors. [G1066-O1109]

The **A. radialis** forms the deep palmar arch (**Arcus palmaris profundus**). It lies below the M. adductor pollicis on the metacarpal bones and joins the R. palmaris profundus of the A. ulnaris. The three **Aa. metacarpales palmares** supply the Mm. interossei and connect distally with the finger arteries.

A. radialis
A. ulnaris
R. carpalis palmaris
R. carpalis palmaris
R. carpalis dorsalis
R. palmaris profundus
R. palmaris superficialis
Arcus palmaris profundus
A. princeps pollicis
Aa. metacarpales palmares
Arcus palmaris superficialis
A. radialis indicis
Aa. digitales palmares communes
Aa. digitales palmares propriae
Aa. digitales palmares propriae

Fig. 3.145 Arteries of the hand, right side; palmar view. [S700]
The palm is supplied by the A. radialis and A. ulnaris, which are normally both involved in the formation of the two deep palmar arches. The **A. radialis** joins the **deep palmar arch** (Arcus palmaris profundus) and sends a connecting branch to the superficial palmar arch. Conversely, the **A. ulnaris** forms the **superficial palmar arch** (Arcus palmaris superficialis) and sends a branch to the Arcus palmaris profundus.

Clinical remarks

The **ALLEN test** is performed prior to the insertion of a catheter into the A. radialis. This test is done to ensure that the A. ulnaris provides a sufficient blood supply to the carpal arterial arches of the hand in case complications occur during the catheterisation. This may include thrombosis with occlusion of the A. radialis by a blood clot. First, the two arteries on both sides of the wrist are compressed to stop the flow of blood until the hand turns pale. If compression on the A. ulnaris ceases, the hand will regain its rosy colour if the blood supply through the A. ulnaris is sufficient.
[S701-L126]

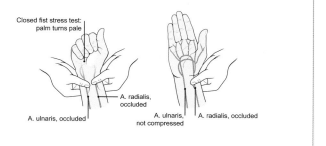

Closed fist stress test: palm turns pale
A. radialis, occluded
A. ulnaris, occluded
A. ulnaris, not compressed
A. radialis, occluded

Veins and lymphatic vessels of the arm

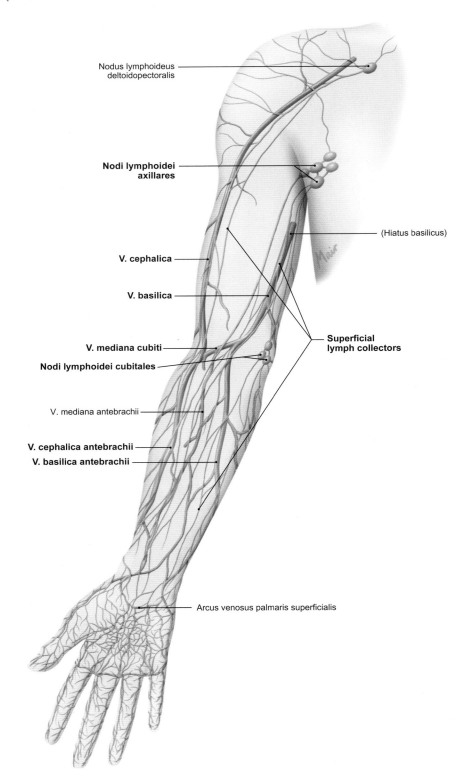

Nodus lymphoideus
deltoidopectoralis

**Nodi lymphoidei
axillares**

(Hiatus basilicus)

V. cephalica

V. basilica

Superficial
lymph collectors

V. mediana cubiti

Nodi lymphoidei cubitales

V. mediana antebrachii

V. cephalica antebrachii

V. basilica antebrachii

Arcus venosus palmaris superficialis

Fig. 3.146 Superficial veins and lymphatic vessels, right side;
ventral view. [S700-L127]

The **superficial venous system** of the arm consists of **two major
trunks** which collect the venous blood from the hand.

On the dorsal side of the thumb, the **V. cephalica antebrachii** collects
the blood from the venous plexus of the back of the hand, and then
passes to the radial flexor side, where it connects in the cubital fossa
via the V. mediana cubiti with the V. basilica antebrachii. In the upper
arm, the V. cephalica runs inside the Sulcus bicipitalis lateralis and then
flows into the V. axillaris in the Trigonum clavipectorale (MOHREN-
HEIM's fossa). In the upper arm, this vessel may be poorly developed
or absent.

The **V. basilica antebrachii** begins on the ulnar side of the back of the
hand, then changes to the ulnar flexor side and finally flows into the Vv.
brachiales, located in the Hiatus basilicus in the lower half of the upper arm.
The **superficial epifascial lymph collectors** form a **radial**, an **ulnar** and
a **medial** bundle in the forearm. In the upper arm, the **medial brachial
bundle** of the V. basilica follows, which drains into the axillary lymph
nodes, while the **dorsolateral brachial bundle** which runs along the V.
cephalica, is additionally linked to the supraclavicular lymph nodes.

The **first regional lymph nodes** of both lymphatic systems are located
predominantly in the axilla (Nodi lymphoidei axillares); single lymph
nodes are, however, also present in the cubital fossa (Nodi lymphoidei
cubitales).

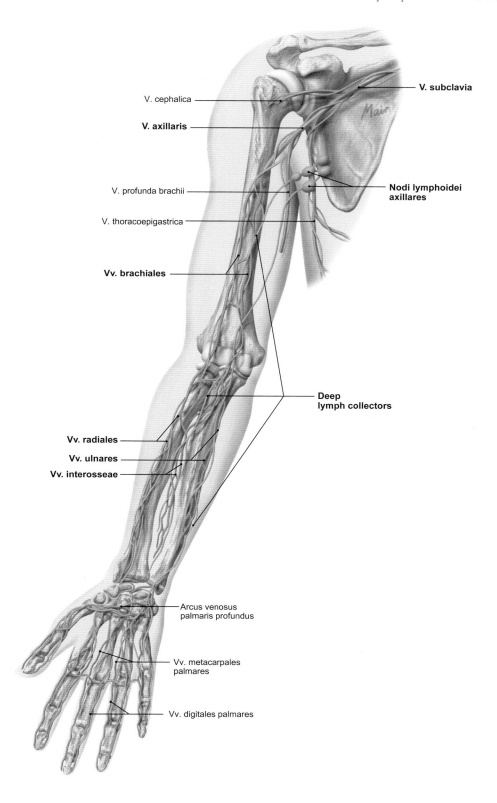

V. cephalica

V. subclavia

V. axillaris

V. profunda brachii

Nodi lymphoidei axillares

V. thoracoepigastrica

Vv. brachiales

Deep lymph collectors

Vv. radiales

Vv. ulnares

Vv. interosseae

Arcus venosus palmaris profundus

Vv. metacarpales palmares

Vv. digitales palmares

Fig. 3.147   Deep veins and lymphatic vessels, right side; ventral view. [S700-L127]
The **deep venous system** and the **deep subfascial lymph collectors** accompany the respective arteries. The deep lymph collectors also drain mainly into the axillary lymph nodes (Nodi lymphoidei axillares), but are also **linked** to the **lymph nodes of the cubital fossa (Nodi lymphoidei cubitales)**.

─ **Clinical remarks** ───────────────────

Skin tumours and infections on the hand and forearm require an inspection of lymph nodes in the cubital region.

Lymph nodes and lymphatic vessels of the axilla

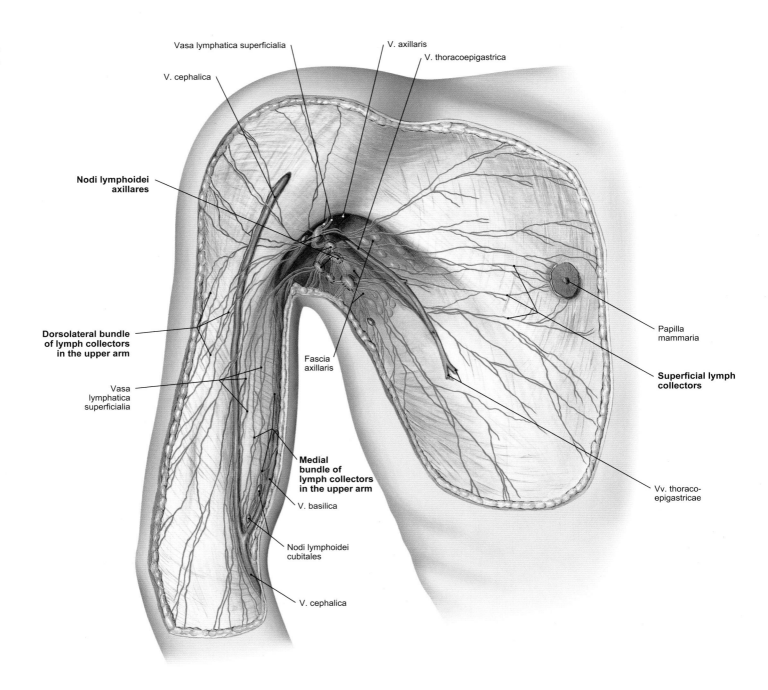

Vasa lymphatica superficialia

V. axillaris

V. thoracoepigastrica

V. cephalica

**Nodi lymphoidei
axillares**

**Dorsolateral bundle
of lymph collectors
in the upper arm**

Vasa
lymphatica
superficialia

Fascia
axillaris

**Medial
bundle of
lymph collectors
in the upper arm**

V. basilica

Nodi lymphoidei
cubitales

V. cephalica

Papilla
mammaria

**Superficial lymph
collectors**

Vv. thoraco-
epigastricae

**Fig. 3.148   Superficial lymphatic vessels and lymph nodes in the
axilla, Fossa axillaris, and the lateral chest wall, Regio thoracica
lateralis, right side;** ventral view. [S700]
In the upper arm, the superficial epifascial lymph collectors form a medial bundle along the V. basilica and a dorsolateral bundle along the

V. cephalica, both of which are mainly linked to the axillary lymph nodes.
The axillary lymph nodes (Nodi lymphoidei axillares) are not only the
regional lymph nodes for the arm, but also collect the lymph of the upper quadrants of the dorsal and ventral chest walls.

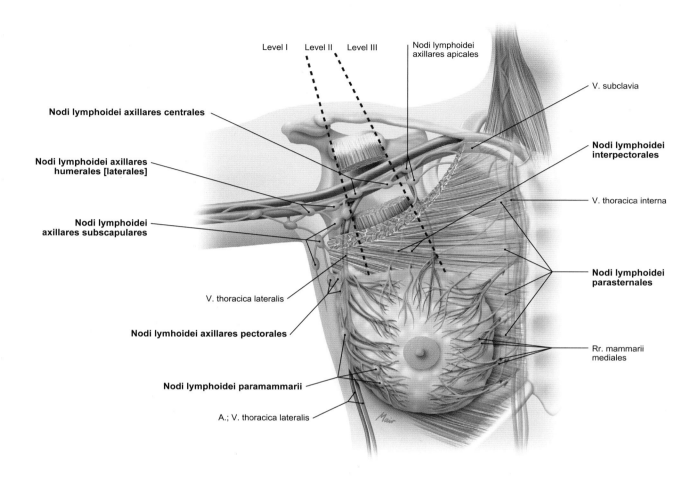

Level I   Level II   Level III   Nodi lymphoidei axillares apicales

V. subclavia

Nodi lymphoidei axillares centrales

Nodi lymphoidei interpectorales

Nodi lymphoidei axillares humerales [laterales]

V. thoracica interna

Nodi lymphoidei axillares subscapulares

Nodi lymphoidei parasternales

V. thoracica lateralis

Nodi lymhoidei axillares pectorales

Rr. mammarii mediales

Nodi lymphoidei paramammarii

A.; V. thoracica lateralis

Fig. 3.149 Levels of lymph nodes in the axilla, Fossa axillaris, right side; ventral view. [S700-L127]

Up to **50 lymph nodes** (Nodi lymphoidei axillares) lie in the adipose tissue of the axilla. These collect the lymph of the arm, the upper thoracic wall including the breast, and of the upper back. The lymph nodes are organised into **three levels** which are clinically important for the treatment of breast cancer. This division is based on the topographical relationship to the **M. pectoralis minor.** Superficial and deep lymph nodes are present in all three levels, but often cannot be attributed clearly to one of these two groups. However, the apical lymph nodes of level III collect the lymph of all other groups and serve as the last lymph node station prior to the Truncus subclavius which drains into the Ductus thoracicus (left side) or into the Ductus lymphaticus dexter (right side; topography of the axillary lymph nodes → Fig. 3.160).

Levels of axillary lymph nodes, level I, inferior group, lateral of the M. pectoralis minor:
* Nodi lymphoidei paramammarii (lateral of the mammary gland)
* Nodi lymphoidei axillares pectorales (along the A. and V. thoracica lateralis)
* Nodi lymphoidei axillares subscapulares (along the A. and V. subscapularis as well as the A. and V. thoracodorsalis)
* Nodi lymphoidei axillares laterales (along the A. and V. axillaris).

Level II, middle or median group, on and under the M. pectoralis minor:
* Nodi lymphoidei interpectorales (between the M. pectoralis minor and M. pectoralis major)
* Nodi lymphoidei axillares centrales (under the M. pectoralis minor).

Level III, superior group, medial of the M. pectoralis minor:
* Nodi lymphoidei axillares apicales (subfascial in the Trigonum clavipectorale = MOHRENHEIM's fossa).

Clinical remarks

Palpation of the lymph nodes is part of a complete physical examination. The physician should be aware that the axillary lymph nodes represent the regional lymph nodes for both the arm and the upper thoracic wall. Due to the frequency of breast cancer (approx. one in ten women will suffer from this once in her lifetime, but men can also be affected), each palpable enlarged axillary lymph node in women should be suspected as a sign of possible breast cancer. Currently, the surgical removal of axillary lymph nodes **(lymphadenectomy)** as part of the surgical treatment in breast cancer pa-

tients is controversial, since it is not proven that this procedure, in addition to removal of the primary tumour, increases the survival rates. However, the diagnostic lymphadenectomy to determine the tumour growth and spreading (staging) is of great importance and requires knowledge of the topography of axillary lymph nodes. Rather than removing level I lymph nodes, the injection of a contrast medium into the tumour is now used to identify **sentinel lymph nodes** for removal.

Superficial blood vessels and nerves of the axilla

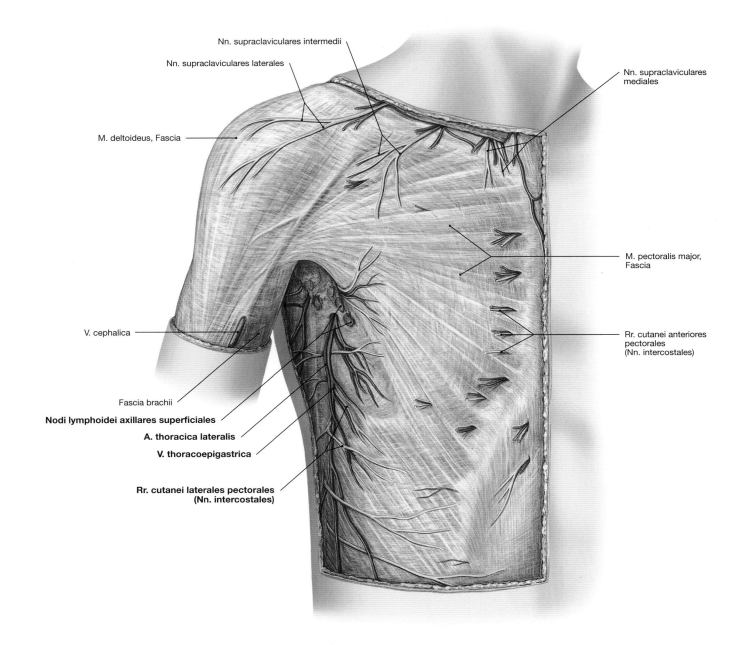

Nn. supraclaviculares intermedii

Nn. supraclaviculares laterales

Nn. supraclaviculares mediales

M. deltoideus, Fascia

M. pectoralis major, Fascia

V. cephalica

Rr. cutanei anteriores pectorales (Nn. intercostales)

Fascia brachii

Nodi lymphoidei axillares superficiales

A. thoracica lateralis

V. thoracoepigastrica

Rr. cutanei laterales pectorales (Nn. intercostales)

Fig. 3.150   Epifascial blood vessels and nerves in the axilla, Fossa axillaris, and the lateral thoracic wall, Regio thoracica lateralis, right side; ventral view. [S700]
Next to the superficial axillary lymph nodes (Nodi lymphoidei axillares superficiales), epifascial blood vessels and nerves are located in the axilla and the lateral thoracic wall. The V. thoracoepigastrica is very vari-
ably developed and lies approximately at the level of the anterior axillary fold, which is formed by the M. pectoralis major. It is sometimes accompanied by a branch of the A. thoracica lateralis. In the respective intercostal spaces, the lateral cutaneous branches of the Nn. intercostales leave from the axilla (Rr. cutanei laterales pectorales).

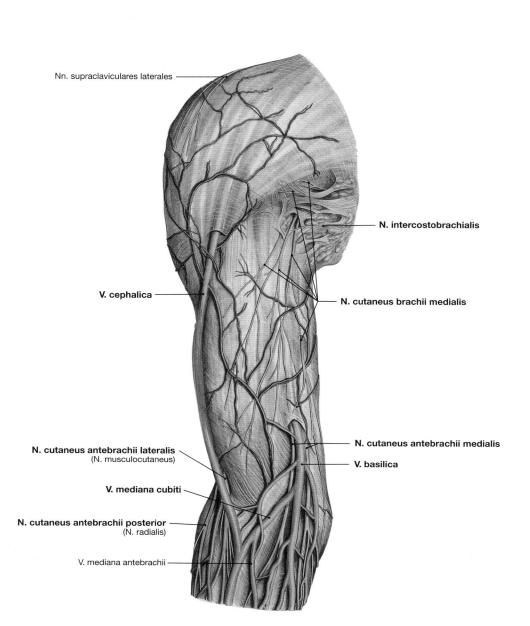

Nn. supraclaviculares laterales

N. intercostobrachialis

V. cephalica

N. cutaneus brachii medialis

N. cutaneus antebrachii medialis

N. cutaneus antebrachii lateralis
(N. musculocutaneus)

V. basilica

V. mediana cubiti

N. cutaneus antebrachii posterior
(N. radialis)

V. mediana antebrachii

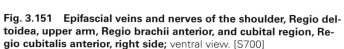

Fig. 3.151 Epifascial veins and nerves of the shoulder, Regio deltoidea, upper arm, Regio brachii anterior, and cubital region, Regio cubitalis anterior, right side; ventral view. [S700]
In the upper arm, the **V. cephalica** ascends in the Sulcus bicipitalis lateralis and lies in the shoulder region between the origins of the M. deltoideus and M. pectoralis major. In the cubital fossa it is usually connected via a **V. mediana cubiti** to the V. basilica. In the Sulcus bicipitalis medialis in the lower half of the upper arm, the **V. basilica** passes through the Fascia brachii and flows into one of the two Vv. brachiales. The **N. cutaneus brachii medialis** passes through the fascia in the axillary region with several thin cutaneous nerves, which radiate along the medial upper arm. These connect in part with the **Nn. intercostobrachiales** from the Nn. intercostales. In the distal part of the upper arm, the cutaneous branches for the forearm pass through the fascia. The **N. cutaneus antebrachii medialis** accompanies the V. basilica, and the **N. cutaneus antebrachii lateralis** accompanies the V. cephalica. As the N. cutaneus antebrachii lateralis is the sensory terminal branch of the N. musculocutaneus, it emerges between the M. biceps brachii and the M. brachialis lying below it, with the N. musculocutaneus running between them. The **N. cutaneus antebrachii posterior** appears further laterally.

Clinical remarks

Due to its good accessibility, the **V. cephalica** is frequently used for the implantation of **pacemakers** or **ports** (for the application of chemotherapies or parenteral nutrition). There are also **central venous catheters (CVCs)** which can be introduced into the upper vena cava via the V. cephalica.

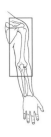

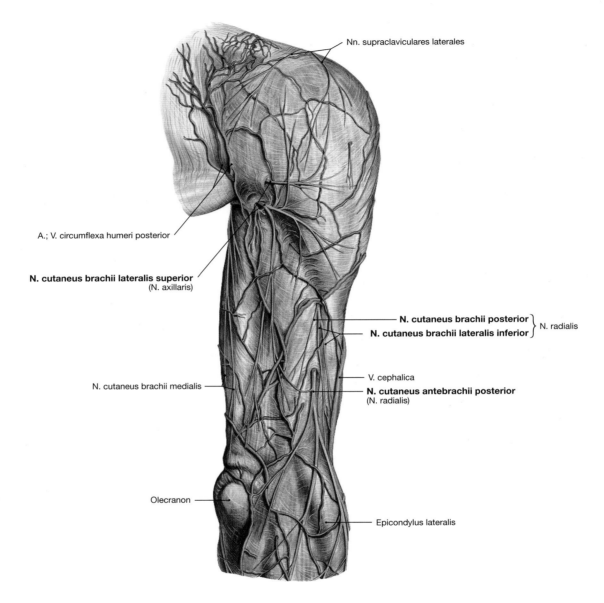

Nn. supraclaviculares laterales

A.; V. circumflexa humeri posterior

N. cutaneus brachii lateralis superior
(N. axillaris)

N. cutaneus brachii posterior ⎫
N. cutaneus brachii lateralis inferior ⎭ N. radialis

N. cutaneus brachii medialis

V. cephalica

N. cutaneus antebrachii posterior
(N. radialis)

Olecranon

Epicondylus lateralis

Fig. 3.152 Epifascial blood vessels and nerves of the shoulder, Regio deltoidea, upper arm, Regio brachii posterior, and elbow, Regio cubitalis posterior, right side; dorsolateral view. [S700]
The **N. cutaneus brachii lateralis superior** is the sensory terminal branch of the N. axillaris. It passes through the fascia at the lower edge of the M. deltoideus, which is innervated by the N. axillaris. The **N. cu-** taneus brachii lateralis inferior, N. cutaneus brachii posterior and **N. cutaneus antebrachii posterior,** however, are branches of the N. radialis and push through the fascia lateral of the M. triceps brachii. The exit of the N. cutaneus antebrachii posterior can usually be found between the M. triceps brachii and the ventrally located M. brachialis.

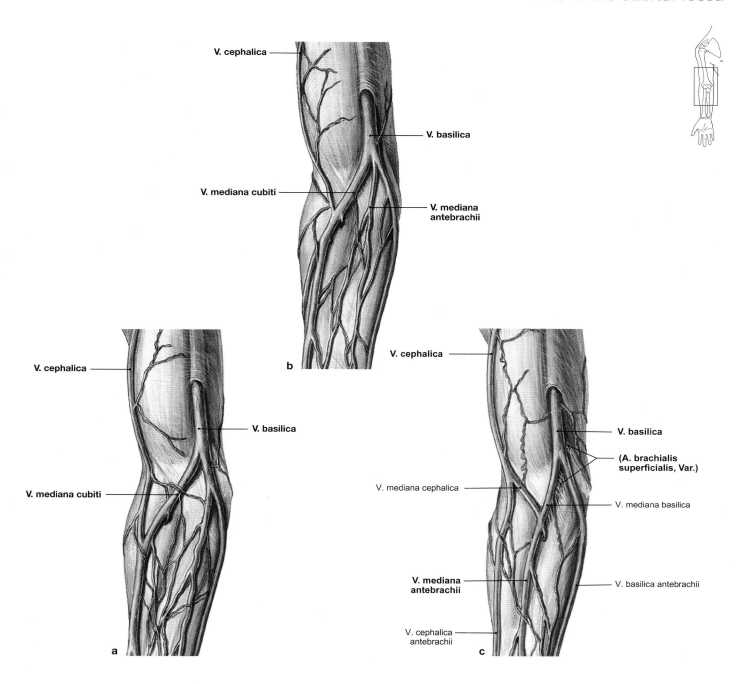

V. cephalica

V. basilica

V. mediana cubiti

V. mediana antebrachii

b

V. cephalica

V. cephalica

V. basilica

V. mediana cubiti

V. cephalica

V. basilica

(A. brachialis superficialis, Var.)

V. mediana cephalica

V. mediana basilica

V. mediana antebrachii

V. basilica antebrachii

V. cephalica antebrachii

a

c

Fig. 3.153a–c Variations of epifascial veins in the cubital fossa, Regio cubitalis anterior, right side; ventral view. [S700]
a, b A **V. mediana cubiti** usually connects the **V. cephalica** with the **V. basilica**. But the **V. cephalica** may vary substantially in the upper arm and can even be absent.

c The V. mediana cubiti is sometimes missing, but the V. cephalica antebrachii and the V. basilica antebrachii communicate indirectly via their connections with a V. mediana antebrachii on the front of the forearm. Special attention should be paid to the possibility of an additional A. brachialis superficialis being present in the cubital fossa which may be situated directly next to the veins.

Clinical remarks

The veins in the cubital fossa are important for **taking blood** and for the **intravenous administration** of drugs. Usually the **V. mediana cubiti** is selected for this purpose. Because of their great variability, the pathway of the veins needs to be examined carefully and palpat-

ed. If an arterial pulse can be felt, a superficial A. brachialis should be considered. Drugs should not be injected into the artery, because with intra-arterial injections some substances may have toxic effects due to insufficient dilution.

Upper limb

3

Superficial blood vessels and nerves of the forearm

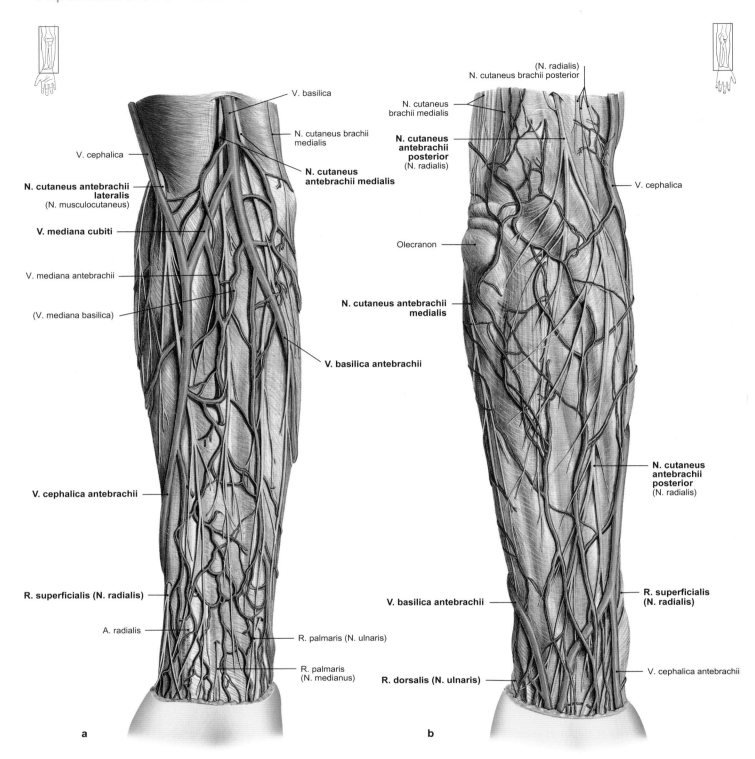

V. basilica

V. cephalica

N. cutaneus brachii medialis

N. cutaneus antebrachii lateralis (N. musculocutaneus)

N. cutaneus antebrachii medialis

V. mediana cubiti

V. mediana antebrachii

(V. mediana basilica)

V. basilica antebrachii

V. cephalica antebrachii

R. superficialis (N. radialis)

A. radialis

R. palmaris (N. ulnaris)

R. palmaris (N. medianus)

a

(N. radialis)
N. cutaneus brachii posterior

N. cutaneus brachii medialis

N. cutaneus antebrachii posterior (N. radialis)

V. cephalica

Olecranon

N. cutaneus antebrachii medialis

N. cutaneus antebrachii posterior (N. radialis)

R. superficialis (N. radialis)

V. basilica antebrachii

R. dorsalis (N. ulnaris)

V. cephalica antebrachii

b

Fig. 3.154a and b Epifascial veins and nerves of the forearm, Regio antebrachii anterior and Regio antebrachii posterior, and of the cubital region, Regio cubitalis anterior, right side. [S700]
a Ventral view. The **V. cephalica antebrachii** originates from the superficial venous plexus on the dorsal side of the thumb (Rete venosum dorsale manus), and then switches onto the radial ventral side of the forearm, while the **V. basilica antebrachii** passes from the ulnar back of the hand to the ulnar ventral side. In the cubital fossa, both veins usually communicate via the **V. mediana cubiti.** The cutaneous nerves and their branches fan out on the forearm. The **N. cutaneus antebra-chii medialis** runs adjacent to the V. basilica, while the **N. cutaneus antebrachii lateralis** initially runs with the V. cephalica.
b Dorsal view. The **N. cutaneus antebrachii posterior** exits between the M. triceps brachii and M. brachialis. On the distal forearm, the **R. superficialis of the N. radialis** penetrates the fascia below the tendon of the M. brachioradialis before reaching the back of the hand. Similarly, the **R. dorsalis of the N. ulnaris** passes beneath the tendon of the M. flexor carpi ulnaris onto the dorsal side. The palmar branches of the N. medianus and N. ulnaris, which are located proximal to the wrists, can generally not be exposed well in dissections.

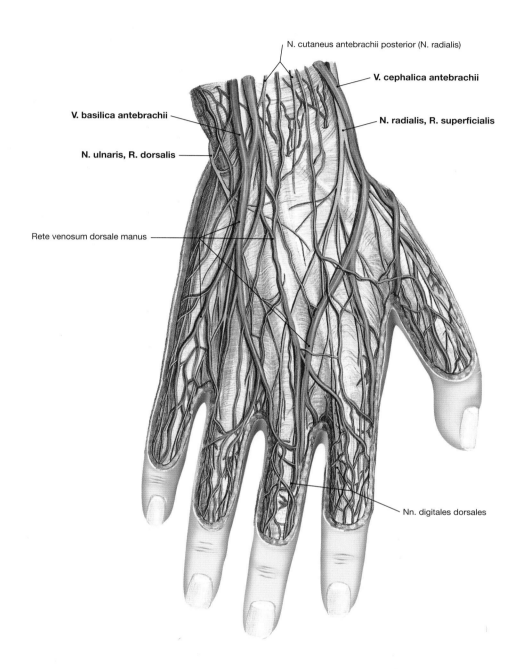

N. cutaneus antebrachii posterior (N. radialis)

V. cephalica antebrachii

N. radialis, R. superficialis

V. basilica antebrachii

N. ulnaris, R. dorsalis

Rete venosum dorsale manus

Nn. digitales dorsales

Fig. 3.155 Epifascial vessels and nerves of the back of the hand, Dorsum manus, right side; dorsal view. [S700]

The **V. cephalica antebrachii** originates from the superficial venous plexus on the dorsal side of the thumb, while the **V. basilica antebrachii** is supplied by ulnar veins on the back of the hand. Above the proximal wrist, the **R. superficialis of the N. radialis** passes beneath the tendon of the M. brachioradialis through the fascia onto the back of the hand. It divides into the Nn. digitales dorsales, which supply sensory innervation to the radial 2½ fingers dorsally. The ulnar 2½ fingers are innervated by the **R. dorsalis of the N. ulnaris,** which passes below the tendon of the M. flexor carpi ulnaris to the dorsal side.

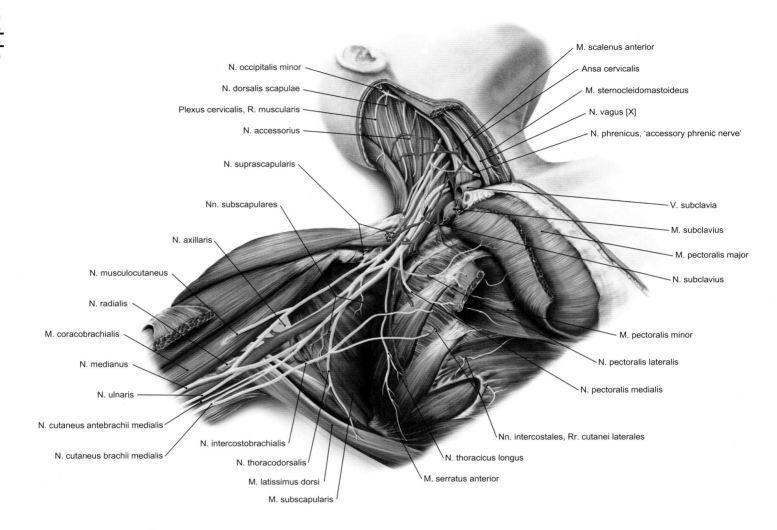

N. occipitalis minor

N. dorsalis scapulae

Plexus cervicalis, R. muscularis

N. accessorius

N. suprascapularis

Nn. subscapulares

N. axillaris

N. musculocutaneus

N. radialis

M. coracobrachialis

N. medianus

N. ulnaris

N. cutaneus antebrachii medialis

N. intercostobrachialis

N. cutaneus brachii medialis

N. thoracodorsalis

M. latissimus dorsi

M. subscapularis

M. scalenus anterior

Ansa cervicalis

M. sternocleidomastoideus

N. vagus [X]

N. phrenicus, 'accessory phrenic nerve'

V. subclavia

M. subclavius

M. pectoralis major

N. subclavius

M. pectoralis minor

N. pectoralis lateralis

N. pectoralis medialis

Nn. intercostales, Rr. cutanei laterales

N. thoracicus longus

M. serratus anterior

Fig. 3.156 Axilla, Fossa axillaris, with nerves from the Plexus brachialis and arterial branches of the A. axillaris, right side; ventral view after severing the Mm. pectorales major and minor near their insertions. [S700-L266]

The **N. dorsalis scapulae** pierces the M. scalenus medius at a relatively high cranial level and is only visible ventrally as shown here, if the head is greatly extended backwards and can be turned to the opposite side. It passes dorsally below the M. levator scapulae **(key muscle!).** The **A. transversa cervicis/colli** passes above the Plexus brachialis to the lower part of the M. trapezius. The **N. suprascapularis** turns laterally after leaving the Truncus superior and runs adjacent to the **A. suprascapularis.** While the nerve below the Lig. transversum scapulae superius passes through the Incisura scapulae, the artery crosses the ligament. The **N. subclavius** is usually inconspicuous and difficult to expose. It runs medially to reach the M. subclavius, and sometimes sends a branch to the N. phrenicus ('accessory phrenic nerve'). Underneath it, the **A. thoracica superior** passes to the chest wall. The **N. thoracicus longus** originates from the supraclavicular part of the Plexus brachialis, but then crosses underneath the plexus on its way to the chest wall, where it terminates on the M. serratus anterior.

The **A. thoracoacromialis** originates in the Trigonum clavipectorale and the **Nn. pectorales medialis and lateralis** originate from the respec-

tive fascicles of the Plexus brachialis and innervate the pectoral muscles. The **A. thoracica lateralis** descends caudally at the lateral margin of the M. pectoralis minor. Then the **A. subscapularis** branches off from the A. axillaris and divides into the **A. circumflexa scapulae,** which passes through the medial axillary space, and into the **A. thoracodorsalis,** which run adjacent to the **N. thoracodorsalis** and descends at the anterior margin of the M. latissimus dorsi.

The **Nn. subscapulares** leave the posterior fascicle of the Plexus brachialis and run medially to join the eponymously named muscle, whereas the **N. axillaris** branches off in the lateral direction and turns dorsally with the **A. circumflexa humeri posterior** to pass through the lateral axillary space. This blood vessel connects with the A. circumflexa humeri anterior, which is the last branch of the A. axillaris.

The arm nerves of the infraclavicular part of the Plexus brachialis originate directly from the fascicles. The **N. radialis** continues the pathway of the posterior fascicle and passes through the triangular interval onto the back of the upper arm. The **N. musculocutaneus** originates from the lateral fascicle, passes laterally and usually penetrates the M. coracobrachialis. The remaining nerve fibres form the lateral portion of the **N. medianus,** of which the medial portion originates from the medial fascicle, which first provides the **N. ulnaris** and the sensory **Nn. cutanei brachii and antebrachii mediales** to the medial upper arm.

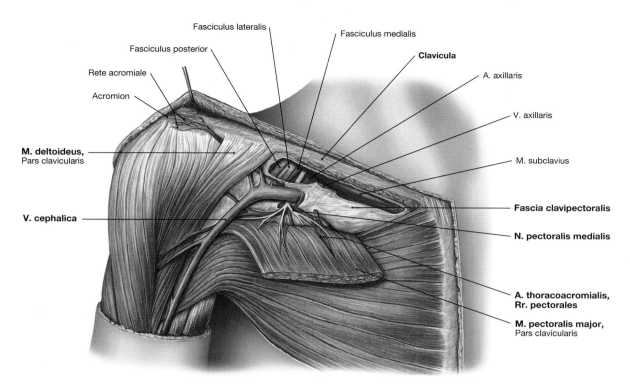

Fasciculus lateralis
Fasciculus posterior
Rete acromiale
Acromion
M. deltoideus, Pars clavicularis
V. cephalica
Fasciculus medialis
Clavicula
A. axillaris
V. axillaris
M. subclavius
Fascia clavipectoralis
N. pectoralis medialis
A. thoracoacromialis, Rr. pectorales
M. pectoralis major, Pars clavicularis

Fig. 3.157 Trigonum clavipectorale (MOHRENHEIM's fossa), right side. [S700]
The Trigonum clavipectorale is the narrow triangular space between the clavicle and the origins of the M. pectoralis major and M. deltoideus. To expose the Trigonum clavipectorale in a dissection, the point of origin of the M. pectoralis major is detached from the clavicle and folded to the side, and the Fascia clavipectoralis is removed. In this triangle, the

V. cephalica flows into the V. axillaris, and the **Nodi lymphoidei axillares apicales** are also located there. The **A. thoracoacromialis** also originates anteriorly from the A. axillaris and divides into its four terminal branches. The **Nn. pectorales medialis and lateralis** originate from the respective fascicles and pass together with the arterial branches to the pectoral muscles, which they supply.

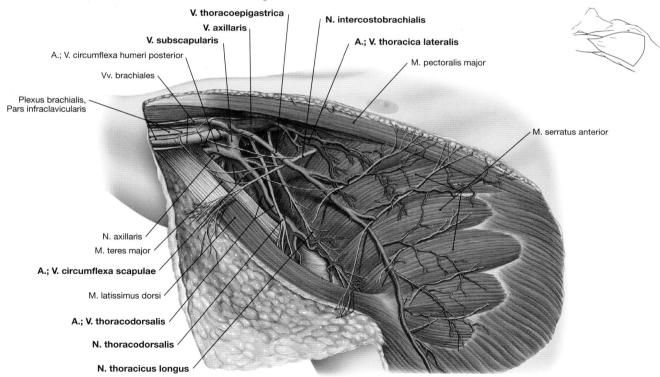

V. thoracoepigastrica
V. axillaris
V. subscapularis
A.; V. circumflexa humeri posterior
Vv. brachiales
Plexus brachialis, Pars infraclavicularis
N. intercostobrachialis
A.; V. thoracica lateralis
M. pectoralis major
M. serratus anterior
N. axillaris
M. teres major
A.; V. circumflexa scapulae
M. latissimus dorsi
A.; V. thoracodorsalis
N. thoracodorsalis
N. thoracicus longus

Fig. 3.158 Axilla, Fossa axillaris, right side; laterocaudal view. [S700]
The axilla is bordered by the M. pectoralis major at the front and by the M. latissimus dorsi from behind, forming the two axillary folds. In the axilla, the three fascicles of the Pars infraclavicularis of the **Plexus brachialis** surround the **A. axillaris** and are covered ventrally by the **V. ax-**

illaris. The **Nn. intercostobrachiales** from the **Nn. intercostales** cross the axilla and join the N. cutaneus brachii medialis. The **N. thoracodorsalis** passes with the eponymously named blood vessels to the medial margin of the M. latissimus dorsi. Ventral thereof, the **N. thoracicus longus** descends on the M. serratus anterior and innervates it.

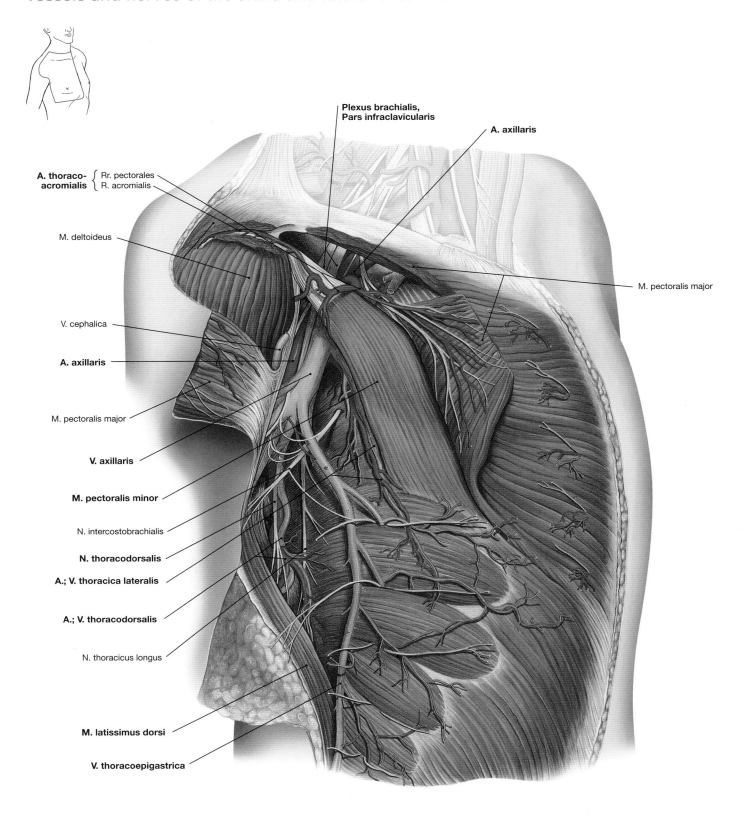

A. thoraco-
acromialis { Rr. pectorales
R. acromialis

M. deltoideus

V. cephalica

A. axillaris

M. pectoralis major

V. axillaris

M. pectoralis minor

N. intercostobrachialis

N. thoracodorsalis

A.; V. thoracica lateralis

A.; V. thoracodorsalis

N. thoracicus longus

M. latissimus dorsi

V. thoracoepigastrica

Plexus brachialis,
Pars infraclavicularis

A. axillaris

M. pectoralis major

Fig. 3.159   Axilla, Fossa axillaris, and lateral chest wall, Regio thoracica lateralis, right side; lateral view. [S700]
Compared to → Fig. 3.158, the M. pectoralis major was split to expose the underlying **M. pectoralis minor** and the anatomical structures emerging from the Trigonum clavipectorale. On the superior margin of the M. pectoralis minor, the **A. thoracoacromialis** is shown with its branches. Together with the Nn. pectorales of the Plexus brachialis, the Rr. pectorales join up with the Mm. pectorales major and minor, which

they supply. The M. pectoralis minor serves as an important landmark for the classification of axillary lymph nodes (→ Fig. 3.149). The **A. and V. thoracica lateralis** run along its lateral margin. Lateral thereof, the **A., V. and N. thoracodorsalis** descend to the inner surface of the M. latissimus dorsi, which they supply together. The V. thoracoepigastrica is not accompanied by an artery, and exhibits a very variable calibre and pathway (here it is relatively well-developed) in the subcutaneous adipose tissue of the lateral chest wall.

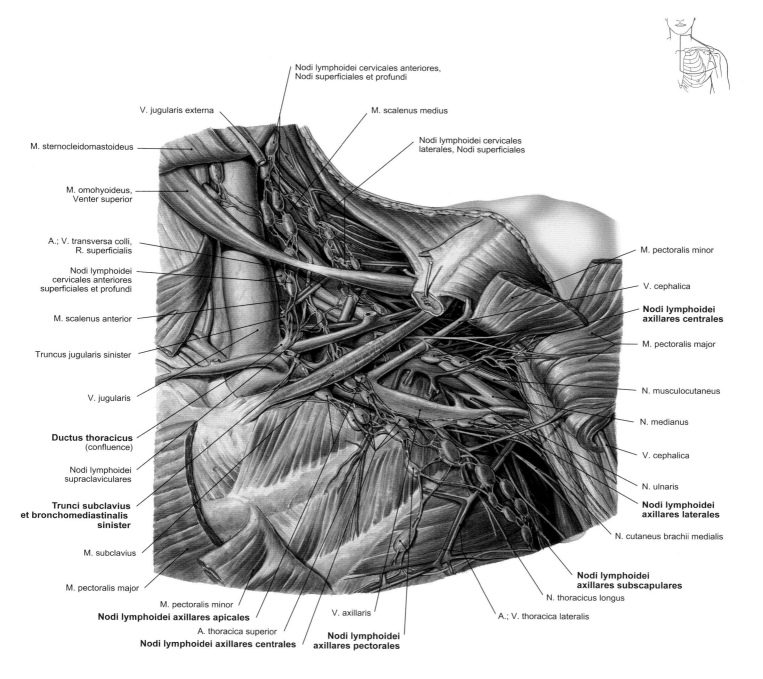

Nodi lymphoidei cervicales anteriores,
Nodi superficiales et profundi

V. jugularis externa

M. scalenus medius

M. sternocleidomastoideus

Nodi lymphoidei cervicales
laterales, Nodi superficiales

M. omohyoideus,
Venter superior

A.; V. transversa colli,
R. superficialis

M. pectoralis minor

Nodi lymphoidei
cervicales anteriores
superficiales et profundi

V. cephalica

**Nodi lymphoidei
axillares centrales**

M. scalenus anterior

M. pectoralis major

Truncus jugularis sinister

N. musculocutaneus

N. medianus

V. jugularis

V. cephalica

Ductus thoracicus
(confluence)

N. ulnaris

Nodi lymphoidei
supraclaviculares

**Nodi lymphoidei
axillares laterales**

**Trunci subclavius
et bronchomediastinalis
sinister**

N. cutaneus brachii medialis

M. subclavius

**Nodi lymphoidei
axillares subscapulares**

M. pectoralis major

N. thoracicus longus

M. pectoralis minor

A.; V. thoracica lateralis

Nodi lymphoidei axillares apicales

V. axillaris

A. thoracica superior

**Nodi lymphoidei
axillares centrales**

**Nodi lymphoidei
axillares pectorales**

**Fig. 3.160   Axilla, Fossa axillaris, and lateral chest wall, Regio
thoracica lateralis, left side;** ventral view. [S700]
In contrast to → Fig. 3.159, the left side of the body is shown here, to
expose the **axillary lymphatic vessels** draining into the Ductus thoracicus, and their openings in the left venous angle, since this is often
damaged in dissections. The M. pectoralis minor has been severed, so
that the axillary lymph nodes can be seen. According to their topographical relationship to the M. pectoralis minor, the axillary lymph nodes are
grouped into **three levels** (→ Fig. 3.149). The first level (lateral of the M.

pectoralis minor) includes the Nodi lymphoidei axillares pectorales
along the A. and V. thoracica lateralis, as well as, further lateral, the Nodi
lymphoidei axillares subscapulares and the Nodi lymphoidei axillares
laterales along the V. axillaris. The second level (at the level of the
M. pectoralis minor) includes the Nodi lymphoidei axillares centrales
beneath the muscle. The third level (medial of the M. pectoralis minor)
is the last station prior to the **Truncus subclavius,** which drains the
lymph via the Ductus thoracicus on the left side into the left venous
angle between the V. jugularis interna and V. subclavia.

Clinical remarks

Before its opening into the left venous angle, the **Ductus thoracicus**
collects the lymph of the entire inferior body half (including abdominal and pelvic organs), and additionally drains the lymph of the left
thorax via the Truncus bronchomediastinalis sinister, as well as the
lymph of the left arm via the Truncus subclavius sinister and the

lymph of the left-sided head/neck region via the Truncus jugularis
sinister.
Malignant tumours in the abdominal and pelvic region can therefore
spread with metastases into the left supraclavicular lymph nodes
(so-called **VIRCHOW's nodes**).

Vessels and nerves of the axilla and medial upper arm

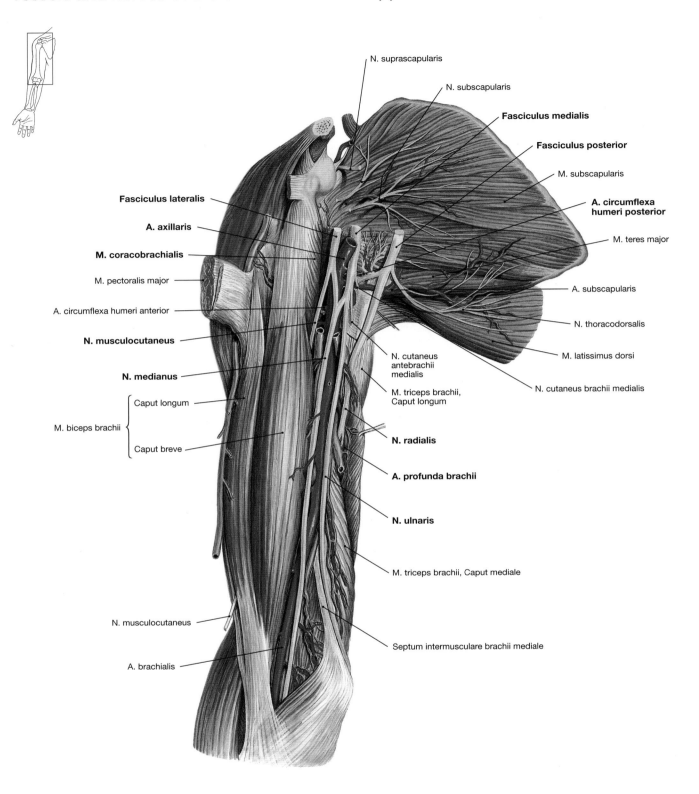

N. suprascapularis

N. subscapularis

Fasciculus medialis

Fasciculus posterior

M. subscapularis

A. circumflexa humeri posterior

M. teres major

A. subscapularis

N. thoracodorsalis

M. latissimus dorsi

N. cutaneus brachii medialis

Fasciculus lateralis

A. axillaris

M. coracobrachialis

M. pectoralis major

A. circumflexa humeri anterior

N. musculocutaneus

N. medianus

Caput longum

M. biceps brachii

Caput breve

M. bicorps brachii

N. musculocutaneus

A. brachialis

N. cutaneus antebrachii medialis

M. triceps brachii, Caput longum

N. radialis

A. profunda brachii

N. ulnaris

M. triceps brachii, Caput mediale

Septum intermusculare brachii mediale

Fig. 3.161 Vessels and nerves of the axilla, Fossa axillaris, and of the medial side of the upper arm, Regio brachii anterior, right side; ventromedial view. [S700]

The M. pectoralis major was severed near its insertion point on the Crista tuberculi majoris, so that the infraclavicular part of the **Plexus brachialis** can be seen. The three fascicles lie proximally. **The Fasciculus lateralis** and **Fasciculus medialis** lie on both sides of the A. axillaris, and along with their nerves they form an M-shaped structure, which is helpful for orientation when dissecting the Plexus brachialis. The lateral arm of the 'M' is formed by the N. musculocutaneus, which is easily identified as it penetrates the M. coracobrachialis. The middle

part is formed by the medial and lateral roots of the N. medianus. The medial arm of the 'M' is formed by the N. ulnaris. In contrast to the N. medianus, which runs in the Sulcus bicipitalis medialis and reaches the cubital fossa medially, the N. ulnaris reaches the dorsal side of the Epicondylus medialis. The **Fasciculus posterior** was mobilised from its position behind the A. axillaris. It provides the N. axillaris proximally, passing together with the A. circumflexa humeri posterior through the lateral axillary space, and then continues as N. radialis, which ultimately arrives at the back of the humerus after crossing the triangular interval along with the A. profunda brachii.

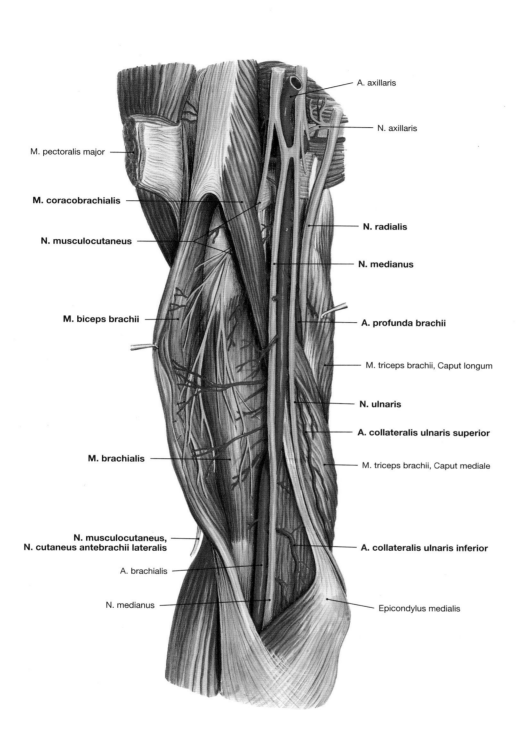

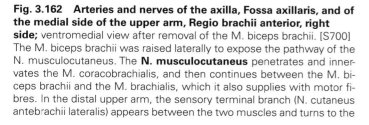

A. axillaris

N. axillaris

M. pectoralis major

M. coracobrachialis

N. radialis

N. musculocutaneus

N. medianus

M. biceps brachii

A. profunda brachii

M. triceps brachii, Caput longum

N. ulnaris

A. collateralis ulnaris superior

M. brachialis

M. triceps brachii, Caput mediale

**N. musculocutaneus,
N. cutaneus antebrachii lateralis**

A. collateralis ulnaris inferior

A. brachialis

N. medianus

Epicondylus medialis

Fig. 3.162 Arteries and nerves of the axilla, Fossa axillaris, and of the medial side of the upper arm, Regio brachii anterior, right side; ventromedial view after removal of the M. biceps brachii. [S700] The M. biceps brachii was raised laterally to expose the pathway of the N. musculocutaneus. The **N. musculocutaneus** penetrates and innervates the M. coracobrachialis, and then continues between the M. biceps brachii and the M. brachialis, which it also supplies with motor fibres. In the distal upper arm, the sensory terminal branch (N. cutaneus antebrachii lateralis) appears between the two muscles and turns to the radial side of the forearm. The **N. medianus** accompanies the A. brachialis inside the Sulcus bicipitalis medialis and further into the cubital fossa. The **N. ulnaris** arrives together with the A. collateralis ulnaris superior on the dorsal side of the Epicondylus medialis. In contrast, the A. collateralis ulnaris inferior is in most cases a thin blood vessel, originating proximal to the elbow from the A. brachialis. The **N. axillaris** leaves the Fasciculus posterior proximally and exits through the lateral axilla, while the **N. radialis** passes with the A. profunda brachii via the triangular interval.

Axillary spaces and triangular interval

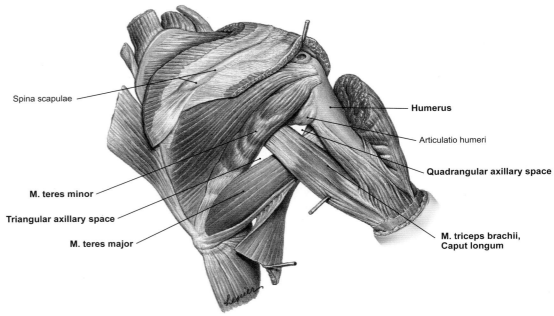

Spina scapulae

Humerus

Articulatio humeri

Quadrangular axillary space

M. teres minor

Triangular axillary space

M. teres major

M. triceps brachii, Caput longum

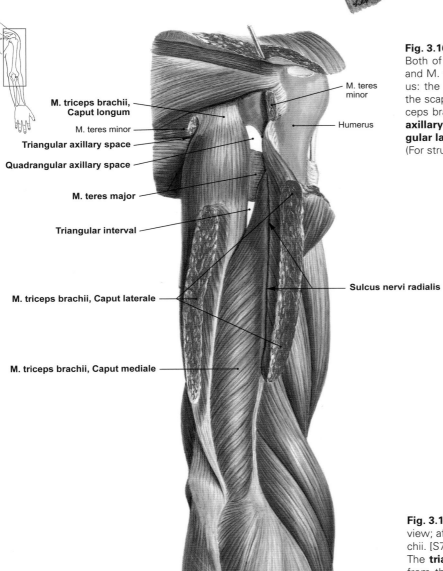

M. triceps brachii, Caput longum

M. teres minor

Triangular axillary space

Quadrangular axillary space

M. teres major

Triangular interval

M. teres minor

Humerus

M. triceps brachii, Caput laterale

Sulcus nervi radialis

M. triceps brachii, Caput mediale

Fig. 3.163 Axillary spaces, right side; dorsal view. [S700] Both of the axillary spaces lie between the M. teres major and M. teres minor and are bordered laterally by the humerus: the two muscles diverge V-shaped from their origins at the scapula and leave a gap. The Caput longum of the M. triceps brachii subdivides this gap into the **triangular medial axillary space** (Spatium axillare mediale) and the **quadrangular lateral axillary space** (Spatium axillare laterale). (For structures passing through → Fig. 3.165.)

Fig. 3.164 Triangular interval, right side; dorsal lateral view; after splitting the Caput laterale of the M. triceps brachii. [S700]

The **triangular interval,** which is an important passageway from the axilla to the dorsal upper arm, is situated distally from the insertion point of the M. teres major and thus caudally of the axillary spaces. The triangular interval is bordered medially by the Caput longum and laterally by the Caput laterale of the M. triceps brachii. (For structures passing through → Fig. 3.165.)

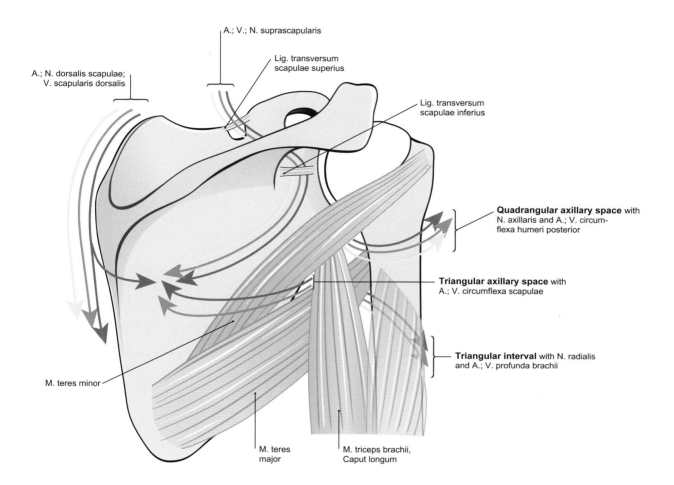

A.; V.; N. suprascapularis

Lig. transversum
scapulae superius

A.; N. dorsalis scapulae;
V. scapularis dorsalis

Lig. transversum
scapulae inferius

Quadrangular axillary space with
N. axillaris and A.; V. circumflexa humeri posterior

Triangular axillary space with
A.; V. circumflexa scapulae

Triangular interval with N. radialis
and A.; V. profunda brachii

M. teres minor

M. teres
major

M. triceps brachii,
Caput longum

Fig. 3.165 Axillary spaces and triangular interval, right side;
schematic representation in the dorsal view. [S702-L126]
Both of the axillary spaces lie between the M. teres major and M. teres
minor and are bordered laterally by the humerus. The Caput longum of
the M. triceps brachii separates the **triangular medial axillary space**
from the **quadrangular lateral axillary space.** Crossing the axillary
spaces are:
- the **medial axillary space:** A. and V. circumflexa scapulae
- the **lateral axillary space:** N. axillaris, A. and V. circumflexa humeri
posterior.
The A. circumflexa scapulae anastomoses with the A. suprascapularis in
the Fossa infraspinata, and via thin branches with the A. dorsalis scapulae

(scapular anastomoses). The A. suprascapularis passes **over** the
Lig. transversum scapulae superius into the Fossa supraspinata and
below the Lig. transversum scapulae inferius into the Fossa infraspinata.
The A. circumflexa humeri posterior anastomoses with the A. circumflexa humeri anterior (**brachial anastomoses, →** Fig. 3.137).
The **triangular interval** is located caudally of the axillary spaces and is
bordered by the Caput longum and the Caput laterale of the M. triceps
brachii.
The following structures cross through the **triangular interval:** N. radialis, A. and V. profunda brachii.

Vessels and nerves of the lateral upper arm

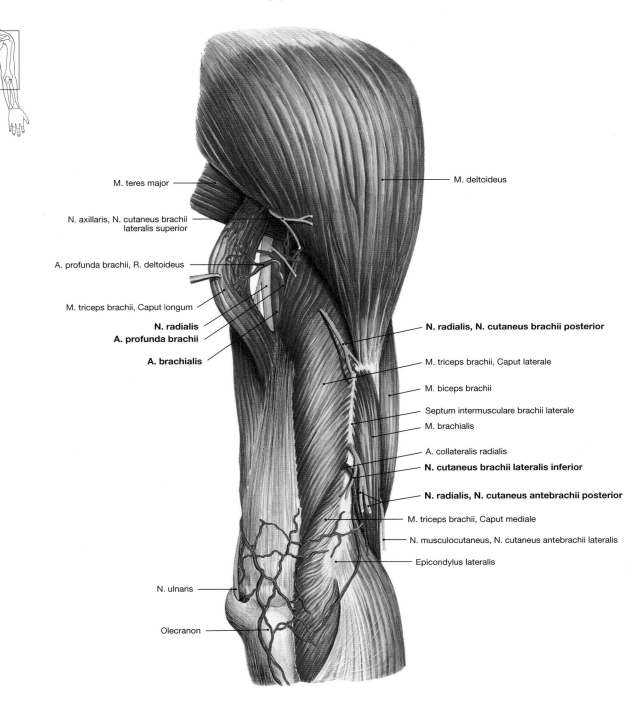

M. teres major

N. axillaris, N. cutaneus brachii lateralis superior

A. profunda brachii, R. deltoideus

M. triceps brachii, Caput longum

N. radialis
A. profunda brachii

A. brachialis

M. deltoideus

N. radialis, N. cutaneus brachii posterior

M. triceps brachii, Caput laterale

M. biceps brachii

Septum intermusculare brachii laterale

M. brachialis

A. collateralis radialis

N. cutaneus brachii lateralis inferior

N. radialis, N. cutaneus antebrachii posterior

M. triceps brachii, Caput mediale

N. musculocutaneus, N. cutaneus antebrachii lateralis

Epicondylus lateralis

N. ulnaris

Olecranon

Fig. 3.166 Arteries and nerves on the lateral side of the upper arm, Regio brachii posterior, right side; dorsolateral view. [S700]
The Caput longum and Caput laterale of the M. triceps brachii have been pushed apart to better identify the **triangular interval,** which is bordered by both muscle heads; the **N. radialis** and the **A. profunda brachii** cross the split dorsally, to reach the humeral shaft inside the

Sulcus nervi radialis. As can be seen, as soon as it passes through the triangular interval, the N. radialis provides branches which innervate the M. triceps and also the N. cutaneus brachii posterior. However, along with the N. cutaneus antebrachii posterior, the N. cutaneus brachii lateralis inferior only branches off in the region of the Sulcus nervi radialis.

Clinical remarks

In the case of a **humeral shaft fracture** with a radial nerve lesion, the M. triceps brachii remains generally intact, as the N. radialis already innervates the M. triceps and also the N. cutaneus brachii posterior when passing through the triangular interval. Since the N. cu-

taneus brachii lateralis inferior, along with the N. cutaneus antebrachii posterior, branch off in the region of the Sulcus nervi radialis, it is at risk of being damaged.

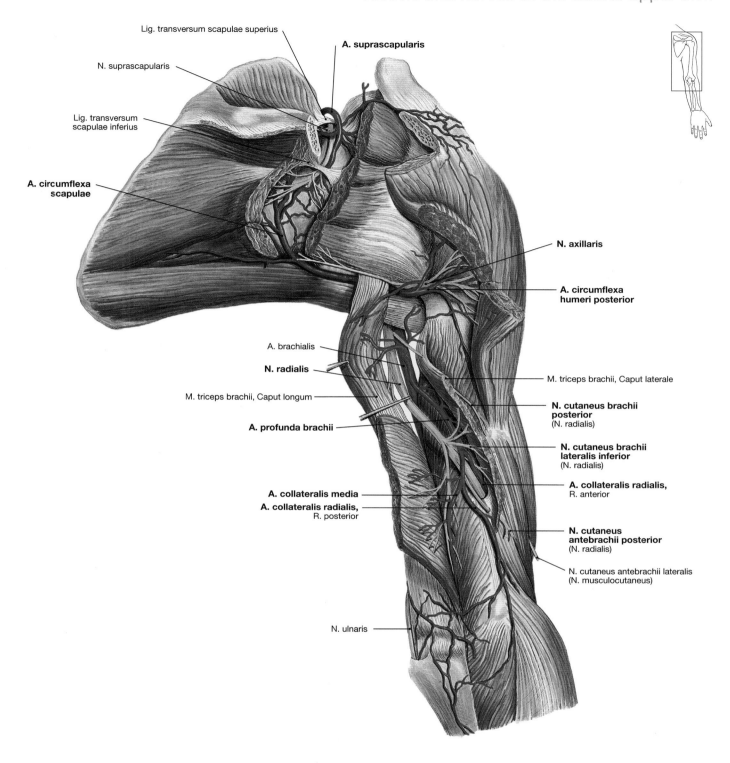

Lig. transversum scapulae superius

A. suprascapularis

N. suprascapularis

Lig. transversum scapulae inferius

A. circumflexa scapulae

N. axillaris

A. circumflexa humeri posterior

A. brachialis

M. triceps brachii, Caput laterale

N. radialis

M. triceps brachii, Caput longum

N. cutaneus brachii posterior (N. radialis)

A. profunda brachii

N. cutaneus brachii lateralis inferior (N. radialis)

A. collateralis media

A. collateralis radialis, R. anterior

A. collateralis radialis, R. posterior

N. cutaneus antebrachii posterior (N. radialis)

N. cutaneus antebrachii lateralis (N. musculocutaneus)

N. ulnaris

Fig. 3.167 Arteries and nerves of the shoulder, Regio deltoidea, and lateral side of the upper arm, Regio brachii dorsalis, right side; dorsolateral view. [S700]

Here we see the branching sequence again of the **N. radialis.** The **triangular interval** has been extended by sharply separating the Caput longum and Caput laterale of the M. triceps brachii from each other. The branches innervating the M. triceps brachii and the N. cutaneus brachii posterior already branch off when passing through the triangular interval. However, the N. cutaneus brachii lateralis inferior and the N. cutaneus antebrachii posterior are only provided inside the Sulcus nervi radialis. The N. radialis runs along with the A. profunda brachii, which divides into the A. collateralis media (to the Epicondylus medialis) and into the A. collateralis radialis (accompanying the nerve).

Additionally, this illustration shows the **axillary spaces** with the structures passing through. The N. axillaris passes through the lateral axillary

space along with the A. circumflexa humeri posterior. The A. circumflexa scapulae passes through dorsally via the medial axillary space. In the Fossa infraspinata, the A. circumflexa scapulae (circulatory area of the A. axillaris) forms an important anastomosis with the A. suprascapularis (circulatory area of the A. subclavia). With this arterial circle, which is often supplemented by anastomoses with the A. dorsalis scapulae (also in the circulatory area of the A. subclavia, not shown here), a bypass or collateral circulation for the blood supply of the arm can be maintained, if the A. axillaris is obstructed proximally.

The A. suprascapularis then passes above the Lig. transversum scapulae superius into the Fossa supraspinata of the scapula, while the N. suprascapularis passes below the ligament through the Incisura scapulae. On their way into the Fossa infraspinata, the nerve and artery are bridged by the Lig. transversum scapulae inferius.

Upper limb

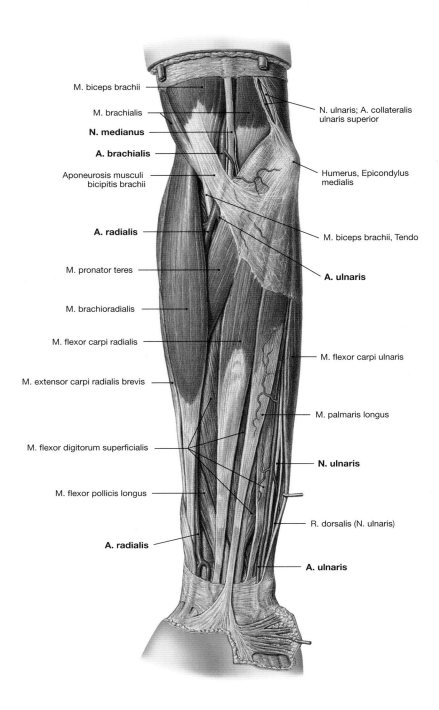

M. biceps brachii

M. brachialis

N. medianus

A. brachialis

Aponeurosis musculi
bicipitis brachii

A. radialis

M. pronator teres

M. brachioradialis

M. flexor carpi radialis

M. extensor carpi radialis brevis

M. flexor digitorum superficialis

M. flexor pollicis longus

A. radialis

N. ulnaris; A. collateralis
ulnaris superior

Humerus, Epicondylus
medialis

M. biceps brachii, Tendo

A. ulnaris

M. flexor carpi ulnaris

M. palmaris longus

N. ulnaris

R. dorsalis (N. ulnaris)

A. ulnaris

**Fig. 3.168 Superficial arteries and nerves of the forearm, Regio
antebrachii anterior, right side;** ventral view. [S700]
Together with the A. brachialis, the **N. medianus** enters the cubital
fossa medially. The A. brachialis divides into the A. radialis and the A. ulnaris, both of which descend to the respective sides of the wrists. The
pulse of the A. radialis is preferably palpated just proximal to the wrist.
The A. ulnaris is accompanied by the N. ulnaris, which is also covered
by the M. flexor carpi ulnaris, as can be seen on the distal forearm.

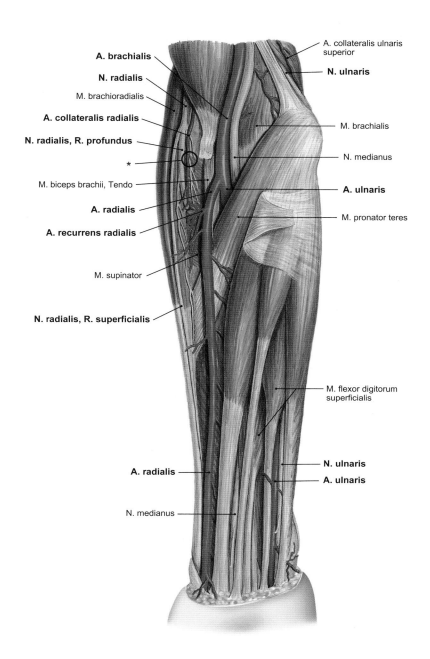

Fig. 3.169 Arteries and nerves of the superficial layer of the forearm, Regio antebrachii anterior, right side; ventral view; after removal of the M. brachioradialis and the Aponeurosis bicipitis antebrachii. [S700]
The M. brachioradialis and the insertion point of the M. biceps brachii in the Fascia antebrachii (Aponeurosis musculi bicipitis antebrachii) have been removed to expose the bifurcation of the **A. brachialis** and the pathway of the A. and N. radialis. After the bifurcation of the A. brachialis, the **A. radialis** continues, passing beneath the M. brachioradialis onto the radial side of the wrist. Beneath the M. brachioradialis, the A. recurrens radialis also ascends to the vascular plexus of the elbow (Rete articulare cubiti), where it anastomoses with the A. collateralis

radialis (*). The **A. ulnaris** branches off dorsally from the M. pronator teres, joins the N. ulnaris below the cubital fossa, and passes beneath the M. flexor carpi ulnaris onto the ulnar side of the wrist. Between the M. brachioradialis and M. brachialis **(radial sulcus),** the **N. radialis** passes laterally into the cubital fossa and divides up into the R. superficialis and R. profundus. The **R. superficialis** accompanies the A. radialis up to the lower third of the forearm, before it changes to the dorsal side. The **R. profundus** innervates and penetrates the M. supinator **(supinator canal).** At the entrance to the muscle there is often a sharp-edged tendinous arch **(arcade of FROHSE),** which can compress the nerve.

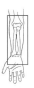

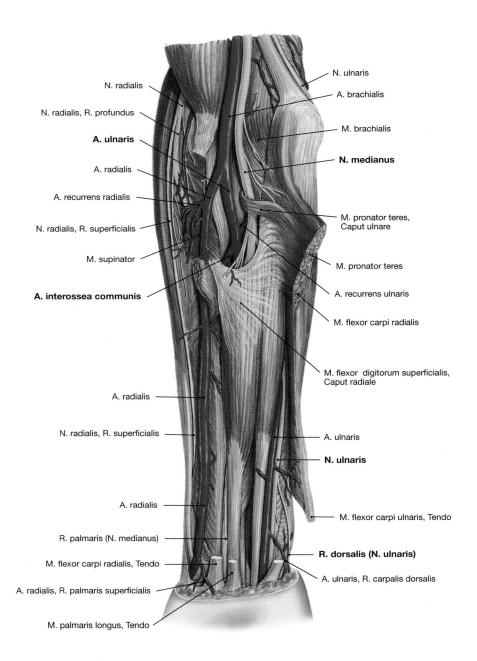

N. radialis

N. radialis, R. profundus

A. ulnaris

A. radialis

A. recurrens radialis

N. radialis, R. superficialis

M. supinator

A. interossea communis

A. radialis

N. radialis, R. superficialis

A. radialis

R. palmaris (N. medianus)

M. flexor carpi radialis, Tendo

A. radialis, R. palmaris superficialis

M. palmaris longus, Tendo

N. ulnaris

A. brachialis

M. brachialis

N. medianus

M. pronator teres,
Caput ulnare

M. pronator teres

A. recurrens ulnaris

M. flexor carpi radialis

M. flexor digitorum superficialis,
Caput radiale

A. ulnaris

N. ulnaris

M. flexor carpi ulnaris, Tendo

R. dorsalis (N. ulnaris)

A. ulnaris, R. carpalis dorsalis

Fig. 3.170 Arteries and nerves of the deep layer of the forearm, Regio antebrachii anterior, right side; ventral view; after splitting the M. pronator teres and the M. flexor carpi radialis, as well as removal of the M. palmaris longus. [S700]
When the flexor muscles of the superficial layer of the forearm are split, the proximal branches of the **A. ulnaris** become visible: the A. interossea communis is a short strong descending vessel, whereas the A. re-currens ulnaris ascends below the M. pronator teres. The **N. medianus** passes between the two heads of the M. pronator teres into the layer between the middle and deep flexor muscles of the forearm.
On the distal forearm, the tendon of the M. flexor carpi ulnaris has been severed to expose the bifurcation of the **R. dorsalis of the N. ulnaris** and its pathway to the back of the hand.

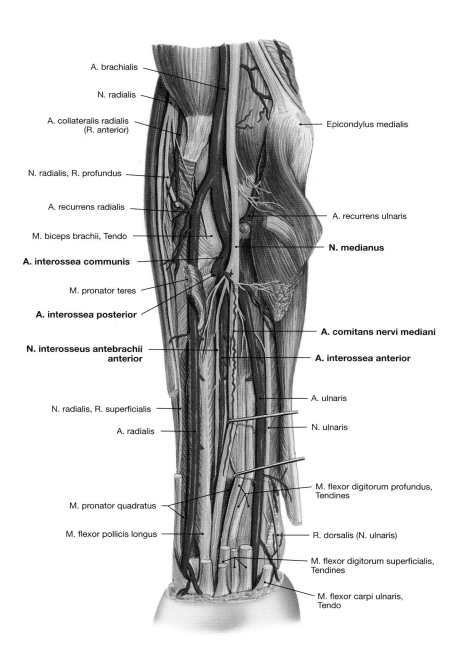

A. brachialis

N. radialis

A. collateralis radialis
(R. anterior)

N. radialis, R. profundus

A. recurrens radialis

M. biceps brachii, Tendo

A. interossea communis

M. pronator teres

A. interossea posterior

**N. interosseus antebrachii
anterior**

N. radialis, R. superficialis

A. radialis

M. pronator quadratus

M. flexor pollicis longus

Epicondylus medialis

A. recurrens ulnaris

N. medianus

A. comitans nervi mediani

A. interossea anterior

A. ulnaris

N. ulnaris

M. flexor digitorum profundus,
Tendines

R. dorsalis (N. ulnaris)

M. flexor digitorum superficialis,
Tendines

M. flexor carpi ulnaris,
Tendo

**Fig. 3.171 Arteries and nerves of the deep layer of the forearm,
Regio antebrachii anterior, right side;** ventral view; after removal of
all superficial flexor muscles. [S700]
When all superficial flexor muscles, including the M. flexor digitorum
superficialis, have been removed, the complete pathway of the **N. medianus** becomes visible. It passes distally between the superficial and
deep flexor muscles in the midline of the forearm, and is often accom-

panied by its own thin blood vessel (A. comitans nervi mediani). On the
proximal forearm, the N. interosseus antebrachii anterior branches off,
providing motor fibres to the deep flexors and sensory fibres to the
wrists. The nerve is accompanied by the A. interossea anterior, while
the A. interossea posterior penetrates the Membrana interossea antebrachii and runs dorsally.

Vessels and nerves of the cubital fossa and elbow

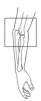

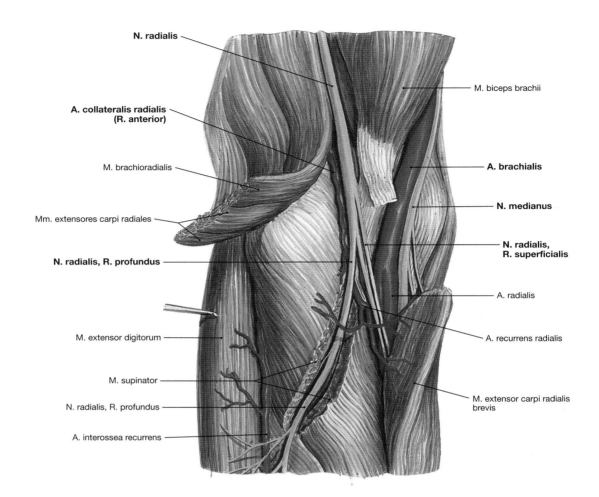

N. radialis

A. collateralis radialis
(R. anterior)

M. brachioradialis

Mm. extensores carpi radiales

N. radialis, R. profundus

M. extensor digitorum

M. supinator

N. radialis, R. profundus

A. interossea recurrens

M. biceps brachii

A. brachialis

N. medianus

N. radialis,
R. superficialis

A. radialis

A. recurrens radialis

M. extensor carpi radialis
brevis

Fig. 3.172 Arteries and nerves of the cubital fossa, Regio cubitalis anterior, right side; lateral (radial) view. [S700]
The illustration shows the pathway of the arm nerves in the area of the cubital fossa and elbow after the splitting of various superficial flexor and extensor muscles. The **N. medianus** arrives from medially with the A. brachialis in the cubital fossa, while the **N. radialis** along with the A.

collateralis radialis passes laterally between the M. brachioradialis and M. brachialis **(radial sulcus)** into the cubital fossa, where it divides into its two terminal branches. The R. superficialis continues below the M. brachioradialis. The R. profundus reaches the dorsal side by passing through the M. supinator **(supinator canal)**.

Clinical remarks

The **N. radialis** can be damaged when compressed in the elbow region. While the radial sulcus only serves as an anatomical landmark for the pathway and the nerve is seldom damaged in this location, the nerve is often damaged when entering the M. supinator. The R. profundus of the N. radialis can also be stretched at the side where the nerve enters the fascia of the M. supinator. This fascial location contains a semicircular thickening **(arcade of FROHSE).** Alternatively, the nerve can be compressed where it enters through

the muscle in the **supinator canal.** Clinically in both cases, the result is a **supinator syndrome** with the inability to extend the thumb and fingers, but without wrist drop occurring. This is explained by the fact that those nerve endings of the N. radialis for the radial group of muscles, which are important for the stabilisation of the joints in the hand, branch off proximal of the M. supinator from the main nerve or the R. profundus of the N. radialis.

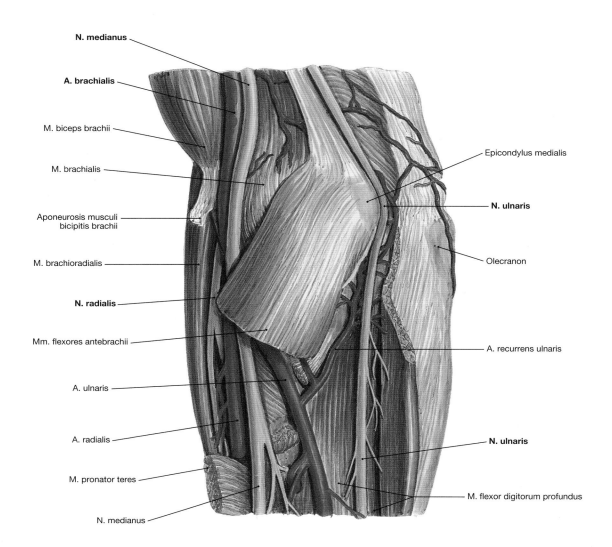

N. medianus

A. brachialis

M. biceps brachii

M. brachialis

Aponeurosis musculi bicipitis brachii

M. brachioradialis

N. radialis

Mm. flexores antebrachii

A. ulnaris

A. radialis

M. pronator teres

N. medianus

Epicondylus medialis

N. ulnaris

Olecranon

A. recurrens ulnaris

N. ulnaris

M. flexor digitorum profundus

Fig. 3.173 Arteries and nerves of the elbow, Regio cubitalis posterior, right side; medial (ulnar) view. [S700]
On the elbow, the **N. ulnaris** is directly adjacent to the bone in the Sulcus nervi ulnaris **(cubital tunnel),** where it is easily irritated on compression **('funny bone').** Then the N. ulnaris passes below the M. flexor carpi ulnaris to the flexor side of the forearm, where it is joined by the A. ulnaris.

Clinical remarks

A momentary compression of the N. ulnaris causes tingling sensations in the innervation area of the nerve **('funny bone')** which subsides within seconds. Permanent ulnar entrapment in the cubital tunnel can result in impaired nerve function **(cubital tunnel syndrome).**

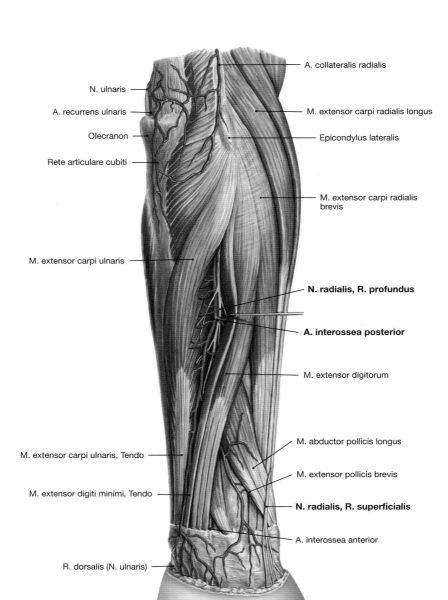

A. collateralis radialis

N. ulnaris

A. recurrens ulnaris

Olecranon

Rete articulare cubiti

M. extensor carpi radialis longus

Epicondylus lateralis

M. extensor carpi radialis brevis

M. extensor carpi ulnaris

N. radialis, R. profundus

A. interossea posterior

M. extensor digitorum

M. abductor pollicis longus

M. extensor carpi ulnaris, Tendo

M. extensor pollicis brevis

M. extensor digiti minimi, Tendo

N. radialis, R. superficialis

A. interossea anterior

R. dorsalis (N. ulnaris)

Fig. 3.174 Arteries and nerves of the deep layer of the forearm, Regio antebrachii posterior, right side; radial view. [S700]
The M. extensor digiti minimi is pushed to the side to show the pathway of the **R. profundus of the N. radialis,** which descends with the A. interossea posterior between the superficial and deep extensor muscles. At the radial side of the wrist, the **R. superficialis of the N. radialis** emerges from the M. brachioradialis and reaches the back of the hand.

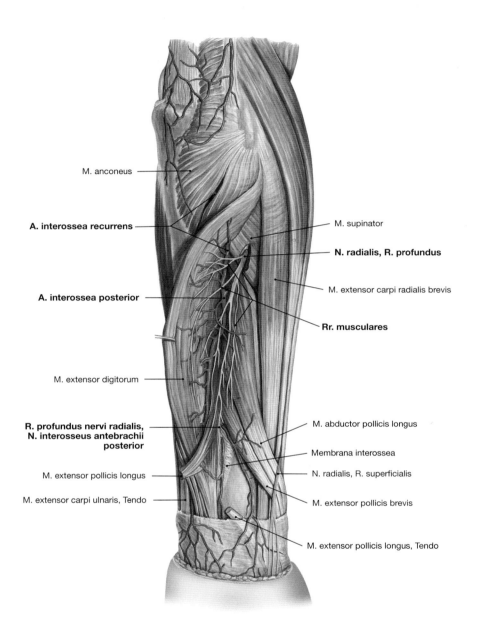

M. anconeus

A. interossea recurrens

A. interossea posterior

M. extensor digitorum

R. profundus nervi radialis,
N. interosseus antebrachii
posterior

M. extensor pollicis longus

M. extensor carpi ulnaris, Tendo

M. supinator

N. radialis, R. profundus

M. extensor carpi radialis brevis

Rr. musculares

M. abductor pollicis longus

Membrana interossea

N. radialis, R. superficialis

M. extensor pollicis brevis

M. extensor pollicis longus, Tendo

Fig. 3.175 Arteries and nerves of the deep layer of the forearm, Regio antebrachii posterior, right side; radial view. [S700]
The M. extensor digitorum has been folded over to expose the branches of the **R. profundus of the N. radialis** and of the **A. interossea posterior.** After its passage through the M. supinator, the R. profundus of the N. radialis innervates all superficial and deep extensor muscles on the forearm, before it runs into the sensory N. interosseus antebrachii posterior on the wrists. The A. interossea posterior, after its passage through the Membrana interossea antebrachii, provides the A. interossea recurrens which ascends below the M. anconeus to the vascular plexus of the elbow (Rete articulare cubiti).

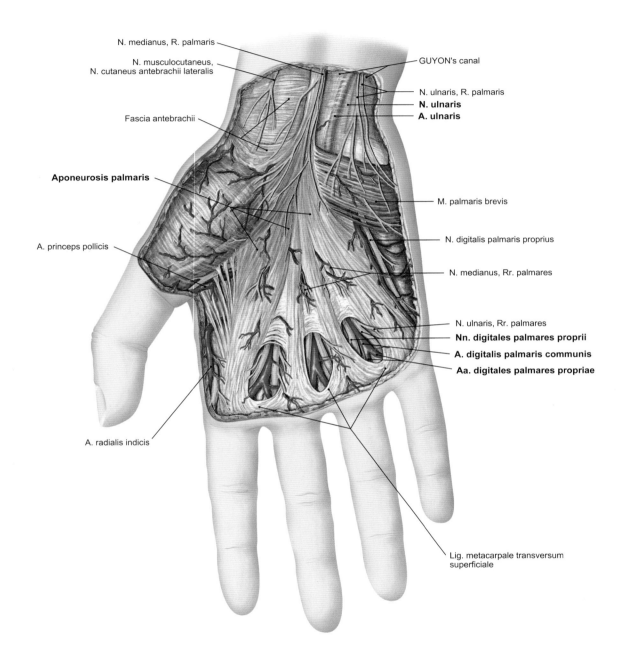

N. medianus, R. palmaris

N. musculocutaneus,
N. cutaneus antebrachii lateralis

Fascia antebrachii

Aponeurosis palmaris

A. princeps pollicis

A. radialis indicis

GUYON's canal

N. ulnaris, R. palmaris

N. ulnaris
A. ulnaris

M. palmaris brevis

N. digitalis palmaris proprius

N. medianus, Rr. palmares

N. ulnaris, Rr. palmares
Nn. digitales palmares proprii
A. digitalis palmaris communis
Aa. digitales palmares propriae

Lig. metacarpale transversum
superficiale

**Fig. 3.176   Arteries and nerves of the superficial layer of the palm
of the hand, Palma manus, right side;** palmar view. [S700]
The blood vessels and nerves in the palm are covered by the **palmar
aponeurosis** (Aponeurosis palmaris) and are therefore well protected.
Proximal to the metacarpophalangeal joints and between the longitudinal tracts of the aponeurosis, the Nn. digitales palmares from the
N. medianus and the N. ulnaris are visible, as well as the bifurcations of
the Aa. digitales palmares communes into the terminal branches for the
individual fingers. As the N. ulnaris and A. ulnaris lie superficially in the
wrist region in the **GUYON's canal,** they are prone to injury and compression.

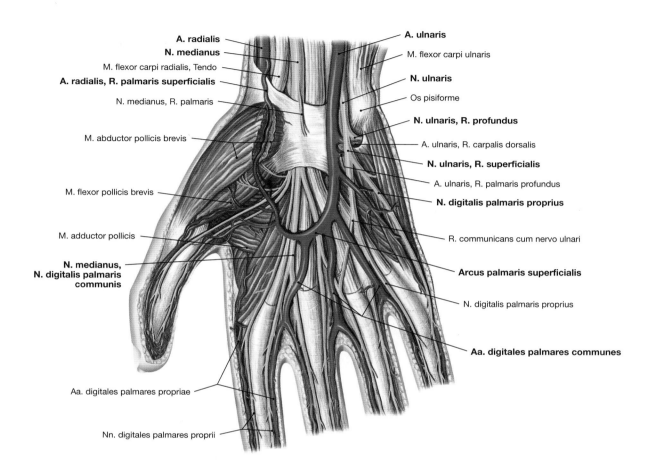

A. radialis
N. medianus
M. flexor carpi radialis, Tendo
A. radialis, R. palmaris superficialis
N. medianus, R. palmaris
M. abductor pollicis brevis
M. flexor pollicis brevis
M. adductor pollicis
N. medianus,
N. digitalis palmaris
communis
Aa. digitales palmares propriae
Nn. digitales palmares proprii

A. ulnaris
M. flexor carpi ulnaris
N. ulnaris
Os pisiforme
N. ulnaris, R. profundus
A. ulnaris, R. carpalis dorsalis
N. ulnaris, R. superficialis
A. ulnaris, R. palmaris profundus
N. digitalis palmaris proprius
R. communicans cum nervo ulnari
Arcus palmaris superficialis
N. digitalis palmaris proprius
Aa. digitales palmares communes

Fig. 3.177 Arteries and nerves of the middle layer of the palm of the hand, Palma manus, right side; palmar view; after removal of the palmar aponeurosis. [S700]
The **superficial palmar arch** (Arcus palmaris superficialis) is largely formed by the A. ulnaris, which usually anastomoses with a branch (R. palmaris superficialis) of the A. radialis. The Aa. digitales palmares for the ulnar 3½ fingers are provided by the superficial palmar arterial arch which crosses over the tendons of the long flexor muscles of the fingers.

The **N. ulnaris** accompanies the A. ulnaris through the **GUYON's canal,** which has been opened here. Distally of the Os pisiforme, the N. ulnaris already divides into the R. profundus and the R. superficialis, which continues in the same direction. The **R. superficialis** bifurcates into the Nn. digitales palmares for the sensory innervation of the ulnar 1½ fingers. The radial 3½ fingers are innervated by respective branches of the **N. medianus,** which enter the palm of the hand through the **carpal tunnel** (Canalis carpi) below the Retinaculum musculorum flexorum.

Clinical remarks

A **compression of the N. medianus or N. ulnaris** can result in an acute impairment of sensory functions in the innervation area and particularly in the autonomous area of the nerves. In the longer term, it can lead to a functional loss as well as atrophy of the innervated muscles.
a Entrapment of the N. medianus in the carpal tunnel **(carpal tunnel syndrome)** results in atrophy of the thenar muscles **(thenar atrophy)**. [G056]
b A lesion of the N. ulnaris in the GUYON's canal **(GUYON's canal syndrome)** can result in atrophy of the hypothenar muscles **(hypothenar atrophy)**. [G720]

Atrophy of the thenar muscle

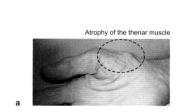

a

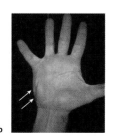

b

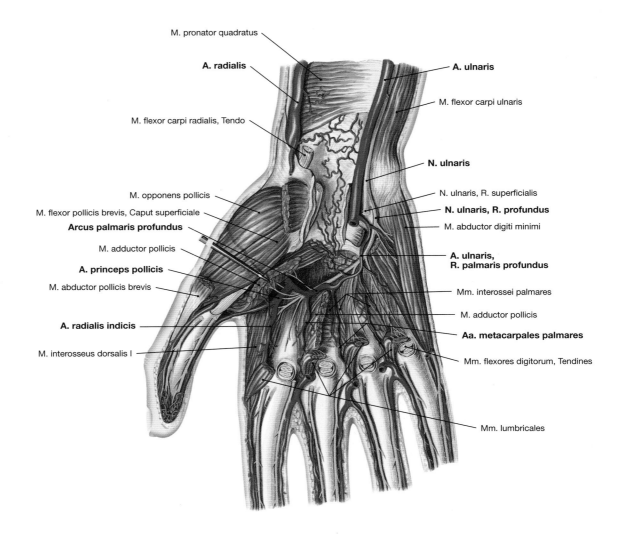

M. pronator quadratus

A. radialis

M. flexor carpi radialis, Tendo

M. opponens pollicis

M. flexor pollicis brevis, Caput superficiale

Arcus palmaris profundus

M. adductor pollicis

A. princeps pollicis

M. abductor pollicis brevis

A. radialis indicis

M. interosseus dorsalis I

A. ulnaris

M. flexor carpi ulnaris

N. ulnaris

N. ulnaris, R. superficialis

N. ulnaris, R. profundus

M. abductor digiti minimi

A. ulnaris, R. palmaris profundus

Mm. interossei palmares

M. adductor pollicis

Aa. metacarpales palmares

Mm. flexores digitorum, Tendines

Mm. lumbricales

Fig. 3.178 Arteries and nerves of the deep layer of the palm of the hand, Palma manus, right side; palmar view; after removal of the long flexor tendons and the Mm. lumbricales, as well as splitting the M. adductor pollicis. [S700]

The **deep palmar arch** (Arcus palmaris profundus) originates from the A. radialis and anastomoses mainly with the R. palmaris profundus of the A. ulnaris. This arch is positioned **beneath** the M. adductor pollicis and on the bases of the Ossa metacarpi; it therefore lies further proxi-

mally than the superficial palmar arterial arch. The deep palmar arterial arch provides the usually rather thin Aa. metacarpales palmares. On its way via the Mm. interossei it is accompanied by the **R. profundus of the N. ulnaris,** which provides the motor innervation of muscles, including those of the little finger, the Mm. interossei, and the two ulnar Mm. lumbricales. The arteries supplying the thumb (A. princeps pollicis) and the radial side of the index finger (A. radialis indicis) are also branches of the A. radialis.

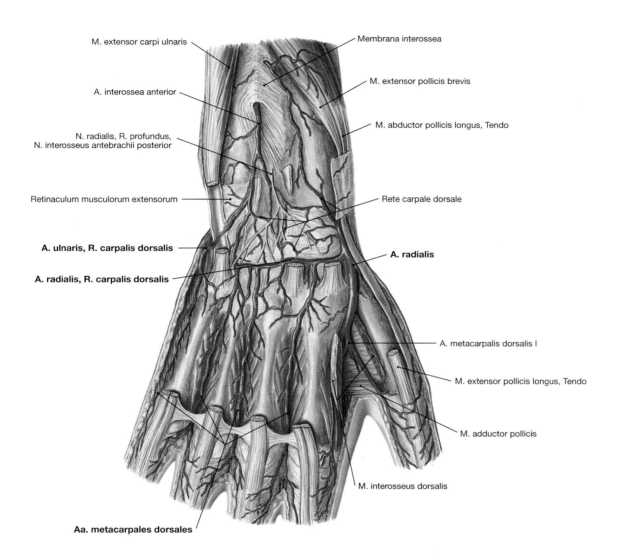

M. extensor carpi ulnaris

A. interossea anterior

N. radialis, R. profundus,
N. interosseus antebrachii posterior

Retinaculum musculorum extensorum

A. ulnaris, R. carpalis dorsalis

A. radialis, R. carpalis dorsalis

Aa. metacarpales dorsales

Membrana interossea

M. extensor pollicis brevis

M. abductor pollicis longus, Tendo

Rete carpale dorsale

A. radialis

A. metacarpalis dorsalis I

M. extensor pollicis longus, Tendo

M. adductor pollicis

M. interosseus dorsalis

Fig. 3.179 Arteries and nerves of the back of the hand, Dorsum manus, right side; dorsal view; after removal of the long extensor tendons. [S700]
In the wrist region, both the **A. radialis** as well as the **A. ulnaris** provide one **R. carpalis dorsalis** each to the back of the hand, which anastomose with each other. The radial branch is usually stronger and contributes greatly to the Aa. metacarpales dorsales that supply the back of the hand, and, as Aa. digitales dorsales, supply the fingers up to the proximal interphalangeal joints. The middle and distal phalanges of the fingers are supplied by the palmar digital arteries. The A. metacarpalis dorsalis I is a direct branch of the A. radialis, which passes between the heads of the M. interosseus dorsalis I into the palm of the hand.

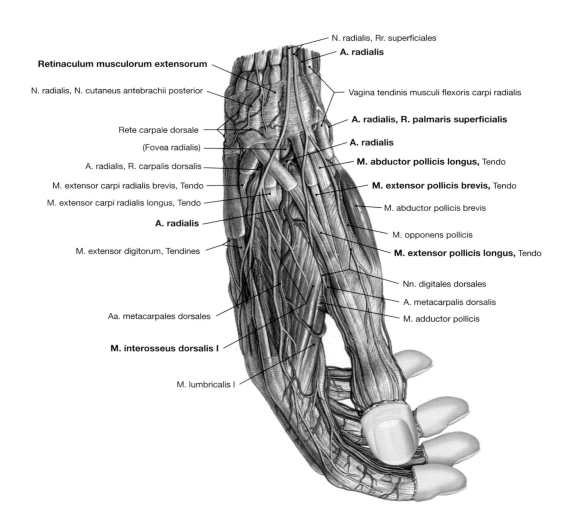

N. radialis, Rr. superficiales

A. radialis

Vagina tendinis musculi flexoris carpi radialis

A. radialis, R. palmaris superficialis

A. radialis

M. abductor pollicis longus, Tendo

M. extensor pollicis brevis, Tendo

M. abductor pollicis brevis

M. opponens pollicis

M. extensor pollicis longus, Tendo

Nn. digitales dorsales

A. metacarpalis dorsalis

M. adductor pollicis

Retinaculum musculorum extensorum

N. radialis, N. cutaneus antebrachii posterior

Rete carpale dorsale

(Fovea radialis)

A. radialis, R. carpalis dorsalis

M. extensor carpi radialis brevis, Tendo

M. extensor carpi radialis longus, Tendo

A. radialis

M. extensor digitorum, Tendines

Aa. metacarpales dorsales

M. interosseus dorsalis I

M. lumbricalis I

Fig. 3.180   Arteries and nerves of the back of the hand, Dorsum manus, right side; radial view. [S700]
This illustration shows the **pathway of the A. radialis** in the wrist region. At the proximal wrist, the A. radialis runs between the tendons of the M. brachioradialis and M. flexor carpi radialis. First, it crosses underneath the Retinaculum musculorum extensorum and provides the R. palmaris superficialis, which joins the superficial palmar arterial arch. The A. radialis then passes beneath the tendons of the two extensor muscles of the first tendon compartment (M. abductor pollicis longus and M. extensor pollicis brevis, → Fig. 3.82) to reach the **Fovea radialis (snuffbox;** between the tendons of the Mm. extensores pollicis brevis and longus), where it provides the R. carpalis dorsalis. After crossing beneath the tendon of the M. extensor pollicis longus, the A. radialis releases the A. metacarpalis dorsalis to the thumb and passes between the two heads of the M. interosseus dorsalis I into the palm of the hand. Sometimes, however, there is also a superficial variation where the artery passes over the extensor tendons.

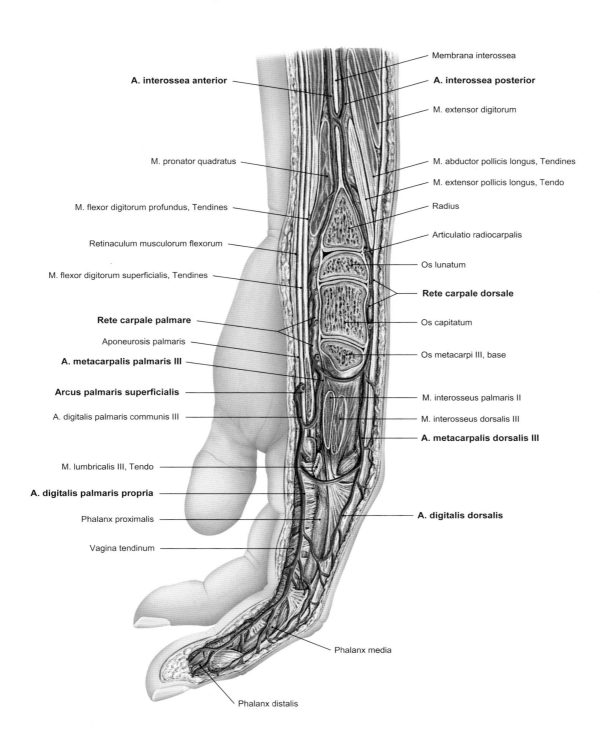

A. interossea anterior

A. interossea posterior

Membrana interossea

M. extensor digitorum

M. pronator quadratus

M. abductor pollicis longus, Tendines

M. extensor pollicis longus, Tendo

M. flexor digitorum profundus, Tendines

Radius

Articulatio radiocarpalis

Retinaculum musculorum flexorum

Os lunatum

M. flexor digitorum superficialis, Tendines

Rete carpale dorsale

Rete carpale palmare

Os capitatum

Aponeurosis palmaris

A. metacarpalis palmaris III

Os metacarpi III, base

Arcus palmaris superficialis

M. interosseus palmaris II

A. digitalis palmaris communis III

M. interosseus dorsalis III

A. metacarpalis dorsalis III

M. lumbricalis III, Tendo

A. digitalis palmaris propria

A. digitalis dorsalis

Phalanx proximalis

Vagina tendinum

Phalanx media

Phalanx distalis

Fig. 3.181 Arteries of the hand, Manus, right side; ulnar view; sagittal section at the level of the ulnar plane of the middle finger. [S700] Along the distal forearm, the Aa. interosseae anterior and posterior run on both sides of the Membrana interossea antebrachii. The carpus of the hand is supplied by palmar and dorsal vascular plexuses (Rete carpale palmare and Rete carpale dorsale), which are fed by the A. radialis and A. ulnaris. The metacarpal and digital arteries on the back of the hand originate from the Rete carpale dorsale. The metacarpal arteries in the palm of the hand originate from the deep palmar arch and the digital arteries from the superficial palmar arch. Each finger is supplied by a total of four digital arteries (palmar and dorsal arteries at the radial and ulnar side, respectively). The dorsal digital arteries only extend up to the middle phalanx. The middle and distal phalanges are supplied by branches of the palmar digital arteries.

Upper limb · 3

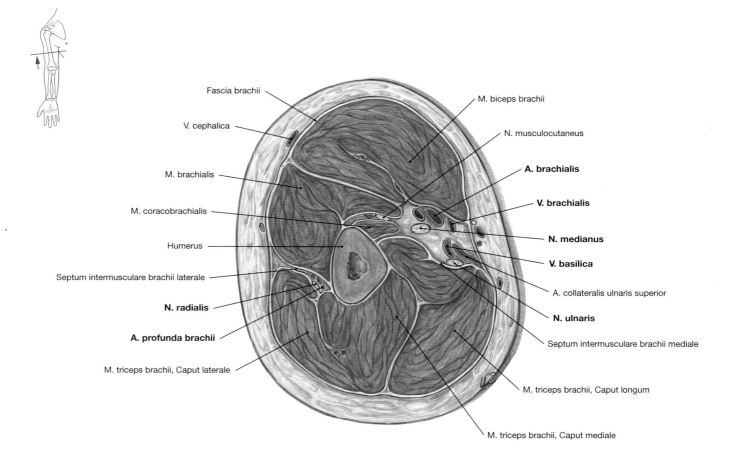

Fascia brachii

V. cephalica

M. brachialis

M. coracobrachialis

Humerus

Septum intermusculare brachii laterale

N. radialis

A. profunda brachii

M. triceps brachii, Caput laterale

M. biceps brachii

N. musculocutaneus

A. brachialis

V. brachialis

N. medianus

V. basilica

A. collateralis ulnaris superior

N. ulnaris

Septum intermusculare brachii mediale

M. triceps brachii, Caput longum

M. triceps brachii, Caput mediale

Fig. 3.182 Upper arm, Brachium, right side; distal view; cross-section in the middle of the upper arm. [S700]

In the cross-section, it is particularly evident that there are **two muscle groups** in the upper arm. The flexor muscles of the elbow joint lie ventrally. The M. biceps brachii covers the M. brachialis, which originates a bit further laterally. The insertion of the M. coracobrachialis on the medial humeral shaft is also clearly delineated. The back of the upper arm is occupied by the heads of the M. triceps brachii. There are two **neurovascular pathways.** The N. medianus, accompanied by the A. brachia-

lis and the Vv. brachiales, runs medially in the Sulcus bicipitalis medialis in front of the Septum intermusculare brachii mediale (medial neurovascular pathway). The V. basilica has already pierced the fascia and has arrived here just before draining into the V. brachialis. The N. ulnaris penetrates the Septum intermusculare brachii mediale further distally and arrives on the dorsal side of the Epicondylus medialis. Laterally, the N. radialis, along with the A. profunda brachii, loops around the humeral shaft (dorsal neurovascular pathway) in the Sulcus nervi radialis and descends between the M. brachialis and M. triceps brachii.

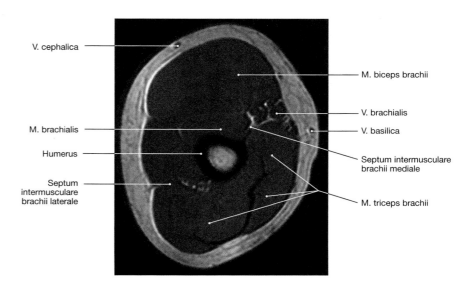

V. cephalica

M. brachialis

Humerus

Septum intermusculare brachii laterale

M. biceps brachii

V. brachialis

V. basilica

Septum intermusculare brachii mediale

M. triceps brachii

Fig. 3.183 Upper arm, Brachium, right side; distal view; magnetic resonance imaging (axial MRI scan) at the middle level of the upper arm. [S700]

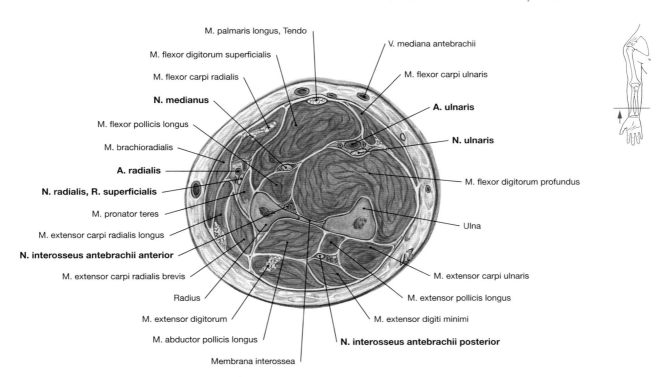

M. palmaris longus, Tendo

V. mediana antebrachii

M. flexor digitorum superficialis

M. flexor carpi ulnaris

M. flexor carpi radialis

N. medianus

A. ulnaris

M. flexor pollicis longus

N. ulnaris

M. brachioradialis

A. radialis

M. flexor digitorum profundus

N. radialis, R. superficialis

M. pronator teres

Ulna

M. extensor carpi radialis longus

N. interosseus antebrachii anterior

M. extensor carpi radialis brevis

M. extensor carpi ulnaris

Radius

M. extensor pollicis longus

M. extensor digitorum

M. extensor digiti minimi

M. abductor pollicis longus

N. interosseus antebrachii posterior

Membrana interossea

Fig. 3.184   Forearm, Antebrachium, right side; distal view; cross-section at the level of the distal third of the forearm. [S700]
On the forearm, there are **five neurovascular pathways** interposed between the groups of the superficial and deep flexor and extensor muscles. Underneath the M. brachioradialis, the A. and V. radialis run together with the R. superficialis of the N. radialis (radial neurovascular pathway).
The N. medianus and its thin accompanying artery (A. comitans nervi mediani) are located between the superficial and middle layers of flexor

muscles in the midline of the forearm (middle neurovascular pathway); under the M. flexor carpi ulnaris lie the A., V. and N. ulnaris (ulnar neurovascular pathway). The A. and V. interossea anterior and the N. interosseus anterior (interosseous neurovascular pathway) pass in front of the Membrana interossea antebrachii. The A. and V. interossea posterior and the N. interosseus posterior (dorsal neurovascular pathway) lie dorsally between the superficial and deep layers of the extensor muscles.

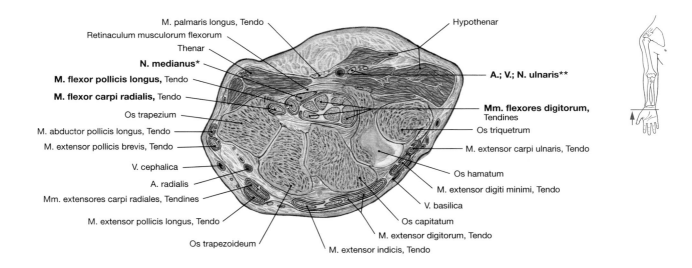

M. palmaris longus, Tendo

Hypothenar

Retinaculum musculorum flexorum

Thenar

N. medianus*

A.; V.; N. ulnaris**

M. flexor pollicis longus, Tendo

M. flexor carpi radialis, Tendo

Mm. flexores digitorum, Tendines

Os trapezium

Os triquetrum

M. abductor pollicis longus, Tendo

M. extensor carpi ulnaris, Tendo

M. extensor pollicis brevis, Tendo

Os hamatum

V. cephalica

M. extensor digiti minimi, Tendo

A. radialis

V. basilica

Mm. extensores carpi radiales, Tendines

Os capitatum

M. extensor pollicis longus, Tendo

M. extensor digitorum, Tendo

Os trapezoideum

M. extensor indicis, Tendo

Fig. 3.185   Wrist, Carpus, right side; distal view; cross-section at the level of the distal row of the carpal bones. [S700]
On the palmar side of the wrist, there are **two neurovascular pathways** which have great clinical significance. The carpal bones together with the Retinaculum musculorum flexorum form the **carpal tunnel** (Canalis carpi), through which the N. medianus together with the tendons of the long finger extensors pass. Any swelling of the tendon sheaths can therefore lead to compression of the N. medianus (carpal

tunnel syndrome, → Fig. 3.128). The N., A. and V. ulnaris lie on the retinaculum in the **GUYON's canal,** and due to this superficial position, they are at risk of external compression (distal lesion of the N. ulnaris → Fig. 3.132).

*   carpal tunnel
** GUYON's canal

Metacarpus and middle finger, cross-sections

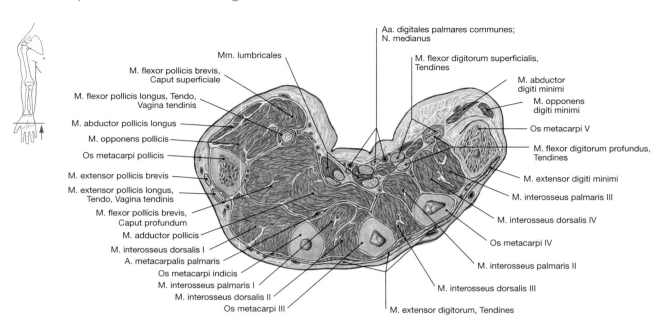

Mm. lumbricales

M. flexor pollicis brevis, Caput superficiale

M. flexor pollicis longus, Tendo, Vagina tendinis

M. abductor pollicis longus

M. opponens pollicis

Os metacarpi pollicis

M. extensor pollicis brevis

M. extensor pollicis longus, Tendo, Vagina tendinis

M. flexor pollicis brevis, Caput profundum

M. adductor pollicis

M. interosseus dorsalis I

A. metacarpalis palmaris

Os metacarpi indicis

M. interosseus palmaris I

M. interosseus dorsalis II

Os metacarpi III

Aa. digitales palmares communes; N. medianus

M. flexor digitorum superficialis, Tendines

M. abductor digiti minimi

M. opponens digiti minimi

Os metacarpi V

M. flexor digitorum profundus, Tendines

M. extensor digiti minimi

M. interosseus palmaris III

M. interosseus dorsalis IV

Os metacarpi IV

M. interosseus palmaris II

M. interosseus dorsalis III

M. extensor digitorum, Tendines

Fig. 3.186 Metacarpus; cross-section at the level of the middle of the third metacarpal bone. [S700]

The cross-section shows the position of the muscles in the palm of the hand, which are organised in three layers (→ Fig. 3.86, → Fig. 3.87, → Fig. 3.88, → Fig. 3.89). **Superficially,** the M. abductor pollicis and M. flexor pollicis brevis, as well as the M. abductor digiti minimi cover the other muscles of the thenar and hypothenar eminence, respectively. The tendons of the long flexor muscles of the fingers run in the **middle layer.** The Mm. lumbricales originate from the tendons of the M. flexor

digitorum profundus. The Mm. interossei palmares and dorsales form the **deep layer** of the palmar muscles. In this muscle group it can be seen that the bellies of the palmar muscles are actually facing the palm of the hand to a greater extent than the dorsal muscles. In addition to the muscles, this illustration also clearly shows the positions of the digital arteries (Aa. digitales palmares communes) and the sensory terminal branches of the N. medianus, which cover the tendons of the finger flexor muscles (→ Fig. 3.177).

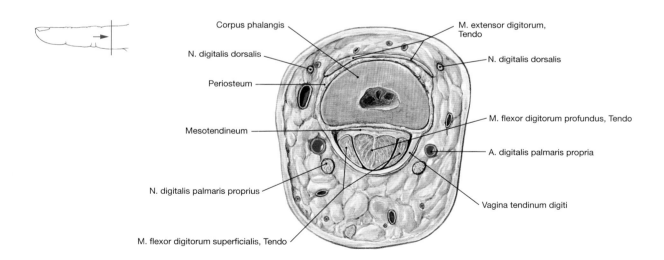

Corpus phalangis

N. digitalis dorsalis

Periosteum

Mesotendineum

N. digitalis palmaris proprius

M. flexor digitorum superficialis, Tendo

M. extensor digitorum, Tendo

N. digitalis dorsalis

M. flexor digitorum profundus, Tendo

A. digitalis palmaris propria

Vagina tendinum digiti

Fig. 3.187 Middle finger, Digitus medius [III]; cross-section through the shaft of the middle phalanx. [S700]

The tendon of the M. flexor digitorum profundus has penetrated the inserting tendon of the M. flexor digitorum superficialis and both tendons then share a common tendon sheath (Vagina tendinum digiti). The

dorsal digital arteries and nerves are already much thinner at the middle phalanges than the corresponding palmar blood vessels and nerves. This explains why the middle phalanges are predominantly (and the distal phalanges exclusively) supplied by the **palmar branches** (A. digitalis palmaris propria and N. digitalis palmaris proprius) (→ Fig. 3.181).

Sample exam questions

To check that you are completely familiar with the content of this chapter, sample questions from an oral anatomy exam are listed here.

Show the sections and most important structures of the humerus on the skeleton:

- Where are the Sulcus nervi radialis and the Sulcus nervi ulnaris?
- What clinical importance do they have?

Explain the structure of the elbow joint in a joint model:

- Which skeletal elements articulate with each other? Which ligaments stabilise the wrist?
- Which types of joints can be found at the wrist?
- Which movements are possible, and with which ranges of motion?
- How are axes of movement performed?
- Which muscles are important for the individual movements?

Show the most important flexor muscles of the fingers:

- Which muscles act predominantly on the individual joints?
- Describe the course of the Mm. interossei with their origins and insertions.
- How do the individual muscles function in relation to their movement axes?
- How are these muscles innervated and which movements are affected when they fail?

Show the N. medianus and explain its pathway on the dissection:

- Explain its innervation area.
- Where is it damaged most often?
- What does the clinical picture look like in the case of a lesion in the wrist region, e.g. in carpal tunnel syndrome?

What arterial pulses can you palpate on the upper limb during a clinical examination?

- Show the blood vessels branching off the Truncus thyrocervicalis and explain their supply areas.
- Explain the pathway of the A. ulnaris and the A. radialis on a dissection.

How is the venous system of the arm organised?

- Where can the physician take a blood sample most easily?

Explain the lymphatic drainage on the arm:

- How are the lymph nodes in the axilla organised?
- Which regions of the body do they drain?

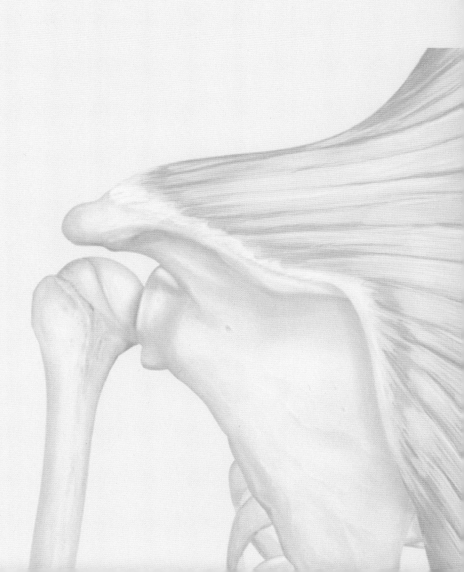

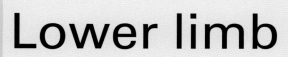

Lower limb

Surface. 346

Skeleton. 348

Musculature. 414

Neurovascular pathways 452

Topography 476

Cross-sectional images. 500

4

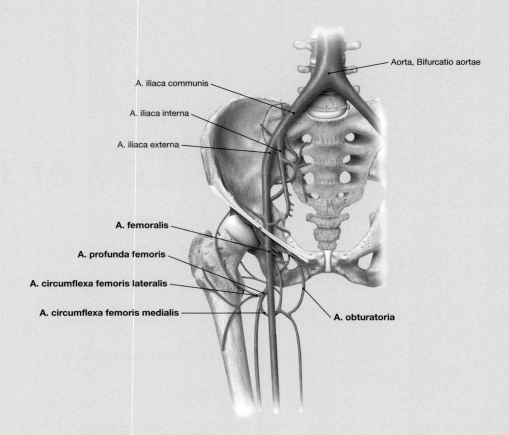

A. iliaca communis

A. iliaca interna

A. iliaca externa

A. femoralis

A. profunda femoris

A. circumflexa femoris lateralis

A. circumflexa femoris medialis

Aorta, Bifurcatio aortae

A. obturatoria

Overview

The **lower limb** can be divided into the **pelvic girdle and the leg.** The pelvic girdle consists of the sacrum and the two hip bones. The leg is divided according to its joints into the thigh, the lower leg and the foot.

The lower limb functions as a **locomotor and a supporting (or weight-bearing) organ.** The long bones of the legs enable a greater length of stride to accelerate locomotion. The individual joints of the lower limb are reinforced by a stable ligamentous apparatus to ensure a safe upright stance and to reduce the load of the muscle groups in the buttock, knee and calf region, which have an important support function.

The human foot acts to stabilise the **upright stance.** In contrast to the hand, the muscles of the foot are less involved in finely regulating dis-

tinct toe movements than in the active stabilisation of the foot and the tension of its arches.

The muscles of the lower limb are innervated by two nerve plexuses that are joined in the **Plexus lumbosacralis.** The plexuses are fed by the anterior branches of the spinal nerves from the spinal cord segments T12–S5, Co1. Different nerves to the pelvic girdle, the perineal and gluteal regions, as well as to the leg emerge from the Plexus lumbosacralis. The lower limb is primarily supplied by the **A. and V. iliaca externa** and their consecutive vascular segments. The lymphatic vessels largely run along the veins and are connected to the **lymph nodes of the groin,** which also drain the abdominal wall, including the external genitalia and certain pelvic organs.

Main topics

After working through this chapter, you should be able to:

- name basic principles of limb development and the clinically relevant variations and malformations;
- describe the bony structures of the pelvic girdle and the leg as well as their joints and range of motion on a skeleton;
- explain the course of the ligaments in the joints, as well as the origin, insertion (attachment) and function of all muscles of the hip, thigh and lower leg, and to show these on a skeleton or dissection; in the case of the foot muscles, basic information about their pathway, function and innervation are generally sufficient;
- describe the structure of the Plexus lumbosacralis and explain the symptoms associated with plexus lesions;
- describe the pathway, function and precise symptoms associated with nerve lesions in the lower limb and show these on a dissection;
- name all the arteries of the lower limb with their most important branches and identify them on the dissection;
- specify the locations for pulse measurement;

- explain vascular anastomoses in the hip region;
- understand the basic principle of the venous flow in the lower limb;
- name the large epifascial veins and show them on the dissection specimen;
- explain the principles of the lymph flow in the lower limb;
- explain the regional lymph nodes of the leg and pelvis with their drainage areas;
- show the borders and contents of the Lacuna musculorum and Lacuna vasorum;
- explain the content and structure of the femoral triangle, the obturator canal and the adductor canal;
- explain the structure of the gluteal region, and identify the neurovascular structures passing through the Foramina suprapiriforme and infrapiriforme and the Foramen ischiadicum minus;
- explain the structure of the popliteal fossa (back of the knee) and the arrangement of the neurovascular pathways crossing it.

Clinical relevance

In order not to lose touch with prospective everyday clinical life with so many anatomical details, the following describes a typical case that shows why the content of this chapter is so important.

Femoral neck fracture

Case study
A 94-year-old lady had a fall in her apartment. When her daughter found her, she was conscious and responsive. She could stand up if assisted. However, she could not put any weight on her right leg and her hip was so painful that standing for any length of time was impossible. The daughter called the paramedics and the old lady explained to them that she had fallen sideways when getting out of a chair. She assured them that she had not been knocked unconscious.

Result of examination
The patient is conscious, awake and fully orientated. She has severe pain in the right hip region; a fresh haemorrhage is visible under the skin. The right leg appears shortened and is rotated outwards (→ Fig. a). Her cardiac (100/min) and respiratory rates (30/min) are increased, but her blood pressure is low (80/40 mm Hg). The patient is brought to the trauma ward of the nearby hospital by ambulance.

Diagnostic procedure
The X-ray of the pelvis and the upper thigh that was taken shows a fracture in the neck area of the right femoral bone. Further fractures cannot be detected.

Diagnosis
Femoral neck fracture (→ Fig. b).

Treatment
Since it is likely that the blood vessels supplying the femoral neck were also damaged by the fracture (→ Fig. b), surgical treatment is carried out immediately in order to prevent shock due to severe haemorrhage. Since the healing of bone fragments is uncertain and lingering even after operative stabilisation, a hip prosthesis is inserted. In doing so, the head and neck of the femur as well as the socket on the hip bone are completely replaced by a total hip endoprosthesis.

Further developments
As the prosthesis is stable, weight-bearing mobilisation can be started the following day. Then follows a week of short-term care. After four weeks, discharge from the hospital is possible and the patient is able to return home where she can continue to look after herself.

This clinical picture is a common diagnosis. The physical examination already indicates a suspected diagnosis of femoral neck fracture. It is important to understand the blood supply to the hip joint in order to fully comprehend the therapeutic procedure – the preparations in the dissection lab help with this.

Dissection lab
The **thigh bone (femur)** consists of a body or shaft (Corpus femoris), from which the neck (Collum femoris) and head of the femur (Caput femoris) are angled medially. The head forms an articular surface embedded in the socket. The angle between the shaft and the neck is referred to as the centrum-collum-diaphyseal (CCD) angle and measures 126°. Because of this angle formation, the femur bears the weight of the upper half of the body asymmetrically. As a result, the bone is not uniformly exposed to compressive stress, but is also exposed to bending or tensile stress (increased risk of fracture!). In the area of the shaft, flexion is reduced by the traction force of the **Tractus iliotibialis** (iliotibial band) on the lateral side of the leg, into which the M. gluteus maximus and the M. tensor fasciae latae radiate. The external hip muscles are the most important extensors, rotators, and abductors of the hip joint.

 This 3–5 cm wide fascial reinforcement must not be damaged during dissection!

The femoral head in a child is mainly nourished by a branch of the A. obturatoria (R. acetabularis) which runs from the hip socket to the head of the femur via the Lig. capitis femoris (→ Fig. 4.52). In adults, this branch supplies only a small proportion of the femur. The nutrition of the femur is now ensured by the Aa. circumflexa femoris medialis and lateralis, both of which commonly originate from the **A. profunda femoris.**

 This artery and its branches are clearly visible deep inside the thigh with a frontal view!

It originates below the inguinal ligament from the A. femoralis and represents the main supplying vessel of the thigh (→ Fig. 4.155 and → Fig. 4.157).

Back to the clinic
The femoral neck fracture of the patient has also caused a rupture of the branches of the Aa. circumflexae femoris medialis and lateralis. Due to the traction of the gluteal muscles at the Trochanter major, the femur is abducted and rotated outwards – recognisable in a shortening of the patient's leg. The risk of fracture in this area increases with age, as the CCD angle increasingly reduces in size (Coxa vara). Due to a decrease in bone mass (osteoporosis), the bone stability is reduced in general. As a result of impaired blood supply, the chance of healing is reduced and secondary complications (vein thrombosis, pneumonia) may follow. Therefore, at this age, everything indicates the need for a total hip endoprosthesis. In younger patients, partial prostheses are increasingly being used. It is important in these surgical interventions to take care of the Aa. circumflexae femoris medialis and lateralis as well as of the surrounding hip muscles. Of course, the anatomical conditions must also be considered in the various surgical approaches.

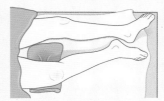

Fig. a Clinical situation after a femoral neck fracture on the right. [S700-L126]
Note the shortened appearance of the leg and its external rotation.

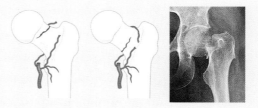

Fig. b Femoral neck fracture with vascular ruptures on the left; with ruptured vessels.
Ventral view [S700-L126]; on the right: X-ray image (AP). [R234]

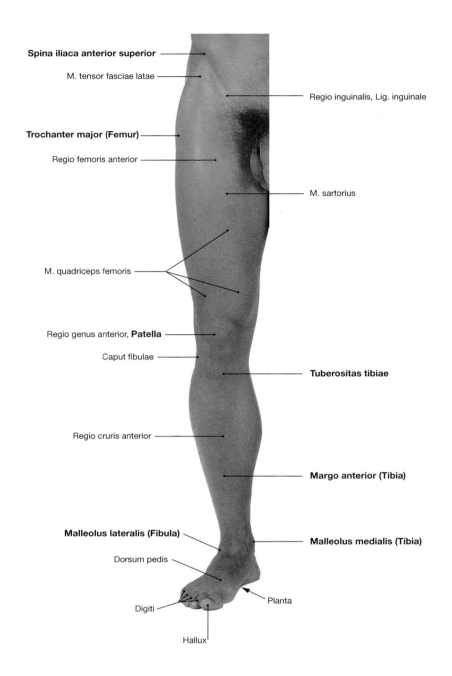

Spina iliaca anterior superior

M. tensor fasciae latae

Regio inguinalis, Lig. inguinale

Trochanter major (Femur)

Regio femoris anterior

M. sartorius

M. quadriceps femoris

Regio genus anterior, Patella

Caput fibulae

Tuberositas tibiae

Regio cruris anterior

Margo anterior (Tibia)

Malleolus lateralis (Fibula)

Malleolus medialis (Tibia)

Dorsum pedis

Planta

Digiti

Hallux

Fig. 4.1 Surface anatomy of the leg, right side; ventral view. [S700]

The surface anatomy of the leg is determined by the muscles and by some of the skeletal elements.

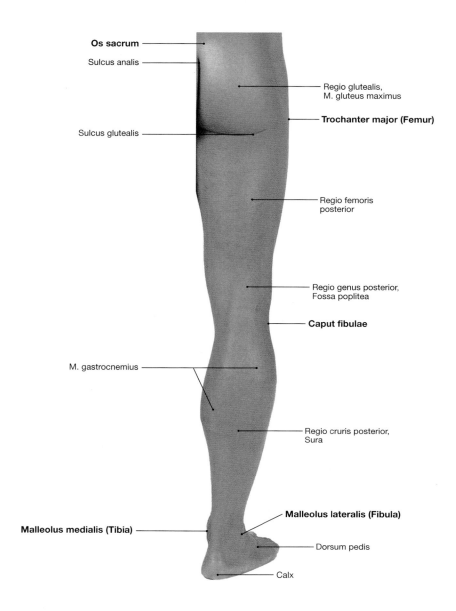

Os sacrum

Sulcus analis

Regio glutealis,
M. gluteus maximus

Trochanter major (Femur)

Sulcus glutealis

Regio femoris
posterior

Regio genus posterior,
Fossa poplitea

Caput fibulae

M. gastrocnemius

Regio cruris posterior,
Sura

Malleolus lateralis (Fibula)

Malleolus medialis (Tibia)

Dorsum pedis

Calx

Fig. 4.2 Surface anatomy of the leg, right side; dorsal view. [S700]

Skeleton of the lower limb

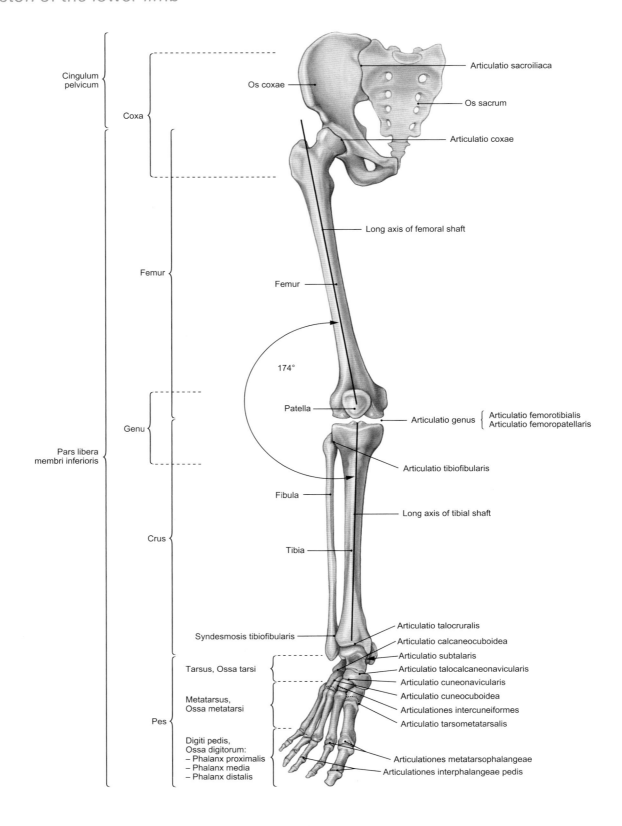

Cingulum
pelvicum

Coxa

Os coxae

Articulatio sacroiliaca

Os sacrum

Articulatio coxae

Long axis of femoral shaft

Femur

Femur

Pars libera
membri inferioris

Genu

174°

Patella

Articulatio genus { Articulatio femorotibialis
Articulatio femoropatellaris

Articulatio tibiofibularis

Fibula

Long axis of tibial shaft

Crus

Tibia

Syndesmosis tibiofibularis

Articulatio talocruralis
Articulatio calcaneocuboidea
Articulatio subtalaris
Articulatio talocalcaneonavicularis
Articulatio cuneonavicularis
Articulatio cuneocuboidea
Articulationes intercuneiformes
Articulatio tarsometatarsalis

Tarsus, Ossa tarsi

Metatarsus,
Ossa metatarsi

Pes

Digiti pedis,
Ossa digitorum:
– Phalanx proximalis
– Phalanx media
– Phalanx distalis

Articulationes metatarsophalangeae
Articulationes interphalangeae pedis

**Fig. 4.3   Bones and joints of the lower limb, Membrum inferius,
right side;** ventral view. [S700]

Whereas the shoulder girdle consists of two bones (scapula and clavicle), the pelvic girdle (Cingulum pelvicum) is formed by two hip bones
(Ossa coxae) and the sacrum (Os sacrum). The thigh and leg form a
laterally open angle of 174°, referred to as the **Q-angle** (abduction angle).

With a **knock-knee deformity** (Genu valgum), the Q-angle is smaller,
and in the **bow-leg deformity** (Genu varum) it is larger. For the development of the lower limbs (→ Fig. 3.3, → Fig. 3.4, → Fig. 3.5).

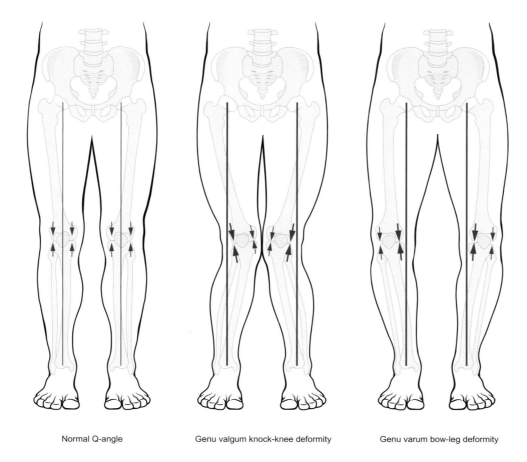

Normal Q-angle   Genu valgum knock-knee deformity   Genu varum bow-leg deformity

Fig. 4.4 Mechanical axis of the leg (MIKULICZ line). [S700-L126]/
[G1067]
Normally, the large joints of the leg lie in a straight line **(MIKULICZ
line)**, which is known as the mechanical axis. This is the connecting line
between the centre of the femoral head in the hip joint and the middle
of the malleolar fork in the talocrural joint.

In the case of a **knock-knee** deformity (Genu valgum), the knee is shifted **medially** from the **mechanical axis;** in the case of a **bow-leg** deformity (Genu varum), the knee is shifted laterally.
The size of the arrows illustrates the ratio of stress on the medial and
lateral joint sections depending on the pathway of the mechanical axis.

Clinical remarks

Since the whole body weight is transferred via the mechanical axis
(MIKULICZ line) to the soles of the feet, the load on the joints is
evenly distributed if the joints are aligned along this mechanical axis.
Abnormalities of the knee joint in the case of a **knock-knee** (Genu
valgum) or **bow-leg** (Genu varum) deformity results in an uneven
load on both compartments of the knee joint (red arrows, → Fig. 4.4).
This can lead to degenerative osteoarthritis in the knee joint **(knee**

arthritis) due to the wear and tear of menisci and joint cartilage. In
the case of a **Genu valgum** this type of arthritis affects the **lateral
compartment** and in the case of a **Genu varum** it affects **the medial compartment.** Substantial deviations from the mechanical axis
may require surgical corrections, including the removal of a bony
wedge (calcaneal osteotomy).

Lower limb

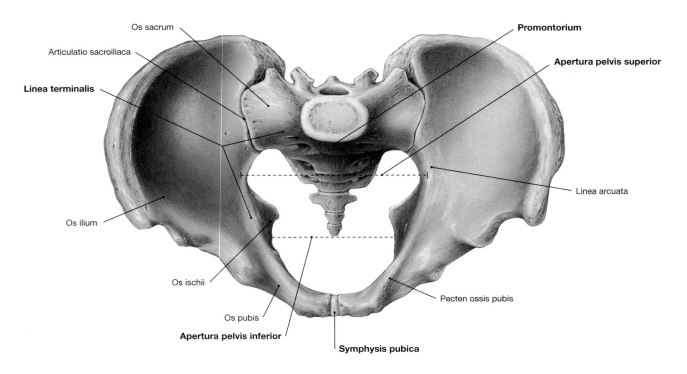

Fig. 4.5   Pelvis; ventrocranial view. [S700]

The pelvis consists of three bones. The sacroiliac joint (Articulatio sacro-iliaca) and the pubic symphysis (Symphysis pubica) connect the two hip bones (Ossa coxae) and the sacrum (Os sacrum) to form a stable ring construction. This bony ring is collectively referred to as the pelvic girdle (Cingulum pelvicum). Together with the paired iliac wings, the pelvic girdle covers the intestines and transfers the body weight onto the legs. At the caudal end of the sacrum is the coccyx or tailbone (Os coccygis) which represents a rudimentary tail. The coccyx has no role in the stability of the pelvis and is therefore not considered a pelvic bone.

The **Linea terminalis** is formed by the Pecten ossis pubis at the front, starting from the pubic symphysis, and by the Linea arcuata at the back, ending on the **promontory.** It includes the pelvic inlet **(Apertura pelvis superior)** and separates the **cranially** positioned **larger pelvis** (Pelvis major) from the **caudally** positioned **lesser pelvis** (Pelvis minor). The promontory is the furthest protruding part of the spine in the pelvic inlet. The pelvic outlet **(Apertura pelvis inferior)** is bordered at the front by the lower rim of the pubic symphysis and by the inferior pubic ramus, on both sides by the ischial tuberosities and at the back by the tip of the coccyx.

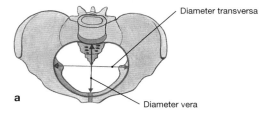

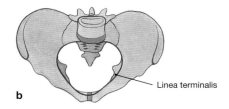

Fig. 4.6a and b   Pelvis of a woman and a man. [S700]
a Pelvis of a woman.
b Pelvis of a man.

The shape of the pelvis shows **specific differences** between the sexes: in **men** the pelvic inlet is **heart-shaped.** The somewhat smaller pubic angle is referred to as the **Angulus subpubicus** (→ Fig. 4.9, → Fig. 4.41a). In contrast, the pelvic inlet is usually a **transverse oval** shape in **women.** In addition, the angle between the inferior pubic rami (**Arcus pubicus,** → Fig. 4.41b) and the distance between the ischial tuberosities, as well as the wings of the ilium, are larger than in men.

The **inner pelvic dimensions** are used to determine the width of the pelvic inlet: the obstetric conjugate diameter **(Diameter vera)** between the posterior aspect of the pubic symphysis and the promontory, the **transverse diameter (Diameter transversa)** between the most later-ally located points of the Linea terminalis on both sides, the diagonal diameter **(Diameter diagonalis,** → Fig. 4.7) between the lower rim of the pubic symphysis and the promontory, and the anatomic diameter **(Diameter anatomica,** → Fig. 4.7) between the upper rim of the pubic symphysis and the promontory.

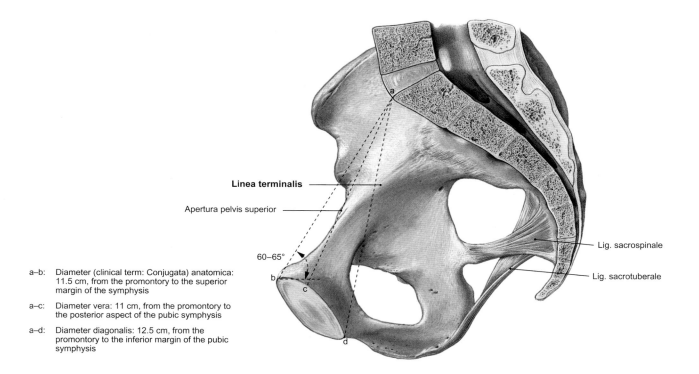

Linea terminalis

Apertura pelvis superior

Lig. sacrospinale

Lig. sacrotuberale

60–65°

a–b: Diameter (clinical term: Conjugata) anatomica: 11.5 cm, from the promontory to the superior margin of the symphysis

a–c: Diameter vera: 11 cm, from the promontory to the posterior aspect of the pubic symphysis

a–d: Diameter diagonalis: 12.5 cm, from the promontory to the inferior margin of the pubic symphysis

Fig. 4.7 Pelvis of the woman; medial view; median section with depiction of the internal pelvic diameters. [S700]
The inner pelvic dimensions vary greatly between individuals. The most important diameter is the **Diameter vera** connecting the posterior aspect of the pubic symphysis and the promontory. The **Diameter ana-** **tomica** and the **Diameter diagonalis** indicate the distance from the promontory to the upper and lower rims of the pubic symphysis. The level of the pelvic inlet along with the horizontal level form the pelvic inclination angle of approx. 60–65°.

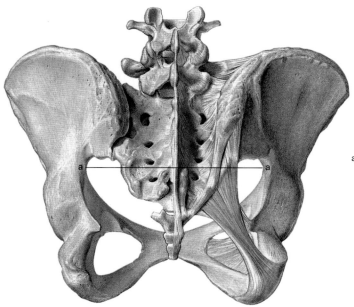

a–a: Diameter transversa: 13.5 cm, distance between the most laterally positioned points on each end of the Linea terminalis.

Fig. 4.8 Pelvis of the woman with pelvic dimensions; dorsal view. [S700]
A further internal diameter of some relevance is the **transverse diameter (Diameter transversa).** The various outer diameters (Distantiae), on the other hand, are of less practical importance and therefore not shown here.

Clinical remarks

Because the pelvic inlet and the lesser pelvis encompass the birth canal, assessment of the pelvic diameter is of great importance during **pregnancy** to determine whether a vaginal birth is possible. The most important diameter for the passage of the fetal head is the **conjugate diameter** (clin. Conjugata vera; at least 11 cm). It can be assessed by vaginal examination of the diagonal diameter, which spans the inferior side of the pubic symphysis to the promontory and is 1.5 cm longer than the Conjugata vera. The Conjugata vera is measured mostly by magnetic resonance imaging (MRI) when a vaginal birth is planned but the size of the child is suspected of being disproportionate to the maternal birth canal. In the case of a caesarean section, the conjugate diameter is directly measured routinely, in order to determine whether future vaginal births may be possible. During pregnancy, the pubic symphysis and sacroiliac joints are loosened by the relaxin hormone which is released from the placenta and the ovary, so that the Conjugata vera expands by approx. 1 cm during childbirth.

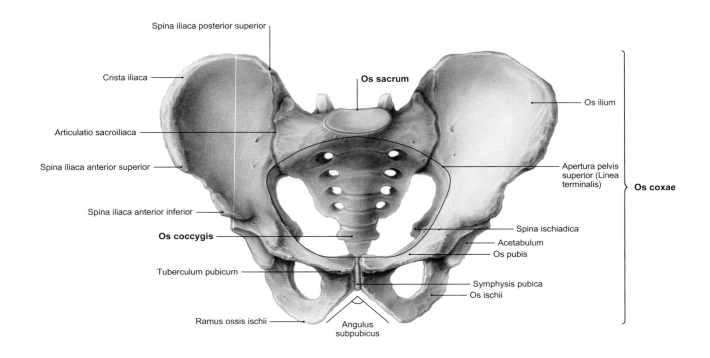

Fig. 4.9 Pelvis of the man; ventral view. [S701-L285]
Sex differences of the pelvis are most obvious at the level of the pelvic aperture and the angle between the lower pubic rami.
The **pelvic inlet** is formed by the bilateral hip bones, ventrally connecting in the pubic symphysis. At the dorsal pelvic side, the **Promontorium** of the sacrum protrudes furthest ventrally. The pelvic inlet in men is heart-shaped, whereas in women it has a transverse oval shape. (→ Fig. 4.6). The lower pubic rami form an acute angle **(Angulus subpubicus)** in men, while in women they form an arch **(Arcus pubicus)**. In women, the pelvic outlet is also wider and, along with the pelvic inlet, restricts the size of the birth canal.

Structure and function

The pelvis consists of three bones (two iliac bones and one sacrum) which are connected by very tight joints to form the **pelvic girdle.** It is not possible to understand the pelvis without a knowledge of its joints. The **symphysis (Symphysis pubica)** is an immobile joint (synarthrosis) with a disc of fibrous cartilage (Discus interpubicus) and a superior and inferior ligament for added stabilisation (→ Fig. 4.41). The symphysis forms the ventral connection between the paired pubic bones. Dorsally, two **sacroiliac joints (Articulatio sacroiliaca)** connect the sacrum with the iliac bones. This typical amphiarthrosis is a true joint with a joint space (diarthrosis) but the tight ligamentous apparatus only permits minimal movements. During labour, the pubic ligaments slightly relax temporarily to enlarge the birth canal. Otherwise, the pelvic joints are very stable and are rarely subject to injury.

Clinical remarks

X-ray images of the pelvis in an anteroposterior (AP) projection are a common diagnostic procedure. This includes the diagnosis of **fractures** or **deformities** of the skeletal elements of the hip joint and pelvic girdle as well as degenerative **arthritis** or local changes in the bone, e.g. caused by the spreading of malignant tumour cells **(me-** **tastases). Inflammatory changes to the sacroiliac joints,** e.g., as part of rheumatoid diseases, can be diagnosed with X-ray images of the pelvis. Clinically, the sacroiliac joint is more frequently referred to as the iliosacral joint.

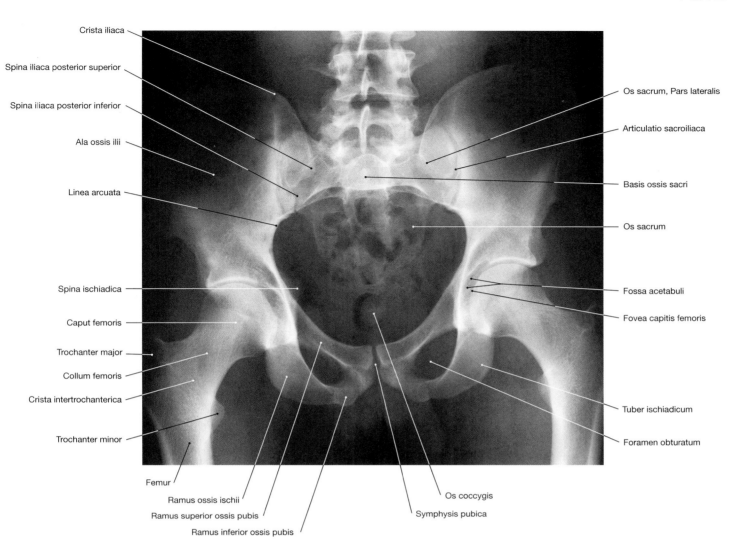

Crista iliaca

Spina iliaca posterior superior

Spina iliaca posterior inferior

Ala ossis ilii

Linea arcuata

Spina ischiadica

Caput femoris

Trochanter major

Collum femoris

Crista intertrochanterica

Trochanter minor

Femur

Ramus ossis ischii

Ramus superior ossis pubis

Ramus inferior ossis pubis

Os sacrum, Pars lateralis

Articulatio sacroiliaca

Basis ossis sacri

Os sacrum

Fossa acetabuli

Fovea capitis femoris

Tuber ischiadicum

Foramen obturatum

Os coccygis

Symphysis pubica

Fig. 4.10 Pelvis of a man; X-ray image with anteroposterior (AP) projection; upright stance. [S700-T895]

Clinical remarks

Anteroposterior (AP) X-ray images are used to diagnose pelvic fractures.

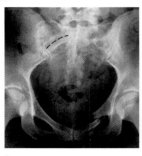

a

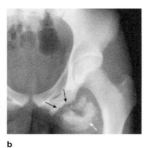

b

a Pelvic fractures are inflicted mainly as a result of **massive compression** forces impacting on the pelvis during serious vehicle accidents or a fall from a great height. Fractures of the pelvic ring usually lead to deformations of the pelvic inlet and outlet. [G198]

b Additionally, strong contractions of the hip musculature, including the adductor muscle group during sports activities, can tear away the bony pelvic insertion sites of these muscles, and are known as **avulsion fractures.** [E513-002]

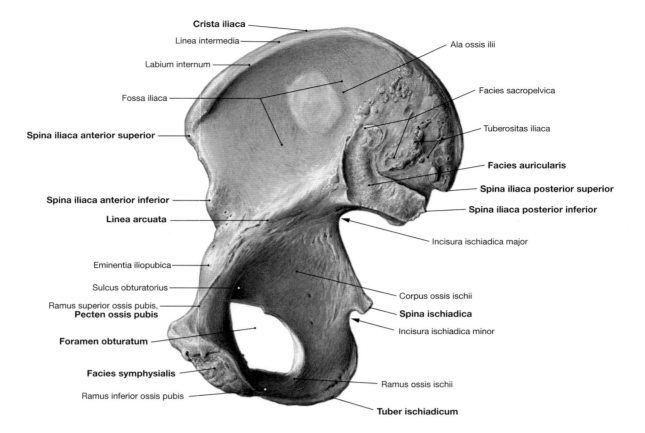

Fig. 4.11 Hip bone, Os coxae, right side; medial view. [S700]
The hip bone consists of three parts, the **ilium (Os ilium)**, the **ischium (Os ischii)** and the **pubis (Os pubis)**. The ilium (above) forms the iliac wing, the ischium (below, rear) and pubis (below, in front) form the bony ring around the Foramen obturatum. The **Facies auricularis** serves as the articular surface of the sacroiliac joint. The Discus interpubicus of the pubic symphysis is attached to the **Facies symphysialis**.

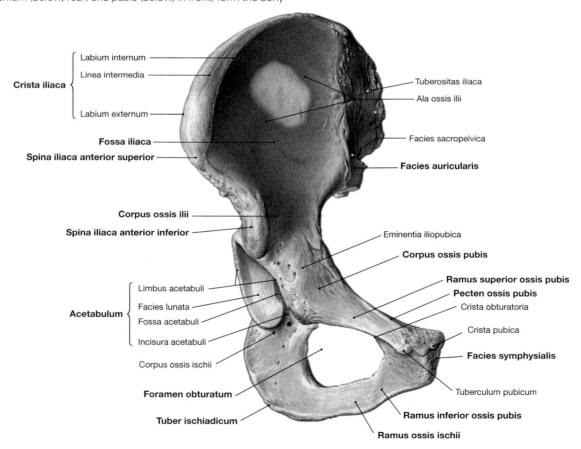

Fig. 4.12 Hip bone, Os coxae, right side; ventral view. [S700]

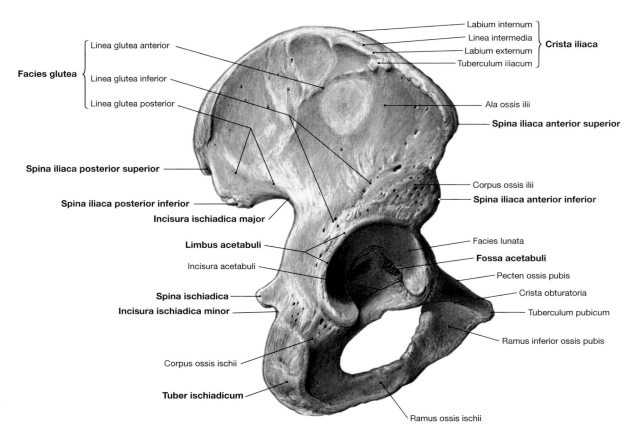

Facies glutea {
  Linea glutea anterior
  Linea glutea inferior
  Linea glutea posterior
}

Labium internum
Linea intermedia
Labium externum
Tuberculum iliacum
} **Crista iliaca**

Ala ossis ilii

Spina iliaca anterior superior

Spina iliaca posterior superior

Spina iliaca posterior inferior

Incisura ischiadica major

Corpus ossis ilii
Spina iliaca anterior inferior

Limbus acetabuli

Incisura acetabuli

Facies lunata
Fossa acetabuli

Spina ischiadica

Incisura ischiadica minor

Pecten ossis pubis

Crista obturatoria

Tuberculum pubicum

Ramus inferior ossis pubis

Corpus ossis ischii

Tuber ischiadicum

Ramus ossis ischii

Fig. 4.13 Hip bone, Os coxae, right side; dorsolateral view. [S700]

The three parts of the hip bone, namely the ilium (Os ilium), the ischium (Os ischii), and the pubis (Os pubis) form the hip socket (acetabulum).

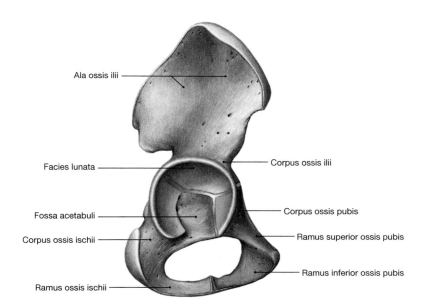

Ala ossis ilii

Corpus ossis ilii

Facies lunata

Corpus ossis pubis

Fossa acetabuli

Corpus ossis ischii

Ramus superior ossis pubis

Ramus inferior ossis pubis

Ramus ossis ischii

Fig. 4.14 Hip bone, Os coxae, of a six-year-old child, right side; lateral view. [S700]

The three parts of the hip bone (Os ilium, Os ischii, Os pubis) are linked by a Y-shaped cartilaginous junction (synchondrosis) of the acetabulum. The cartilaginous junction ossifies between the 13th and 18th year of life.

Clinical remarks

In the case of severe trauma, such as the impaction of outstretched legs in a car accident, a fracture of the acetabulum with dislocation of the femoral head **(central hip dislocation)** may occur.

During childhood and adolescence, the development of an endochondral ossification in the area of the acetabulum must be consid-

ered in X-ray examinations of the pelvic bones in children, in order to avoid the risk of confusing a cartilaginous junction with a fracture gap.

Lower limb

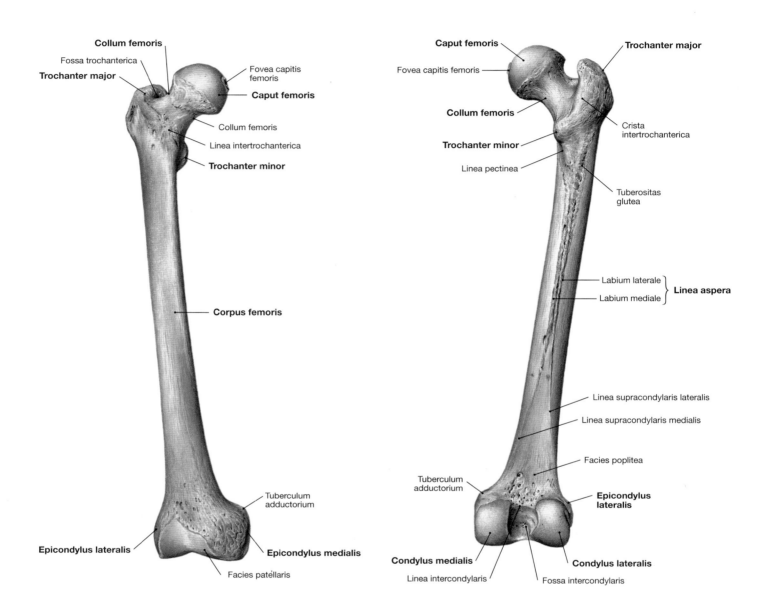

Fig. 4.15 Femur, right side; ventral view. [S700]
On the proximal shaft of the femur, the Trochanter major is located later-ally and the Trochanter minor dorsomedially.

Fig. 4.16 Femur, right side; dorsal view. [S700]
The Linea aspera serves as apophysis for the origin of the M. quadri-ceps femoris and for the insertion of other muscles of the adductor group.

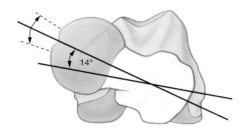

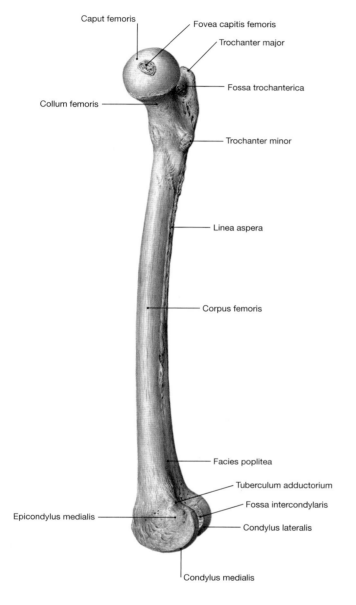

Caput femoris

Fovea capitis femoris

Trochanter major

Fossa trochanterica

Collum femoris

Trochanter minor

Linea aspera

Corpus femoris

Facies poplitea

Tuberculum adductorium

Fossa intercondylaris

Epicondylus medialis

Condylus lateralis

Condylus medialis

Fig. 4.17 Femur, right side; medial view. [S700]

Fig. 4.18 Femur, right side; proximal view; the proximal and distal ends of the femur are projected on top of each other. [S700]
Against the axis connecting both femoral condyles (= transverse axis of the knee joint), the femoral neck is rotated by **12–14°** anteriorly **(torsion angle of the femur).** In infants, this angle is approximately 30°.
If the torsion angle of the femur is more pronounced, this results in an internal rotation of the toes (pointing inwards) when walking. If the angle of antetorsion is smaller than 12°, the toes point outwards.

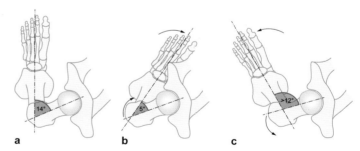

Fig. 4.19a–c Deviations of the antetorsion angle of the femoral neck, left side; schematic representation. [S701-L231]
a In a normal hip joint, the femoral neck is rotated forward by 12–14° from the transverse axis and this is called the antetorsion angle.
b A smaller angle is called **anteversion of the femoral neck.** As a result, the tip of the foot and toes are rotated inwards ('in-toeing' or 'pigeon toe').
c A larger antetorsion angle causes **retroversion of the femoral neck** with toes pointing outwards ('out-toeing' or 'duck walk').

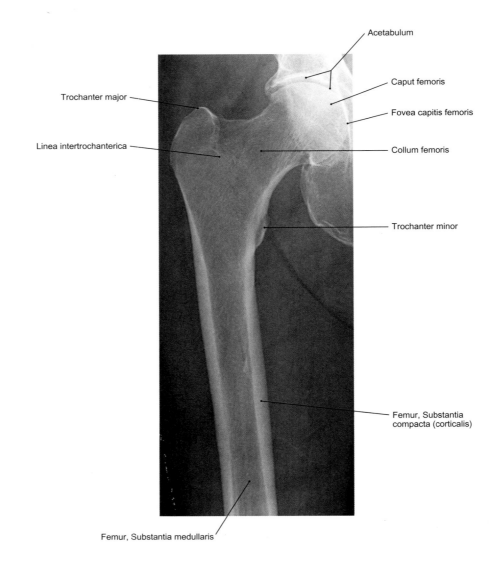

Acetabulum

Caput femoris

Fovea capitis femoris

Trochanter major

Collum femoris

Linea intertrochanterica

Trochanter minor

Femur, Substantia compacta (corticalis)

Femur, Substantia medullaris

Fig. 4.20 Proximal end of the femoral bone, femur, right side;
X-ray image in anteroposterior (AP) projection. [F264-004]

Clinical remarks

Fractures of the hip are located in the proximal third of the femur. Fractures of the femur can occur as a result of a simple fall when walking and are most common in elderly people with an unsteady gait and reduced bone density (osteoporosis). The frequency of hip fractures increases as people get older and doubles after the age of 50 for every decade of life.

a Most often, clinically, a leg appears shorter. The diagnosis is confirmed by X-ray imaging. [R110-20]

b Femoral fractures occur at the femoral neck **(femoral neck fracture)** or at the section between the Trochanter major and minor (intertrochanteric fracture). [S701-L126]

c Fractures within the joint capsule can impair the blood supply to the femoral neck and femoral head due to ruptured branches of the A. circumflexa femoris medialis and lateralis. In addition to a marked loss of blood, an **avascular necrosis** can occur and prevent the fracture from healing. The risk is higher with a femoral neck fracture than with an intertrochanteric fracture because the latter is located outside the joint capsule. [S701-L266]

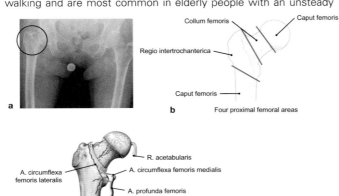

Collum femoris

Caput femoris

Regio intertrochanterica

Caput femoris

Four proximal femoral areas

a

b

R. acetabularis

A. circumflexa femoris lateralis

A. circumflexa femoris medialis

A. profunda femoris

c

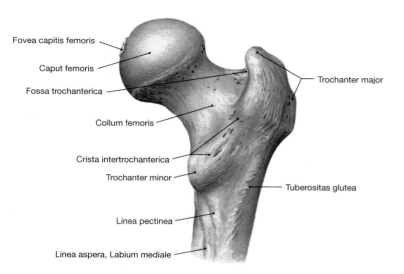

Fovea capitis femoris

Caput femoris

Fossa trochanterica

Collum femoris

Crista intertrochanterica

Trochanter minor

Linea pectinea

Linea aspera, Labium mediale

Trochanter major

Tuberositas glutea

Fig. 4.21 Proximal end of the femur, right side; dorsal view. [S700]

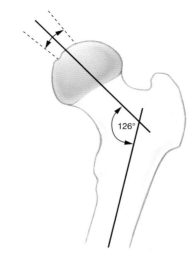

126°

Fig. 4.22 Proximal end of the femur, right side; with illustration of the femoral neck-shaft angle. [S700]
The femoral neck forms an angle of **126°** with the longitudinal axis of the femoral shaft. This angle is referred to as the **centrum-collum-dia-physeal angle (CCD angle).** In a newborn, the CCD angle measures 150°. An **increased CCD angle** is referred to as a **Coxa valga** deformity, and a **decreased CCD angle** as **Coxa vara.**

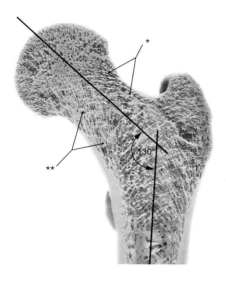

*

**

130°

Fig. 4.23 Proximal end of the femur, right side; illustrating the spongy bone structure with an increased femoral neck-shaft angle (Coxa valga). The section is at the level of the antetorsion angle. [S700]
The **spongy bone trabeculae** are arranged in **curved lines,** i. e. along the lines of maximum traction and compression forces (so-called trajectories). With Coxa valga the **compressive** loads increase. Therefore, the medially located 'traction bundle' (**) of the spongy bone trabeculae is more developed, while the size of the laterally located 'compression bundle' (*) of the spongy bone is reduced.

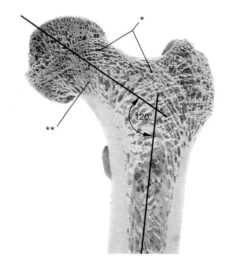

*

**

120°

Fig. 4.24 Proximal end of the femur, right side; illustrating the spongy bone structure with a decreased femoral neck-shaft angle (Coxa vara). Section at the level of the antetorsion angle. [S700]
The **tensile** stresses increase in the Coxa vara. The lateral 'traction bundle' (*) of the spongy bone is strengthened and the medial 'pressure bundle' (**) is less pronounced. Because of the high **stress when bending,** the cortical bone on the medial side of the femoral neck is particularly strong.

Clinical remarks

Changes in the femoral neck-shaft angle can restrict the range of motion. In Coxa vara in particular, the abduction is reduced. Changing the stress on the articular surfaces in the case of **Coxa vara** or **Coxa valga** may cause increased wear and tear, resulting in degenerative arthritis of the hip joint **(coxarthrosis)** or the knee joint. In addition, **Coxa vara** predisposes to **fractures of the femoral neck due to increased stress when bending.**

Angle of inclination

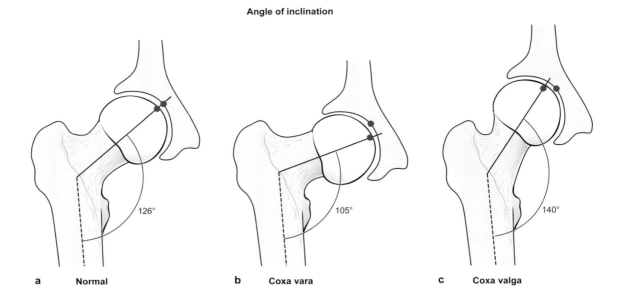

a   Normal   b   Coxa vara   c   Coxa valga

Fig. 4.25a–c   Coxa vara and Coxa valga. Proximal ends of the femur; ventral view. [S701-L126]
a The femoral neck-shaft angle and femoral shaft (centrum-collum-diaphyseal angle) is ususally approx. 126°.

b When the angle is smaller, it is called a **Coxa vara.**
c When the angle is wider, it is called a **Coxa valga.**

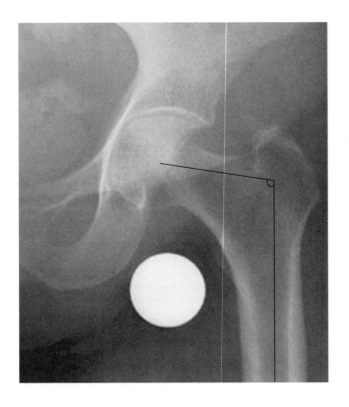

Fig. 4.26   Coxa vara, left side; X-ray image in anteroposterior projection. [R333]

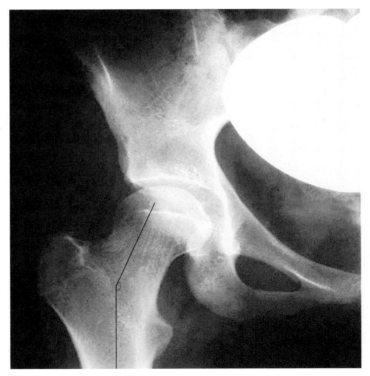

Fig. 4.27   Coxa valga, right side; X-ray image in anteroposterior projection. [R333]

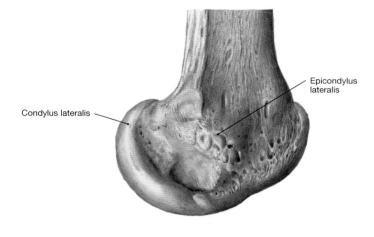

Condylus lateralis

Epicondylus lateralis

Fig. 4.28 Distal end of the femur, right side; lateral view. [S700]
To understand the flexion-extension movement in the knee joint (→ Fig. 4.72), the shape of the articular surfaces of the femoral condyles is important. The articular surfaces are shifted dorsally in relation to the median axis of the shaft **(retroposition).** In addition, the condyles have a **greater curvature at the back** (smaller radius of curvature) than at the front (larger radius of curvature). Their curvature is therefore **spiral-shaped.** This phenomenon is more distinct at the medial than at the lateral condyle (→ Fig. 4.54b).

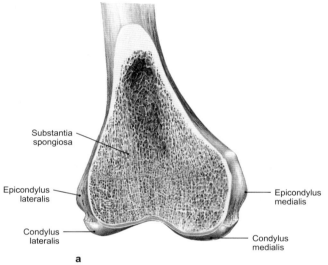

Substantia spongiosa

Epicondylus lateralis

Epicondylus medialis

Condylus lateralis

Condylus medialis

a

Facies patellaris

Epicondylus lateralis

Epicondylus medialis

Condylus lateralis

Condylus medialis

Fossa intercondylaris

b

Fig. 4.29a and b Distal end of the femur, right side. [S700]
a Frontal section through the body of the joint; ventral view.
b Distal view.

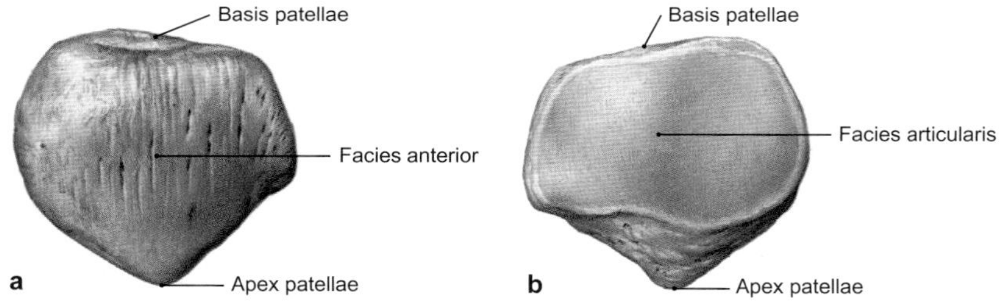

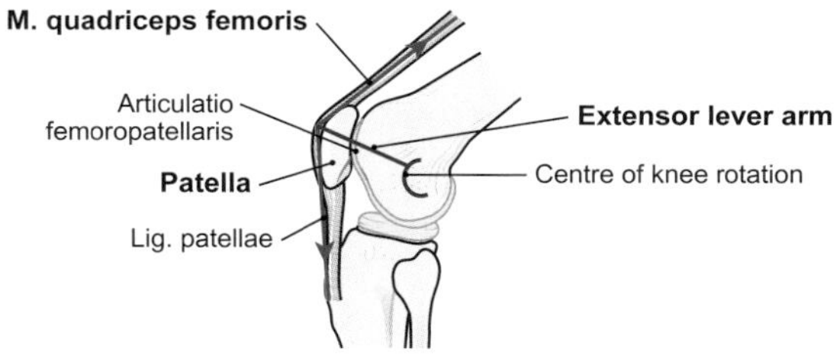

Basis patellae

Facies anterior

Apex patellae

a

Basis patellae

Facies articularis

Apex patellae

b

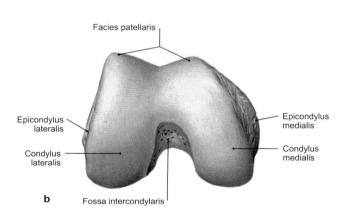

M. quadriceps femoris

Articulatio femoropatellaris

Extensor lever arm

Patella

Centre of knee rotation

Lig. patellae

Fig. 4.30a and b Patella, right side. [S700]
a Ventral view.
b Dorsal view.
The patella is a **sesamoid bone** (Os sesamoideum) within the tendon of the M. quadriceps femoris.

Fig. 4.31 Function of the patella. [S701-L126]
The patella serves as a **hypomochlion** and guides the tendon over the distal end of the femur to its insertion site at the Tuberositas tibiae. This raises the virtual lever arm of the M. quadriceps femoris and almost doubles its torque.

Clinical remarks

Since arthritis of the knee joints **(knee arthritis)** is a common disease and frequently requires prosthetic surgery on both articular surfaces **(total knee replacement,** TKR), anatomical knowledge of the articulating bones is of utmost importance. Recent studies have shown that the shape of the articular surfaces and the radius of curvature of both femoral condyles differ slightly on either side. In knee prosthetics therefore, every attempt is made to reproduce the shape of the articular surfaces as precisely as possible, so that the prostheses allow similar motion patterns as in a healthy knee.

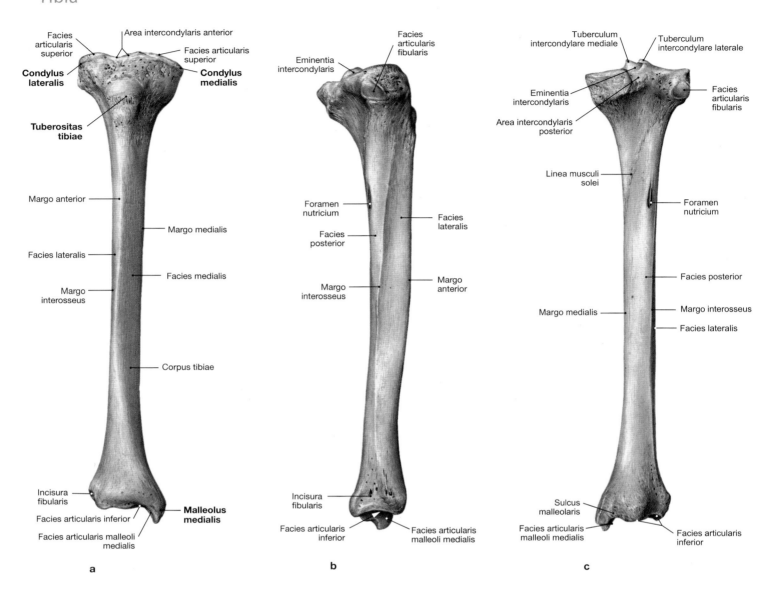

Facies articularis superior
Area intercondylaris anterior
Facies articularis superior
Condylus lateralis
Condylus medialis
Tuberositas tibiae
Margo anterior
Margo medialis
Facies lateralis
Facies medialis
Margo interosseus
Corpus tibiae
Incisura fibularis
Facies articularis inferior
Facies articularis malleoli medialis
Malleolus medialis

a

Facies articularis fibularis
Eminentia intercondylaris
Foramen nutricium
Facies posterior
Facies lateralis
Margo interosseus
Margo anterior
Incisura fibularis
Facies articularis inferior
Facies articularis malleoli medialis

b

Tuberculum intercondylare mediale
Tuberculum intercondylare laterale
Eminentia intercondylaris
Facies articularis fibularis
Area intercondylaris posterior
Linea musculi solei
Foramen nutricium
Facies posterior
Margo medialis
Margo interosseus
Facies lateralis
Sulcus malleolaris
Facies articularis malleoli medialis
Facies articularis inferior

c

Fig. 4.32a–c Tibia, right side. [S700]
a Ventral view.
b Lateral view.
c Dorsal view.

The proximal articular surface is shifted dorsally from the median axis of the shaft **(retroposition)**. In addition, the articular surface is tilted slightly dorsally by 3°–7° **(retroversion)**. The retroversion is more pronounced at the medial condyle than at the lateral condyle and especially affects the medial rim of the articular surface here.

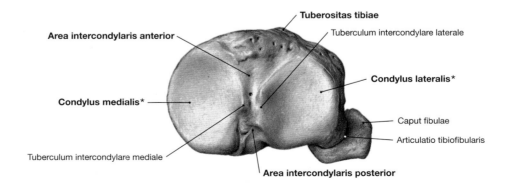

Tuberositas tibiae
Tuberculum intercondylare laterale
Area intercondylaris anterior
Condylus lateralis*
Condylus medialis*
Caput fibulae
Articulatio tibiofibularis
Tuberculum intercondylare mediale
Area intercondylaris posterior

Fig. 4.33 Tibia and fibula, right side; proximal view. [S700]

The articular surfaces of the condyles (*) are collectively referred to as **Facies articularis superior**.

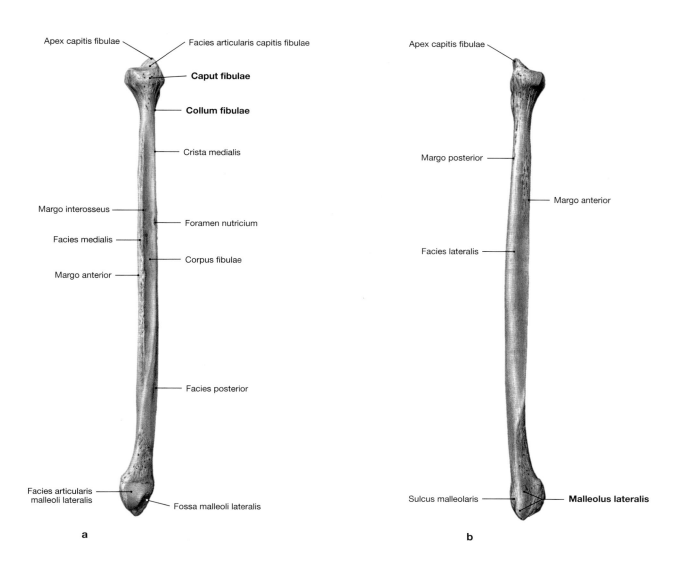

Apex capitis fibulae

Facies articularis capitis fibulae

Caput fibulae

Collum fibulae

Crista medialis

Margo interosseus

Foramen nutricium

Facies medialis

Corpus fibulae

Margo anterior

Facies posterior

Facies articularis malleoli lateralis

Fossa malleoli lateralis

a

Apex capitis fibulae

Margo posterior

Margo anterior

Facies lateralis

Sulcus malleolaris

Malleolus lateralis

b

Fig. 4.34a and b   Fibula, right side. [S700]
a Medial view.
b Lateral view.

For proper positioning of an isolated fibula, both the articular surface of the fibula head and that of the ankle should be facing medially.

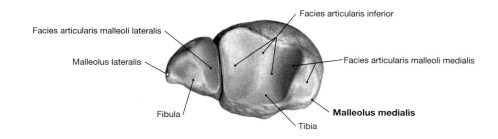

Facies articularis inferior

Facies articularis malleoli lateralis

Malleolus lateralis

Facies articularis malleoli medialis

Fibula

Malleolus medialis

Tibia

Fig. 4.35   Tibia and fibula, right side; distal view. [S700]

Bones of the foot

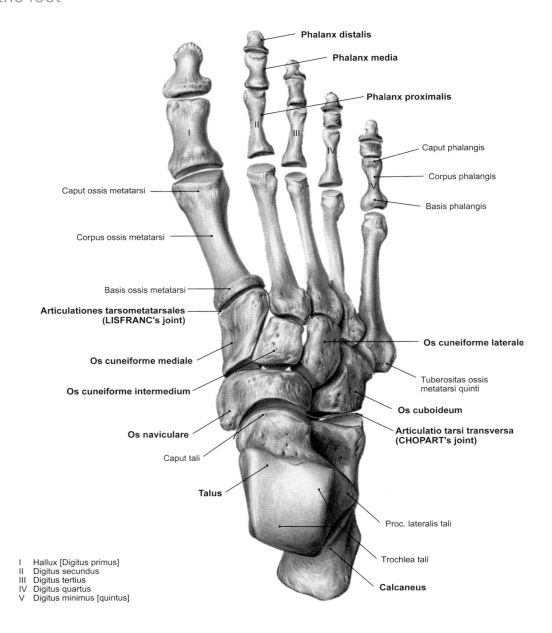

Phalanx distalis

Phalanx media

Phalanx proximalis

Caput phalangis

Corpus phalangis

Basis phalangis

Caput ossis metatarsi

Corpus ossis metatarsi

Basis ossis metatarsi

**Articulationes tarsometatarsales
(LISFRANC's joint)**

Os cuneiforme mediale

Os cuneiforme intermedium

Os naviculare

Caput tali

Talus

Os cuneiforme laterale

Tuberositas ossis
metatarsi quinti

Os cuboideum

**Articulatio tarsi transversa
(CHOPART's joint)**

Proc. lateralis tali

Trochlea tali

Calcaneus

I   Hallux [Digitus primus]
II Digitus secundus
III Digitus tertius
IV Digitus quartus
V   Digitus minimus [quintus]

Fig. 4.36 Bones of foot, Ossa pedis, right side; dorsal view. [S700] The foot **(Pes)** can be divided into the **tarsus** with tarsal bones, Ossa tarsi, the **metatarsus** with the metatarsal bones (Ossa metatarsi) and the toes (Digiti pedis), which consist of several phalanges. The tarsus includes **the ankle or talus, the heel or calcaneus, the navicular** **bone (Os naviculare), the cuboid bone (Os cuboideum)** and the three **cuneiform bones (Ossa cuneiformia).** Clinically, there is a distinction between the hindfoot and forefoot. The articular line in the tarsometatarsal joints is mostly considered the line that separates the two parts of the foot.

Clinical remarks

The Articulatio tarsi transversa (clin.: **CHOPART's joint;** blue) and the Articulationes tarsometatarsales (clin.: **LISFRANC's joint;** red) are preferred locations for surgical amputations in the case of injuries, frostbite, or circulatory disorders associated with necrosis. **Dislocations** occur very rarely in these joints.

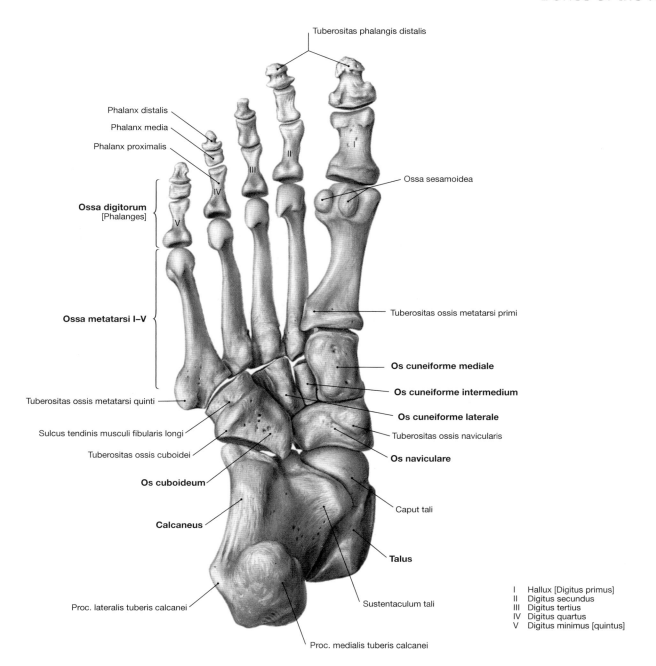

Tuberositas phalangis distalis

Phalanx distalis

Phalanx media

Phalanx proximalis

Ossa digitorum
[Phalanges]

Ossa metatarsi I–V

Tuberositas ossis metatarsi quinti

Sulcus tendinis musculi fibularis longi

Tuberositas ossis cuboidei

Os cuboideum

Calcaneus

Proc. lateralis tuberis calcanei

Ossa sesamoidea

Tuberositas ossis metatarsi primi

Os cuneiforme mediale

Os cuneiforme intermedium

Os cuneiforme laterale

Tuberositas ossis navicularis

Os naviculare

Caput tali

Talus

Sustentaculum tali

Proc. medialis tuberis calcanei

I	Hallux [Digitus primus]
II	Digitus secundus
III	Digitus tertius
IV	Digitus quartus
V	Digitus minimus [quintus]

Fig. 4.37 Bones of the foot, Ossa pedis, right side; plantar view.
[S700]

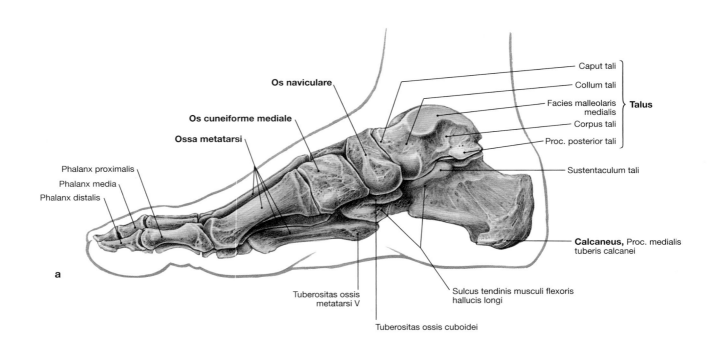

Caput tali
Collum tali
Facies malleolaris medialis
Corpus tali
Proc. posterior tali

Talus

Os naviculare

Os cuneiforme mediale

Ossa metatarsi

Phalanx proximalis
Phalanx media
Phalanx distalis

Sustentaculum tali

Calcaneus, Proc. medialis tuberis calcanei

Sulcus tendinis musculi flexoris hallucis longi

Tuberositas ossis metatarsi V

Tuberositas ossis cuboidei

a

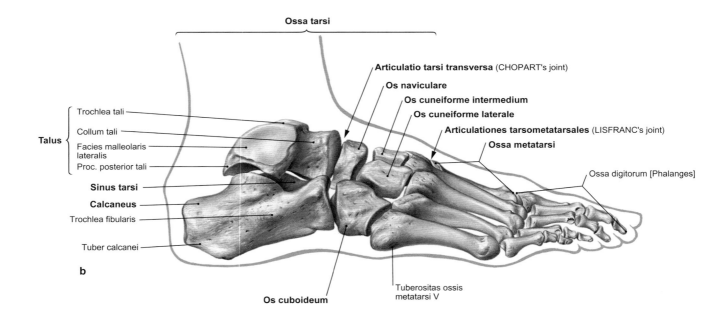

Ossa tarsi

Articulatio tarsi transversa (CHOPART's joint)

Os naviculare

Os cuneiforme intermedium

Os cuneiforme laterale

Articulationes tarsometatarsales (LISFRANC's joint)

Ossa metatarsi

Ossa digitorum [Phalanges]

Trochlea tali
Collum tali
Facies malleolaris lateralis
Proc. posterior tali

Talus

Sinus tarsi

Calcaneus

Trochlea fibularis

Tuber calcanei

b

Os cuboideum

Tuberositas ossis metatarsi V

Fig. 4.38a and b   Bones of the foot, Ossa pedis, right side. [S700]
a Medial view.
b Lateral view.

The Sinus tarsi is a hollow space which is formed by both the Sulcus tali and the Sulcus calcanei.

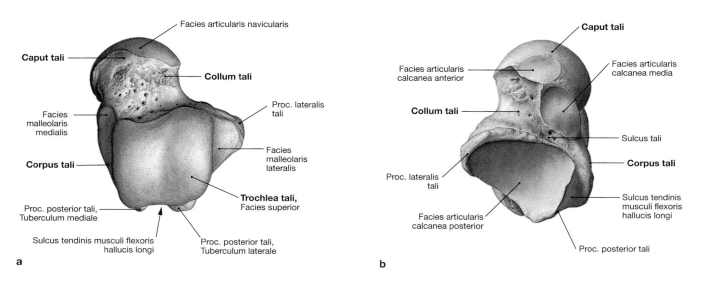

Facies articularis navicularis

Caput tali

Collum tali

Facies
malleolaris
medialis

Proc. lateralis
tali

Corpus tali

Facies
malleolaris
lateralis

Trochlea tali,
Facies superior

Proc. posterior tali,
Tuberculum mediale

Sulcus tendinis musculi flexoris
hallucis longi

Proc. posterior tali,
Tuberculum laterale

a

Caput tali

Facies articularis
calcanea anterior

Facies articularis
calcanea media

Collum tali

Sulcus tali

Proc. lateralis
tali

Corpus tali

Facies articularis
calcanea posterior

Sulcus tendinis
musculi flexoris
hallucis longi

Proc. posterior tali

b

Fig. 4.39a and b   Talus, right side. [S700]
a Dorsal view. The Trochlea tali is wider at the front than at the back.
b Plantar view.

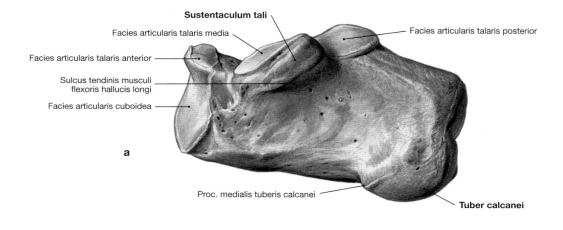

Sustentaculum tali

Facies articularis talaris media

Facies articularis talaris posterior

Facies articularis talaris anterior

Sulcus tendinis musculi
flexoris hallucis longi

Facies articularis cuboidea

a

Proc. medialis tuberis calcanei

Tuber calcanei

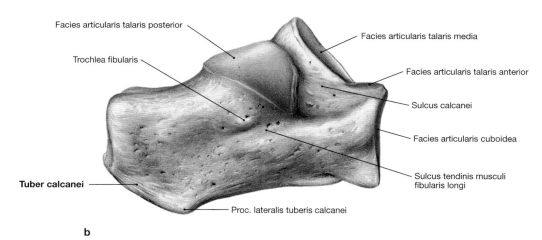

Facies articularis talaris posterior

Facies articularis talaris media

Trochlea fibularis

Facies articularis talaris anterior

Sulcus calcanei

Facies articularis cuboidea

Sulcus tendinis musculi
fibularis longi

Tuber calcanei

Proc. lateralis tuberis calcanei

b

Fig. 4.40a and b   Calcaneus, right side. [S700]
a Medial view.
b Lateral view.

Joints and ligaments of the pelvis

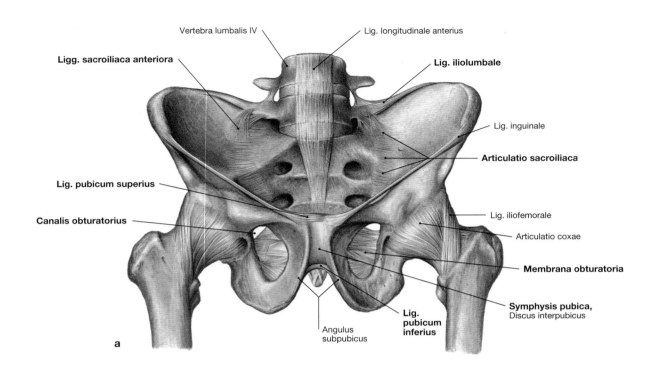

Vertebra lumbalis IV — Lig. longitudinale anterius

Ligg. sacroiliaca anteriora — **Lig. iliolumbale**

Lig. inguinale

Articulatio sacroiliaca

Lig. pubicum superius

Lig. iliofemorale

Canalis obturatorius

Articulatio coxae

Membrana obturatoria

Symphysis pubica, Discus interpubicus

Angulus subpubicus — **Lig. pubicum inferius**

a

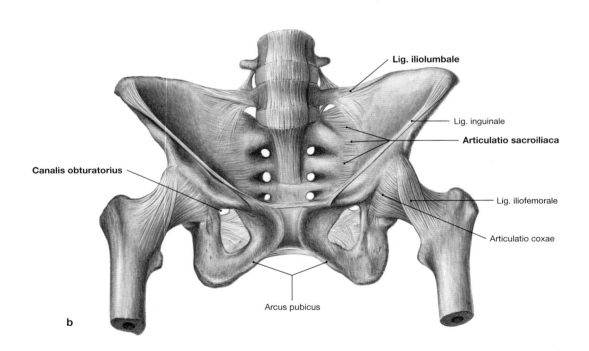

Lig. iliolumbale

Lig. inguinale

Articulatio sacroiliaca

Canalis obturatorius

Lig. iliofemorale

Articulatio coxae

Arcus pubicus

b

Fig. 4.41a and b   Joints and ligaments of the pelvis; ventral view. [S700]
a View of the male pelvis.
b View of the female pelvis.
The pelvic girdle (Cingulum pelvicum) is connected dorsally by the two amphiarthroses of the sacroiliac joints **(Articulationes sacroiliacae)** and ventrally by the pubic symphysis **(Symphysis pubica)** to form a ring structure. Each sacroiliac joint is stabilised ventrally by the **Ligg. sacroiliaca anteriora** and superiorly by the **Lig. iliolumbale** that runs from the Proc. costalis of the fourth and fifth lumbar vertebrae to the

Crista iliaca (at the dorsal ligaments, → Fig. 4.43). This strong ligamentous apparatus only allows small tilting movements of the pelvis of about 10°.
The pubic symphysis is bridged by the **Lig. pubicum superius** above and the **Lig. pubicum inferius** below.
In both sexes, the Foramen obturatum is almost completely closed off by the **Membrana obturatoria** so that only the **Canalis obturatorius** remains open for the neurovascular pathways to pass through to the medial side of the thigh (A./V. obturatoria, N. obturatorius).

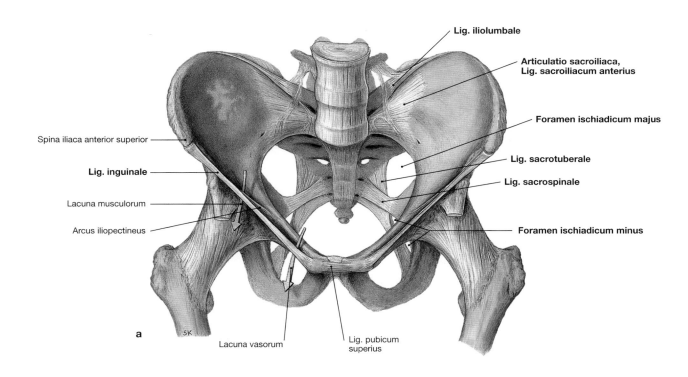

Lig. iliolumbale

Articulatio sacroiliaca,
Lig. sacroiliacum anterius

Foramen ischiadicum majus

Lig. sacrotuberale

Lig. sacrospinale

Foramen ischiadicum minus

Spina iliaca anterior superior

Lig. inguinale

Lacuna musculorum

Arcus iliopectineus

a

Lacuna vasorum

Lig. pubicum
superius

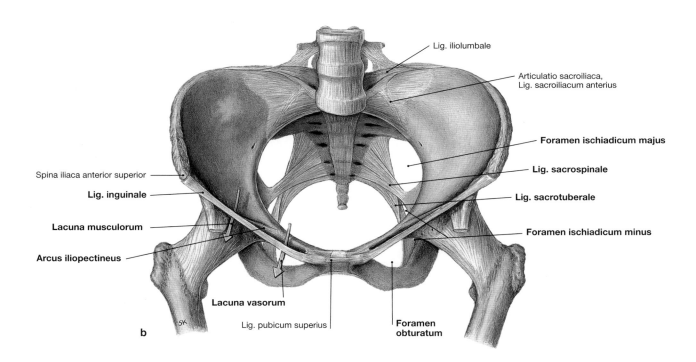

Lig. iliolumbale

Articulatio sacroiliaca,
Lig. sacroiliacum anterius

Foramen ischiadicum majus

Lig. sacrospinale

Lig. sacrotuberale

Foramen ischiadicum minus

Spina iliaca anterior superior

Lig. inguinale

Lacuna musculorum

Arcus iliopectineus

Lacuna vasorum

Lig. pubicum superius

Foramen
obturatum

b

Fig. 4.42a and b   Joints and ligaments of the pelvis; ventrocranial view. [S700-L238]
a View of the male pelvis.
b View of the female pelvis.
The almost horizontal course of the **Lig. sacrospinale** connects the sacrum with the Spina ischiadica, and dorsally, the oblique course of the **Lig. sacrotuberale** runs to the Tuber ischiadicum. Both ligaments complete the Incisurae ischiadicae major and minor to the **Foramen**

ischiadicum majus and the **Foramen ischiadicum minus.** These openings are significant passageways for the blood vessels and nerves of the Plexus sacralis to pass to the gluteal region (Regio glutealis). The space below the groin or inguinal ligament **(Lig. inguinale)** is divided by the Arcus iliopectineus into the lateral Lacuna musculorum and the medial Lacuna vasorum (→ Fig. 4.175) through which the neurovascular pathways pass to the anterior side of the thigh.

Joints and ligaments of the pelvis

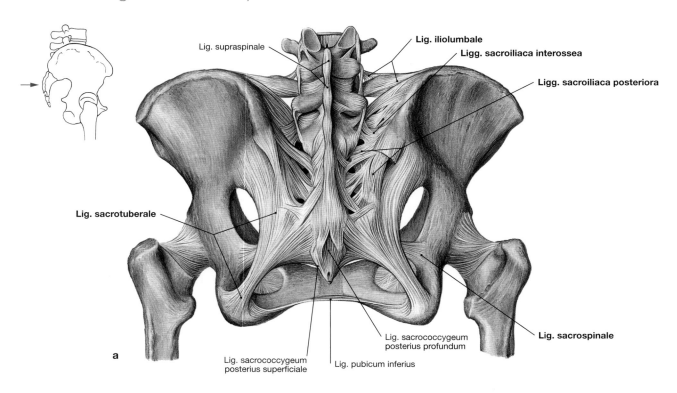

Lig. supraspinale

Lig. iliolumbale

Ligg. sacroiliaca interossea

Ligg. sacroiliaca posteriora

Lig. sacrotuberale

Lig. sacrospinale

Lig. sacrococcygeum posterius profundum

Lig. sacrococcygeum posterius superficiale

Lig. pubicum inferius

a

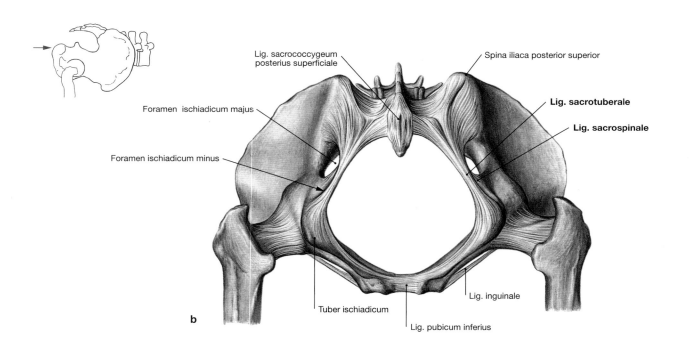

Lig. sacrococcygeum posterius superficiale

Spina iliaca posterior superior

Foramen ischiadicum majus

Lig. sacrotuberale

Foramen ischiadicum minus

Lig. sacrospinale

Tuber ischiadicum

Lig. inguinale

Lig. pubicum inferius

b

Fig. 4.43a and b   Joints and ligaments of the pelvis in females.
[S700]
a Dorsal view.
b Caudal view.
On the dorsal side, the sacroiliac joint is stabilised by the **Ligg. sacro-iliaca posteriora and interossea** (for the ligaments at the front, → Fig. 4.41). Due to the strongly developed ligaments, particularly on

the posterior side, only small tilting movements of the pelvis of up to 10° are possible.
The almost horizontal **Lig. sacrospinale** connects the sacrum with the Spina ischiadica, and dorsally the oblique **Lig. sacrotuberale** runs to the Tuber ischiadicum. Both ligaments confine the **Foramina ischiadi-ca majus and minus** which are passageways for the blood vessels and nerves of the Plexus sacralis to the gluteal region.

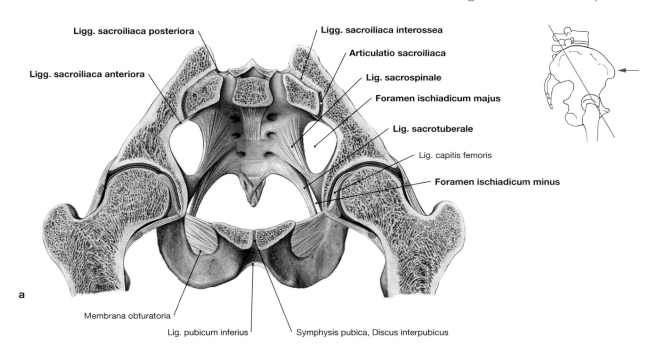

Ligg. sacroiliaca posteriora

Ligg. sacroiliaca anteriora

Ligg. sacroiliaca interossea

Articulatio sacroiliaca

Lig. sacrospinale

Foramen ischiadicum majus

Lig. sacrotuberale

Lig. capitis femoris

Foramen ischiadicum minus

a

Membrana obturatoria

Lig. pubicum inferius

Symphysis pubica, Discus interpubicus

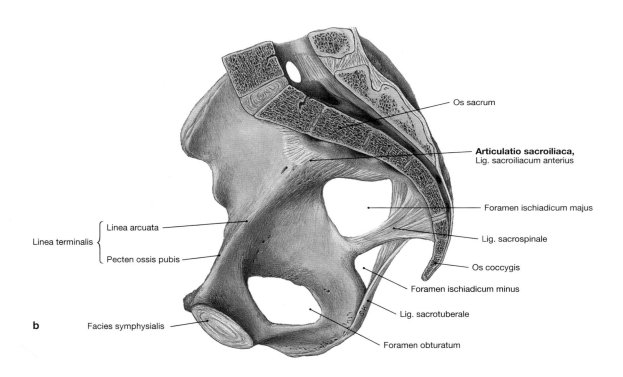

Os sacrum

Articulatio sacroiliaca,
Lig. sacroiliacum anterius

Foramen ischiadicum majus

Linea terminalis { Linea arcuata

Pecten ossis pubis

Lig. sacrospinale

Os coccygis

Foramen ischiadicum minus

Lig. sacrotuberale

b Facies symphysialis

Foramen obturatum

Fig. 4.44a and b   Joints and ligaments of the pelvis in females.
a Oblique cross-section; ventrocaudal view. [S700]
b Median section; view from the left side. [S700-L238]
The sacroiliac joint is illustrated here with its ligaments (**Ligg. sacroiliaca anteriora, posteriora** and **interossea** as well as the **Lig. sacrospi-**
nale and the **Lig. sacrotuberale**). Only the **Lig. iliolumbale** is not visible. The Lig. sacrospinale and Lig. sacrotuberale confine the **Foramina**
ischiadica majus and **minus** which are passageways for the blood
vessels and nerves of the Plexus sacralis to the gluteal region.

Joints and ligaments of the pelvis

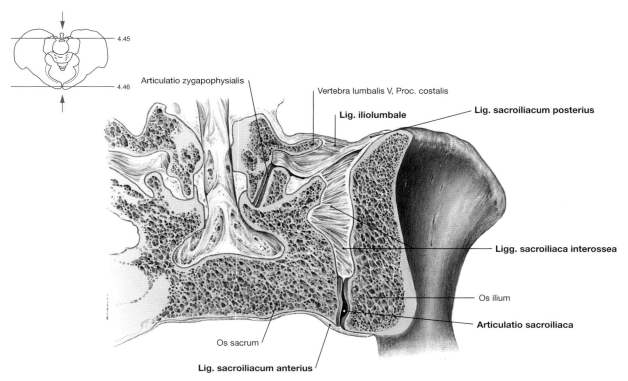

Fig. 4.45 Sacroiliac joint, Articulatio sacroiliaca; frontal section; dorsal view. [S700]
The strong ligaments, of which the **Ligg. sacroiliaca anteriora and interossea,** as well as the **Lig. iliolumbale** can be seen here, stabilise the sacroiliac joint and enable a transfer of weight from the trunk to the pelvic girdle. In particular, the dorsal **Ligg. sacroiliaca interossea** and **posteriora** broadly connect the sacrum and ilium.

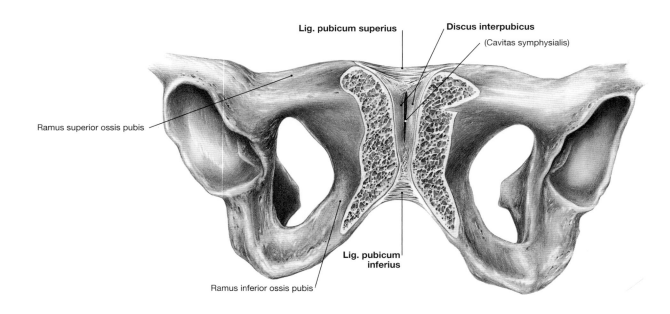

Fig. 4.46 Pubic symphysis, Symphysis pubica; oblique section; ventrocaudal view. [S700]
The pubic symphysis is a cartilaginous fixed joint (symphysis). The **Discus interpubicus** consists of fibrous cartilage; only the boundaries of the Facies symphysiales of both the pubic bones consist of hyaline cartilage. From the first decade of life, an elongated gap (Cavitas symphysialis) often begins to develop. This gap is bridged by the **Lig. pubicum superius** above and the **Lig. pubicum inferius** below.

Clinical remarks

Pain in the sacroiliac joint can be caused by **injury** and **degenerative osteoarthritis** as well as rheumatic diseases, which in part tend to primarily affect this joint (Morbus BECHTEREW). Since the sacroiliac joint is located directly below the nerve branches of the Plexus lumbosacralis, pain may radiate into the leg (→ Fig. 4.142).

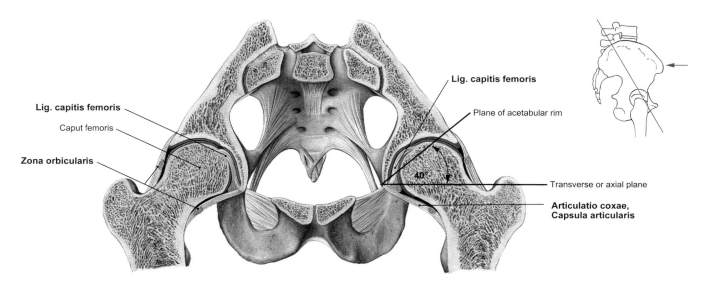

Fig. 4.47   Hip joints, Articulationes coxae; oblique cross-section; ventrocranial view. [S700]

In the **hip joint,** the acetabulum forms the socket. The head of the joint is the proximal end of the femur.

Together with the Labrum acetabuli, the acetabulum covers more than half of the femoral head (Caput femoris). Thus, the hip joint is a special form of a ball-and-socket joint, referred to as the **cotyloid joint** (Articulatio cotylica, enarthrosis). The **angle** between the **acetabular rim**

plane and the horizontal line is **40°.** The hip joint transfers the whole body weight onto the legs. Therefore, the joint capsule **(Capsula articularis)** is reinforced by a strong ligamentous apparatus. Circular fibres of the joint capsule surround the femoral neck, in particular on the dorsal side, and are referred to as **Zona orbicularis.** The ligaments of the capsule also radiate into this zone. The Lig. capitis femoris has no mechanical function.

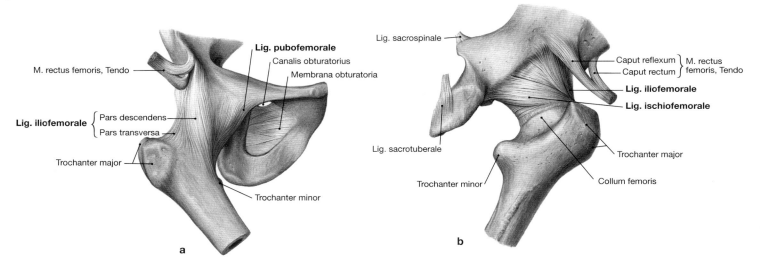

Fig. 4.48a and b   Hip joint, Articulatio coxae, right side. [S700]
a Ventral view.
b Dorsal view.

The ligamentous apparatus of the hip joint essentially consists of three ligaments that spiral around the femoral head and neck. **Their main function** is to confine the **extension** and to **prevent the tilting** of the pelvis in a **dorsal direction,** since the ligaments become stretched by extension and thereby clamp the femoral head as if in a vice:

- **Lig. iliofemorale** (in front, above): inhibits not only extension, but also in particular the adduction, which lessens the load on the small gluteal muscles
- **Lig. pubofemorale** (in front, below): inhibits extension, abduction and external rotation
- **Lig. ischiofemorale** (at the back): inhibits extension, and in particular internal rotation and adduction.

Clinical remarks

Orthopaedic studies show that the position and shape of the acetabulum and femoral head are important factors in the development of osteoarthritis in the hip joint **(coxarthrosis).** Premature degenerative changes may be induced by the socket not fully covering the ball portion of the upper thighbone **(hip dysplasia),** characterised by a

lower than usual **angle of the acetabular rim plane,** as well as it covering the hip joint more than usual. The covering can be too extensive if the acetabular rim projects forwards, with the hip socket tilted dorsally **(retroversion of the acetabulum),** or if the articular surface is located deep inside the acetabulum **(Coxa profunda).**

Structure and movement of the hip joint

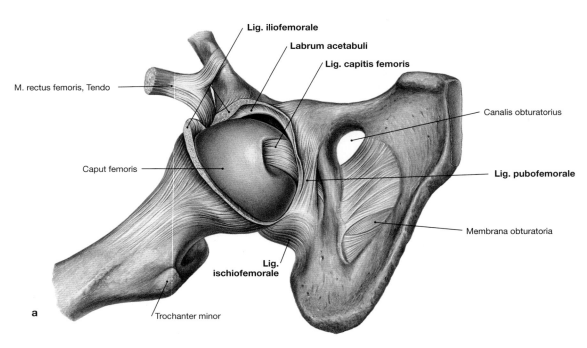

M. rectus femoris, Tendo

Lig. iliofemorale

Labrum acetabuli

Lig. capitis femoris

Canalis obturatorius

Caput femoris

Lig. pubofemorale

Membrana obturatoria

Lig. ischiofemorale

Trochanter minor

a

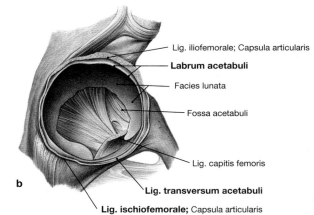

Lig. iliofemorale; Capsula articularis

Labrum acetabuli

Facies lunata

Fossa acetabuli

Lig. capitis femoris

b

Lig. transversum acetabuli

Lig. ischiofemorale; Capsula articularis

Fig. 4.49a and b Hip joint, Articulatio coxae, right side; ventral view. [S700]
a With a capsulotomy and partial exarticulation of the femoral head.
b With removal of the femoral head.
In addition to the external ligaments **(Lig. iliofemorale, Lig. pubofem-orale, Lig. ischiofemorale),** the **Lig. capitis femoris** is also visible inside the joint, which lacks any support function. The **Lig. transversum acetabuli** completes the acetabulum below by forming a ring and, along with the **Labrum acetabuli,** which also consists of fibrous connective tissue, guides the femoral head.

Structure and function

The hip joint is a **ball-and-socket joint** with a restricted range of movement because the femoral head articulates in a deep socket of the acetabulum. The socket is enlarged to such an extent by a rim of interstitial tissue, the Labrum acetabuli, that it surrounds more than half of the diameter of the femoral head. Stabilised by the **Lig. ili-** **ofemorale, Lig. pubofemorale and Lig. ischiofemorale,** the hip joint is well protected from most injuries, except from massive trauma such as a severe car accident when the legs of the passengers are compressed into the hip joint.

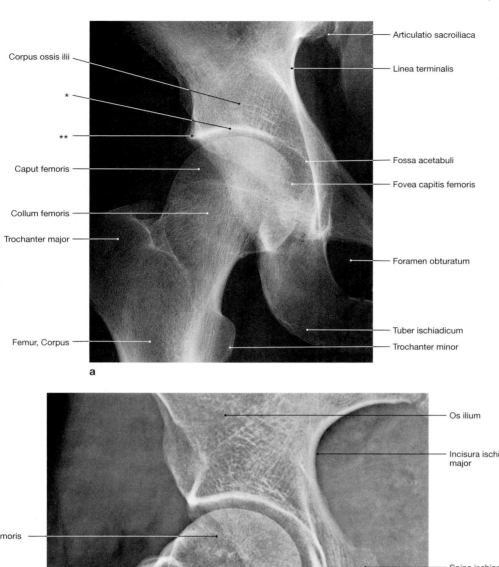

Corpus ossis ilii

*

**

Caput femoris

Collum femoris

Trochanter major

Femur, Corpus

a

Articulatio sacroiliaca

Linea terminalis

Fossa acetabuli

Fovea capitis femoris

Foramen obturatum

Tuber ischiadicum

Trochanter minor

Os ilium

Incisura ischiadica major

Caput femoris

Trochanter major

Spina ischiadica

Incisura ischiadica minor

Foramen obturatum

Trochanter minor

Tuber ischiadicum

b

Fig. 4.50a and b   Hip joint, Articulatio coxae, right side; X-ray images.
a X-ray in anteroposterior (AP) projection; upright stance. [S700-T902]

b X-ray in the so-called LAUENSTEIN projection (abduction and flexion of the thigh; supine position). [S700]
*   clin.: acetabular roof
** clin.: acetabular notch

Clinical remarks

If a disease of the hip joint is suspected, special X-ray images are taken in various joint positions, such as the **LAUENSTEIN projec-tion** in abduction and flexion of the thigh, for allowing a better assessment of the joint bodies.

Hip joint, X-ray

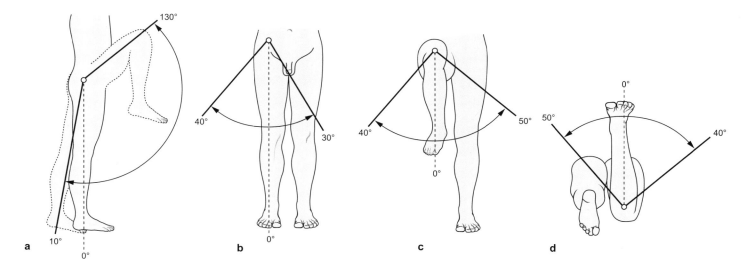

Fig. 4.51a–d Range of movement in the hip joint, Articulatio coxae. [S700-L126]/[S002-5]

The hip joint is a **cotyloid joint** (Articulatio cotylica, enarthrosis), which as a ball-and-socket joint has three degrees of freedom. All its movement axes run through the centre of the femoral head. The range of movement is limited by the strict bony guidance in the acetabulum and by the strong ligamentous apparatus. The ligaments work in unison to limit the extension (retroversion) by surrounding the femoral head like a vice to ensure a stable stance. Flexion (anteversion), however, which is

important when running, has a great degree of freedom and is inhibited only by soft tissue.
Internal and external rotation, abduction and adduction are also limited by the ligaments.

Range of motion:

a Extension–flexion: 10°–0°–130°
b Abduction–adduction: 40°–0°–30°
c and **d** Lateral rotation–medial rotation: 50°–0°–40°

The most important muscles for movements of the hip joint	
Movement	**Muscles**
Anteversion	M. iliopsoas
Retroversion	M. gluteus maximus
Abduction	M. gluteus medius and M. gluteus minimus
Adduction	M. adductor magnus
External rotation	M. gluteus maximus
Internal rotation	M. gluteus medius and M. gluteus minimus

Clinical remarks

The position and shape of the hip socket and the femoral head may induce the development of **osteoarthritis of the hip**. Risk factors include obesity and repeated stress on the joint, as is prevalent with extreme sports (weight-lifting and body-building).

a Destruction of the joint cartilage with hip arthritis can be visualised indirectly by a change in the contours of the femoral head. Additionally, bony spurs (osteophytes) can form at the hip joint (arrows).
b If a conservative treatment with pain medication is ineffective, the hip joint needs to be replaced with a hip prosthesis which can, as shown here, include the replacement of both the femoral head and joint socket (total endoprosthesis, TEP).
[R110-20]

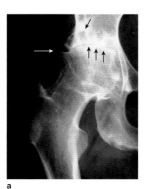

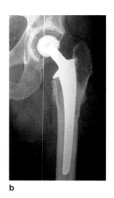

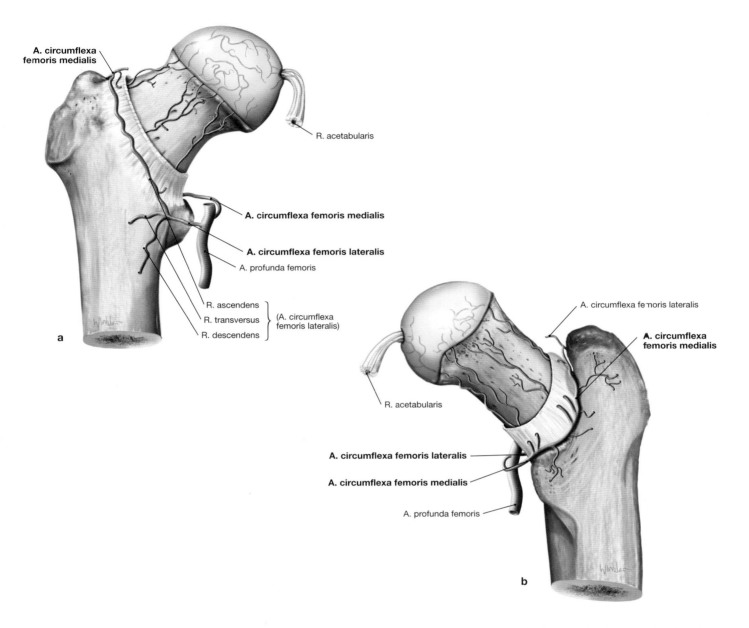

Fig. 4.52a and b   Blood supply to the hip joint, right side.
[S700-L266]
a Ventral view.
b Dorsal view.
In adults, the **A. circumflexa femoris medialis** is the main supplying vessel of the femoral head. While the **R. acetabularis** (from the A. obturatoria and A. circumflexa femoris medialis) which passes through the Lig. capitis femoris, supplies a large proportion of the femoral head in infants, it supplies only one-fifth to one-third of the proximal epiphysis in adults. However, the A. circumflexa femoris medialis supplies the femoral head and neck via several smaller branches running on the posterior side of the neck within the joint capsule. The **A. circumflexa femoris lateralis** primarily supplies the femoral neck on the anterior side. The acetabulum is supplied ventrally and dorsally by the A. obturatoria, and cranially by the A. glutea superior.

Clinical remarks

Arterial blood supply is crucial for the maintenance of the femoral head. Oxygen deficiency (ischaemia) results in **necrosis of the femoral head,** which, in the worst case scenario, requires the replacement of the femoral head by an **endoprosthesis.** Therefore, the supplying arteries must be treated with the utmost care in surgical interventions on the hip joint. It has to be noted that the A. circumflexa femoris medialis runs on the posterior side of the femoral neck, where it is covered and protected by the short hip muscles of the pelvitrochanteric group. These muscles should therefore be left alone in order to avoid injury to the artery.

Because the Aa. circumflexae femoris medialis and lateralis run between the layers of the joint capsule, the supplying arteries may be damaged in the case of intracapsular **femoral neck fractures.** Immediately replacing the femoral head with a prosthesis is therefore increasingly being performed as the treatment of choice. The spontaneous necrosis of the femoral head during early puberty **(PERTHES' disease)** also appears to be mainly caused by an insufficient arterial blood supply to the femoral head.

Lower limb

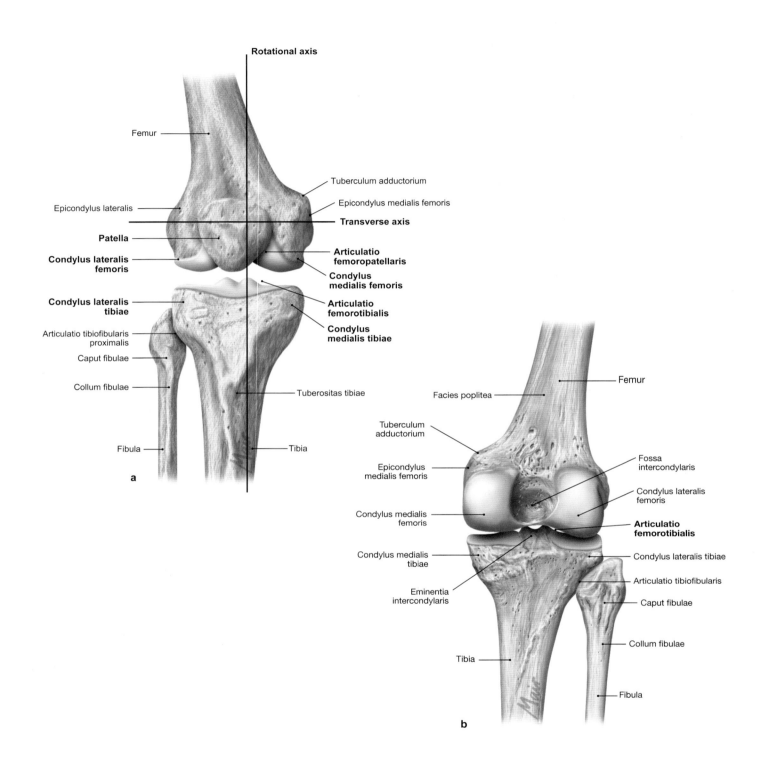

Fig. 4.53a and b   Knee joint, Articulatio genus, right side.
[S700-L127]
a Ventral view.
b Dorsal view.
In the knee joint, the femur articulates with the tibia **(Articulatio femo-rotibialis)** and with the patella **(Articulatio femoropatellaris;** → Fig. 4.197). All the bones are ensheathed by a common joint capsule. In the Articulatio femorotibialis, the femoral condyles constitute the head, and the upper articular surface (Facies articularis superior) of both

tibial condyles forms the socket of the joint. The knee joint is a **bicon-dylar joint** (Articulatio bicondylaris) which functions as a **pivot-hinge joint** (trochoginglymus) and possesses two degrees of freedom in movement. The instantaneous transverse axis of movement for **exten-sion** and **flexion** runs through the trochlea of the femoral condyles. The longitudinal axis of rotational movements runs perpendicularly off-cen-tre through the Tuberculum intercondylare mediale. For the range of motion in the knee joint → Fig. 4.72.

Structure and function

The knee joint is the **most complex large joint** of the human body. This joint contains two menisci and a highly complex and versatile ligamentous apparatus of collateral and cruciate ligaments. Depending on which position the knee joint is in, these components experience different levels of twisting and stress. The knee is a modified **hinge joint** which allows a small degree of medial and lateral rotation. In an extended position, this joint structure allows the transfer of the body weight onto the lower leg without needing to use any muscles for a secure stance. In a flexed position, rotational movements are possible but the knee joint is significantly less stable. Physical work and sport activities can make great demands on a flexed knee, which explains the high frequency of knee injuries, particularly in sport and athletics, where these injuries frequently require reconstructive surgery of the ligamentous apparatus in the knee.

Clinical remarks

In addition to the hip joint, the knee joint bears the body weight. Degeneration of the knee joint **(knee arthritis)** is a common disease and frequently requires prosthetic replacement of the joint. The diagnosis is commonly made by simple X-ray imaging. The clinical staging depends on the severity of the degenerative changes. Moderate to severe degenerative changes include an apparent narrowing of the joint space (arrows). This is caused by a loss of cartilage which is not visible on the X-ray image and therefore appears to be part of the joint space.

Since the knee joint is not well stabilised by muscles, **injuries to the ligamentous apparatus** and the **menisci** occur frequently. These can partially be treated with minimally invasive interventions **(arthroscopy),** requiring a good anatomical knowledge of the knee joint. Malformations of the patella or of the Facies patellaris of the femur may result in repeated **dislocations of the patella.** In addition to physical exercises or training of the respective M. vastus medialis or lateralis, surgical correction with tightening of the joint capsule (capsulorrhaphy) or transfer of the Lig. patellae is the treatment of choice. [R110-20]

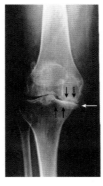

4

Lower limb

Knee joint, X-ray

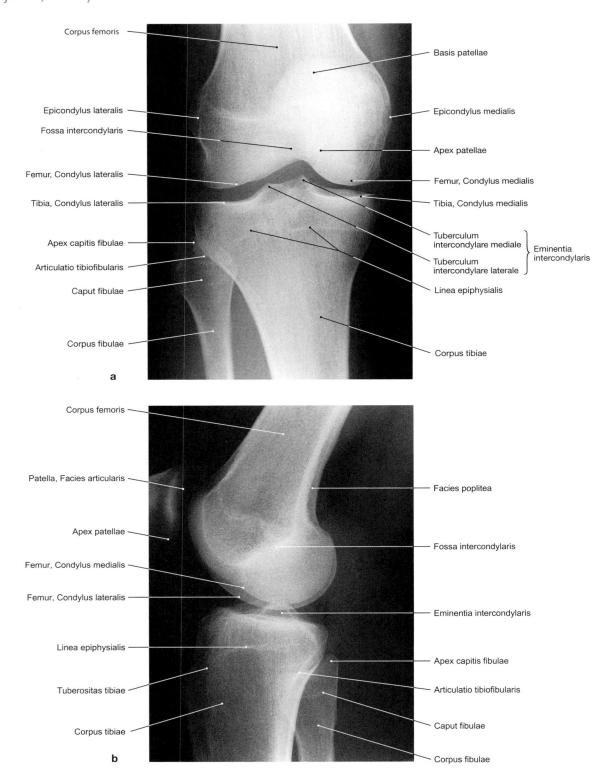

Corpus femoris

Basis patellae

Epicondylus lateralis

Epicondylus medialis

Fossa intercondylaris

Apex patellae

Femur, Condylus lateralis

Femur, Condylus medialis

Tibia, Condylus lateralis

Tibia, Condylus medialis

Apex capitis fibulae

Tuberculum intercondylare mediale

Eminentia intercondylaris

Articulatio tibiofibularis

Tuberculum intercondylare laterale

Caput fibulae

Linea epiphysialis

Corpus fibulae

Corpus tibiae

a

Corpus femoris

Patella, Facies articularis

Facies poplitea

Apex patellae

Fossa intercondylaris

Femur, Condylus medialis

Femur, Condylus lateralis

Eminentia intercondylaris

Linea epiphysialis

Apex capitis fibulae

Tuberositas tibiae

Articulatio tibiofibularis

Corpus tibiae

Caput fibulae

b

Corpus fibulae

Fig. 4.54a and b   Knee joint, Articulatio genus, X-ray image; supine position. [S700-T902]
a X-ray image with anteroposterior (AP) projection.

b X-ray image with lateral projection. Note the fact that the contours of the medial and lateral femoral condyles are not congruent.

Clinical remarks

With diseases of the knee joint, X-ray images are generally taken in two planes. The joint space and socket of the tibia can be better assessed with an anteroposterior (AP) projection, while the femoral condyles are better displayed in lateral views. In addition to fractures, misalignments and degenerative diseases such as osteoarthritis of the knee can also be diagnosed easily.

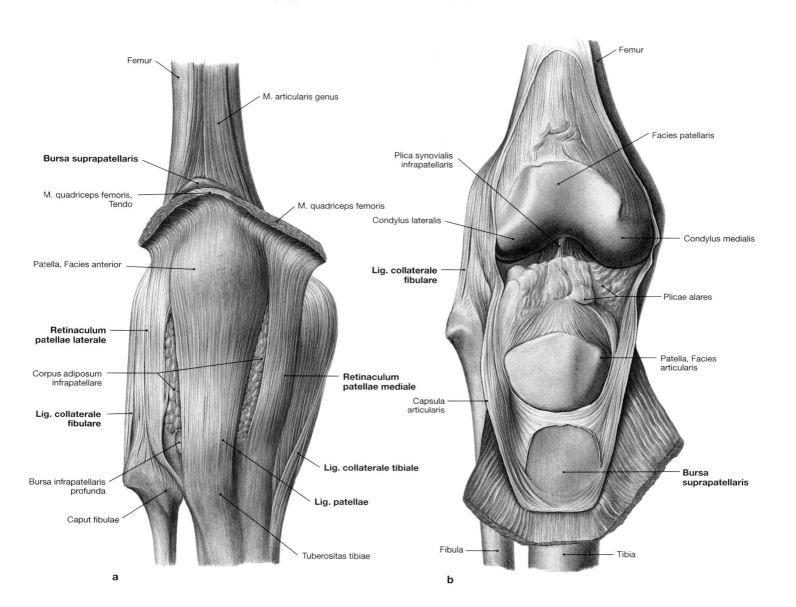

Femur

M. articularis genus

Bursa suprapatellaris

M. quadriceps femoris, Tendo

M. quadriceps femoris

Patella, Facies anterior

Retinaculum patellae laterale

Corpus adiposum infrapatellare

Lig. collaterale fibulare

Bursa infrapatellaris profunda

Caput fibulae

Retinaculum patellae mediale

Lig. collaterale tibiale

Lig. patellae

Tuberositas tibiae

a

Femur

Plica synovialis infrapatellaris

Condylus lateralis

Lig. collaterale fibulare

Facies patellaris

Condylus medialis

Plicae alares

Patella, Facies articularis

Capsula articularis

Bursa suprapatellaris

Fibula

Tibia

b

Fig. 4.55a and b   Knee joint, Articulatio genus, right side; ventral view. [S700]
a View with closed joint capsule.
b View after capsulotomy.
The knee joint is surrounded by **external ligaments** which stabilise the joint and reinforce the capsule from outside, and by **internal ligaments** (→ Fig. 4.64) which lie within the Capsula fibrosa. This is an illustration of the external ligaments. Anteriorly, these include the **Lig. patellae,** which is an extension of the tendon of the M. quadriceps femoris, as well as the **Retinacula patellae mediale** and **laterale,** both of which have superficial longitudinal and deep transverse fibres. They are also

considered to be parts of the inserting tendon of the M. quadriceps femoris (Mm. vasti medialis and lateralis). Medially and laterally, there are two collateral ligaments **(Ligg. collateralia tibiale** and **fibulare)** which insert on the respective bones of the lower leg. The joint capsule follows the joint surfaces at a short distance. The **HOFFA's fat pad (Corpus adiposum infrapatellare),** lying anteriorly between the Membrana fibrosa and Membrana synovialis, is connected to the anterior cruciate ligament via a fold, the Plica synovialis infrapatellaris, and has Plicae alares on both sides. The knee joint is associated with several **bursae,** some of which communicate with the joint capsule, as shown here for the Bursa suprapatellaris.

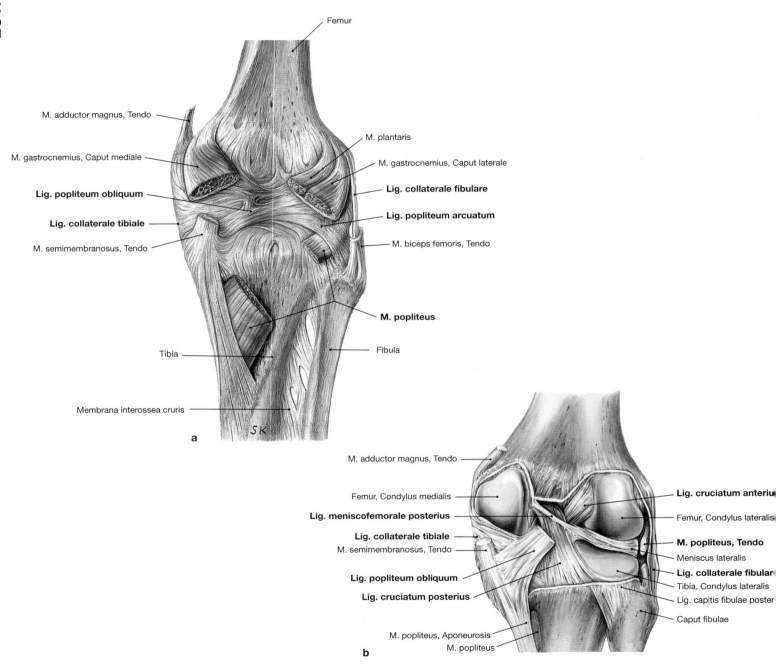

Femur

M. adductor magnus, Tendo

M. plantaris

M. gastrocnemius, Caput mediale

M. gastrocnemius, Caput laterale

Lig. popliteum obliquum

Lig. collaterale fibulare

Lig. collaterale tibiale

Lig. popliteum arcuatum

M. semimembranosus, Tendo

M. biceps femoris, Tendo

M. popliteus

Tibia

Fibula

Membrana interossea cruris

a

M. adductor magnus, Tendo

Femur, Condylus medialis

Lig. cruciatum anteriu

Lig. meniscofemorale posterius

Femur, Condylus lateralis

Lig. collaterale tibiale

M. semimembranosus, Tendo

M. popliteus, Tendo

Meniscus lateralis

Lig. popliteum obliquum

Lig. collaterale fibular

Lig. cruciatum posterius

Tibia, Condylus lateralis

Lig. capitis fibulae poster

Caput fibulae

M. popliteus, Aponeurosis

M. popliteus

b

Fig. 4.56a and b Knee joint, Articulatio genus, right side; dorsal view.

a View of closed joint capsule of the knee. The posterior side of the knee joint contains additional **external ligaments** which reinforce the joint capsule. The **Lig. popliteum obliquum** passes from the lateral femoral condyle medially downwards, while the **Lig. popliteum arcuatum** runs in the opposite direction, thereby bridging the M. popliteus. Of the two collateral ligaments, only the **Lig. collaterale tibiale** is attached to the joint capsule. The **Lig. collaterale fibulare,** however, has **no** attachment to the capsule and is separated from the capsule by the tendon of the M. popliteus. [S700-L238]

b View after capsulotomy. Upon surgical opening of the joint capsule or capsulotomy, several **internal ligaments** are visible. The anterior cruciate ligament **(Lig. cruciatum anterius)** runs from the inner surface of the lateral femoral condyle in an anterior direction to the Area intercondylaris anterior of the tibia. The posterior cruciate ligament **(Lig. cruciatum posterius)** runs in the opposite direction from the inner surface of the medial femoral condyle to the Area intercondylaris posterior of the tibia. The **Lig. meniscofemorale anterius** (not visible here) and the **Lig. meniscofemorale posterius** connect the posterior horn of the lateral meniscus (Meniscus lateralis) with the medial condyle anterior and posterior to the posterior cruciate ligament and thereby support the function of the posterior cruciate ligament. [S700]

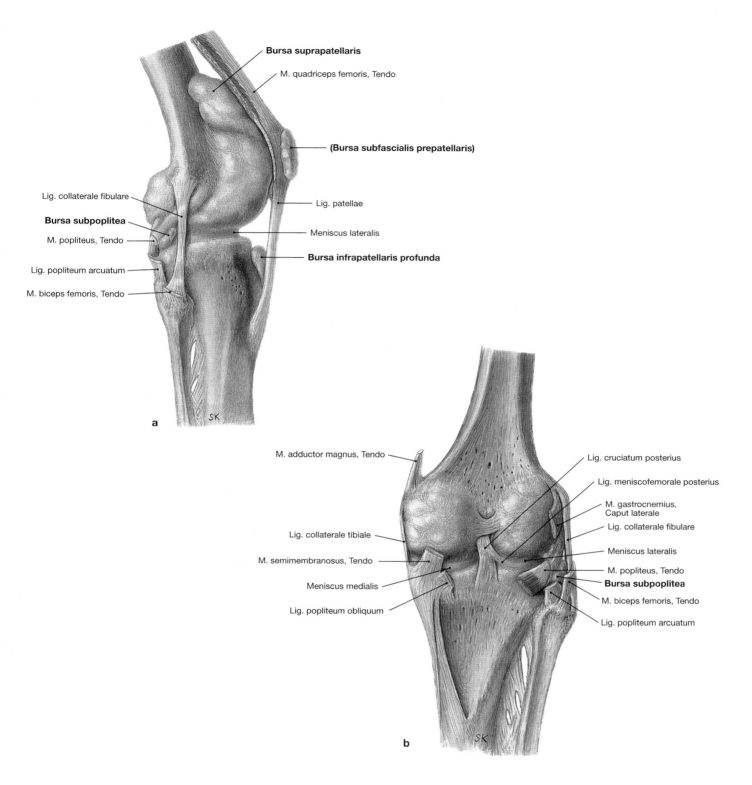

Bursa suprapatellaris

M. quadriceps femoris, Tendo

(Bursa subfascialis prepatellaris)

Lig. collaterale fibulare

Bursa subpoplitea

M. popliteus, Tendo

Lig. popliteum arcuatum

M. biceps femoris, Tendo

Lig. patellae

Meniscus lateralis

Bursa infrapatellaris profunda

a

M. adductor magnus, Tendo

Lig. collaterale tibiale

M. semimembranosus, Tendo

Meniscus medialis

Lig. popliteum obliquum

Lig. cruciatum posterius

Lig. meniscofemorale posterius

M. gastrocnemius, Caput laterale

Lig. collaterale fibulare

Meniscus lateralis

M. popliteus, Tendo

Bursa subpoplitea

M. biceps femoris, Tendo

Lig. popliteum arcuatum

b

Fig. 4.57a and b Knee joint, Articulatio genus, right side, with synovial bursae; illustration of the articular cavity after injection of plastic moulding. [S700-L238]
a Lateral view.
b Dorsal view.

The knee joint is surrounded by up to 30 **synovial bursae (Bursae synoviales).** Some bursae communicate with the joint capsule, such as the **Bursa suprapatellaris** (in front, above) beneath the quadriceps tendon, or the **Bursa subpoplitea** (at the back, below) beneath the tendon of the M. popliteus.

Clinical remarks

Intense mechanical loading of the knee (in bending activities) can cause an inflammation of the bursae **(bursitis).**

Skeleton

Knee joint with synovial bursae

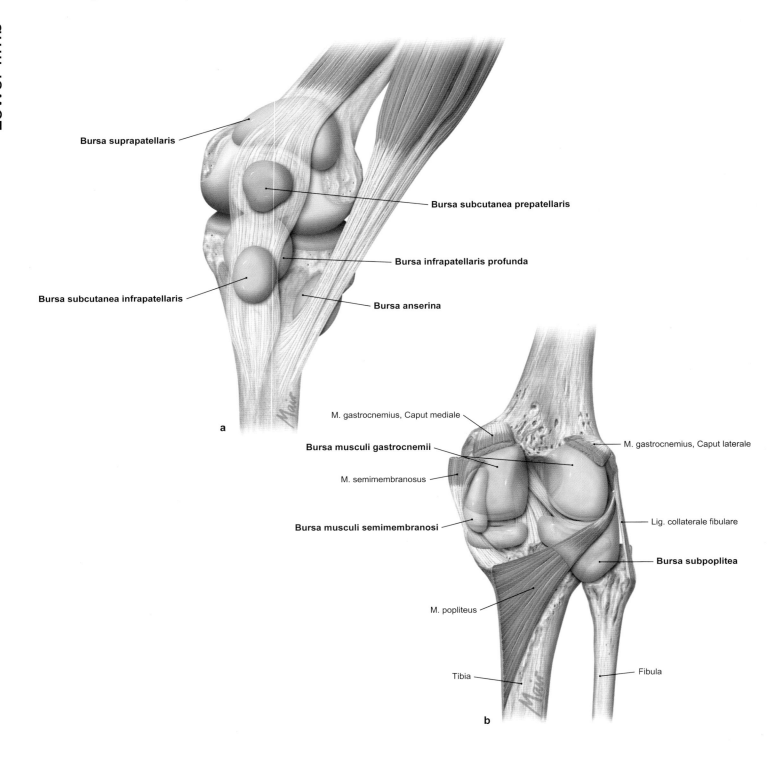

Bursa suprapatellaris

Bursa subcutanea prepatellaris

Bursa infrapatellaris profunda

Bursa subcutanea infrapatellaris

Bursa anserina

a

M. gastrocnemius, Caput mediale

Bursa musculi gastrocnemii

M. semimembranosus

M. gastrocnemius, Caput laterale

Bursa musculi semimembranosi

Lig. collaterale fibulare

Bursa subpoplitea

M. popliteus

Tibia

Fibula

b

Fig. 4.58a and b   Knee joint, Articulatio genus, right side, with synovial bursae. [S700-L127]
a Anterior medial view.
b Dorsal view.
Bursae which communicate with the joint capsule, such as the **Bursa suprapatellaris** (anterosuperior beneath the quadriceps tendon) or the **Bursa subpatellaris** (posterolateral beneath the M. popliteus), take on synovial fluid from the joint cavity when the knee joint swells up as a result of injury or also rheumatoid disease.

Other bursae are located in places exposed to increased compressive loading (e.g. when kneeling), such as the **Bursa prepatellaris** or the **Bursa infrapatellaris,** or serve as gliding surfaces underneath muscle tendons at their insertion sites, such as the **Bursa musculi semimembranosi** or the **Bursae subtendineae musculorum gastrocnemii medialis and lateralis**.

Clinical remarks

Chronic inflammatory joint effusions, such as those occurring in rheumatic diseases (e.g. rheumatoid arthritis), can lead to enlargement and fusion of the bursae which appear as a swelling in the popliteal fossa. Such a fusion of the Bursa musculi semimembranosi with the Bursa subtendinea musculi gastrocnemii medialis is called a **BAKER's cyst**.

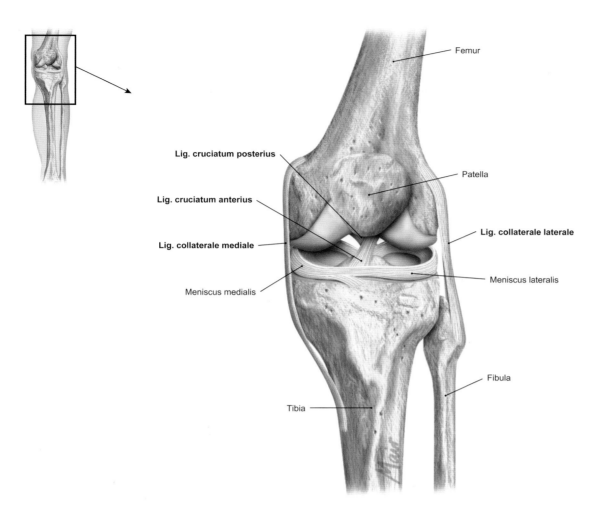

Lig. cruciatum posterius

Lig. cruciatum anterius

Lig. collaterale mediale

Meniscus medialis

Femur

Patella

Lig. collaterale laterale

Meniscus lateralis

Fibula

Tibia

Fig. 4.59 Knee joint, Articulatio genus, left side, with collateral ligaments and cruciate ligaments; ventral view. [S701-L127]
Structurally, the knee joint is the most complex of the large joints in the human body. This joint is stabilised by several **external ligaments**

(→ Fig. 4.55, → Fig. 4.56) and internal ligaments located within the joint cavity. For joint stability, the key structures are medial and lateral **collateral ligaments** and anterior and posterior **cruciate ligaments** within the joint cavity.

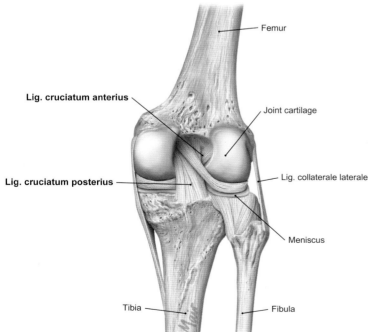

Lig. cruciatum anterius

Lig. cruciatum posterius

Tibia

Femur

Joint cartilage

Lig. collaterale laterale

Meniscus

Fibula

Fig. 4.60 Knee joint, Articulatio genus, left side, with collateral ligaments and cruciate ligaments; dorsal view. [S701-L127]

Collateral ligaments of the knee joint

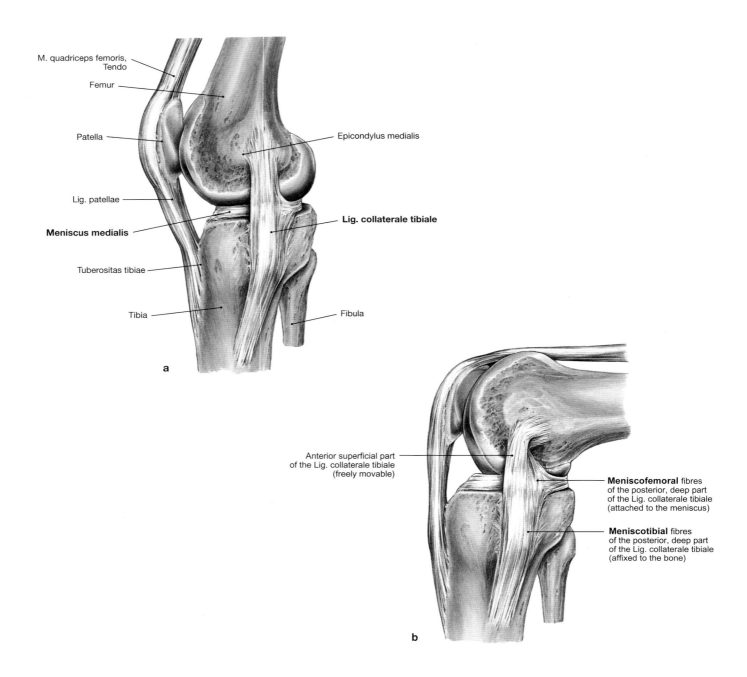

Fig. 4.61a and b   Medial ('inner') collateral ligament (Lig. collaterale tibiale); medial view. [S700]

a View of an extended knee position.
The medial collateral ligament **(Lig. collaterale tibiale)** is relatively broad and passes from the Epicondylus medialis of the femur to below the medial condyle of the tibia. Only its posterior fibres are attached firmly to the Meniscus medialis. In contrast, the outer (lateral) collateral ligament **(Lig. collaterale fibulare)** is not merged with the Meniscus

lateralis (→ Fig. 4.62). Because the anterior radius of curvature of the femoral condyles is larger, the collateral ligaments will be tensed with extension of the knee. Therefore, no rotation is possible in this position.
b View of a flexed knee position. During knee flexion, the Lig. collaterale tibiale is twisted and causes the Meniscus medialis to be fixed in place. The ligament is relaxed during knee flexion because the posterior parts of the femur condyles have a smaller radius of curvature to allow rotational movements in the flexed knee.

Clinical remarks

The collateral ligaments stabilise the knee joint medially and laterally. The medial collateral ligament (clin.: **MCL**) in particular stabilises against **abduction,** the lateral collateral ligament (clin.: **LCL**) against **adduction.** In the case of damaged ligaments (ligament rupture), the

joint has a greater hinging capacity. This phenomenon is utilised during physical examination to assess potential lesions of the collateral ligaments.

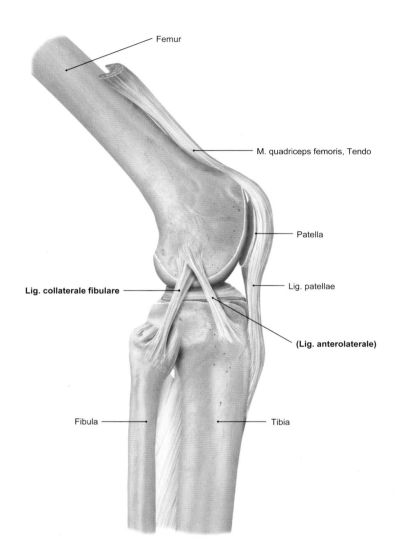

Femur

M. quadriceps femoris, Tendo

Patella

Lig. patellae

Lig. collaterale fibulare

(Lig. anterolaterale)

Fibula

Tibia

Fig. 4.62 Lateral collateral ligament (Lig. collaterale fibulare), and anterolateral ligament in extended position; lateral view. [S700-L280]

The lateral collateral ligament **(Lig. collaterale fibulare)** runs from the Epicondylus lateralis of the femur to the head of the fibula and is thus not only significantly narrower than the medial collateral ligament, but also shorter. An additional ligament passing from the lateral epicondylus of the femur to the Condylus lateralis of the tibia is the 'anterolateral ligament' (clin.: ALL). New studies have shown that structures characterised as ALL are, in fact, not a separate ligament but rather a part of the aponeurosis of the M. biceps femoris.

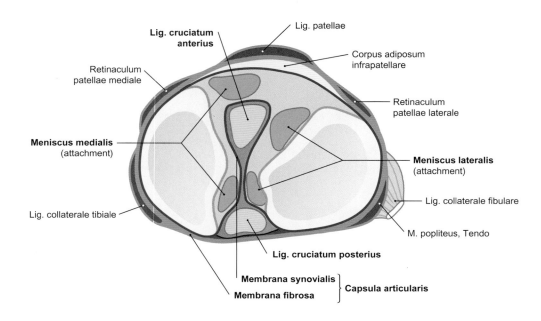

Fig. 4.63 Schematic representation of the capsule of the knee joint, right side; cranial view. [S702-L126]

As with other joints, the capsule of the knee joint **(Capsula articularis)** consists of an external layer of dense fibrous tissue (Membrana fibrosa) and an internal lining, the Membrana synovialis. Notably, the two layers are only ventrally and laterally in direct contact. In contrast, the Membrana synovialis diverges dorsally inwards and covers the **cruciate ligaments (Ligg. cruciata anterius et posterius).** The cruciate ligaments are therefore not within the joint cavity. Their location is described as **extrasynovial** but **intracapsular.**

The illustration also shows the different **attachments of the collateral ligaments** to the joint capsule. While the medial collateral ligament has fused directly with the joint capsule and the medial meniscus, the lateral collateral ligament is separated from the joint capsule by the tendon of origin of the M. popliteus.

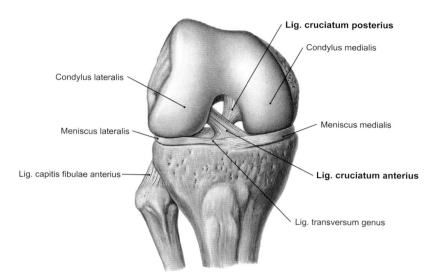

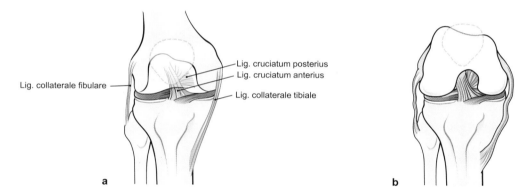

Fig. 4.64   Knee joint, Articulatio genus, right side, in 90° flexion; ventral view; after removal of the joint capsule and the collateral ligaments. [S700]
The most important internal ligaments are the two cruciate ligaments. The **anterior cruciate ligament (Lig. cruciatum anterius)** runs from the inner surface of the lateral femoral condyle to the Area intercondylaris anterior of the tibia (descending from superior posterior lateral in

an anterior direction). The **posterior cruciate ligament (Lig. cruciatum posterius)** runs downwards from the inner surface of the medial femoral condyle to the Area intercondylaris posterior of the tibia in the opposite direction (descending from superior anterior medial in a posterior direction). The cruciate ligaments are located inside the Capsula fibrosa **(intracapsular),** but outside the Capsula synovialis, and thus they are **extrasynovial.**

Fig. 4.65a and b   Stabilisation of the knee joint, Articulatio genus, right side, by collateral and cruciate ligaments; ventral view. [S702-L216]
a Stabilisation in the extended position. The cruciate and collateral ligaments form a functional unit. The **collateral ligaments** are **tensed only**

during extension of the knee and stabilise the knee joint in this position against rotational and abduction/adduction movements.
b Stabilisation in the flexed position. In contrast to the collateral ligaments, the cruciate ligaments are tensed during all positions of the knee joint: the medial part during extension, and the lateral part during flexion.

Clinical remarks

Injuries to the anterior cruciate ligament are the most common knee injury. It occurs frequently as a sports injury during soccer or handball when the flexed knee bears the full body weight and engages in rotational movements. (→ Fig. a).
With an **injury to the cruciate ligaments,** the lower leg can slide in a sagittal direction similar to a drawer: forwards with injury to the anterior cruciate ligament (clin.: ACL, the **anterior drawer** test), backwards with injury to the posterior cruciate ligament (clin.: PCL, the **posterior drawer** test). This is tested with the patient in a supine position: the examiner fixes the knee in a flexed position of 90° by sitting on the foot and pulling the lower leg forwards or pushing it backwards. This frequently permits the diagnosis of an injury to the cruciate ligament. Magnetic resonance imaging (MRI) is necessary to assess the extent of damage to the menisci and collateral ligaments (→ Fig. b).
A ruptured cruciate ligament cannot heal by itself and requires surgical intervention. However, there is a high increased risk of subse-

quent degenerative changes, such as arthritis of the knee. For every second patient, this is the cause of a renewed cruciate ligament rupture within the ensuing 20 years.

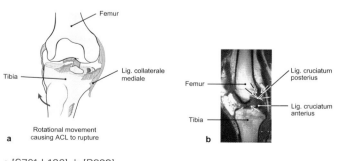

a [S701-L126], b [R333]

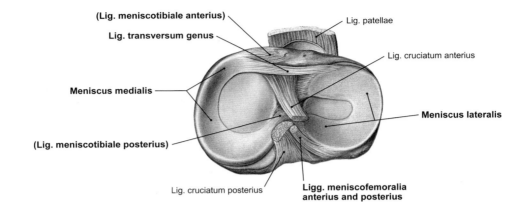

Fig. 4.66 labels:
(Lig. meniscotibiale anterius)
Lig. transversum genus
Lig. patellae
Lig. cruciatum anterius
Meniscus medialis
Meniscus lateralis
(Lig. meniscotibiale posterius)
Lig. cruciatum posterius
Ligg. meniscofemoralia anterius and posterius

Fig. 4.66 Menisci of the knee joint, right side; cranial view. [S700] Both menisci are roughly C-shaped and appear wedge-shaped in cross-sections. The **medial meniscus** is larger and anchored via the **Ligg. meniscotibialia anterius** and **posterius** to the respective Area intercondylaris of the tibia. In addition, the medial meniscus is fixed to the medial collateral ligament. In contrast, the **lateral meniscus** is fixed to the medial femoral condyle via the **Ligg. meniscofemoralia anterius** and **posterius,** but not attached to the lateral collateral ligament,

from which it is separated by the tendon of the M. popliteus (→ Fig. 4.63). The posterior horn of the lateral meniscus is only indirectly as well as flexibly connected to the tibia via the M. popliteus. Anteriorly, both menisci are interconnected through the **Lig. transversum genus.** This results in a significantly increased range of motion of the lateral condyle when bending the knee.

Both menisci are composed of fibrous cartilage inside and dense connective tissue outside.

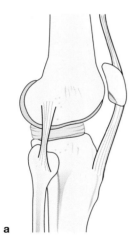

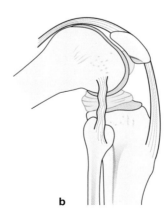

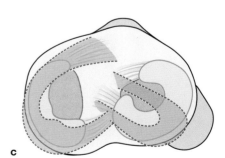

Fig. 4.67a–c Movability of the menisci during flexion. a, b [S700-L126]/[G1061], c [S700-L126]/[B500]
a Extended position.
b, c Flexed position.

During flexion, both menisci are pushed posteriorly over the sides of the tibial condyles. The mobility of the lateral meniscus is considerably higher because it is less fixed.

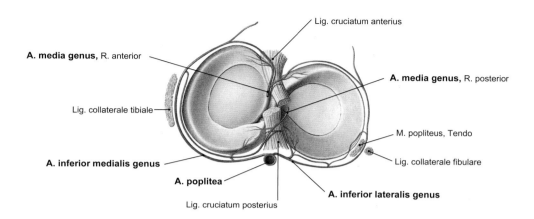

Fig. 4.68 Arterial blood supply to the menisci, right side; cranial view. [S700]

The **outer portions** are supplied with blood via a **perimeniscal capillary plexus,** which is fed by the Aa. inferiores medialis and lateralis genus and by the A. media genus (branches of the **A. poplitea**). In contrast, the **inner portions** are devoid of blood vessels and are supplied by diffusion from the **synovial fluid**.

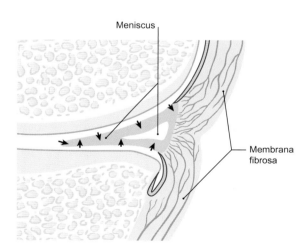

Fig. 4.69 Blood supply of the menisci. [S702-L126]/[G1060-001]

Both menisci are composed of **fibrous cartilage inside** and **dense connective tissue outside.** The supply of the menisci has a major influence on their regenerative capacity. The **peripheral portion** of the menisci is supplied directly with **blood** from the perimeniscal capillary plexus of the A. poplitea and therefore it can regenerate relatively well after injury. In contrast, the **central portion** of the menisci is supplied indirectly by diffusion via the **synovial fluid,** and therefore its metabolism and regenerative capacities are restricted.

Injury to the menisci

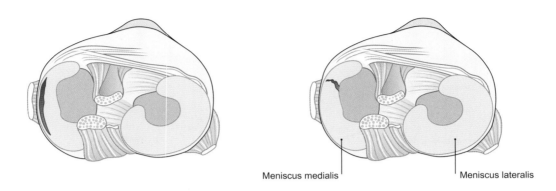

Meniscus medialis   Meniscus lateralis

Fig. 4.70a and b   Lesions of the medial meniscus, right side; cranial view. [S702-L126]
As the medial meniscus is connected directly to the medial collateral ligament through the joint capsule, **lesions of the medial meniscus occur much more frequently** than lesions of the lateral meniscus. These might include partial ruptures or even avulsion of parts of the meniscus.

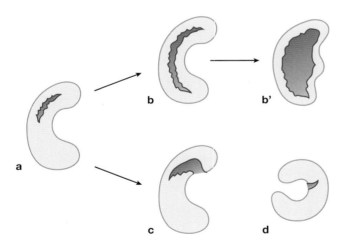

Fig. 4.71a–d   Developmental stages of meniscal ruptures. [S700-L126]
a Occurrence of a longitudinal rupture or tear.
b Prolongation of the rupture (tear) from the posterior horn to the anterior horn and displacement into the joint (= bucket handle tears, **b'**).
c Additional transverse rupture (mostly avulsion of the anterior or posterior horn).
d Transverse rupture (tear), of the lateral C-shaped meniscus in most cases.

Clinical remarks

Meniscal injuries are common. It is mostly the **medial meniscus that is affected due to its stronger attachment to bone and capsule.** Acute injuries occur with sudden rotational movements of the flexed knee while bearing weight, which and cause a painful restriction on active and passive extension movements. Chronic degenerative changes are often caused by a misalignment. If injuries affect the well-perfused peripheral areas of the menisci, spontaneous healing is possible. Rupture of the inner portions, on the other hand, typically require an arthroscopic partial removal (meniscectomy) in order to restore the freedom of movement. However, it can often result in degenerative **osteoarthritis of the knee** joint.

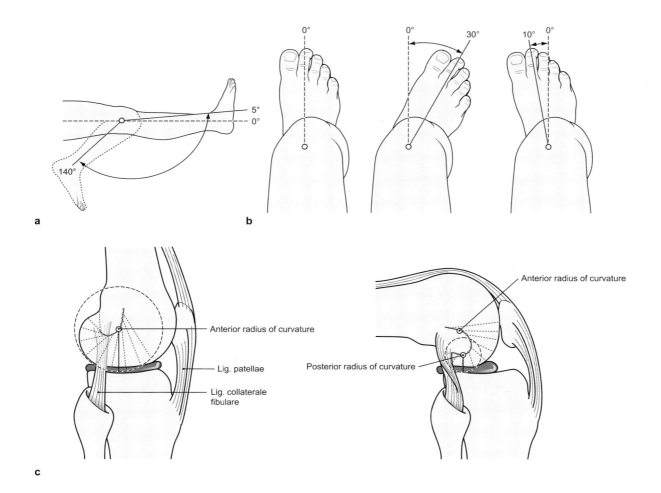

Fig. 4.72a–c   Range of motion of the knee joint, Articulatio genus. [S702-L126]

a Active knee flexion to 120° can be increased to 140° if the ischiocrucal muscles are warmed up. Passively, flexion to 160° is possible before soft tissue inhibits further flexion. Extension to the neutral position is possible but can be 5°–10° with passive movement. The range of motion at extension and flexion is 5°–0°–140°.

b Rotational movements are only possible when the knee is flexed. In the extended knee, the collateral ligaments are tensed which prevents rotations. External rotation is more extensive than internal rotation because the cruciate ligaments wind around each other during internal rotation. Abduction and adduction are almost completely blocked by the strong collateral ligaments. The range of motion for lateral rotation and medial rotation is: 30°–0°–10°.

c The knee joint is a **bicondylar joint** (Articulatio bicondylaris) which acts like a **pivot-hinge joint** (trochoginglymus) and possesses two degrees of freedom of movement. The transverse axis for **extension** and **flexion movements** runs through the trochlea of both femoral condyles. The **longitudinal axis** of the **rotational movements** is slightly shifted medially and therefore it runs perpendicularly off-centre through the Tuberculum intercondylare mediale of the tibia. Due to the smaller posterior radius of curvature of the femoral condyles, the **transverse axis** does not remain in a constant position, but moves on a convex line up towards the back during flexion. The flexion of the knee is therefore a **combined rolling and sliding movement,** in which the condyles roll up to 20° posteriorly and then turn on this spot. Since the medial and lateral condyles of the femur and of the tibia are not identically shaped, it is predominantly the lateral femoral condyle that rocks back and forth (similar to a rocking chair), whereas the medial condyle rotates on the spot (similar to a ball-and-socket joint). At the same time, the femur turns slightly outwards. In the terminal phase of the extension movement, the tension of the anterior cruciate ligament also induces a forced lateral rotation of 5°–10°, during which the medial condyle of the femur actually loses contact with the medial meniscus.

Most important muscles for movement in the knee joint	
Movement	**Muscles**
Flexion	M. semimembranosus
Extension	M. quadriceps femoris
External rotation	M. biceps femoris
Internal rotation	M. semimembranosus

Knee joint, clinical examination

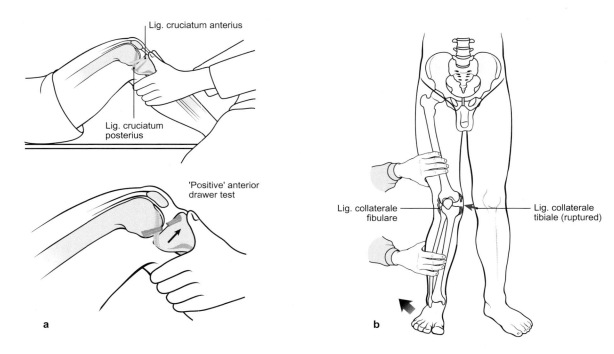

Lig. cruciatum anterius

Lig. cruciatum posterius

'Positive' anterior drawer test

a

Lig. collaterale fibulare

Lig. collaterale tibiale (ruptured)

b

Fig. 4.73a and b   Clinical examinations for assessing ligament functions at the knee joint. [S702-L126]/[R234]
a Examination of the anterior cruciate ligament (drawer test). When the anterior cruciate ligament is ruptured, the lower leg can be pulled forward in the sagittal plane from the upper leg, like a drawer.

b Examination of the medial collateral ligament (MCL). When the medial collateral ligament is ruptured, the lower leg can be slightly bent out to the side from an upper leg position ('flipped out').

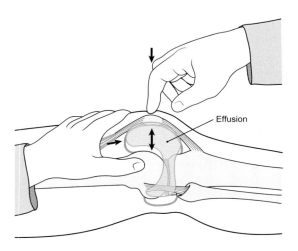

Effusion

Fig. 4.74   Clinical examination of a knee joint effusion; lateral view, right side. [S702-L126]
For an explanation → Clinical remarks.

Clinical remarks

Injuries to menisci and ligaments of the knee joint generally lead to an acute knee joint effusion. This is often obvious because of the swelling (lump). In order to confirm the findings, the phenomenon of the **floating patella** is triggered. This is done by stroking the Recessus suprapatellaris with one hand from the thigh towards the knee joint. In the case of downwards pressure, the patella seems to move around as if on a water pillow (→ Fig. 4.74).

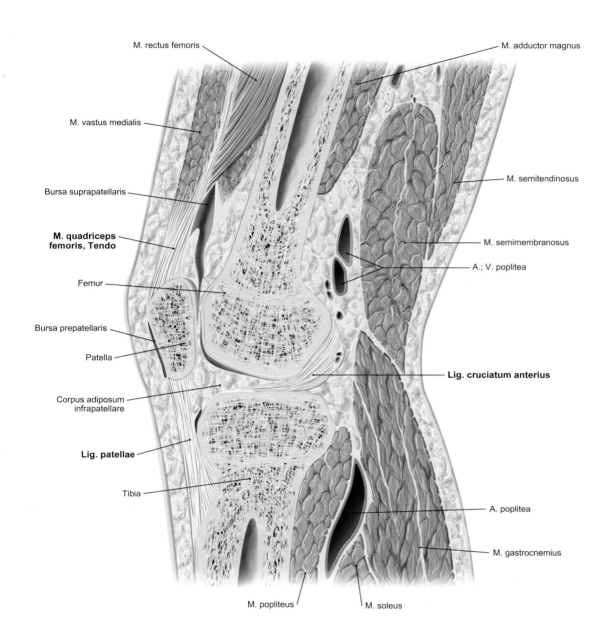

M. rectus femoris

M. adductor magnus

M. vastus medialis

M. semitendinosus

Bursa suprapatellaris

M. semimembranosus

M. quadriceps femoris, Tendo

A.; V. poplitea

Femur

Bursa prepatellaris

Patella

Lig. cruciatum anterius

Corpus adiposum infrapatellare

Lig. patellae

Tibia

A. poplitea

M. gastrocnemius

M. popliteus

M. soleus

Fig. 4.75   Knee joint, Articulatio genus, right side; sagittal section; lateral view. [S700-L127]/[G1060-001]
This sagittal section through the knee joint shows segments of ligaments and menisci. Visualising the positions of the individual structures in these sectional images is critically important for MRI diagnostics of the knee joint (MRI, → Fig. 4.77 and → Fig. 4.78).

Section through the knee joint

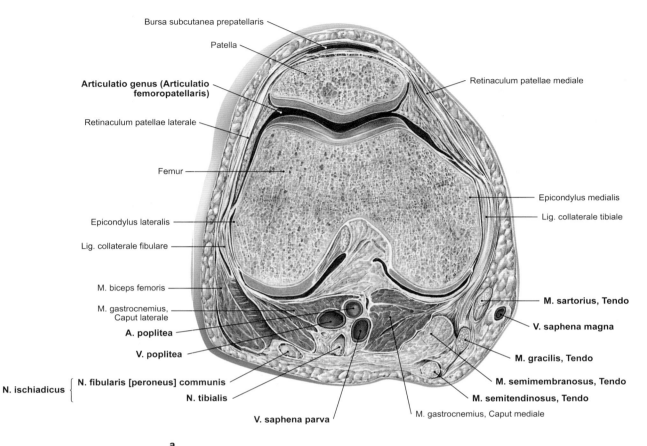

Bursa subcutanea prepatellaris

Patella

Articulatio genus (Articulatio femoropatellaris)

Retinaculum patellae mediale

Retinaculum patellae laterale

Femur

Epicondylus medialis

Epicondylus lateralis

Lig. collaterale tibiale

Lig. collaterale fibulare

M. biceps femoris

M. gastrocnemius, Caput laterale

A. poplitea

M. sartorius, Tendo

V. saphena magna

V. poplitea

M. gracilis, Tendo

N. ischiadicus { **N. fibularis [peroneus] communis**

N. tibialis

M. semimembranosus, Tendo

M. semitendinosus, Tendo

M. gastrocnemius, Caput mediale

V. saphena parva

a

b

Patellar opening or facet angle

Fig. 4.76a and b   Knee joint, Articulatio genus.
a Right knee, cross-section, distal view. The cross-section through the knee joint shows the articular surfaces of the **Articulatio femoropatellaris.** The **M. biceps femoris** lies laterally on the posterior side, and is therefore the most important external rotator. On the medial side, however, several muscles are involved in the medial rotation: the inserting tendons of the **Mm. sartorius, gracilis, and semitendinosus** run superficially. They insert further distally in the common aponeurosis at the medial aspect of the tibia, commonly referred to as the 'Pes anserinus superficialis'. The insertion of the tendon of the **M. semimembranosus** lies underneath it and is referred to as the 'Pes anserinus profundus'.
The **V. saphena magna** is found in the epifascial subcutaneous adipose tissue on the medial side of the knee. On the dorsal side, the terminal branches of the N. ischiadicus (N. fibularis communis and N. tibialis) are located laterally and superficially, while the V. poplitea with the V. saphena parva lie more deeply, and the A. poplitea is the deepest structure. [S700]

b Left knee, X-ray image of the patella and the patella gliding surface of a left knee joint flexed at 60°. The X-rays reach from the tip of the patella via the base of the patella to the X-ray plate. This gives a caudal view of the bent knee joint and it becomes possible to see the patella's opening or facet angle of 130°. One can assess the Facies articularis patellae and the femoral gliding surface, whereby the joint space appears particularly wide, due to the thick articular cartilage. X-ray images in 30° and 60° knee flexions show the pathway of the patella inside the gliding surface of the femur (Facies patellaris femoris). [F1062-001]

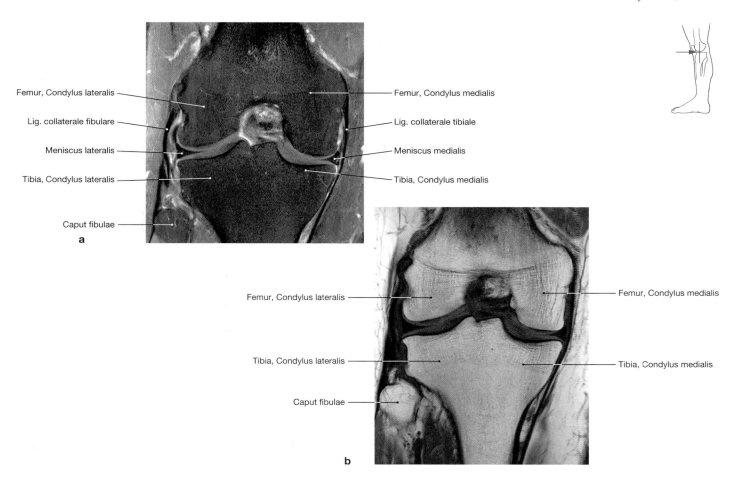

Femur, Condylus lateralis

Lig. collaterale fibulare

Meniscus lateralis

Tibia, Condylus lateralis

Caput fibulae

a

Femur, Condylus medialis

Lig. collaterale tibiale

Meniscus medialis

Tibia, Condylus medialis

Femur, Condylus lateralis

Tibia, Condylus lateralis

Caput fibulae

Femur, Condylus medialis

Tibia, Condylus medialis

b

Fig. 4.77a and b   Knee joint, Articulatio genus, right side; magnetic resonance imaging (MRI), coronary sagittal scan. [S700-T832]

a T1-weighted fat-saturated native MRI image.
b T1-weighted native MRI image.

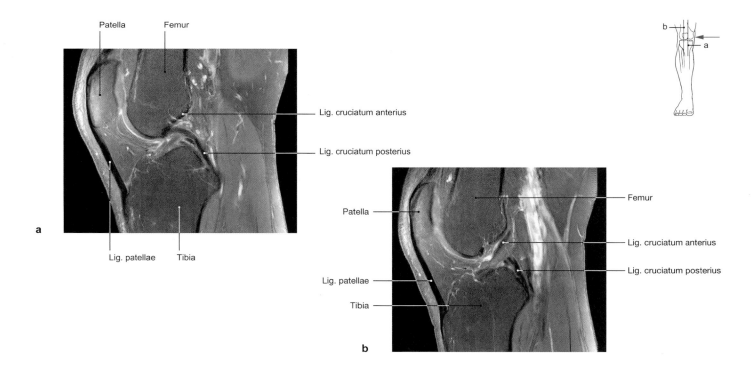

Patella   Femur

Lig. cruciatum anterius

Lig. cruciatum posterius

a

Lig. patellae   Tibia

Femur

Patella

Lig. cruciatum anterius

Lig. cruciatum posterius

Lig. patellae

Tibia

b

Fig. 4.78a and b   Knee joint, Articulatio genus, right side; magnetic resonance imaging (MRI); medial view. [S700-T832]
Compact bone appears black with this MRI technique.

a Sagittal scan through the medial patella.
b Sagittal scan through the lateral patella.

Lower limb

Knee joint, arthroscopy

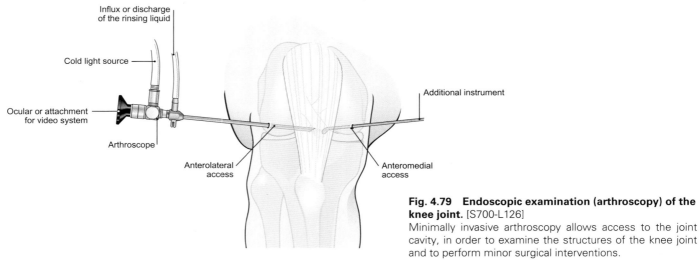

Influx or discharge of the rinsing liquid

Cold light source

Ocular or attachment for video system

Arthroscope

Anterolateral access

Additional instrument

Anteromedial access

Fig. 4.79 Endoscopic examination (arthroscopy) of the knee joint. [S700-L126]
Minimally invasive arthroscopy allows access to the joint cavity, in order to examine the structures of the knee joint and to perform minor surgical interventions.

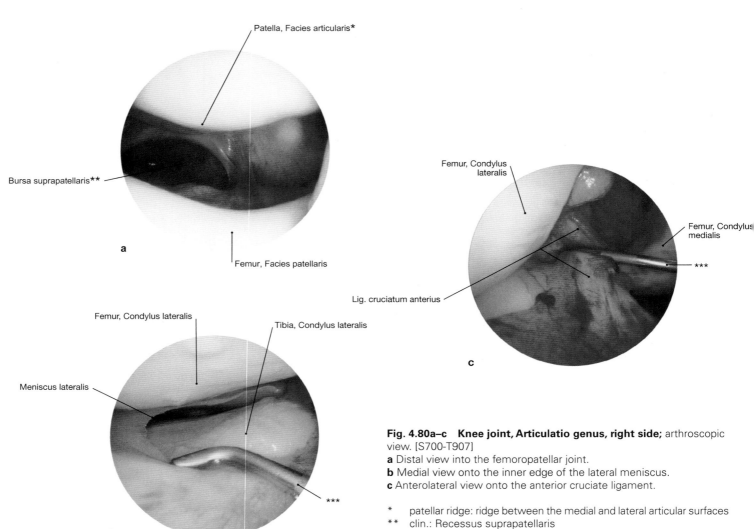

Patella, Facies articularis*

Bursa suprapatellaris**

a

Femur, Facies patellaris

Femur, Condylus lateralis

Femur, Condylus medialis

***

Lig. cruciatum anterius

c

Femur, Condylus lateralis

Tibia, Condylus lateralis

Meniscus lateralis

***

b

Fig. 4.80a–c Knee joint, Articulatio genus, right side; arthroscopic view. [S700-T907]
a Distal view into the femoropatellar joint.
b Medial view onto the inner edge of the lateral meniscus.
c Anterolateral view onto the anterior cruciate ligament.

* patellar ridge: ridge between the medial and lateral articular surfaces
** clin.: Recessus suprapatellaris
*** probe

Clinical remarks

An **arthroscopy** is a procedure that is frequently carried out on the knee joint. On the one hand, they serve as a **diagnostic procedure,** if, for example, the rupture of a meniscus cannot be confirmed or excluded by MRI scans. On the other hand, they are part of the **treatment,** such as the removal of torn meniscus parts, a repair of the cruciate ligaments (cruciate ligament reconstruction), or removal of loose bodies which painfully inhibit movements.

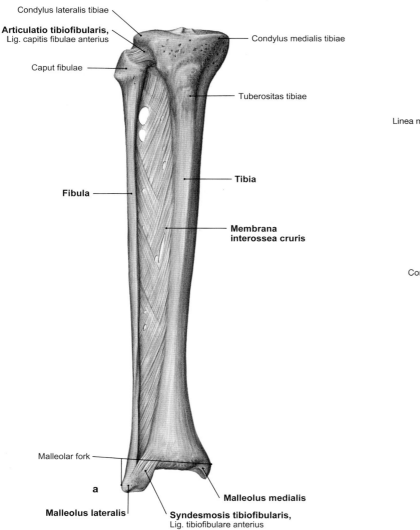

Condylus lateralis tibiae

Articulatio tibiofibularis,
Lig. capitis fibulae anterius

Condylus medialis tibiae

Caput fibulae

Tuberositas tibiae

Tibia

Fibula

**Membrana
interossea cruris**

Malleolar fork

a

Malleolus lateralis

Syndesmosis tibiofibularis,
Lig. tibiofibulare anterius

Malleolus medialis

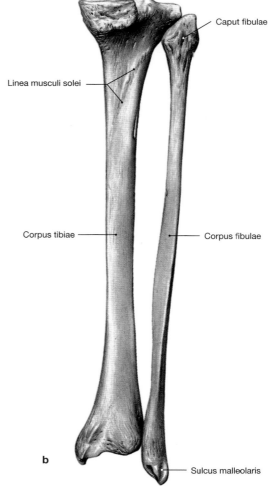

Caput fibulae

Linea musculi solei

Corpus tibiae

Corpus fibulae

b

Sulcus malleolaris

Fig. 4.81a and b Connections (junctions) of the tibia and fibula, right side. [S700]
a Ventral view.
b Dorsal view.
The proximal joint is an amphiarthrosis **(Articulatio tibiofibularis)** with the **Ligg. capitis fibulae anterius and posterius.** Distally, both the bones are firmly connected by the **Ligg. tibiofibularia anterius** and

posterius, and form a syndesmosis **(Syndesmosis tibiofibularis).** The **Membrana interossea cruris** with its fibres of tight connective tissue, primarily running obliquely from the tibia downwards to the fibula, provides further stabilisation. Together with the inferior articular surface of the tibia, the medial and lateral ankle protruberances (malleoli) form the **malleolar fork,** which provides the socket for the talocrural joint.

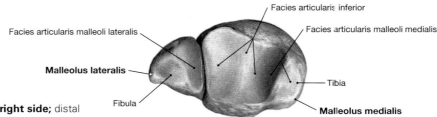

Facies articularis malleoli lateralis

Facies articularis inferior

Facies articularis malleoli medialis

Malleolus lateralis

Tibia

Fibula

Malleolus medialis

Fig. 4.82 Distal end of the tibia and of the fibula, right side; distal view. [S700]

Clinical remarks

Proximal fractures in the head and neck regions of the fibula can result from traumata in the area of the malleolar fork due to excessive rotation called **MAISONNEUVE fractures.**
Fractures of the distal end of the tibia are called **WEBER fractures,** which, depending on the involvement of the Syndesmosis tibiofibu-

laris, are classified into three grades (→ Fig. 4.83 and → Fig. 4.84). Since even minor deformities in the talocrural joint result in degenerative arthritis **(arthrosis, osteoarthritis),** virtually all of these fractures require surgical correction and stabilisation with plates or screws.

Skeleton

Lower thigh bones

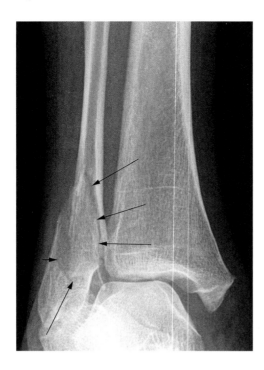

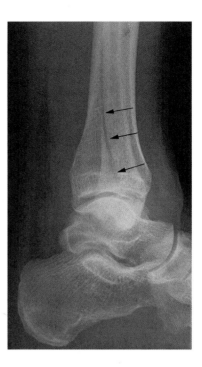

a

b

Fig. 4.83a and b   Distal end of the tibia and of the fibula, right side, with distal fracture of the fibula (WEBER B). [S008-3]
a X-ray image in anteroposterior (AP) projection. The fracture lines are marked with arrows.

b X-ray image in lateral projection. The fracture lines are marked with arrows.

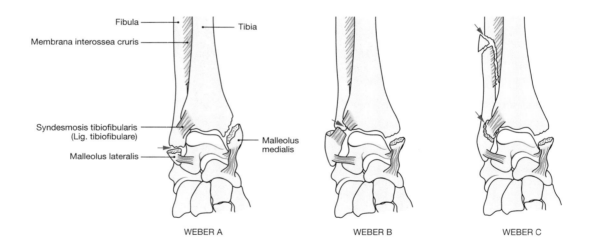

WEBER A   WEBER B   WEBER C

Fig. 4.84   Classification of ankle fractures according to WEBER grades A, B, C. [S700-L126]

Clinical remarks

Fractures of the distal end of the fibula are defined as **WEBER fractures** and classified in three grades of severity, according to the involvement of the Syndesmosis tibiofibularis.
- **WEBER A:** The Malleolus lateralis is broken **below** the syndesmosis, which itself is intact.
- **WEBER B:** The fracture line goes **through** the syndesmosis which may be injured.

- **WEBER C:** The fracture is located **above** the ruptured syndesmosis. This WEBER C fracture is associated with a severe destabilisation of the talocrural joint.

The classification by WEBER is based on the fracture line of the fibula. Particularly WEBER-B and -C fractures can coincide with additional fractures of the Malleolus medialis and/or tibia.

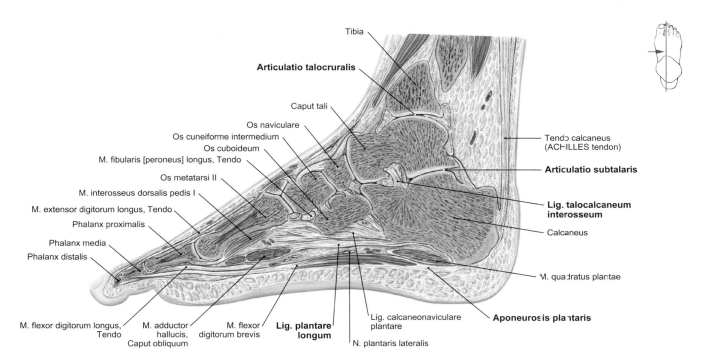

Tibia

Articulatio talocruralis

Caput tali

Os naviculare

Os cuneiforme intermedium

Os cuboideum

M. fibularis [peroneus] longus, Tendo

Os metatarsi II

M. interosseus dorsalis pedis I

M. extensor digitorum longus, Tendo

Phalanx proximalis

Phalanx media

Phalanx distalis

M. flexor digitorum longus, Tendo

Caput obliquum

M. adductor hallucis,

M. flexor digitorum brevis

Lig. plantare longum

N. plantaris lateralis

Lig. calcaneonaviculare plantare

Aponeurosis plantaris

M. quadratus plantae

Calcaneus

Lig. talocalcaneum interosseum

Articulatio subtalaris

Tendo calcaneus (ACHILLES tendon)

Fig. 4.85 Foot, Pes, right side; sagittal section through the second metatarsal bone, for presentation of the ankle joints; medial view. [S700]

Most foot movements occur in both of the ankle joints. The talocrural joint **(Articulatio talocruralis)** includes the joint connections between both lower leg bones which form the malleolar fork and the talus foot bone. The subtalar joint divides into two compartments. The talus and calcaneus form the posterior compartment (Articulatio subtalaris). The anterior compartment (Articulatio talocalcaneonavicularis) has a complex structure. Sagittal sections help to clarify the topography and joint surfaces of the ankle joints.

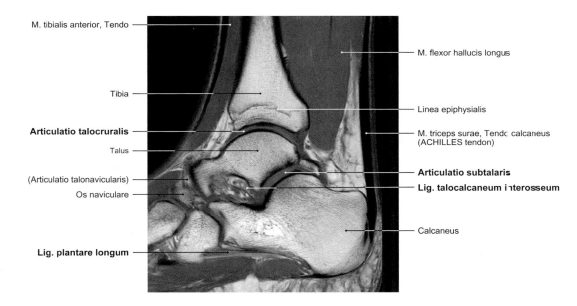

M. tibialis anterior, Tendo

Tibia

Articulatio talocruralis

Talus

(Articulatio talonavicularis)

Os naviculare

Lig. plantare longum

M. flexor hallucis longus

Linea epiphysialis

M. triceps surae, Tendo calcaneus (ACHILLES tendon)

Articulatio subtalaris

Lig. talocalcaneum interosseum

Calcaneus

Fig. 4.86 Foot, Pes, right side, presentation of the ankle joints; magnetic resonance imaging (MRI); medial view. [S700-T832]

Structure and function

It is via the **talocrural joint** that the tightly linked bones of the lower leg are connected to the foot skeleton. This **hinge joint** has medial and lateral ligaments which enable different levels of stabilisation and allow plantar flexion and dorsal flexion of the foot, which enable the rolling movements of the foot which are important for walking (→ Fig. 4.103). Injuries to the ligaments of the ankle joint are the most frequent ligament-related injuries in the human body. The lateral ligaments rupture more quickly because on this side the ligamentous apparatus is weaker than on the medial side. During walking, the talocrural joint and the **subtalar joint** work together. The two compartments of the subtalar joint are functionally connected by plane joints. In this way, the foot can tilt to compensate for uneven ground and forcefully push off the ground during walking.

Talocrural and subtalar joints

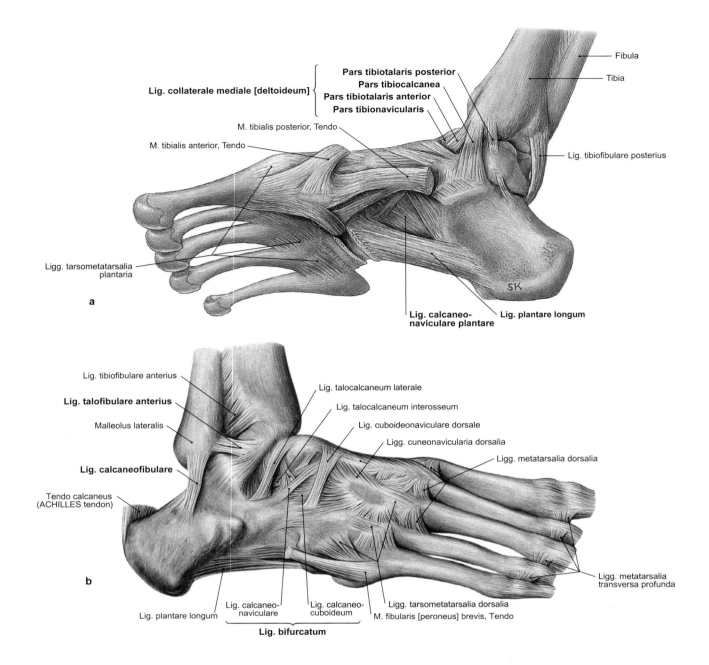

Fibula

Tibia

Lig. collaterale mediale [deltoideum] {
Pars tibiotalaris posterior
Pars tibiocalcanea
Pars tibiotalaris anterior
Pars tibionavicularis

M. tibialis posterior, Tendo

M. tibialis anterior, Tendo

Lig. tibiofibulare posterius

Ligg. tarsometatarsalia plantaria

a

SK

Lig. calcaneo-naviculare plantare   **Lig. plantare longum**

Lig. tibiofibulare anterius

Lig. talofibulare anterius

Malleolus lateralis

Lig. calcaneofibulare

Tendo calcaneus (ACHILLES tendon)

Lig. talocalcaneum laterale

Lig. talocalcaneum interosseum

Lig. cuboideonaviculare dorsale

Ligg. cuneonavicularia dorsalia

Ligg. metatarsalia dorsalia

Ligg. metatarsalia transversa profunda

b

Lig. plantare longum   Lig. calcaneo-naviculare   Lig. calcaneo-cuboideum   Ligg. tarsometatarsalia dorsalia   M. fibularis [peroneus] brevis, Tendo

Lig. bifurcatum

Fig. 4.87a and b Talocrural joint, Articulatio talocruralis, right side, with ligaments.
a Medial view. [S700-L238]
b Lateral view. [S700]
Movements of the foot take place in the talocrural joint and in the subtalar joint. The remaining tarsal and metatarsal joints are amphiarthroses, that can expand the range of motion in the talocalcaneonavicular joint, albeit only slightly. The malleolar fork forms the socket, and

the trochlea of the talus the joint head of the talocrural joint. **Medially** both joints are stabilised by a fan-shaped ligament, known as the **Lig. collaterale mediale (deltoideum),** which is composed of four fibrous tracts (Pars tibiotalaris anterior, Pars tibiotalaris posterior, Pars tibiocalcanea and Pars tibionavicularis), that connect the respective bones. **Laterally,** there are **three separate ligaments (Lig. talofibulare anterius, Lig. talofibulare posterius, Lig. calcaneofibulare).** In addition, these ligaments also stabilise the talocalcaneonavicular joint.

Clinical remarks

Injuries affect the **talocrural joint** more **frequently** than the **subtalar joint,** since the ligaments around the ankle area are not particularly strong. Since the trochlea of the talus is broader in the anterior than the posterior part (→ Fig. 4.39a), secure bony guidance is only guaranteed in dorsiflexion (extension) through the widening of the malleolar fork. The most common ligament injury in humans is the rupture of the lateral ligaments (Lig. talofibulare anterius and Lig. calcaneofibulare) in **supination trauma** (spraining or twisting the ankle) (→ Fig. a, → Fig. b).

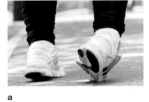

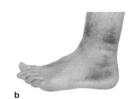

a   **b**

a [G123], **b** [J787]

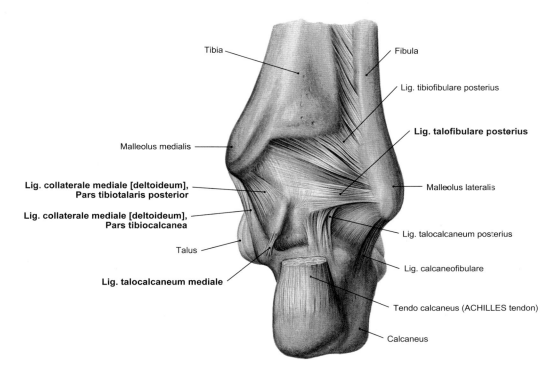

Fig. 4.88 Talocrural joint, Articulatio talocruralis, right side, with ligaments; dorsal view. [S700]

Parts of the Lig. collaterale mediale (Pars tibiotalaris posterior, Pars tibiocalcanea) and the lateral Lig. talofibulare posterius secure the joint at the back.

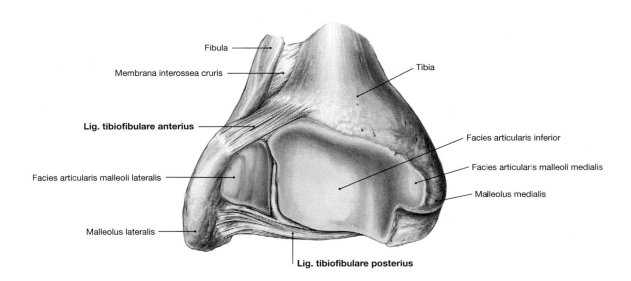

Fig. 4.89 Distal end of the tibia and of the fibula, right side; distal view. [S700]

The tibia and fibula are held together with the Syndesmosis tibiofibularis and form the malleolar fork, the socket of the talocrural joint.

Skeleton

Subtalar joint

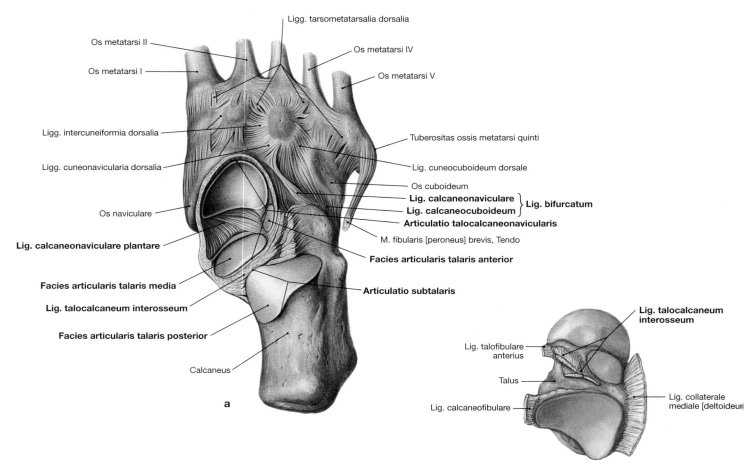

Ligg. tarsometatarsalia dorsalia

Os metatarsi II

Os metatarsi I

Os metatarsi IV

Os metatarsi V

Ligg. intercuneiformia dorsalia

Tuberositas ossis metatarsi quinti

Ligg. cuneonavicularia dorsalia

Lig. cuneocuboideum dorsale

Os cuboideum

Os naviculare

Lig. calcaneonaviculare
Lig. calcaneocuboideum } **Lig. bifurcatum**

Articulatio talocalcaneonavicularis

Lig. calcaneonaviculare plantare

M. fibularis [peroneus] brevis, Tendo

Facies articularis talaris anterior

Facies articularis talaris media

Lig. talocalcaneum interosseum

Articulatio subtalaris

Facies articularis talaris posterior

Calcaneus

a

Lig. talocalcaneum interosseum

Lig. talofibulare anterius

Talus

Lig. collaterale mediale [deltoideur

Lig. calcaneofibulare

Fig. 4.91   Subtalar joint, Articulatio talocalcaneonavicularis, proximal joint bodies, right side; distal view. [S700]

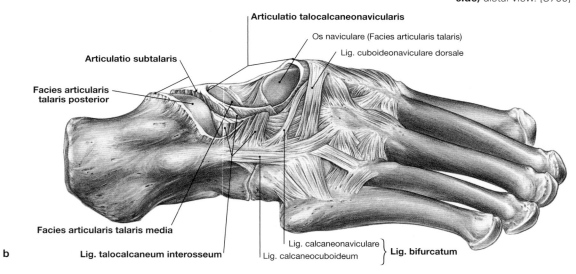

Articulatio talocalcaneonavicularis

Os naviculare (Facies articularis talaris)

Articulatio subtalaris

Lig. cuboideonaviculare dorsale

Facies articularis talaris posterior

Facies articularis talaris media

Lig. talocalcaneum interosseum

Lig. calcaneonaviculare } **Lig. bifurcatum**
Lig. calcaneocuboideum

b

Fig. 4.90a and b   Subtalar joint, Articulatio talocalcaneonavicularis, distal joint bodies, right side; after the removal of the talus. [S700]
a Proximal view.
b Lateral view.

In the subtalar joint, the talus, calcaneus and Os naviculare articulate in two completely separate joints. The posterior joint **(Articulatio subtalaris)** is formed by the posterior corresponding articular surfaces of the talus and calcaneus. This partial joint is separated from the anterior partial joint **(Articulatio talocalcaneonavicularis)** by the **Lig. talocalcaneum interosseum,** which is positioned in the Sinus tarsi. In the anterior partial joint, the anterior articular surfaces of the talus and calcaneus

articulate with each other, as does the head of the talus anteriorly with the Os naviculare, and inferiorly with the spring ligament **(Lig. calcaneonaviculare plantare).** At this point, the ligament usually has an articular surface of hyaline cartilage. It is involved in the tensing of the arches of the foot. Functionally, both partial joints form a single unit. This explains why the term **Articulatio talocalcaneonavicularis** is often used for the entire subtalar joint. Besides the ligaments of the talocrural joint, there are additional ligaments that stabilise the skeletal elements of the subtalar joint. These include the Lig. talocalcaneum interosseum, the Lig. talocalcaneum mediale and the Lig. talocalcaneum laterale (→ Fig. 4.87b and → Fig. 4.88). For the range of motion in the subtalar joint → Fig. 4.100.

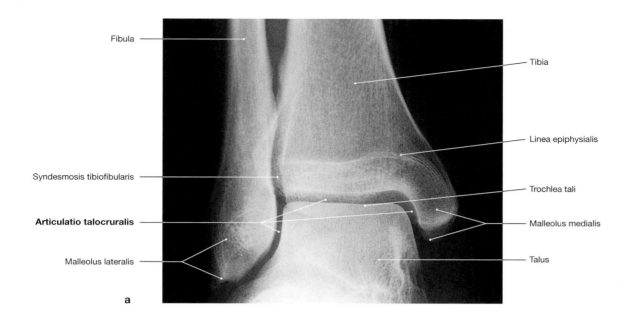

Fibula

Tibia

Linea epiphysialis

Syndesmosis tibiofibularis

Trochlea tali

Articulatio talocruralis

Malleolus medialis

Malleolus lateralis

Talus

a

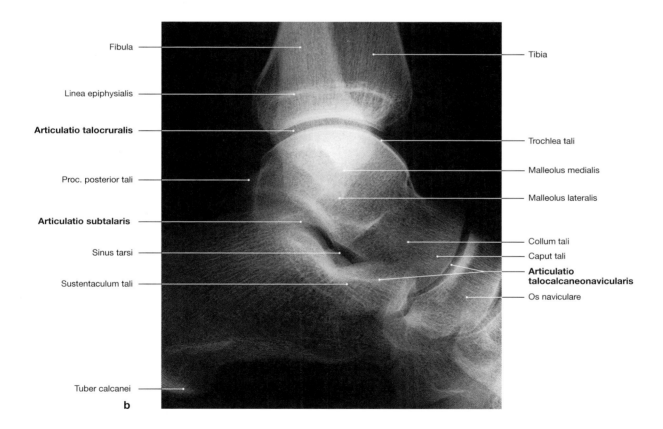

Fibula

Tibia

Linea epiphysialis

Articulatio talocruralis

Trochlea tali

Malleolus medialis

Proc. posterior tali

Malleolus lateralis

Articulatio subtalaris

Sinus tarsi

Collum tali

Caput tali

Sustentaculum tali

Articulatio talocalcaneonavicularis

Os naviculare

Tuber calcanei

b

Fig. 4.92a and b Talocrural joint and subtalar joint, Articulationes talocruralis and talocalcaneonavicularis, right side. [S700-T902]

a X-ray image with anterior-posterior (AP) projection.
b X-ray image with lateral projection.

Lower limb

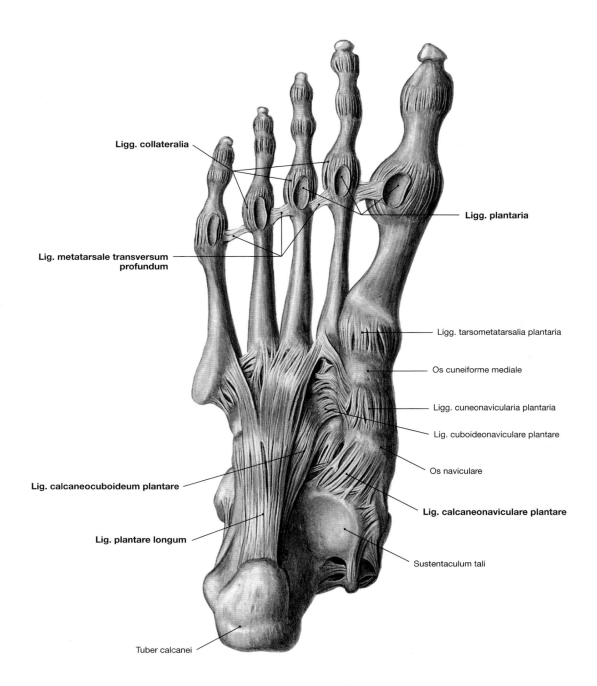

Ligg. collateralia

Ligg. plantaria

Lig. metatarsale transversum profundum

Ligg. tarsometatarsalia plantaria

Os cuneiforme mediale

Ligg. cuneonavicularia plantaria

Lig. cuboideonaviculare plantare

Os naviculare

Lig. calcaneocuboideum plantare

Lig. calcaneonaviculare plantare

Lig. plantare longum

Sustentaculum tali

Tuber calcanei

Fig. 4.93 Joints of the foot, Articulationes pedis, right side, with ligaments; plantar view. [S700]
The remaining tarsal and metatarsal joints are **amphiarthroses,** which are of minor significance for the mobility of the individual joints. Together, however, they enlarge the range of motion in the subtalar joint and connect the bones of the foot to an elastic (springy) base. In the tarsal region, two joints can be singled out for their contribution to the supination and pronation movements of the foot. The **CHOPART's joint** (Articulatio tarsi transversa) is composed of both the Articulatio talonavicularis and the Articulatio calcaneocuboidea (→ Fig. 4.36). The **LISFRANC's joint** (Articulationes tarsometatarsales) serves as the connection to the metatarsus (→ Fig. 4.36). These joint lines have clinical relevance as amputation lines. In addition, the tarsal bones articulate in several distinct joints. The metatarsal bones are connected proximally by the **Articulationes intermetatarsales** and distally by the **Lig. metatarsale trans-**

versum profundum. The joints of the forefoot and midfoot are interlinked by strong plantar, dorsal and interosseous **ligaments.** The CHOPART's joint is stabilised in particular by the dorsal **Lig. bifurcatum,** which splits into two fibrous tracts (Lig. calcaneonaviculare and Lig. calcaneocuboideum) (→ Fig. 4.90a). The opposite ligament on the sole of the foot is the **Lig. calcaneocuboideum plantare.** As well as the spring ligament, the **Lig. plantare longum** helps to maintain the arches of the foot. It is located more superficially than the other plantar ligaments and runs from the calcaneus to the Os cuboideum and to the Ossa metatarsi II–IV. The joints of the **toes** can be divided into **metatarsophalangeal joints** (Articulationes metatarsophalangeae) as well as **proximal and distal joints** (Articulationes interphalangeae proximales and distales). All joints of the toes are restricted in their mobility by strong ligaments on both sides (Ligg. collateralia) and by the Ligg. plantaria from below.

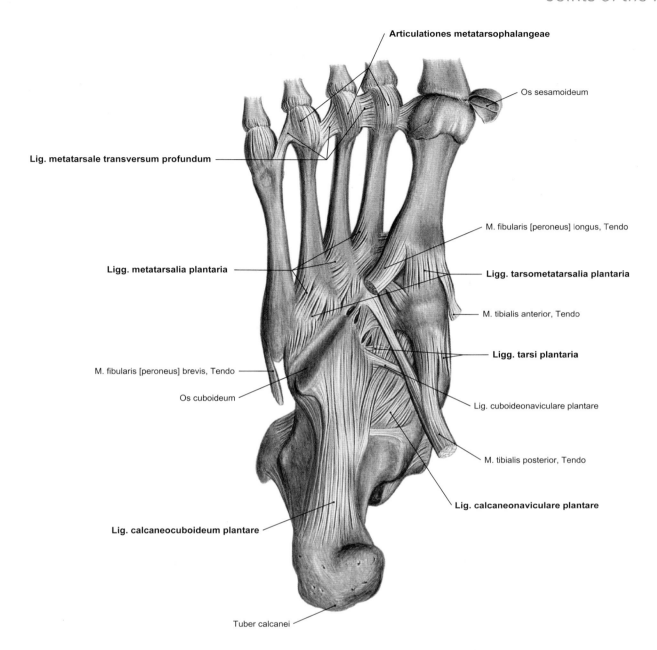

Articulationes metatarsophalangeae

Os sesamoideum

Lig. metatarsale transversum profundum

M. fibularis [peroneus] longus, Tendo

Ligg. metatarsalia plantaria

Ligg. tarsometatarsalia plantaria

M. tibialis anterior, Tendo

Ligg. tarsi plantaria

M. fibularis [peroneus] brevis, Tendo

Os cuboideum

Lig. cuboideonaviculare plantare

M. tibialis posterior, Tendo

Lig. calcaneonaviculare plantare

Lig. calcaneocuboideum plantare

Tuber calcanei

Fig. 4.94 Joints of the foot, Articulationes pedis, right side, with ligaments; plantar view; after removal of the Lig. plantare longum. [S700]

Clinical remarks

One of the most common deformities in the first metatarsophalangeal joint is the **hallux valgus,** in which the head of the first metatarsal bone deviates medially and is markedly prominent, with the big toe (hallux) adducted laterally (→ figure). This may result in severe pain in the affected joint and may cause soft tissue swelling. The hallux valgus deformity often requires surgical revision. New therapeutic approaches attempt to paralyse the adductive muscles (M. adductor hallucis) with injections of botulinum toxin in order to resolve the deformity. In the **hammer toe** deformity, the proximal or distal interphalangeal joints are fixed in a flexed position. In the case of a **claw toe** deformity, the metacarpophalangeal joint is also overextended, with the proximal phalanx even being pushed over the metatarsal bone.
[R110-20]

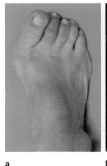
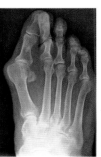

a   b

Arch of the foot

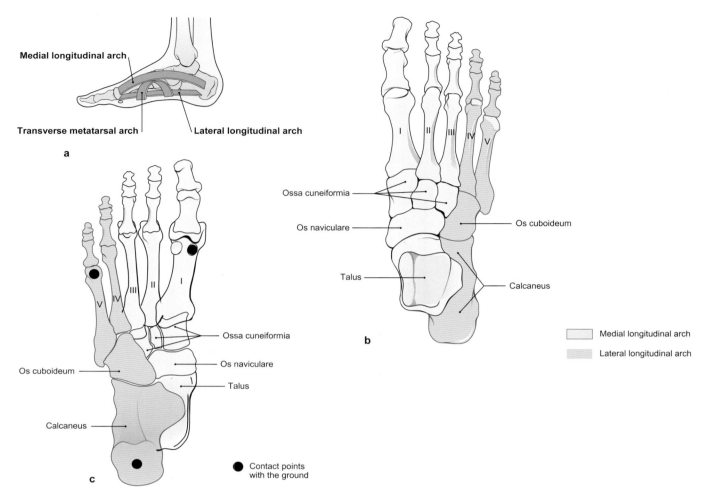

Fig. 4.95a–c   Bones of the arch of the foot, right side; schematic representation.
a Medial view. [S701-L126]
b Dorsal view. [S700-L126]
c Plantar view. [S700-L126]
When standing, the weight of the body is transmitted via **medial and lateral cords.** The medial cord includes the first three metatarsal bones and continues via the Os naviculare, the Os cuneiformia and the Ossa

metatarsi I–III up to the first three toes. The lateral vector is formed by the fourth and fifth metatarsal bones and continues via the calcaneus, Os cuboideum and Ossa metatarsi IV and V to both of the lateral toes. The shape and support system of the tarsal and metatarsal bones form the **longitudinal arch** and the **transverse arch** of the foot. Due to these arches, the foot has only three contact points with the ground: the heads of the metatarsal bones I and V, and the Tuber calcanei.

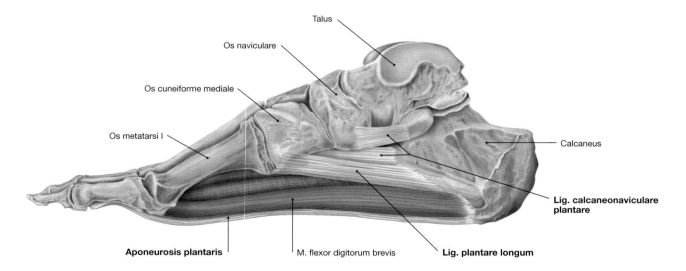

Fig. 4.96   Ligaments of the longitudinal plantar arch, right side;
medial view. [S700-L280]
The **ligaments** of the foot **passively** support the longitudinal arch of the foot. The ligamentous systems can be divided into three levels or layers:

- Upper level: spring ligament (Lig. calcaneonaviculare plantare)
- Middle level: Lig. plantare longum
- Lower level: plantar aponeurosis (Aponeurosis plantaris).

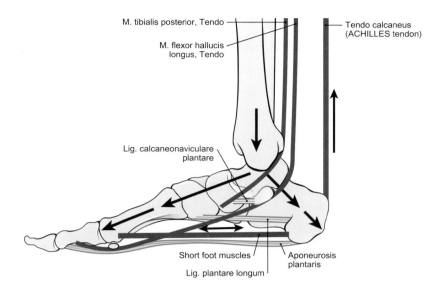

M. tibialis posterior, Tendo

M. flexor hallucis longus, Tendo

Tendo calcaneus (ACHILLES tendon)

Lig. calcaneonaviculare plantare

Short foot muscles

Aponeurosis plantaris

Lig. plantare longum

Fig. 4.97 Longitudinal arch of the foot, right side; schematic drawing, medial view. [S702-L126]/[B500-M282]

The heads of all the metatarsal bones are located in the plantar plane, whereas the Ossa cuneiformia, Os naviculare and the talus increasingly overlay the lateral skeletal parts in the posterior direction, so that the talus is on top of the calcaneus. Thereby the **longitudinal arch opens**

medially. This is **actively** supported by the tendons of the **deep calf muscles** (M. flexor hallucis longus, M. flexor digitorum longus, M. tibialis posterior) and by the **short muscles** in the sole of the foot. This support structure provides a **tension band** which counteracts the body weight.

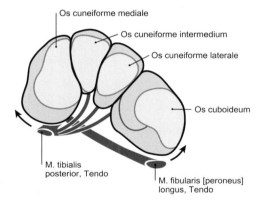

Os cuneiforme mediale

Os cuneiforme intermedium

Os cuneiforme laterale

Os cuboideum

M. tibialis posterior, Tendo

M. fibularis [peroneus] longus, Tendo

Fig. 4.98 Transverse arch of the foot, right side; schematic drawing, dorsal view. [S702-L126]/[G1069]

The **transverse arch** of the foot is formed by the wedge-shaped **cuneiform bones** and the base of the metatarsal bones, and is **passively**

stabilised by the **ligaments** of the foot. In particular, it is **actively** supported by the tendons of the **M. tibialis posterior** and **M. fibularis longus,** and by the **M. adductor hallucis**.

Clinical remarks

Deformities of the feet are very common. High arches (Pes cavus) and flat arches (Pes planus) of the foot can result in excessive pronation and supination of the foot, respectively, which affects the biomechanics of the entire leg (→ Fig. a, → Fig. b). The most common congenital deformity of the extremities is the **congenital clubfoot** in which the foot is fixed in plantar flexion and supination. This is apparently caused by persistence (or insufficient regression) of the intrauterine physiological position of the feet (→ Fig. 3.3). However, deformities are more often secondary to the failure of the tension band system. In the **acquired flatfoot deformity (fallen arches)** the foot is bent medially as the talus 'falls' or drops. Therefore, the metatarsal heads are spread out (splayed), so that the metatarsal bones II–IV come into contact with the ground, which can lead to painful pressure points.
[S701-L126]

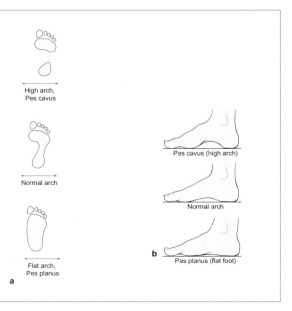

High arch, Pes cavus

Normal arch

Flat arch, Pes planus

a

Pes cavus (high arch)

Normal arch

b   Pes planus (flat foot)

Skeleton

Movements of the ankle and other joints of the feet

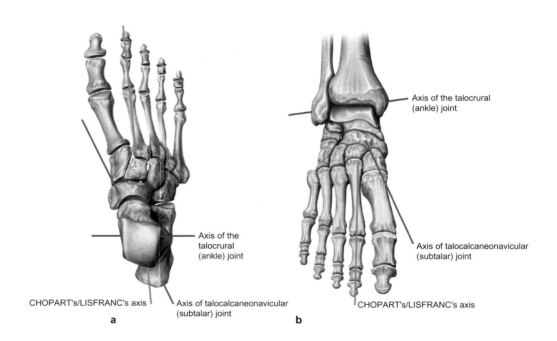

Axis of the talocrural
(ankle) joint

Axis of the
talocrural
(ankle) joint

Axis of talocalcaneonavicular
(subtalar) joint

CHOPART's/LISFRANC's axis

Axis of talocalcaneonavicular
(subtalar) joint

CHOPART's/LISFRANC's axis

a

b

**Fig. 4.99a and b   Axes of the ankle joints as well as the
CHOPART's and LISFRANC's joints.** Red: axis of the talocrural joint,
blue: axis of the subtalar joint, green: axis of the CHOPART's and LIS-
FRANC's joints.
a Cranial view. [S700]
b Ventral view. [S701-L127]
The **talocrural joint** is a classical **hinge joint** (ginglymus). The axis of
the talocrural joint projects through the malleolar fork. In contrast, the
subtalar joint is an **atypical pivot joint** (Articulatio trochoidea), defined by a simplified axis. This virtual axis enters the 'neck' of the talus
and exits through the lateral posterior calcaneus. The joined axis of the
CHOPART's and LISFRANC's joints is aligned with the second phalangeal. While the LISFRANC's joint is considered a typical amphiarthrosis
joint, the range of motion of the CHOPART's joint is even greater, so
that it functions as a pivot joint.

Structure and function

The **CHOPART's joints, LISFRANC's joints** and the subtalar and
talocalcaneonavicular joint add to the range of motion in that a twisting movement of the forefoot is supported by the **rigid hinge joint.**
This enables the entire sole of the foot to tilt during pronation and
supination. The range of motion of the individual phalangeal joints is
largely irrelevant because the toes are fixed, or flexed and extended
in their entirety while standing or walking.

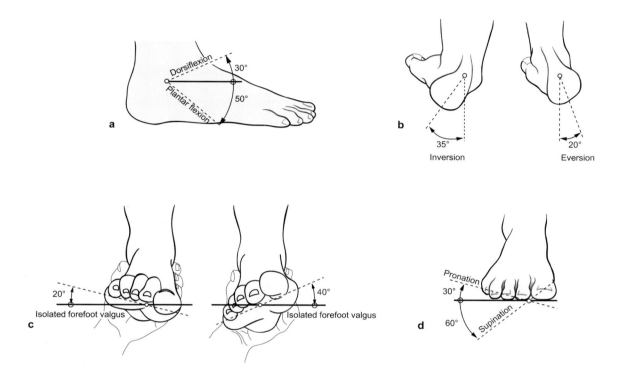

Fig. 4.100a–d   Range of motion of the talocrural joint and the subtalar joint as well as the CHOPART and LISFRANC's joints.
a Lifting of the foot (dorsal extension) and lowering **(plantar flexion)** take place in the talocrural joint. [S700-L126]/[G1070]
b Inversion (medial movement of the hindfoot) and **eversion** (lateral movement of the hindfoot) involve the subtalar joint. [S700-L126]/[B500~M282/L132]
c These movements of the tarsus of the foot are supported by the twisting movement (valgus) of the forefoot in the other joints (CHOPART's and LISFRANC's joint lines). [S700-L303]

d Additionally, **supination** (lifting the medial edge of the foot) and **pronation** (lifting the lateral edge of the foot) support the range of motion of the foot. [S700-L126]/[G1070]
Range of motion:
* Talocrural joint: dorsal extension–plantar flexion: 30°–0°–50°
* Subtalar joint: eversion–inversion: 20°–0°–35°
* CHOPART's/LISFRANC's joints: lateral–medial twisting: 20°–0°–40°
* Subtalar joint and CHOPART's/LISFRANC's joints: pronation–supination: 30°–0°–60°

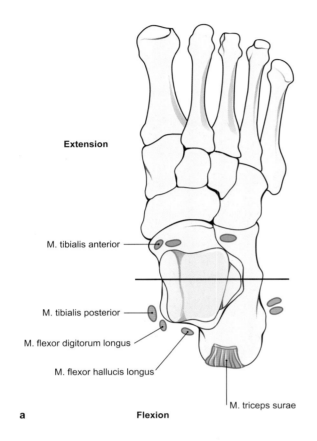

Extension

M. tibialis anterior

M. tibialis posterior

M. flexor digitorum longus

M. flexor hallucis longus

M. triceps surae

a   Flexion

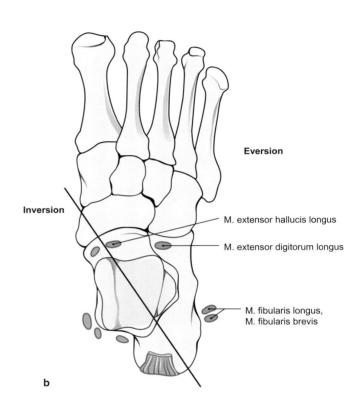

Eversion

Inversion

M. extensor hallucis longus

M. extensor digitorum longus

M. fibularis longus,
M. fibularis brevis

b

Fig. 4.101a and b   **Effect of the muscles of the lower leg on the ankle joints;** schematic dorsal view. [S702-L126]/[B500]
a Course of the inserting tendons in relation to the axis of the talocrural joint.
b Course of the inserting tendons in relation to the axis of the subtalar joint.
All muscles with inserting tendons that run ventrally to the flexion/extension axis of the talocrural joint are **dorsal extensors** (red). Muscles, of which the tendons run dorsally to this axis, are **plantar flexors** (blue).

Muscles that run medially to the axis of the subtalar joint are **supinators** (lifting the medial side of the foot, blue). All muscles with inserting tendons that run laterally to the axis, act as **pronators** (lifting the lateral side of the foot, red). Therefore, the muscles of the anterior group work as dorsal extensors and, with the exception of the M. tibialis anterior, as pronators. The calf muscles are all plantar flexors and strong supinators. The primary function of the fibular muscle group is pronation, but it also supports the plantar flexion.

The most important muscles for movements of the ankle and foot joints		
Mvoement		**Muscle**
Dorsal extension		M. tibialis anterior
Plantar flexion		M. triceps surae
Pronation		M. fibularis longus
Supination		M. triceps surae

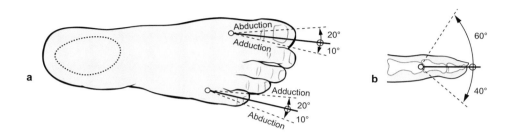

Fig. 4.102a and b   Range of motion in the toe joints.
a The metatarsophalangeal joints are ball-and-socket joints but tight ligaments restrict their movement to two degrees of freedom (rotational movements are not possible). [S700-L126]/[G1070]
b Middle and end phalangeal joints are hinge joints with a small range of movement.

More important than the active movement of the toes is the passive resistance they generate while rolling off the foot when walking. [S700-L126]/[B500-M282]
Range of motion in the metatarsophalangeal joints:
*   Dorsal extension–plantar flexion: 60°–0°–40°
*   Adduction–abduction: 20°–0°–10° (adduction is defined as movement to the midline of the foot!)

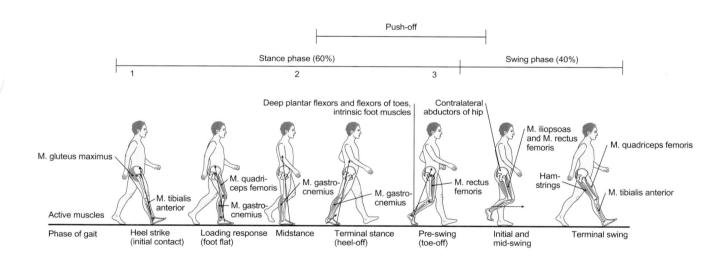

Fig. 4.103   Walking process. [S701-L126]
A walk is composed of a **stance phase** and a **swing phase.** During the stance phase an initial two-legged stance (1) is followed consecutively by a one-legged stance (2) and a terminal two-legged stance (3). This includes a sequence of dorsal flexion combined with pronation when

the heel hits the ground, followed by plantar flexion with supination when pushing off the ground with the toes. As the walking speed accelerates, the individual phases become shorter. When running, the two-legged stance phases are eliminated.

4

Lower limb

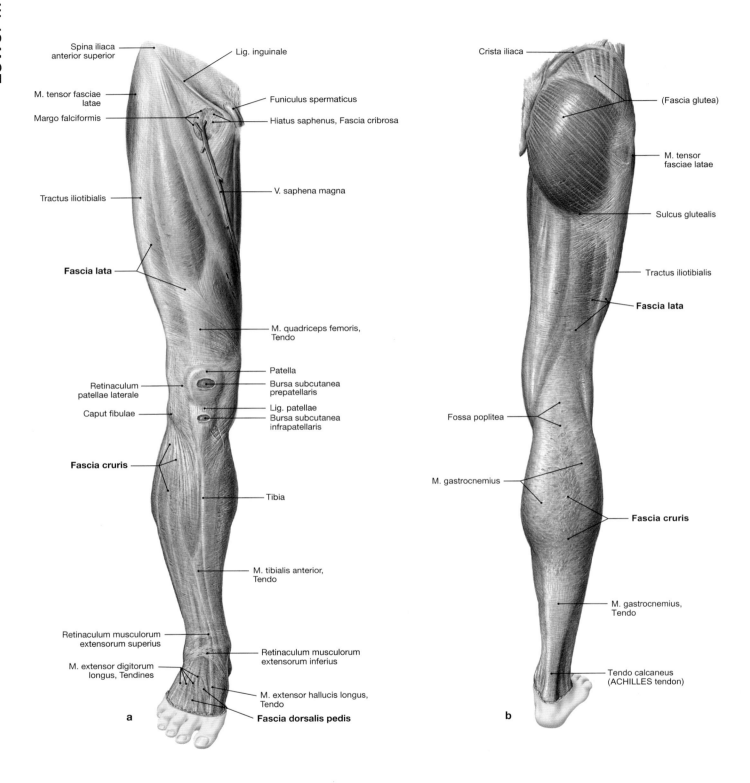

Fig. 4.104a and b   Fascia of the thigh, Fascia lata, of the lower leg, Fascia cruris, and of the dorsum of the foot, Fascia dorsalis pedis, right side. [S700]

a Ventral view.
b Dorsal view.

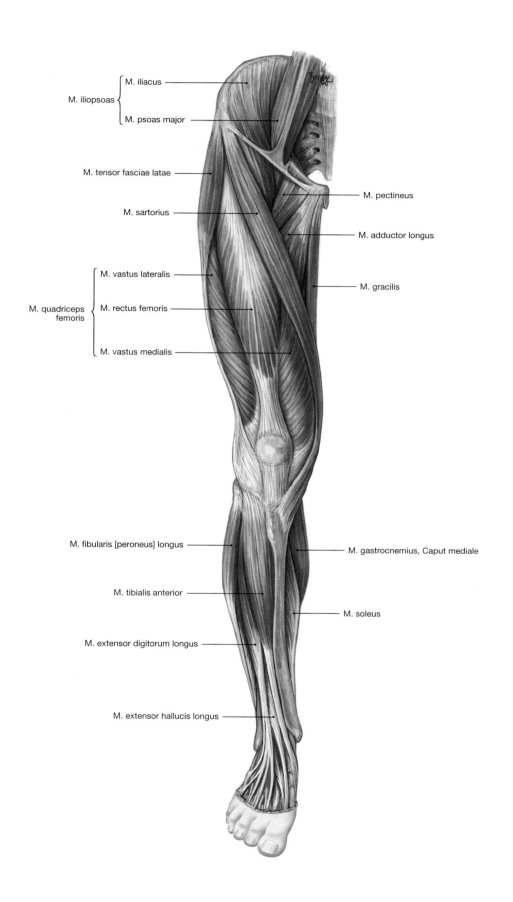

M. iliopsoas {
M. iliacus
M. psoas major
}

M. tensor fasciae latae

M. sartorius

M. quadriceps femoris {
M. vastus lateralis
M. rectus femoris
M. vastus medialis
}

M. pectineus

M. adductor longus

M. gracilis

M. fibularis [peroneus] longus

M. tibialis anterior

M. extensor digitorum longus

M. extensor hallucis longus

M. gastrocnemius, Caput mediale

M. soleus

Fig. 4.105 Ventral muscles of the hip and leg, right side; ventral view. [S700]

→ T 44, T 46, T 47, T 50

4

Lower limb

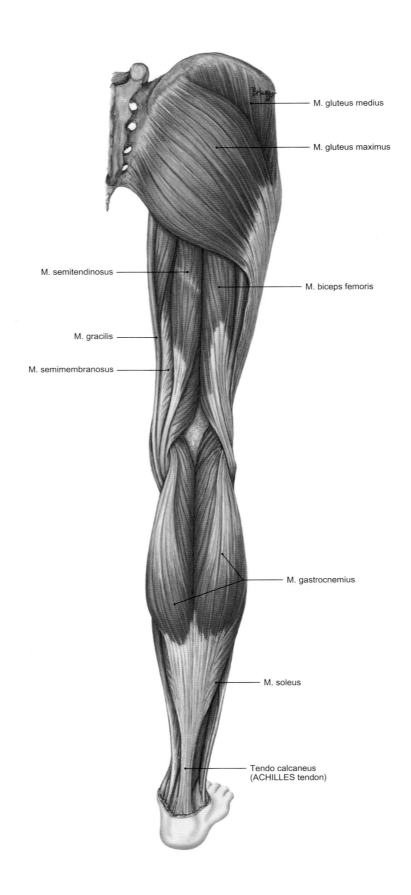

M. gluteus medius

M. gluteus maximus

M. semitendinosus

M. biceps femoris

M. gracilis

M. semimembranosus

M. gastrocnemius

M. soleus

Tendo calcaneus
(ACHILLES tendon)

Fig. 4.106   Dorsal muscles of the hip and leg, right side; dorsal
view. [S700]

→ T 45, T 49, T 52

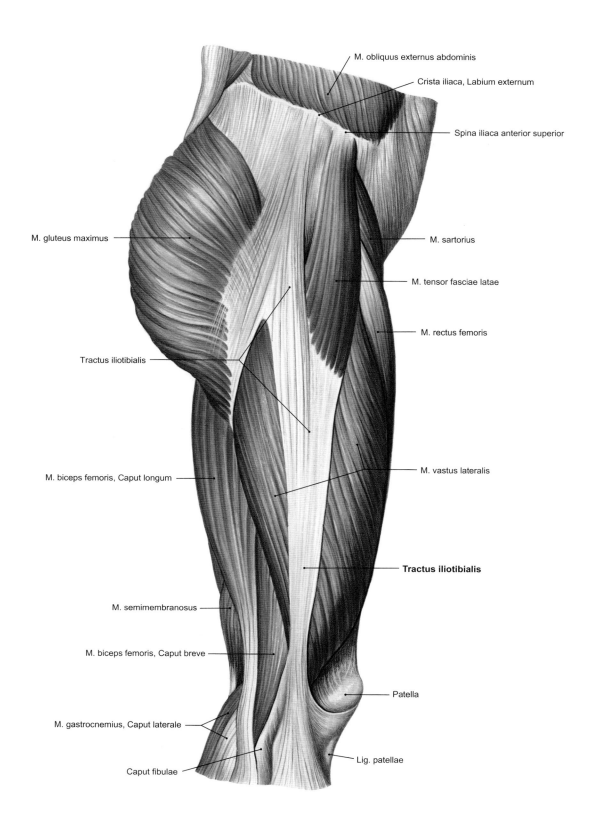

M. obliquus externus abdominis

Crista iliaca, Labium externum

Spina iliaca anterior superior

M. gluteus maximus

M. sartorius

M. tensor fasciae latae

M. rectus femoris

Tractus iliotibialis

M. biceps femoris, Caput longum

M. vastus lateralis

Tractus iliotibialis

M. semimembranosus

M. biceps femoris, Caput breve

Patella

M. gastrocnemius, Caput laterale

Lig. patellae

Caput fibulae

Fig. 4.107 Muscles of the hip and thigh, right side; lateral view. [S700]
The **Tractus iliotibialis** serves as reinforcement of the thigh fascia (Fascia lata), and connects the ilium with the tibia. It counterbalances the medial forces on the thigh bone induced by the weight of the body. This principle is known as a **tension band effect**.

→ T 45

417

Muscles of the hip and thigh

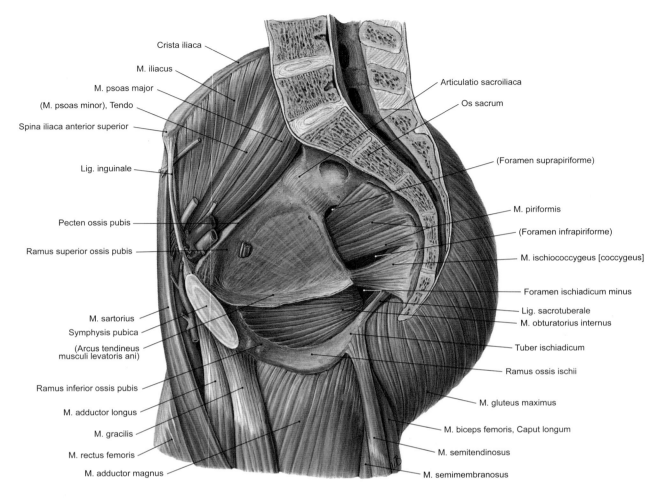

Crista iliaca
M. iliacus
M. psoas major
(M. psoas minor), Tendo
Spina iliaca anterior superior
Lig. inguinale
Pecten ossis pubis
Ramus superior ossis pubis
M. sartorius
Symphysis pubica
(Arcus tendineus musculi levatoris ani)
Ramus inferior ossis pubis
M. adductor longus
M. gracilis
M. rectus femoris
M. adductor magnus

Articulatio sacroiliaca
Os sacrum
(Foramen suprapiriforme)
M. piriformis
(Foramen infrapiriforme)
M. ischiococcygeus [coccygeus]
Foramen ischiadicum minus
Lig. sacrotuberale
M. obturatorius internus
Tuber ischiadicum
Ramus ossis ischii
M. gluteus maximus
M. biceps femoris, Caput longum
M. semitendinosus
M. semimembranosus

Fig. 4.108   Muscles of the hip and thigh, right side; medial view.
[S700]

→ T 44–T 48

Structure and function

The M. psoas major inserts at the lumbar spine and the contraction of this muscle therefore affects the curvature of the lumbar spine (→ Fig. a, → Fig. b). Long hours of sedentary activities can result in **shortening and inflexibility of the psoas muscle** and cause back pain as a result of hyperlordosis of the lumbar spine (→ Fig. b). This pain is most prominent with activities which involve a hyperextension of the hip joint since this stretches the muscle.
[S701-L231]

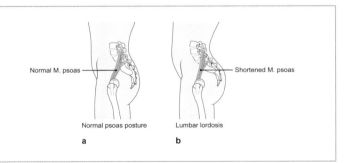

Normal M. psoas

Shortened M. psoas

Normal psoas posture

Lumbar lordosis

a

b

Clinical remarks

The dorsal hip muscles stabilise the hip joint during directional changes in movement and while jumping. Weak gluteal muscles lead to **instability in the hip joint** and can lead to an **increased stress load on the adductor muscles of the knee** (valgus stress; → figure), thereby increasing the load on the anterior cruciate ligament.
[S701-L231]

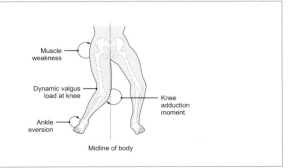

Muscle weakness

Dynamic valgus load at knee

Ankle eversion

Knee adduction moment

Midline of body

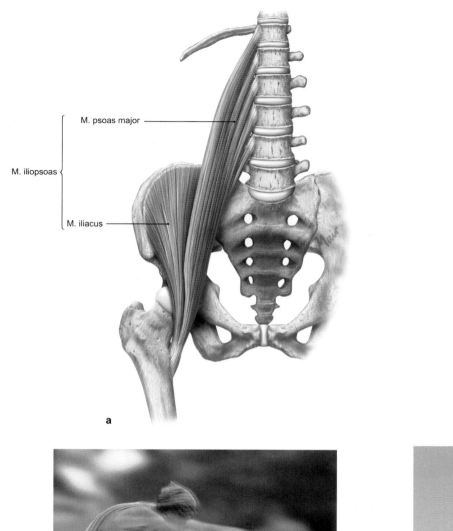

M. psoas major

M. iliopsoas

M. iliacus

a

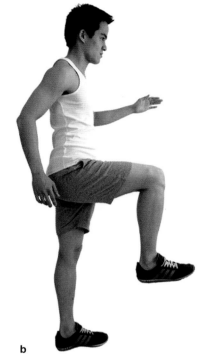

b

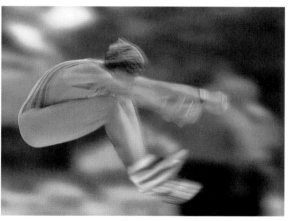

c

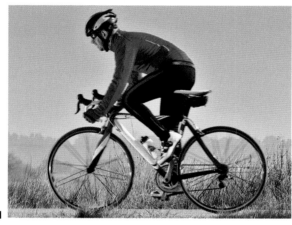

d

Fig. 4.109a–d   Ventral muscles of the hip, right side; ventral view.
The muscles of the hip and upper leg are just as central to the ability to
stand up from a sitting position and to secure a stable stance as to enable walking.
a The **M. iliopsoas** is the **most important flexor** of the hip joint. It is
composed of two separate muscles, the M. psoas major and M. iliacus,
which originate from two different sites but which work as a functional
unit due to using a common tendon that inserts at the Trochanter minor.
Both muscles are innervated by different nerves: the M. psoas major

mainly receives direct motor branches from the Plexus lumbalis which
is embedded within the muscle. By contrast, M. iliacus is innervated by
the N. femoralis.
b–d The M. iliopsoas enables strong flexion in the hip joint (b) and is
particularly used during sports activities such as the long jump and cycling. a [S700-L127], b [S701-L271], c, d [J787]

→ T 44

Clinical remarks

The differences in nerve innervation of the two parts of the M. iliopsoas need to be considered when an injection of Botulinum toxin is
needed to treat **muscle spasms.** Permanent contraction of the iliopsoas results in a flexed hip joint which makes it impossible to assume a stance position on this leg. As a first step, the part of the
muscle close to the inserting tendon at the Trochanter minor can be
injected below the inguinal ligament. These muscle fibres are indeed

mainly derived from the M. iliacus. If unsuccessful in reducing the
flexion in the hip joint, the muscles of the M. psoas major need to be
injected. In a lean adult and in children, injecting into the psoas muscle is certainly possible via the abdominal wall, but this carries an
increased risk of injuring intestinal organs. Alternatively, a dorsal injection next to the lumbar spine and through the musculature of the
back is possible.

Musculature

Muscles of the hip and thigh

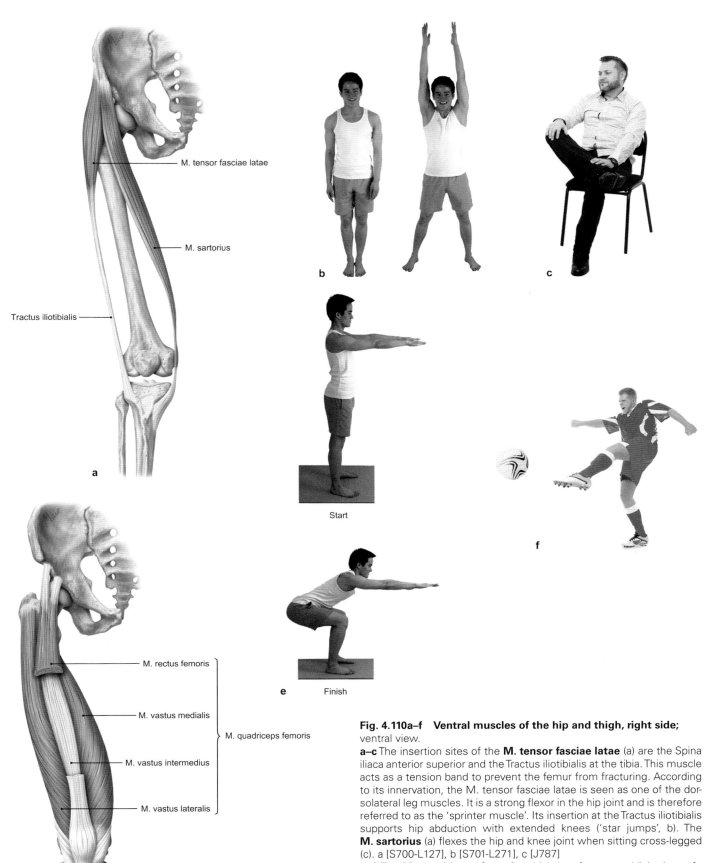

Fig. 4.110a–f Ventral muscles of the hip and thigh, right side; ventral view.

a–c The insertion sites of the **M. tensor fasciae latae** (a) are the Spina iliaca anterior superior and the Tractus iliotibialis at the tibia. This muscle acts as a tension band to prevent the femur from fracturing. According to its innervation, the M. tensor fasciae latae is seen as one of the dorsolateral leg muscles. It is a strong flexor in the hip joint and is therefore referred to as the 'sprinter muscle'. Its insertion at the Tractus iliotibialis supports hip abduction with extended knees ('star jumps', b). The **M. sartorius** (a) flexes the hip and knee joint when sitting cross-legged (c). a [S700-L127], b [S701-L271], c [J787]

d–f The **M. quadriceps femoris** which has four parts (d) is the **only extensor of the knee joint** and is essential for the body to raise itself from a squatting position. Because the M. rectus femoris spans two joints and additionally flexes the hip, the quadriceps muscle is also activated during knee flexion (e) and powerful kicking movements (f). d [S700-L127], e [S701-L271], f [J787]

→ T 45, T 47

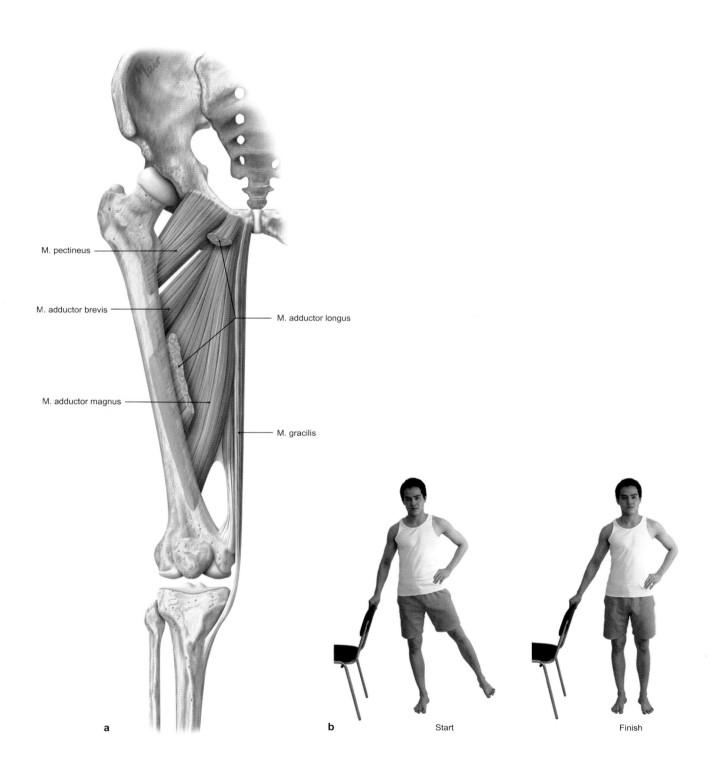

Fig. 4.111a and b Medial muscles of the hip and thigh, right side; ventral view.

a The **adductor muscle group** (Mm. adductores) lies medially on the thigh. [S700-L127]

b The adductor muscles are the most important muscles for adduction in the hip joint. Their actions stabilise the hip during walking and stand-

ing, and prevent the leg, for example, sliding laterally on a slippery surface. A malfunction of the adductors therefore results in an insecure posture and gait. [S701-L271]

→ T 48

Musculature

Muscles of the hip and thigh

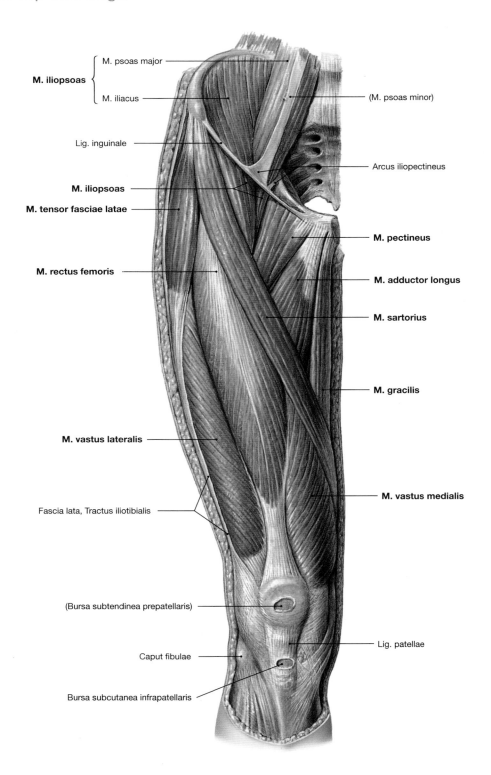

M. psoas major

M. iliopsoas {

M. iliacus

(M. psoas minor)

Lig. inguinale

Arcus iliopectineus

M. iliopsoas

M. tensor fasciae latae

M. pectineus

M. rectus femoris

M. adductor longus

M. sartorius

M. gracilis

M. vastus lateralis

M. vastus medialis

Fascia lata, Tractus iliotibialis

(Bursa subtendinea prepatellaris)

Lig. patellae

Caput fibulae

Bursa subcutanea infrapatellaris

Fig. 4.112 Ventral muscles of the hip and thigh, and medial muscles of the thigh, right side; ventral view; after removal of the Fascia lata ventrally of the Tractus iliotibialis. [S700]

The **M. iliopsoas** is composed of two different muscles which originate from within the lumbar spine (M. psoas major) and from the Fossa iliaca (M. iliacus). Below the inguinal ligament, these two muscles only run a short distance down the thigh to their common insertion point at the Trochanter minor.

The **M. sartorius** is a split portion of the Fascia lata and crosses the thigh medially before inserting on the medial aspect of the tibia posterior to the transverse (flexion) axis of the knee. It can therefore bend the hip joint as well as the knee joint.

Medially, the muscles of the **adductor group** lie in several layers on top of each other, so that only the superficially located M. pectineus, M. adductor longus and M. gracilis are visible. The four heads of the **M. quadriceps femoris** (M. rectus femoris, M. vastus lateralis, medialis, and intermedius) lie distally and laterally of the M. sartorius. Their common inserting tendon incorporates the patella as a sesamoid bone before the fibres continue as the Lig. patellae to the Tuberositas tibiae. The most lateral hip muscle is the **M. tensor fasciae latae,** which radiates into the Tractus iliotibialis. The common insertion of the Mm. sartorius, gracilis, and semitendinosus below the medial tibial condyle is often referred to as the 'Pes anserinus superficialis'.

→ T 44, T 47, T 48

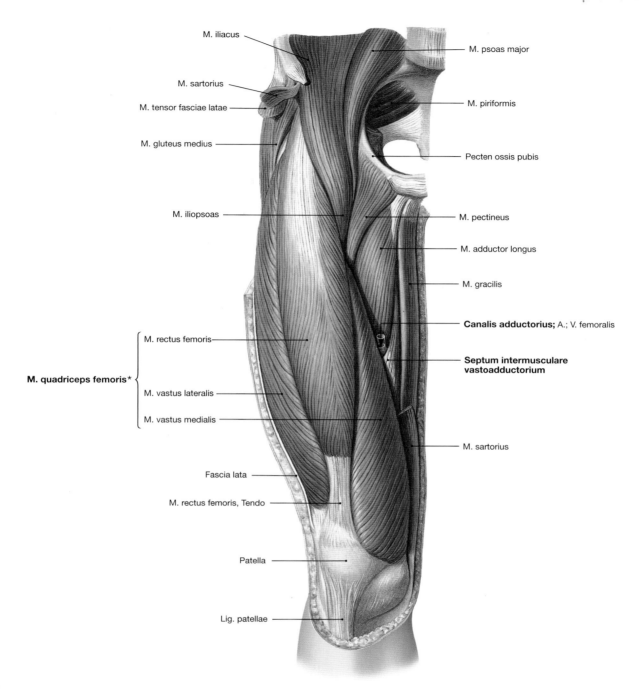

M. iliacus

M. psoas major

M. sartorius

M. piriformis

M. tensor fasciae latae

M. gluteus medius

Pecten ossis pubis

M. iliopsoas

M. pectineus

M. adductor longus

M. gracilis

Canalis adductorius; A.; V. femoralis

M. rectus femoris

Septum intermusculare
vastoadductorium

M. quadriceps femoris*

M. vastus lateralis

M. vastus medialis

M. sartorius

Fascia lata

M. rectus femoris, Tendo

Patella

Lig. patellae

Fig. 4.113 Ventral muscles of the thigh and hip, and medial muscles of the thigh, right side; ventral view; after removal of the Fascia lata as well as the Mm. sartorius and tensor fasciae latae. [S700]
After removal of the M. sartorius, the entrance to the **adductor canal** (Canalis adductorius) is visible where it is bordered dorsally by the M. adductor longus. The adductor canal is covered by the Septum intermusculare vastoadductorium, which connects the fasciae of the M. vastus medialis, the M. adductor longus and the M. adductor magnus.

The four heads of the **M. quadriceps femoris** (M. rectus femoris, Mm. vasti lateralis, medialis, and intermedius) are located laterally to the adductor canal.

* The fourth head of the M. quadriceps femoris – the M. vastus intermedius – lies below the M. rectus femoris.

→ T 44, T 47, T 48

Clinical remarks

With **spasticity** or **dystonia,** if the hip joint is fixed in a flexed position due to permanent contraction of the M. iliopsoas, standing upright is impossible. To treat it, the motor innervation of the muscle is inhibited by the injection of botulinum toxin in order to relax the mus-

cle via a synaptic blockade. Because of the particular course of the muscle, only a small part of it is accessible by injection below the inguinal ligament, so that an additional injection into the lumbar section of the M. psoas major may be required.

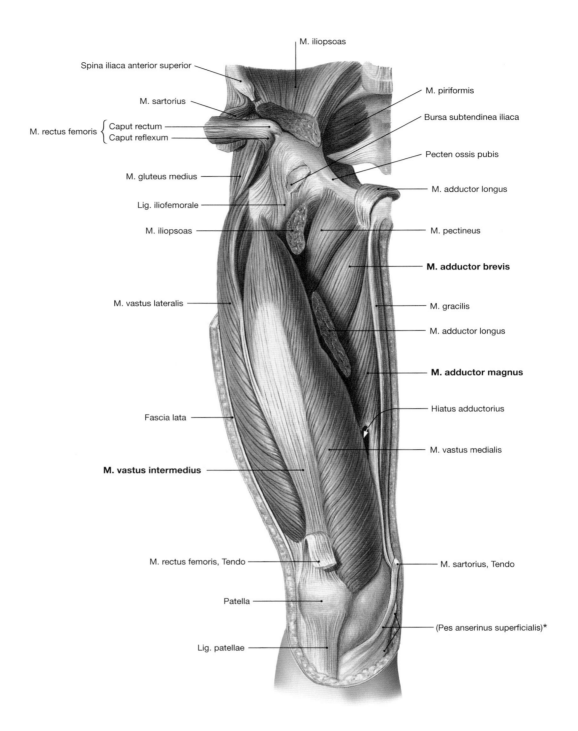

M. iliopsoas

Spina iliaca anterior superior

M. sartorius

M. rectus femoris { Caput rectum / Caput reflexum

M. gluteus medius

Lig. iliofemorale

M. iliopsoas

M. vastus lateralis

Fascia lata

M. vastus intermedius

M. rectus femoris, Tendo

Patella

Lig. patellae

M. piriformis

Bursa subtendinea iliaca

Pecten ossis pubis

M. adductor longus

M. pectineus

M. adductor brevis

M. gracilis

M. adductor longus

M. adductor magnus

Hiatus adductorius

M. vastus medialis

M. sartorius, Tendo

(Pes anserinus superficialis)*

Fig. 4.114 Ventral muscles of the hip and thigh, and deep medial muscles of the thigh, right side; ventral view; after removal of the Fascia lata, of the Mm. sartorius, rectus femoris and adductor longus and partial removal of the M. iliopsoas in the joint area. [S700] The M. rectus femoris and a part of the M. adductor longus are folded back laterally and superiorly. After removal of the M. rectus femoris, the **M. vastus intermedius** of the M. quadriceps femoris is visible. The resection of the M. sartorius and M. adductor longus reveals the deep adductor muscles – the **M. adductor brevis** and parts of the **M. adductor magnus.**

* common insertion of the Mm. sartorius, gracilis and semitendinosus

→ T 47, T 48

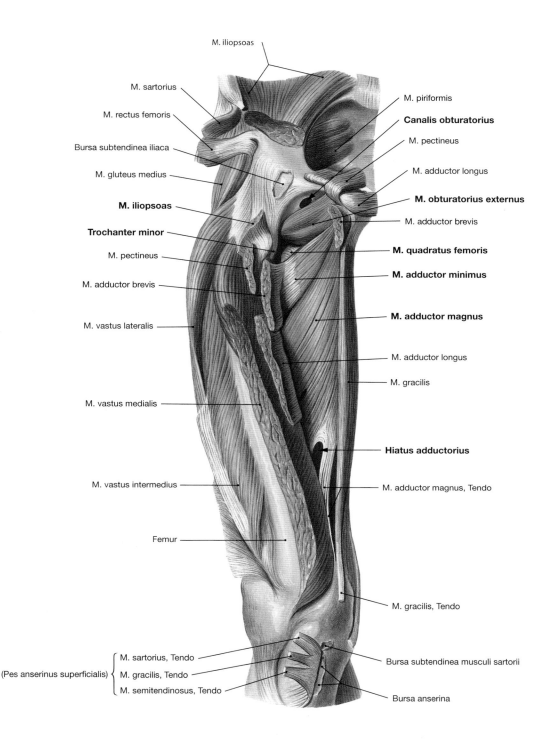

M. iliopsoas

M. sartorius

M. rectus femoris

Bursa subtendinea iliaca

M. gluteus medius

M. iliopsoas

Trochanter minor

M. pectineus

M. adductor brevis

M. vastus lateralis

M. vastus medialis

M. vastus intermedius

Femur

(Pes anserinus superficialis) { M. sartorius, Tendo
M. gracilis, Tendo
M. semitendinosus, Tendo

M. piriformis

Canalis obturatorius

M. pectineus

M. adductor longus

M. obturatorius externus

M. adductor brevis

M. quadratus femoris

M. adductor minimus

M. adductor magnus

M. adductor longus

M. gracilis

Hiatus adductorius

M. adductor magnus, Tendo

M. gracilis, Tendo

Bursa subtendinea musculi sartorii

Bursa anserina

Fig. 4.115 Ventral muscles of the thigh and hip, and deep medial muscles of the thigh, right side; ventral view; after extensive removal of the superficial and some deeper muscles. [S700]

If, in addition to the superficial adductor muscles, the M. adductor brevis is also folded to the side, the **M. adductor magnus** becomes visible, the upper portion of which is also referred to as the M. adductor minimus. The M. adductor magnus and its inserting tendon form the **adductor hiatus** (Hiatus adductorius) through which the blood vessels of the thigh (A./V. femoralis) pass dorsally into the popliteal fossa. Proximally, the insertion of the M. iliopsoas on the Trochanter minor can be identified after resection of the M. pectineus and M. adductor brevis. In

addition, the **Canalis obturatorius** is also exposed as an opening in the Membrana obturatoria, which forms a neurovascular pathway between the lesser pelvis and the thigh. Caudal of this opening, the almost horizontal fibres of the **M. obturatorius externus** and the deeper **M. quadratus femoris** are revealed, both of which belong to the pelvitrochanteric group of the dorsal hip muscles (→ Fig. 4.116). As these two muscles are not displayed very often in dissection classes, it is hard to visualise their course.

→ T 44–T 47

Musculature

Muscles of the hip

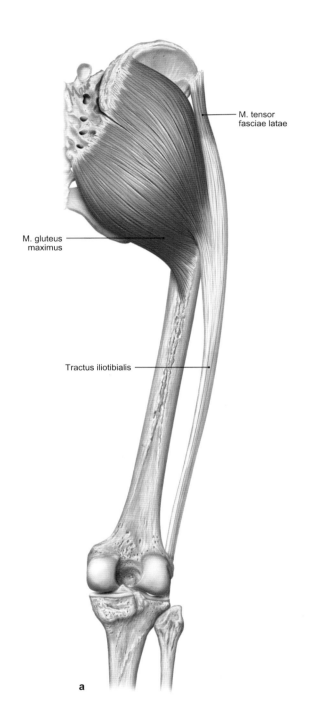

M. tensor
fasciae latae

M. gluteus
maximus

Tractus iliotibialis

a

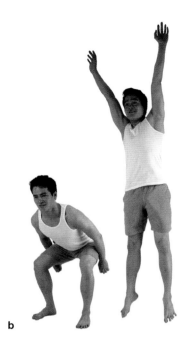

b

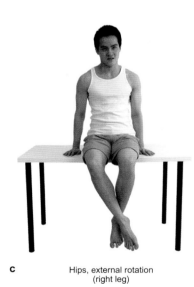

c   Hips, external rotation
(right leg)

Fig. 4.116a–c   Dorsal muscles of the hip, M. gluteus maximus, right side; dorsal view.
a The dorsal muscles of the hip can be divided into either a dorsolateral or a pelvitrochanteric group. The **dorsolateral group** includes the Mm. gluteus maximus, medius and minimus. According to its innervation, the **M. tensor fasciae latae** may also be included in this group. [S700-L127]

b The **M. gluteus maximus** is the most important **extensor** of the hip. This muscle is particularly important for straightening up from a squatting position and for climbing stairs. In addition, jumping becomes impossible without this muscle. [S701-L271]
c The M. gluteus maximus is also the strongest **lateral rotator** of the hip joint. [S701-L271]

→ T 45

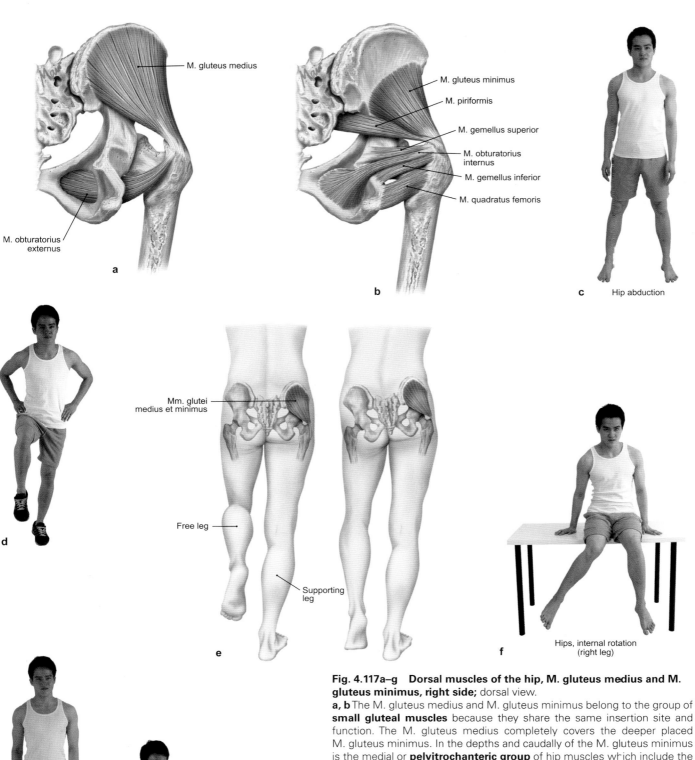

M. gluteus medius

M. obturatorius externus

a

M. gluteus minimus

M. piriformis

M. gemellus superior

M. obturatorius internus

M. gemellus inferior

M. quadratus femoris

b

c Hip abduction

d

Mm. glutei medius et minimus

Free leg

Supporting leg

e

Hips, internal rotation (right leg)

f

g

Fig. 4.117a–g   Dorsal muscles of the hip, M. gluteus medius and M. gluteus minimus, right side; dorsal view.

a, b The M. gluteus medius and M. gluteus minimus belong to the group of **small gluteal muscles** because they share the same insertion site and function. The M. gluteus medius completely covers the deeper placed M. gluteus minimus. In the depths and caudally of the M. gluteus minimus is the medial or **pelvitrochanteric group** of hip muscles which include the M. piriformis, M. obturatorius internus, Mm. gemelli superior and inferior, and the M. quadratus femoris. [S700-L127]

c–f The small gluteal muscles are the most important abductors in the hip joint (c). During standing or walking, they stabilise the hip and prevent tilting of the hip to the opposite side when standing on one leg. This tilting of the hip, known as the TRENDELENBURG sign, is frequently observed with palsy of the N. gluteus superior (e). The M. gluteus medius and M. gluteus minimus are additionally the most important hip **internal rotators** (f), even though their movement is not as significant. c, d, f [S701-L271], e [S700-L127]

g The muscles of the pelvitrochanteric group are innervated by direct motor branches from the Plexus sacralis and support the **external rotation** of the hip which is required for crossing the legs. Although innervated by the N. obturatorius and originating as an adductor muscle, the M. obturatorius externus is also a functional part of this group. [S701-L271]

→ T 45, T 46

427

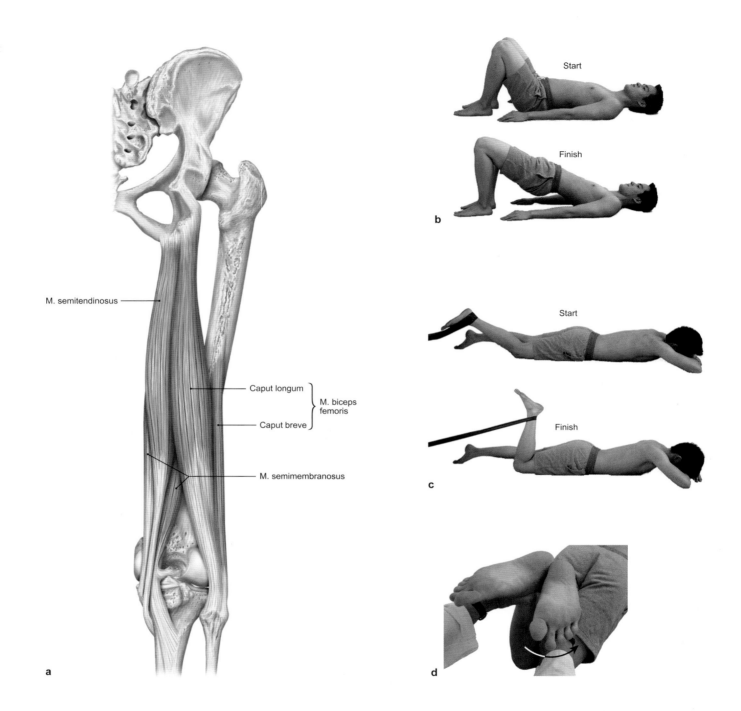

M. semitendinosus

Caput longum ⎤
⎥ M. biceps
⎥ femoris
Caput breve ⎦

M. semimembranosus

a

Start

Finish

b

Start

Finish

c

d

Fig. 4.118a–d   Dorsal (hamstring, ischiocrural) muscles of the thigh, right side; dorsal view.

a–c The dorsal **(hamstring) muscles** are located on the posterior (dorsal) side of the thigh where they originate from the Tuber ischiadicum and insert on both bones of the lower leg (a). These muscles thereby span two joints and extend the hip joint (b), while being the strongest flexors in the knee joint (c).

d The lateral **M. biceps femoris** functions in **lateral rotation** of both the hip and knee joint, whereas the medially located **M. semitendinosus** and **M. semimembranosus** facilitate **internal rotation**.
a [S700-L127], b–d [S701-L271]

→ T 49

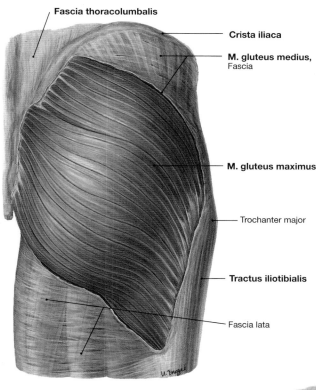

Fascia thoracolumbalis

Crista iliaca

M. gluteus medius,
Fascia

M. gluteus maximus

Trochanter major

Tractus iliotibialis

Fascia lata

a

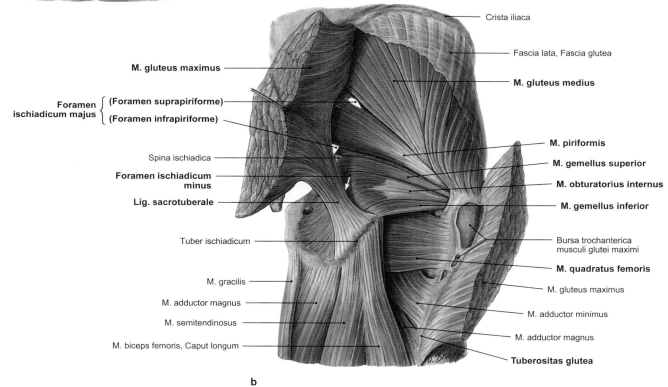

Crista iliaca

Fascia lata, Fascia glutea

M. gluteus maximus

M. gluteus medius

Foramen
ischiadicum majus { **(Foramen suprapiriforme)**

(Foramen infrapiriforme)

M. piriformis

M. gemellus superior

Spina ischiadica

M. obturatorius internus

**Foramen ischiadicum
minus**

M. gemellus inferior

Lig. sacrotuberale

Bursa trochanterica
musculi glutei maximi

Tuber ischiadicum

M. quadratus femoris

M. gracilis

M. gluteus maximus

M. adductor magnus

M. adductor minimus

M. semitendinosus

M. adductor magnus

M. biceps femoris, Caput longum

Tuberositas glutea

b

Fig. 4.119a and b   Dorsal muscles of the hip and thigh, right side;
dorsal view. [S700]

a After splitting open the Fascia lata. The illustration shows the superficial origins and insertions of the **M. gluteus maximus**. The muscle originates superficially from the posterior aspect of the sacrum, the iliac crest and the Fascia thoracolumbalis. These muscle fibres run obliquely, while those of the M. gluteus medius, located deeply under the **M. gluteus maximus,** run almost vertically. The M. gluteus maximus has superficial attachments on the Fascia lata and Tractus iliotibialis.

b After severing the M. gluteus maximus. The illustration depicts the deep origins and insertion points of the **M. gluteus maximus**. The muscle's deep point of origin is the Lig. sacrotuberale and the deep insertion

point is the Tuberositas glutea of the femur. When the M. gluteus maximus is split or folded laterally, the **M. gluteus medius** with its vertical fibre projections and the **pelvitrochanteric muscles** become visible. The **M. piriformis** divides the Foramen ischiadicum majus into the **Foramina suprapiriforme** and **infrapiriforme,** which are important openings for neurovascular pathways from the pelvis. It should be noted that there can be a more tendinous portion of the **M. obturatorius internus** between its fulcrum (hypomochlion) in the Incisura ischiadica minor and its insertion point in the Fossa trochanterica.

→ T 45, T 46, T 49

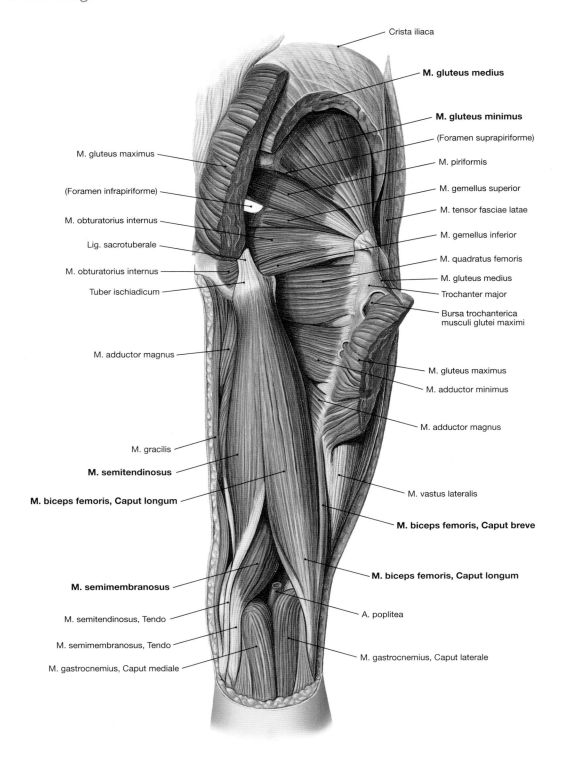

Crista iliaca

M. gluteus medius

M. gluteus minimus

(Foramen suprapiriforme)

M. gluteus maximus

M. piriformis

M. gemellus superior

(Foramen infrapiriforme)

M. tensor fasciae latae

M. obturatorius internus

M. gemellus inferior

Lig. sacrotuberale

M. quadratus femoris

M. obturatorius internus

M. gluteus medius

Tuber ischiadicum

Trochanter major

Bursa trochanterica
musculi glutei maximi

M. adductor magnus

M. gluteus maximus

M. adductor minimus

M. adductor magnus

M. gracilis

M. semitendinosus

M. vastus lateralis

M. biceps femoris, Caput longum

M. biceps femoris, Caput breve

M. biceps femoris, Caput longum

M. semimembranosus

A. poplitea

M. semitendinosus, Tendo

M. semimembranosus, Tendo

M. gastrocnemius, Caput laterale

M. gastrocnemius, Caput mediale

Fig. 4.120 Dorsal muscles of the thigh and hip, right side; dorsal view; after partial removal of the M. gluteus maximus and medius. [S700]
After severing the M. gluteus medius as well as the M. gluteus maximus, the **M. gluteus minimus** becomes visible. Together with the M. gluteus medius, it is seen as part of the group of the **small gluteal muscles.** Both muscles assist in the abduction of the hip and the stabilisation of the pelvis when standing on one leg.

On the dorsal side of the thigh, the **hamstring muscles** have been dissected, which run from the Tuber ischiadicum to the bones of the lower leg. Medially, the **M. semitendinosus** (named after its long tendon of insertion) is located superficially to the **M. semimembranosus** (named after its flat tendon of origin); the lateral **M. biceps femoris** of which the Caput longum also originates from the Tuber ischiadicum, while its Caput breve has a distal origin on the femur (Labium laterale of the Linea aspera).

→ T 45, T 49

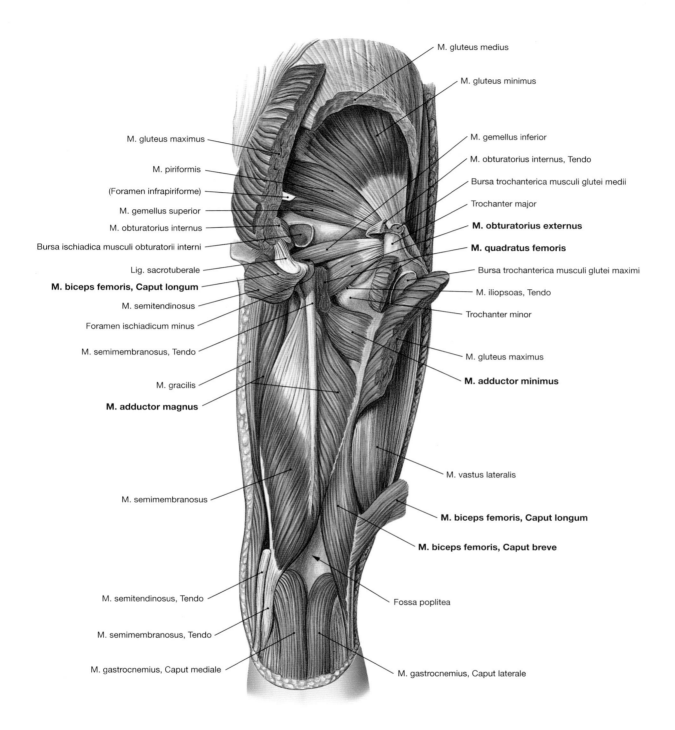

M. gluteus medius

M. gluteus minimus

M. gluteus maximus

M. piriformis

(Foramen infrapiriforme)

M. gemellus superior

M. obturatorius internus

Bursa ischiadica musculi obturatorii interni

Lig. sacrotuberale

M. biceps femoris, Caput longum

M. semitendinosus

Foramen ischiadicum minus

M. semimembranosus, Tendo

M. gracilis

M. adductor magnus

M. semimembranosus

M. semitendinosus, Tendo

M. semimembranosus, Tendo

M. gastrocnemius, Caput mediale

M. gemellus inferior

M. obturatorius internus, Tendo

Bursa trochanterica musculi glutei medii

Trochanter major

M. obturatorius externus

M. quadratus femoris

Bursa trochanterica musculi glutei maximi

M. iliopsoas, Tendo

Trochanter minor

M. gluteus maximus

M. adductor minimus

M. vastus lateralis

M. biceps femoris, Caput longum

M. biceps femoris, Caput breve

Fossa poplitea

M. gastrocnemius, Caput laterale

Fig. 4.121 Deep dorsal muscles of the thigh and hip, right side; dorsal view; after extensive removal of the superficial gluteal and hamstring (ischiocrural) muscles. [S700]
Upon splitting the M. quadratus femoris, the deeper **M. obturatorius externus** is visible; its course is often difficult to visualise. Removal of the long head of the M. biceps femoris exposes the deep components of the adductor group. The **M. adductor magnus** consists of two functionally different muscle parts, which also have a different innervation.

Its major component originates from the inferior pubic ramus (this part is sometimes referred to as the **M. adductor minimus**) and from the ischiopubic ramus. The posterior part, on the other hand, originates from the Tuber ischiadicum, and according to its function and innervation, is ascribed to the hamstring muscles.

→ T 45, T 46, T 48, T 49

Lower limb

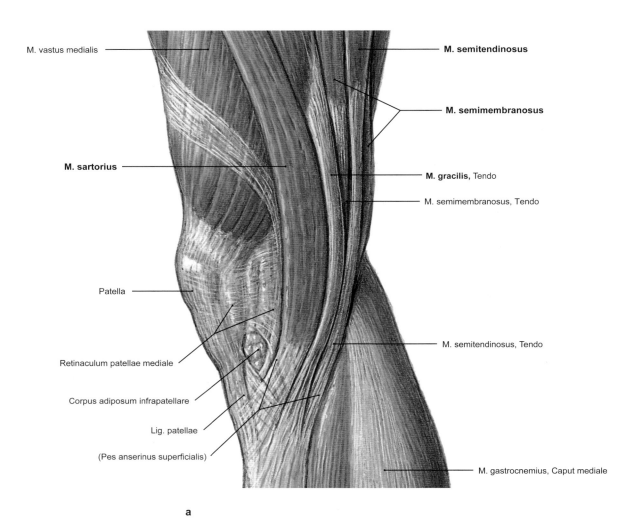

M. vastus medialis

M. semitendinosus

M. semimembranosus

M. sartorius

M. gracilis, Tendo

M. semimembranosus, Tendo

Patella

Retinaculum patellae mediale

M. semitendinosus, Tendo

Corpus adiposum infrapatellare

Lig. patellae

(Pes anserinus superficialis)

M. gastrocnemius, Caput mediale

a

Fig. 4.122a Muscles in the knee joint region, left side; medial view. [S700]
The common insertion point of the Mm. sartorius, gracilis and semi-tendinosus beneath the medial tibial condyle is often referred to as the 'Pes anserinus superficialis'. The deep insertion point of the M. semi-membranosus is often referred to as 'Pes anserinus profundus'.

→ T 47–T 49

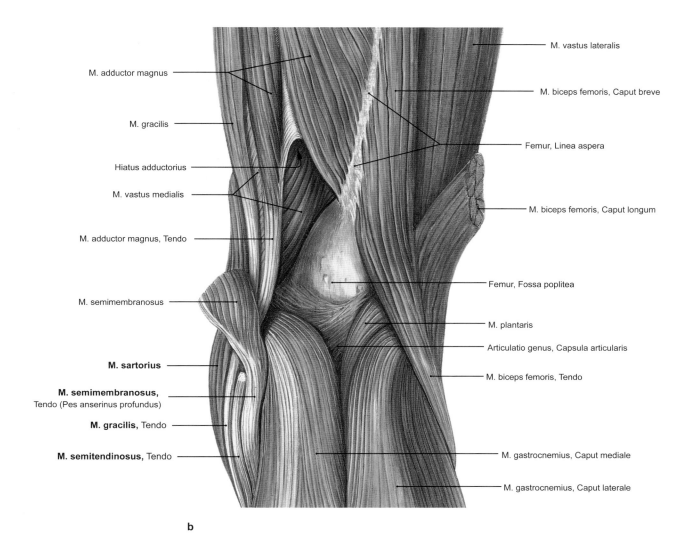

M. adductor magnus

M. gracilis

Hiatus adductorius

M. vastus medialis

M. adductor magnus, Tendo

M. semimembranosus

M. sartorius

M. semimembranosus,
Tendo (Pes anserinus profundus)

M. gracilis, Tendo

M. semitendinosus, Tendo

M. vastus lateralis

M. biceps femoris, Caput breve

Femur, Linea aspera

M. biceps femoris, Caput longum

Femur, Fossa poplitea

M. plantaris

Articulatio genus, Capsula articularis

M. biceps femoris, Tendo

M. gastrocnemius, Caput mediale

M. gastrocnemius, Caput laterale

b

Fig. 4.122b   Muscles in the knee joint region, right side; dorsal view. [S700]
The common insertion point of the Mm. sartorius, gracilis and semi-tendinosus beneath the medial tibial condyle is often referred to as the 'Pes anserinus superficialis'. The deep insertion point of the M. semi-membranosus is often referred to as 'Pes anserinus profundus'.

→ T 47–T 49

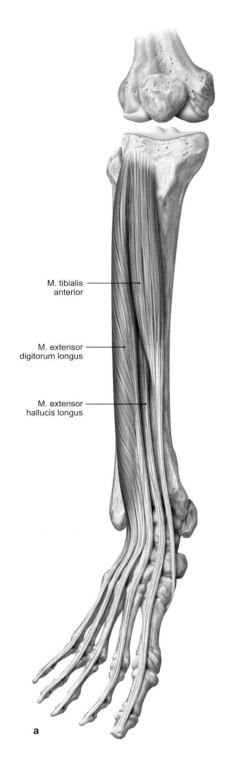

M. tibialis
anterior

M. extensor
digitorum longus

M. extensor
hallucis longus

a

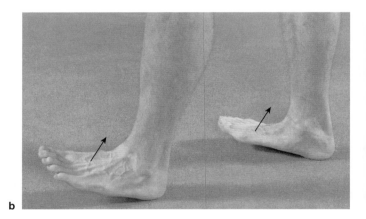

b

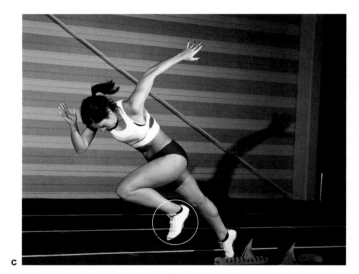

c

Fig. 4.123a–c   Muscles of the lower leg, right side.
a, b Ventral view. In the lower leg region there are three muscle groups. To understand their function, it is important to know their position in relation to the axes of movement of the ankle joints (→ Fig. 4.101). All the muscles lying in front of the transverse axis of the talocrural joint are **extensors** (a). In this group, the **M. tibialis anterior** is the most important extensor in the ankle joint, whereas the **M. extensor digitorum longus** and the **M. extensor hallucis longus** also extend the phalangeal joints of the toes (b). The muscles, of which the tendons lie **medially** to the obliquely running axis of the subtalar joint from medial-

ly superior to laterally inferior, are plantar **supinators** which raise the medial edge of the foot. The M. tibialis anterior is therefore also a weak supinator. In contrast, the **laterally** located M. extensor digitorum longus and hallucis longus raise the lateral side of the foot to support **pronation** of the foot. a [S700-L127], b [E563]
c Extension of the talocrural joint and the phalangeal joints of the toes is necessary for raising the tip of the foot in the swing phase of the leg when walking or running. [J787]

→ T 50

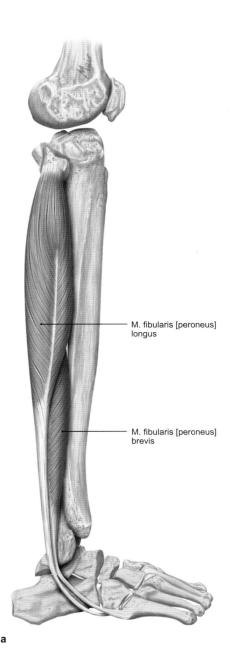

M. fibularis [peroneus] longus

M. fibularis [peroneus] brevis

a

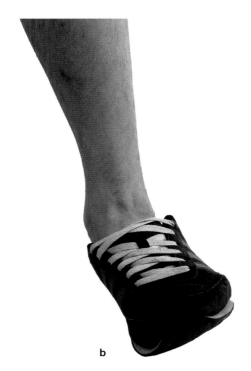

b

Fig. 4.124a and b   Lateral muscles of the lower leg, fibularis muscle group, right side.
a Lateral view. The lateral (fibular) muscles of the lower leg are the **Mm. fibulares longus and brevis** and serve as the most important pronators of the foot. These muscles also act as plantar flexors of the talocrural joint because of their location posterior to the flexion-extension axis. [S700-L127]
b Pronation of the foot is the most important function of the fibularis muscle group. [S701-L271]

→ T 51

Lower limb

Muscles of the lower leg

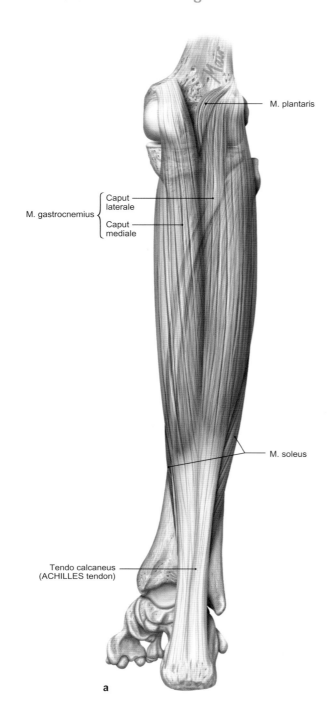

M. plantaris

M. gastrocnemius {
Caput laterale
Caput mediale

M. soleus

Tendo calcaneus (ACHILLES tendon)

a

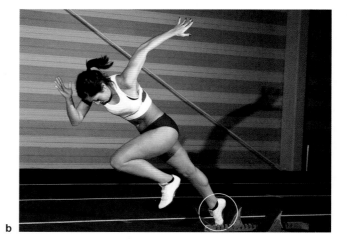

b

Fig. 4.125a and b   Superficial calf muscles, right side.
a Dorsal view. All muscles positioned **posterior** to the transverse axis of the talocrural joint act as **flexors** of the foot. This includes the superficial and deep calf muscles. The **M. triceps surae** belongs to the dorsal superficial muscles and comprises the two-headed **M. gastrocnemius** and the **M. soleus** located deeper below. As the M. triceps surae, in contrast to the M. soleus, originates from the femur condyles, thereby spanning two joints, this muscle also supports flexion of the knee joint.

Besides being the **strongest flexor** of the talocrural joint, the M. triceps surae is also the **strongest supinator** of the foot. In contrast, the **M. plantaris** is insignificant and a weak flexor in the knee joint. [S700-L127]
b Plantar flexion of the foot is important for the foot to push off powerfully when walking and running. [J787]

→ T 52

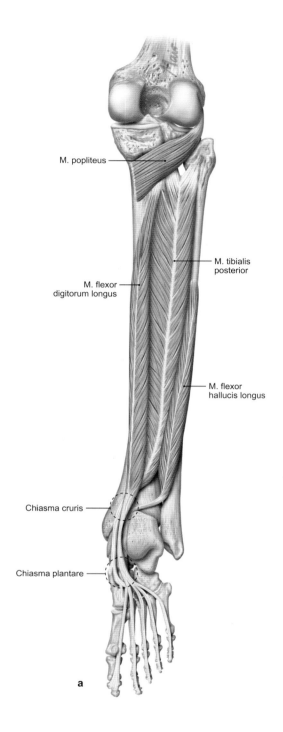

M. popliteus

M. tibialis posterior

M. flexor digitorum longus

M. flexor hallucis longus

Chiasma cruris

Chiasma plantare

a

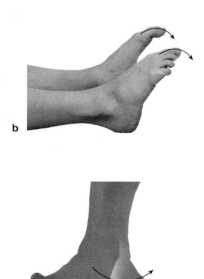

b

c

Fig. 4.126a–c   Deep calf muscles, right side.
a Dorsal view. The deep dorsal calf muscles are largely similar to the extensors on the ventral side (→ Fig. 4.123) but are arranged differently from medial to lateral. The tendon of the M. flexor digitorum longus crosses over the tendon of the M. tibialis posterior and the M. flexor hallucis longus above the inner side of the ankle (Chiasma cruris) and at the underside of the foot (Chiasma plantare), respectively.
The **M. tibialis posterior** is a strong supinator in addition to having a flexing function. The **M. flexor digitorum longus** and the **M. flexor hallucis longus** are flexors of the toes in the phalangeal joints. The **M. popliteus** has a special status as an important stabiliser of the knee joint. The tendon of the M. flexor digitorum longus crosses the tendon of the M. tibialis posterior above the medial malleolus **(Chiasma cruris),** as

well as the tendon of the M. flexor hallucis longus in the sole of the foot **(Chiasma plantare).** The **M. popliteus** has a special role as the most important stabiliser of the knee joint. This muscle initiates flexion in the knee joint by inducing an **internal rotation of the knee.** [S700-L127]
b, c Because of their relative course to the axis of the ankle joint, all muscles of this group act as flexors (b) and support the supination of the foot (c). The **M. flexor digitorum longus** and the **M. flexor hallucis longus** are also flexors of the phalangeal joints of the toes (b). Nestled between both muscles lies the **M. tibialis posterior** which is a strong supinator of the foot (c). [S701-L271]

→ T 53

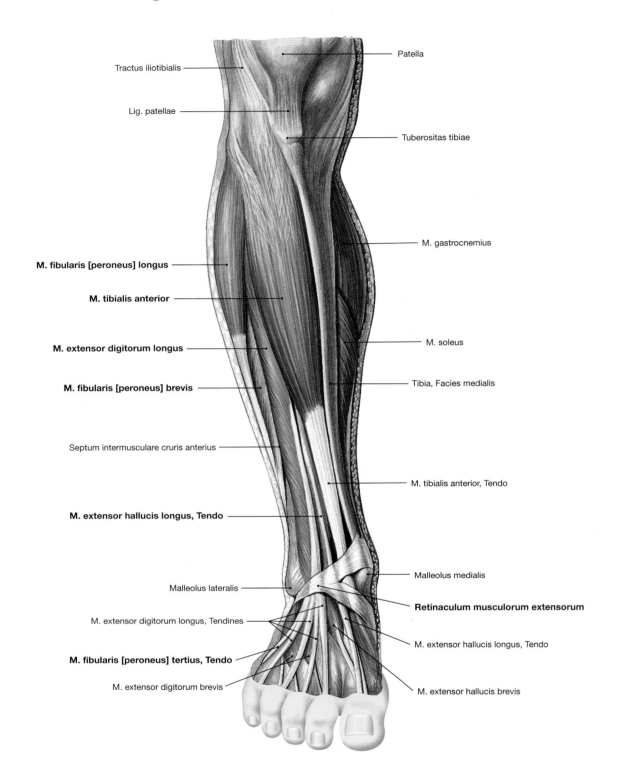

Tractus iliotibialis

Lig. patellae

M. fibularis [peroneus] longus

M. tibialis anterior

M. extensor digitorum longus

M. fibularis [peroneus] brevis

Septum intermusculare cruris anterius

M. extensor hallucis longus, Tendo

Malleolus lateralis

M. extensor digitorum longus, Tendines

M. fibularis [peroneus] tertius, Tendo

M. extensor digitorum brevis

Patella

Tuberositas tibiae

M. gastrocnemius

M. soleus

Tibia, Facies medialis

M. tibialis anterior, Tendo

Malleolus medialis

Retinaculum musculorum extensorum

M. extensor hallucis longus, Tendo

M. extensor hallucis brevis

Fig. 4.127 Ventral and lateral muscles of the lower leg and foot, right side; ventral view. [S700]

The **M. tibialis anterior** of the extensor group can be palpated near the edge of the tibia. As its inserting tendon runs medially to the axis of the subtalar joint, it functions as a (albeit weak) supinator, in contrast to the other extensor muscles. The **M. extensor digitorum longus** originates proximally from the tibia and fibula, whereas the **M. extensor hallucis longus** is located between the other two extensors on the distal leg. Occasionally, the M. extensor digitorum longus splits off and inserts on the Os metatarsi V, which are confusingly called **M. fibularis tertius**. In

the distal part, the tendons are guided by a reinforcement of the fascia of the lower leg, the **Retinaculum musculorum extensorum.** The retinacula of the foot function as retaining ligaments and prevent the tendons from lifting off the bones during extension of the foot. Both fibular muscles **(Mm. fibulares longus** and **brevis)** constitute the lateral group and originate proximally and distally from the fibula. Clinically, they are often referred to by their former name as peroneal muscles (fibula, greek term: perone).

→ T 50, T 51

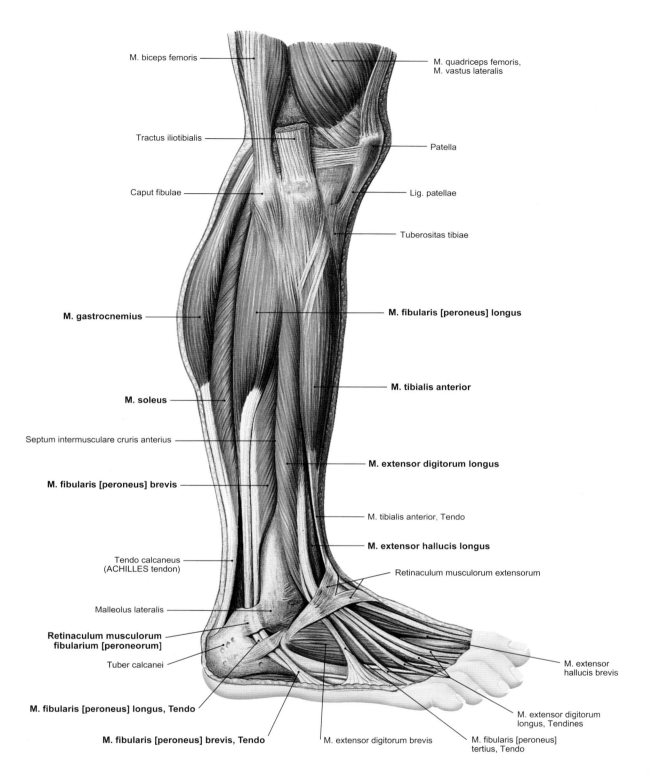

M. biceps femoris

M. quadriceps femoris, M. vastus lateralis

Tractus iliotibialis

Patella

Caput fibulae

Lig. patellae

Tuberositas tibiae

M. gastrocnemius

M. fibularis [peroneus] longus

M. soleus

M. tibialis anterior

Septum intermusculare cruris anterius

M. extensor digitorum longus

M. fibularis [peroneus] brevis

M. tibialis anterior, Tendo

M. extensor hallucis longus

Tendo calcaneus (ACHILLES tendon)

Retinaculum musculorum extensorum

Malleolus lateralis

Retinaculum musculorum fibularium [peroneorum]

Tuber calcanei

M. extensor hallucis brevis

M. fibularis [peroneus] longus, Tendo

M. fibularis [peroneus] brevis, Tendo

M. extensor digitorum brevis

M. extensor digitorum longus, Tendines

M. fibularis [peroneus] tertius, Tendo

Fig. 4.128 Muscles of the lower leg and foot, right side; lateral view. [S700]

In the lateral view, all three muscle groups of the lower leg are visible. The fibular muscles are located laterally, just behind the anterior extensors, and the flexors are located dorsally. As the deep flexors on the dorsal side are directly adjacent to the bones of the leg, only the superficial muscles (M. triceps surae), including the **M. gastrocnemius** and the deeper **M. soleus,** can be seen. The tendons of the fibular muscle group are guided by the **Retinacula musculorum fibularium.** The M. fibularis brevis inserts at the Os metatarsi V, whereas the tendon of the M. fibularis longus passes along the sole of the foot to the Os metatarsi I and the Os cuneiforme mediale, thus actively supporting the arches of the foot. It should be noted that the **M. extensor hallucis longus** is found distally between the M. tibialis anterior and the M. extensor digitorum longus.

→ T 50–T 52, T 54

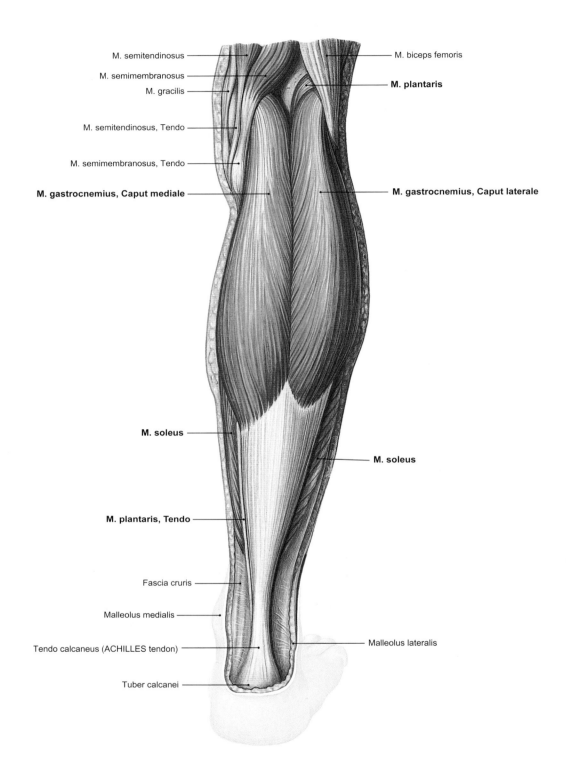

M. semitendinosus

M. semimembranosus

M. gracilis

M. semitendinosus, Tendo

M. semimembranosus, Tendo

M. gastrocnemius, Caput mediale

M. biceps femoris

M. plantaris

M. gastrocnemius, Caput laterale

M. soleus

M. soleus

M. plantaris, Tendo

Fascia cruris

Malleolus medialis

Tendo calcaneus (ACHILLES tendon)

Tuber calcanei

Malleolus lateralis

Fig. 4.129 Superficial layer of the dorsal muscles of the lower leg, right side; dorsal view. [S700]
The superficial flexor group consists of the **M. triceps surae** and the **M. plantaris.** The strong M. triceps surae is composed of the two-headed **M. gastrocnemius** and the deeper **M. soleus** below it. All superficial dorsal muscles insert at the heel bone via the **ACHILLES tendon** (Tendo calcaneus). The M. triceps surae is the strongest flexor of the

talocrural joint and the strongest supinator of the foot, even stronger than the M. tibialis posterior. If it malfunctions (in the case of a herniated disc with lesion of the spinal cord segment S1 or lesion of the N. tibialis), standing on the toes is impossible!

→ T 52

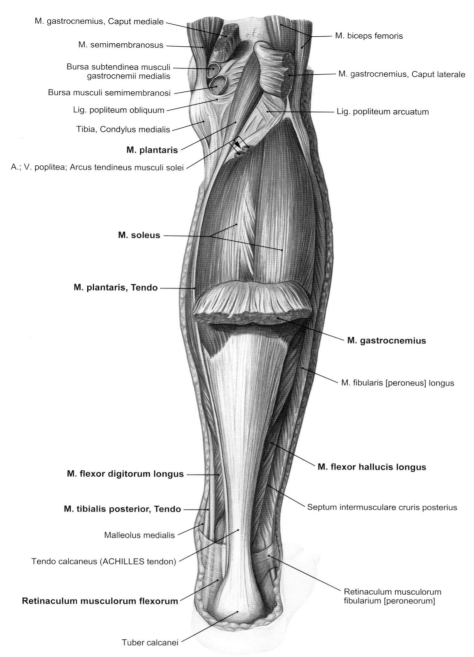

M. gastrocnemius, Caput mediale

M. semimembranosus

Bursa subtendinea musculi gastrocnemii medialis

Bursa musculi semimembranosi

Lig. popliteum obliquum

Tibia, Condylus medialis

M. plantaris

A.; V. poplitea; Arcus tendineus musculi solei

M. soleus

M. plantaris, Tendo

M. flexor digitorum longus

M. tibialis posterior, Tendo

Malleolus medialis

Tendo calcaneus (ACHILLES tendon)

Retinaculum musculorum flexorum

Tuber calcanei

M. biceps femoris

M. gastrocnemius, Caput laterale

Lig. popliteum arcuatum

M. gastrocnemius

M. fibularis [peroneus] longus

M. flexor hallucis longus

Septum intermusculare cruris posterius

Retinaculum musculorum fibularium [peroneorum]

Fig. 4.130 Superficial layer of the dorsal muscles of the lower leg, right side; dorsal view; after severing the origins of the M. gastrocnemius. [S700]
When folding back the **M. gastrocnemius,** the **M. plantaris** becomes visible proximally, lying underneath the **M. soleus.** The muscle bellies of the deep flexors are located further distally and can be found on both sides of the ACHILLES tendon after removal of the Fascia cruris. Their tendons of insertion are guided through the **Retinaculum musculorum flexorum** at the medial malleolus.

→ T 53

Clinical remarks

A **rupture of the ACHILLES tendon** can especially occur when it is exposed to sudden stress when, during dorsal flexion of the foot, the stretched muscle strongly contracts. The diagnosis is mostly done by ultrasound or MRI prior to surgical intervention.
[G729]

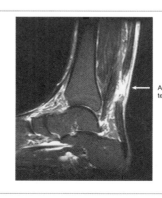

ACHILLES tendon rupture

Musculature

Muscles of the lower leg

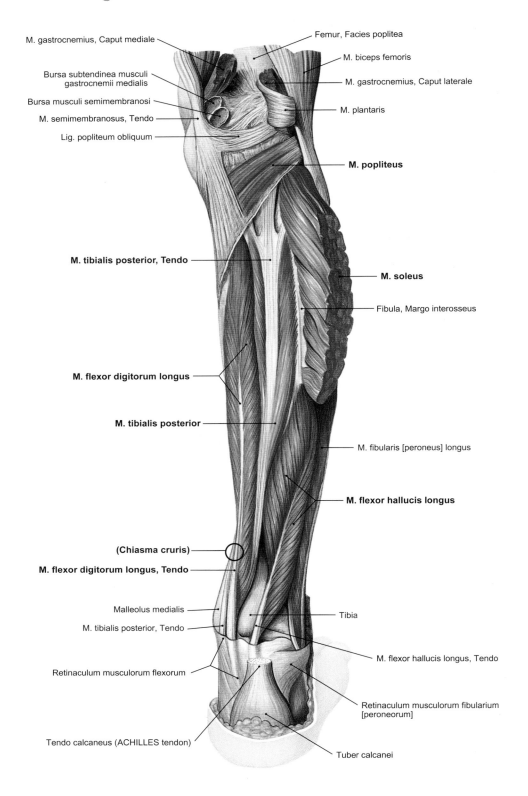

M. gastrocnemius, Caput mediale

Bursa subtendinea musculi gastrocnemii medialis

Bursa musculi semimembranosi

M. semimembranosus, Tendo

Lig. popliteum obliquum

M. tibialis posterior, Tendo

M. flexor digitorum longus

M. tibialis posterior

(Chiasma cruris)

M. flexor digitorum longus, Tendo

Malleolus medialis

M. tibialis posterior, Tendo

Retinaculum musculorum flexorum

Tendo calcaneus (ACHILLES tendon)

Femur, Facies poplitea

M. biceps femoris

M. gastrocnemius, Caput laterale

M. plantaris

M. popliteus

M. soleus

Fibula, Margo interosseus

M. fibularis [peroneus] longus

M. flexor hallucis longus

Tibia

M. flexor hallucis longus, Tendo

Retinaculum musculorum fibularium [peroneorum]

Tuber calcanei

Fig. 4.131 Deep layer of the dorsal muscles of the lower leg, right side; dorsal view; after removing the superficial flexors. [S700] After removal of the superficial flexors, the deep muscles are visible. The **M. tibialis posterior** is located between the two flexor muscles of the toes. The **M. flexor digitorum longus** originates furthest medially, followed laterally by the **M. tibialis posterior** and then distally by the **M. flexor hallucis longus.** Their tendons converge at the medial malleolus where they are bridged by the **Retinaculum musculorum flexorum.** The tendon of the M. flexor digitorum longus crosses the tendon of the M. tibialis posterior on this course **(Chiasma cruris).**

The **M. popliteus,** which originates from the Condylus lateralis and the posterior horn of the Meniscus lateralis, lies proximally. The muscle inserts on the posterior aspect of the proximal tibia and thereby functions as a relatively strong **medial rotator.** The primary function of the M. popliteus is therefore an **active stabilisation** of the knee against an extreme lateral rotation.

→ T 53

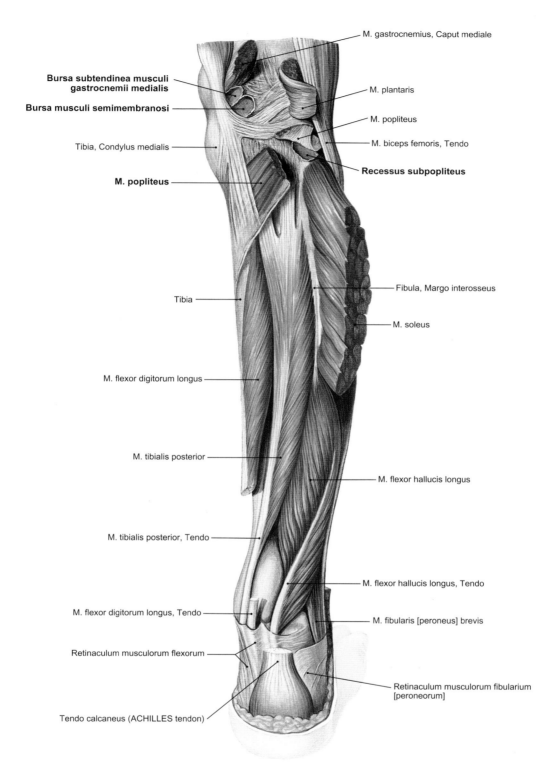

M. gastrocnemius, Caput mediale

Bursa subtendinea musculi gastrocnemii medialis

Bursa musculi semimembranosi

M. plantaris

M. popliteus

Tibia, Condylus medialis

M. biceps femoris, Tendo

Recessus subpopliteus

M. popliteus

Tibia

Fibula, Margo interosseus

M. soleus

M. flexor digitorum longus

M. tibialis posterior

M. flexor hallucis longus

M. tibialis posterior, Tendo

M. flexor hallucis longus, Tendo

M. flexor digitorum longus, Tendo

M. fibularis [peroneus] brevis

Retinaculum musculorum flexorum

Retinaculum musculorum fibularium [peroneorum]

Tendo calcaneus (ACHILLES tendon)

Fig. 4.132 Deep layer of the dorsal muscles of the lower leg, right side; dorsal view; after removal of the superficial flexors and splitting of the M. popliteus. [S700]

After severing the M. popliteus, the Bursa subpoplitea becomes visible, which usually communicates with the knee joint cavity and is therefore also referred to as **Recessus subpopliteus.** Further bursae are found below the tendons of origin and insertion of the dorsal muscles (**Bursa musculi semimembranosi** and **Bursae subtendineae musculorum gastronemii medialis and lateralis**). These can also communicate with the joint cavity (→ Fig. 4.57).

→ T 53

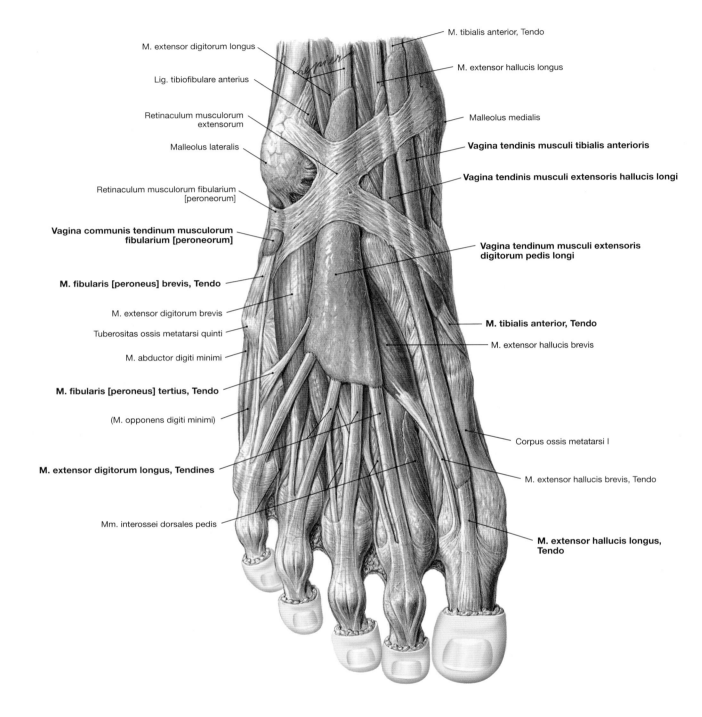

M. extensor digitorum longus

Lig. tibiofibulare anterius

Retinaculum musculorum extensorum

Malleolus lateralis

Retinaculum musculorum fibularium [peroneorum]

Vagina communis tendinum musculorum fibularium [peroneorum]

M. fibularis [peroneus] brevis, Tendo

M. extensor digitorum brevis

Tuberositas ossis metatarsi quinti

M. abductor digiti minimi

M. fibularis [peroneus] tertius, Tendo

(M. opponens digiti minimi)

M. extensor digitorum longus, Tendines

Mm. interossei dorsales pedis

M. tibialis anterior, Tendo

M. extensor hallucis longus

Malleolus medialis

Vagina tendinis musculi tibialis anterioris

Vagina tendinis musculi extensoris hallucis longi

Vagina tendinum musculi extensoris digitorum pedis longi

M. tibialis anterior, Tendo

M. extensor hallucis brevis

Corpus ossis metatarsi I

M. extensor hallucis brevis, Tendo

M. extensor hallucis longus, Tendo

Fig. 4.133 Tendinous sheath, Vaginae tendinum of the foot, right side; dorsal view, in relation to the Dorsum pedis. [S700]
The Fascia cruris has been removed with the exception of the Retinaculum musculorum extensorum. The **retinacula** of the foot serve as retaining ligaments and prevent the tendons lifting off the bones during muscle contractions. Each extensor muscle has its own tendinous sheath (Vagina tendinis), which surround all its tendons of insertion in a 'guiding tube' and additionally serves as a gliding surface. In contrast, the tendons of the M. fibularis longus and M. fibularis brevis have a common synovial sheath.

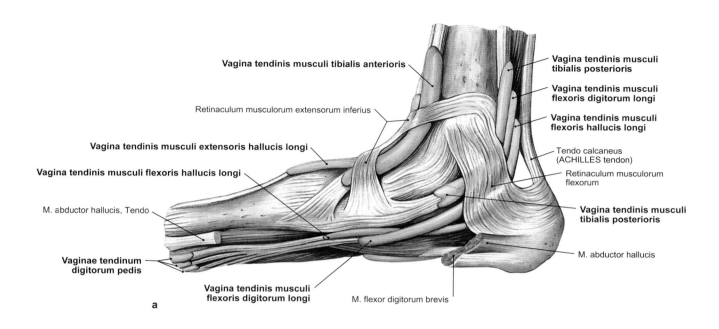

Vagina tendinis musculi tibialis anterioris

Retinaculum musculorum extensorum inferius

Vagina tendinis musculi extensoris hallucis longi

Vagina tendinis musculi flexoris hallucis longi

M. abductor hallucis, Tendo

Vaginae tendinum digitorum pedis

Vagina tendinis musculi flexoris digitorum longi

M. flexor digitorum brevis

Vagina tendinis musculi tibialis posterioris

Vagina tendinis musculi flexoris digitorum longi

Vagina tendinis musculi flexoris hallucis longi

Tendo calcaneus (ACHILLES tendon)

Retinaculum musculorum flexorum

Vagina tendinis musculi tibialis posterioris

M. abductor hallucis

a

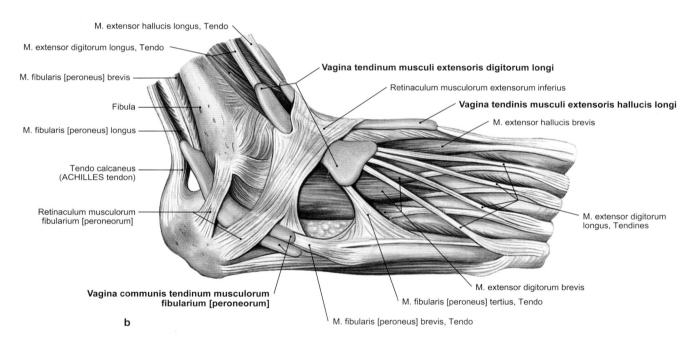

M. extensor hallucis longus, Tendo

M. extensor digitorum longus, Tendo

M. fibularis [peroneus] brevis

Fibula

M. fibularis [peroneus] longus

Tendo calcaneus (ACHILLES tendon)

Retinaculum musculorum fibularium [peroneorum]

Vagina communis tendinum musculorum fibularium [peroneorum]

Vagina tendinum musculi extensoris digitorum longi

Retinaculum musculorum extensorum inferius

Vagina tendinis musculi extensoris hallucis longi

M. extensor hallucis brevis

M. extensor digitorum longus, Tendines

M. extensor digitorum brevis

M. fibularis [peroneus] tertius, Tendo

M. fibularis [peroneus] brevis, Tendo

b

Fig. 4.134a and b Tendinous sheaths, Vaginae tendinum, of the foot, right side. [S700]
a Medial view.
b Lateral view.
The synovial sheaths surround the inserting tendons of all three muscle groups of the (lower) leg, particularly where the tendons are fixed to the

bones by the retinacula. The Retinaculum musculorum flexorum forms the **malleolar canal** on the medial ankle, through which the neurovascular pathways (N. tibialis; A./V. tibialis posterior) also reach the sole of the foot.

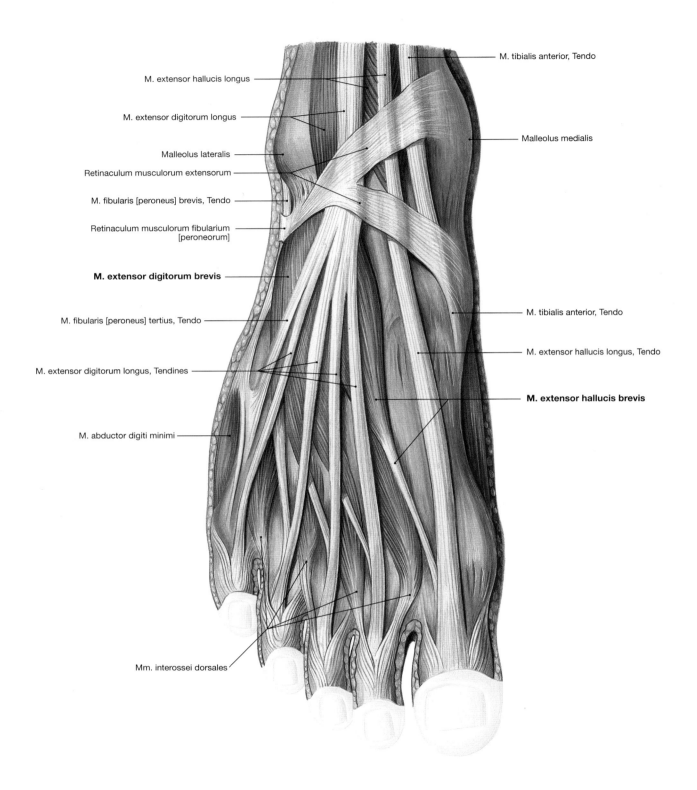

M. tibialis anterior, Tendo

M. extensor hallucis longus

M. extensor digitorum longus

Malleolus medialis

Malleolus lateralis

Retinaculum musculorum extensorum

M. fibularis [peroneus] brevis, Tendo

Retinaculum musculorum fibularium [peroneorum]

M. extensor digitorum brevis

M. fibularis [peroneus] tertius, Tendo

M. tibialis anterior, Tendo

M. extensor hallucis longus, Tendo

M. extensor digitorum longus, Tendines

M. extensor hallucis brevis

M. abductor digiti minimi

Mm. interossei dorsales

Fig. 4.135 Dorsal muscles (dorsum, instep) of the foot, right side; dorsal view. [S700]

Underneath the long extensor tendons of the toes, with their muscle bellies on the ventral lower leg, there are also two short extensors. The **M. extensor digitorum brevis** and the **M. extensor hallucis brevis** originate on the dorsal side of the calcaneus, and their tendons of inser-tion radiate laterally into the long extensor tendons and additionally into the dorsal aponeurosis. Thus they contribute to the extension of the toes and the first metatarsophalangeal joint. The Mm. interossei dor-sales, which are also visible, are regarded as plantar muscles (→ Fig. 4.140, → Fig. 4.141).

→ T 54

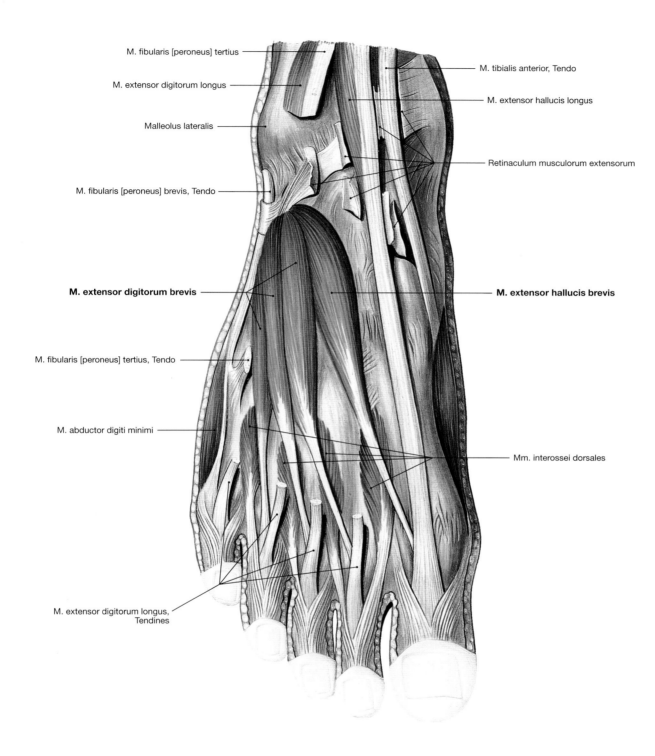

M. fibularis [peroneus] tertius

M. extensor digitorum longus

Malleolus lateralis

M. fibularis [peroneus] brevis, Tendo

M. extensor digitorum brevis

M. fibularis [peroneus] tertius, Tendo

M. abductor digiti minimi

M. extensor digitorum longus, Tendines

M. tibialis anterior, Tendo

M. extensor hallucis longus

Retinaculum musculorum extensorum

M. extensor hallucis brevis

Mm. interossei dorsales

Fig. 4.136 Dorsal muscles of the foot, right side; dorsal view. [S700]
The Retinaculum musculorum extensorum has been split and the tendon of the M. extensor digitorum longus has been partially removed. In this way, the muscles of the dorsum of the foot become visible. They include the short extensor muscles of the toes **(M. extensor digito-** **rum brevis)** and of the big toe **(M. extensor hallucis brevis).** These muscles originate from the dorsal side of the calcaneus and insert into the dorsal aponeurosis of the second to fourth toes or at the dorsal side of the proximal phalanx of the big toe.

→ T 50, T 54, T 56

Lower limb

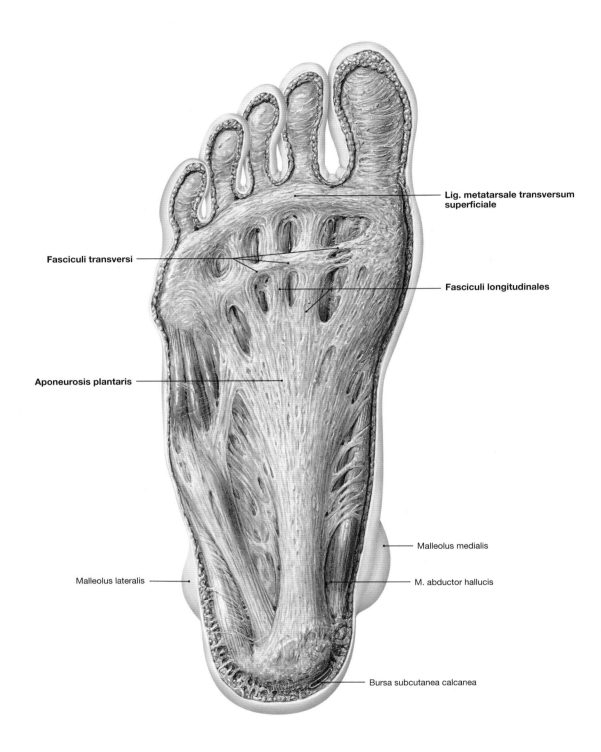

Lig. metatarsale transversum superficiale

Fasciculi transversi

Fasciculi longitudinales

Aponeurosis plantaris

Malleolus medialis

Malleolus lateralis

M. abductor hallucis

Bursa subcutanea calcanea

Fig. 4.137 Plantar aponeurosis, Aponeurosis plantaris, of the foot, right side; plantar view. [S700]
The **plantar aponeurosis** is a membranous layer of dense connective tissue with a strong central and two weaker lateral parts. Its **Fasciculi longitudinales** run from the Tuber calcanei to the ligaments of the metatarsophalangeal joints. Above the Ossa metatarsi they are connected via transverse fibre tracts **(Fasciculi transversi)**. The obliquely running connections via the bases of the proximal phalanges of the toes are collectively referred to as **Lig. metatarsale transversum superficiale**. Two septa run from the plantar aponeurosis to the bones and thereby form three muscle compartments in the sole of the foot.

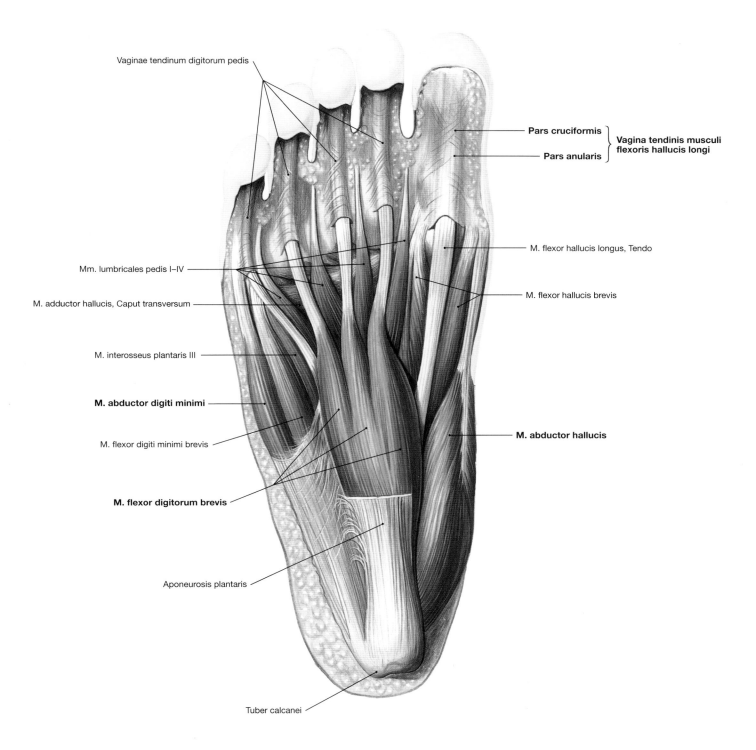

Vaginae tendinum digitorum pedis

Pars cruciformis ⎫ Vagina tendinis musculi
Pars anularis ⎬ flexoris hallucis longi

M. flexor hallucis longus, Tendo

Mm. lumbricales pedis I–IV

M. adductor hallucis, Caput transversum

M. flexor hallucis brevis

M. interosseus plantaris III

M. abductor digiti minimi

M. abductor hallucis

M. flexor digiti minimi brevis

M. flexor digitorum brevis

Aponeurosis plantaris

Tuber calcanei

Fig. 4.138 Superficial muscle layer of the sole of the foot, right side; plantar view; after removal of the plantar aponeurosis. [S700]
Unlike the muscles of the hand, the plantar muscles are not so much involved in the differentiated movements of individual toes, but rather function as an **active tension system for the arches of the foot** and should therefore be viewed as a functional unit. The plantar muscles support the ligaments, which act as a passive stabilisation system. Because of the septa, which run from the plantar aponeurosis to the bones of the foot, the muscles are divided into **three compartments** (the hallux, toes 2–4, the little toe). These compartments are not fully separated from each other and it is therefore more helpful to visualise the dissecting muscles as **four layers.**

The muscles of the **superficial layer** comprise the **M. abductor hallucis,** the **M. flexor digitorum brevis,** and the **M. abductor digiti minimi.** The inserting tendons of the M. flexor digitorum brevis are pierced by the long flexor tendons. The tendons of the digital flexor muscles have their own tendinous sheaths (Vaginae tendinum) which are not connected to those in the tarsal region. These sheaths include reinforcing ligaments, which in part form 'tubes' around the tendons (Pars anularis) and have intersecting fibres in-between (Pars cruciformis).

→ T 54–T 57

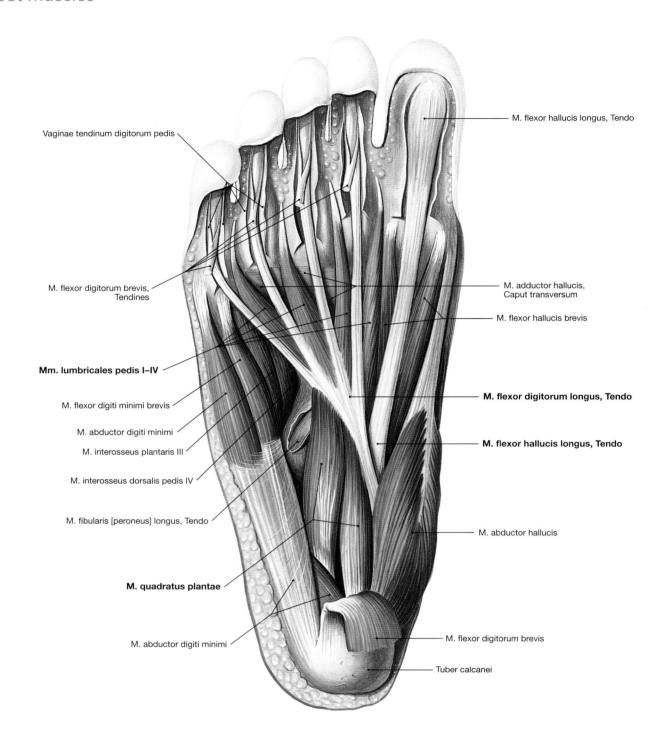

Vaginae tendinum digitorum pedis

M. flexor hallucis longus, Tendo

M. flexor digitorum brevis, Tendines

M. adductor hallucis, Caput transversum

M. flexor hallucis brevis

Mm. lumbricales pedis I–IV

M. flexor digiti minimi brevis

M. flexor digitorum longus, Tendo

M. abductor digiti minimi

M. interosseus plantaris III

M. flexor hallucis longus, Tendo

M. interosseus dorsalis pedis IV

M. fibularis [peroneus] longus, Tendo

M. abductor hallucis

M. quadratus plantae

M. flexor digitorum brevis

M. abductor digiti minimi

Tuber calcanei

Fig. 4.139 Middle muscle layer of the sole of the foot, right side; plantar view; after severing the M. flexor digitorum brevis. [S700]
The muscles lie in **four layers** on top of each other. After removal of the M. flexor digitorum brevis, the muscles and their tendons of insertion in the **second layer** are visible. The **tendons** of the long flexor muscles (**M. flexor hallucis longus** and **M. flexor digitorum longus**) are visible here as well as two muscles of the middle compartment. The tendon of

the M. flexor digitorum longus is the insertion site of the **M. quadratus plantae,** which functionally supports the long flexor digitorum muscle and thus acts as an accessory flexor of the toes. The tendon also serves as the origin for the four **Mm. lumbricales** which insert medially on the proximal phalanges of the toes (II–V).

→ T 55–T 57

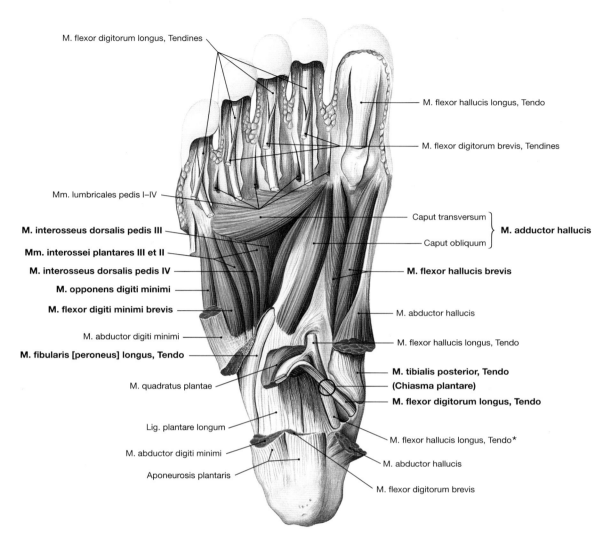

M. flexor digitorum longus, Tendines

M. flexor hallucis longus, Tendo

M. flexor digitorum brevis, Tendines

Mm. lumbricales pedis I–IV

Caput transversum ⎤
⎥ **M. adductor hallucis**
Caput obliquum ⎦

M. interosseus dorsalis pedis III

Mm. interossei plantares III et II

M. interosseus dorsalis pedis IV

M. opponens digiti minimi

M. flexor digiti minimi brevis

M. abductor digiti minimi

M. fibularis [peroneus] longus, Tendo

M. quadratus plantae

Lig. plantare longum

M. abductor digiti minimi

Aponeurosis plantaris

M. flexor hallucis brevis

M. abductor hallucis

M. flexor hallucis longus, Tendo

M. tibialis posterior, Tendo
(Chiasma plantare)

M. flexor digitorum longus, Tendo

M. flexor hallucis longus, Tendo*

M. abductor hallucis

M. flexor digitorum brevis

Fig. 4.140   Deep and deepest muscle layers of the sole of the foot, right side; plantar view; after removal of the two superficial layers and of the long flexor tendons. [S700]
The **M. flexor hallucis brevis** and the **M. adductor hallucis** are located within the **deep (third) layer** in the compartment of the big toe, whereas the **M. flexor digiti minimi brevis** and the inconstant **M. opponens digiti minimi** are located in the compartment of the little toe.

The **deepest (fourth) layer** comprises the three **Mm. interossei plantares** and the four **Mm. interossei dorsales,** as well as the **tendons of the M. tibialis posterior** and of the **M. fibularis longus.**
* The point where the tendon of the M. flexor digitorum longus crosses over the tendon of the M. flexor hallucis longus is also referred to as Chiasma plantare.

→ T 53, T 55–T 57

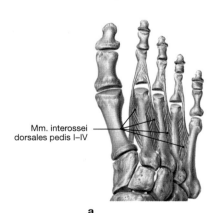

Mm. interossei dorsales pedis I–IV

a

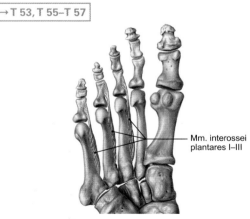

Mm. interossei plantares I–III

b

Fig. 4.141a and b   Mm. interossei dorsales and plantares of the foot, right side. [S700]
a Mm. interossei dorsalis; dorsal view. The four **Mm. interossei dorsales** (I–IV) are two-headed muscles and originate from opposing sides of the bases of the Ossa metatarsi I–V. They insert on the proximal phalanges of the second to fourth toes in such a way that muscles I and II run along the medial and lateral sides of the second toe, whereas the muscles III and IV run laterally along the third and fourth toes. Therefore, not only do these muscles flex the metatarsophalangeal joint, but

they also support lateral **abduction** of **toes II–IV** and **adduction** of the **second toe.**
b Mm. interossei plantares; plantar view. The three **Mm. interossei plantares** (I–III) only have one head and originate from the plantar side of the Ossa metatarsi III–V. They insert on the medial side of the respective toes. In addition to being flexors of the metatarsophalangeal joints, they also **adduct** these toes.

→ T 56

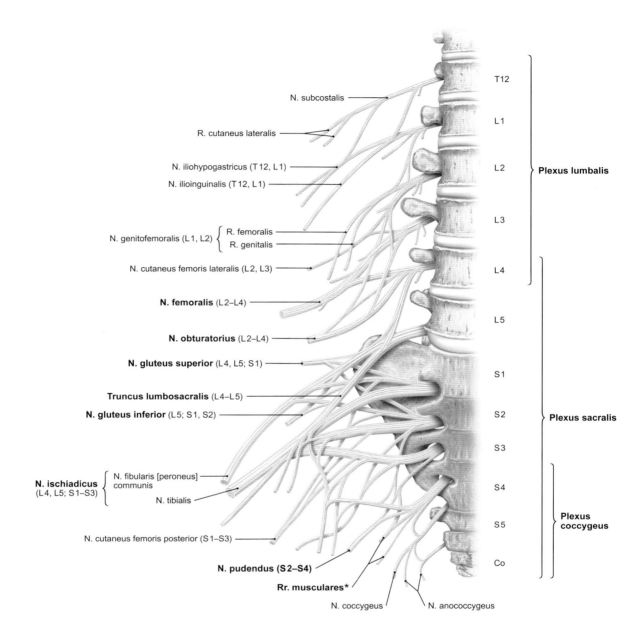

N. subcostalis

R. cutaneus lateralis

N. iliohypogastricus (T 12, L 1)
N. ilioinguinalis (T 12, L 1)

N. genitofemoralis (L 1, L 2) { R. femoralis
R. genitalis

N. cutaneus femoris lateralis (L 2, L 3)

N. femoralis (L 2–L 4)

N. obturatorius (L 2–L 4)

N. gluteus superior (L 4, L 5; S 1)

Truncus lumbosacralis (L 4–L 5)
N. gluteus inferior (L 5; S 1, S 2)

N. ischiadicus
(L 4, L 5; S 1–S 3) { N. fibularis [peroneus] communis
N. tibialis

N. cutaneus femoris posterior (S 1–S 3)

N. pudendus (S 2–S 4)
Rr. musculares*

N. coccygeus   N. anococcygeus

T 12

L 1

L 2

L 3

L 4

L 5

S 1

S 2

S 3

S 4

S 5

Co

} **Plexus lumbalis**

} **Plexus sacralis**

} **Plexus coccygeus**

Fig. 4.142   Plexus lumbosacralis (T12–S5, Co1): segmental arrangement of the nerves, right side; ventral view. [S700-L127]
The lower limb is innervated by the **Plexus lumbosacralis.** The plexus is composed of the Rr. anteriores of the spinal nerves which originate from the lumbar, sacral and coccygeal spinal cord segments and unite to form the **Plexus lumbalis** (T12–L4) and the **Plexus sacralis** (L4–S5, Co1). The segments S4–Co1 are also referred to as Plexus coccygeus. Both plexuses are connected by the **Truncus lumbosacralis** which conveys nerve fibres of the spinal cord segments L4, L5 from the Plexus lumbalis to the lesser pelvis. Functionally, the most important nerves of the Plexus lumbalis are the N. femoralis and the N. obturatorius.
The **N. femoralis** provides motor innervation to the ventral group of the hip and thigh muscles (flexing the hip joint and extending the knee), and sensory innervation to the ventral aspect of the thigh and the anterior-

medial aspect of the lower leg. The **N. obturatorius** provides motor innervation to the adductor group and sensory innervation to the medial thigh. The strongest and longest nerve branch of the Plexus sacralis is the **N. ischiadicus.** With both its divisions (N. tibialis and N. fibularis communis) it provides motor innervation to the hamstring muscles (extensor in the hip joint and flexor in the knee) and to all the muscles of the lower legs and feet. It also provides sensory innervation to the calf and foot. The **Nn. glutei superior and inferior** innervate the gluteal muscles which represent the major extensors, rotators and abductors of the hip. The **N. pudendus** innervates the muscles of the perineal region and provides sensory innervation to the external genitalia. The muscles of the pelvic floor are innervated by direct muscle branches (*).

→ T 42

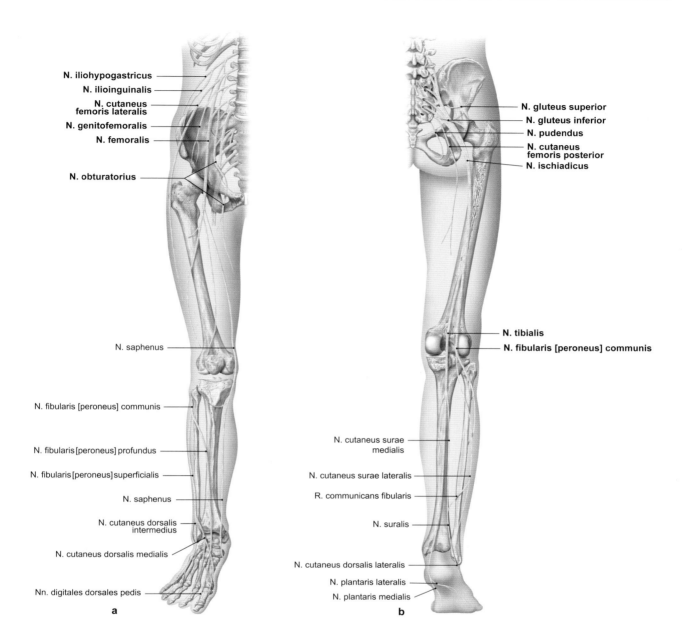

N. iliohypogastricus
N. ilioinguinalis
N. cutaneus femoris lateralis
N. genitofemoralis
N. femoralis

N. obturatorius

N. saphenus

N. fibularis [peroneus] communis

N. fibularis [peroneus] profundus

N. fibularis [peroneus] superficialis

N. saphenus

N. cutaneus dorsalis intermedius

N. cutaneus dorsalis medialis

Nn. digitales dorsales pedis

a

N. gluteus superior
N. gluteus inferior
N. pudendus
N. cutaneus femoris posterior
N. ischiadicus

N. tibialis
N. fibularis [peroneus] communis

N. cutaneus surae medialis

N. cutaneus surae lateralis

R. communicans fibularis

N. suralis

N. cutaneus dorsalis lateralis

N. plantaris lateralis

N. plantaris medialis

b

Fig. 4.143a and b   Plexus lumbosacralis (T12–S5, Co1): nerves of the leg, right side. [S700-L127]
a Ventral view.
b Dorsal view.

The nerves of the **Plexus lumbalis** (T12–L4) run **ventrally** of the hip joint and supply the lower part of the lateral and anterior abdominal wall as well as the anterior side of the thigh. The branches of the **Plexus sacralis** lie on the **dorsal side** of the hip joint. They innervate the dorsal side of the thigh, as well as most of the leg and the entire foot.

Plexus sacralis (L4–S5, Co1)

- Muscle branches to the pelvitrochanteric muscles of the hip (M. obturatorius internus, Mm. gemelli superior and inferior, M. quadratus femoris, M. piriformis; L4–S2)
- N. gluteus superior (L4–S1)
- N. gluteus inferior (L5–S2)
- N. ischiadicus (L4–S3)
- N. cutaneus femoris posterior (S1–S3)
- Cutaneous branches to the skin area of the ischial tuberosity (N. cutaneus perforans, S2, S3) and coccyx (N. anococcygeus, S5–Co1)
- N. pudendus (S2–S4)
- Nn. splanchnici pelvici (preganglionic parasympathetic fibres; S2–S4)
- Muscle branches to the pelvic floor (M. levator ani and M. ischiococcygeus, S3, S4)

Plexus lumbalis (T12–L4)

- Muscle branches to the M. iliopsoas and M. quadratus lumborum (T12–L4)
- N. iliohypogastricus (T12, L1)
- N. ilioinguinalis (T12, L1)
- N. genitofemoralis (L1, L2)
- N. cutaneus femoris lateralis (L2, L3)
- N. femoralis (L2–L4)
- N. obturatorius (L2–L4)

Lower limb

Cutaneous innervation of the lower limb

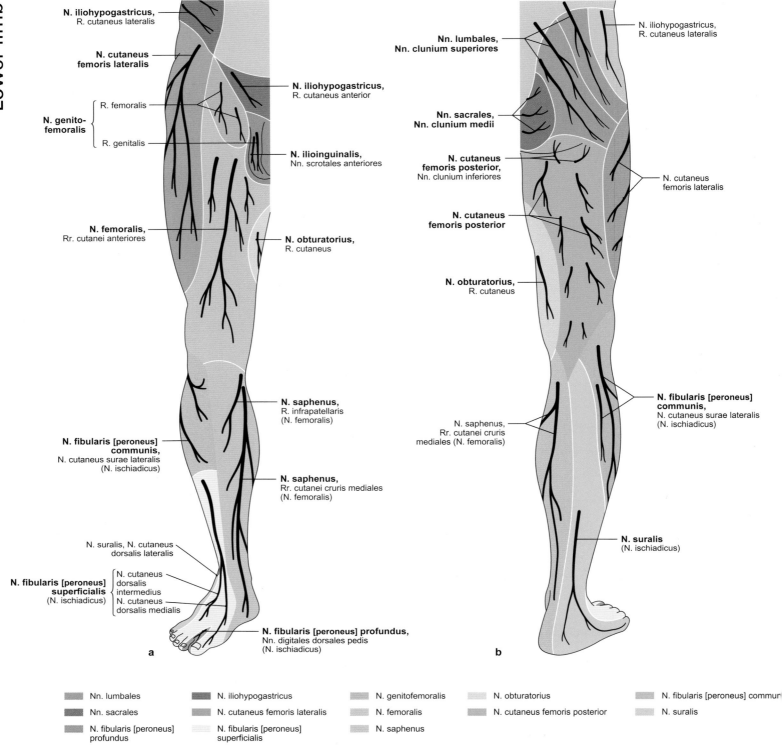

N. iliohypogastricus,
R. cutaneus lateralis

N. cutaneus
femoris lateralis

N. genito-
femoralis — R. femoralis

R. genitalis

N. iliohypogastricus,
R. cutaneus anterior

N. ilioinguinalis,
Nn. scrotales anteriores

N. femoralis,
Rr. cutanei anteriores

N. obturatorius,
R. cutaneus

N. saphenus,
R. infrapatellaris
(N. femoralis)

N. fibularis [peroneus]
communis,
N. cutaneus surae lateralis
(N. ischiadicus)

N. saphenus,
Rr. cutanei cruris mediales
(N. femoralis)

N. suralis, N. cutaneus
dorsalis lateralis

N. fibularis [peroneus]
superficialis
(N. ischiadicus)

N. cutaneus
dorsalis
intermedius
N. cutaneus
dorsalis medialis

N. fibularis [peroneus] profundus,
Nn. digitales dorsales pedis
(N. ischiadicus)

a

Nn. lumbales,
Nn. clunium superiores

N. iliohypogastricus,
R. cutaneus lateralis

Nn. sacrales,
Nn. clunium medii

N. cutaneus
femoris posterior,
Nn. clunium inferiores

N. cutaneus
femoris lateralis

N. cutaneus
femoris posterior

N. obturatorius,
R. cutaneus

N. fibularis [peroneus]
communis,
N. cutaneus surae lateralis
(N. ischiadicus)

N. saphenus,
Rr. cutanei cruris
mediales (N. femoralis)

N. suralis
(N. ischiadicus)

b

Nn. lumbales	N. iliohypogastricus	N. genitofemoralis
Nn. sacrales	N. cutaneus femoris lateralis	N. femoralis
N. fibularis [peroneus] profundus	N. fibularis [peroneus] superficialis	N. saphenus

N. obturatorius · N. cutaneus femoris posterior · N. fibularis [peroneus] commur · N. suralis

Fig. 4.144a and b   Cutaneous nerves of the lower limb, right side.
[S700-L127]
a Ventral view.
b Dorsal view.
The sensory innervation of the **inguinal region** and the **ventral side** of the leg is supplied by **all the nerves** of the **Plexus lumbalis.** The lateral aspect of the lower leg and the dorsum of the foot are innervated by branches of the Plexus sacralis. The **gluteal region** is innervated by the **Rr. posteriores** of the lumbar (Nn. clunium superiores) and sacral (Nn. clunium medii) spinal nerves, whereas the dorsal side of the entire leg and the sole of the foot are innervated by branches of the Plexus sacralis.

Clinical remarks

Referred or radiated pain generated in the area of the plexus is influenced by the pathway of the nerves originating from the Plexus lumbalis and Plexus sacralis. If the **Plexus lumbalis** is compressed by a haematoma or a tumour, the pain typically radiates into the **an**terior aspect of the thigh. With compression of the **Plexus sacralis,** the pain radiates into the **dorsal side** of the thigh **(ischialgia)** and often down into the lower leg.

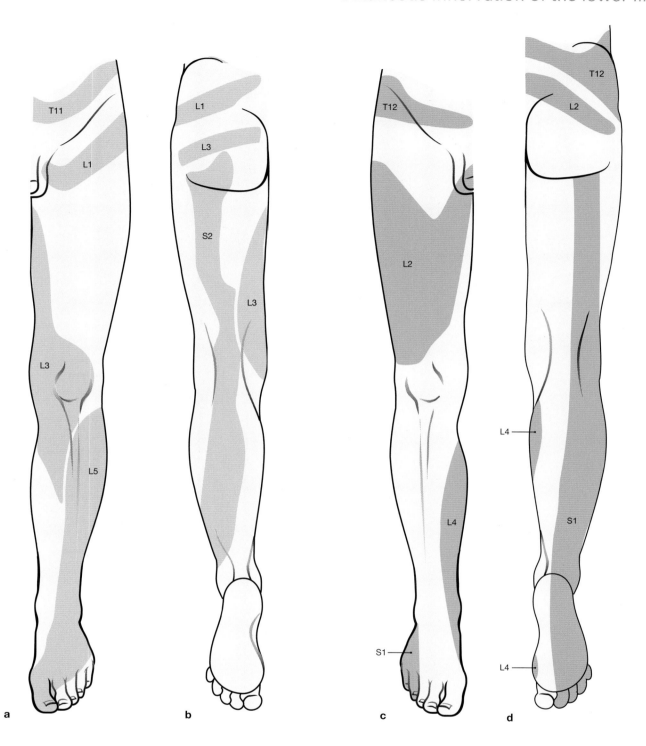

a
b
c
d

Fig. 4.145a–d Segmental cutaneous innervation (dermatomes) of the lower limb, right side. [S700-L126]/[F1067-001]
a Ventral view, dermatomes T11, L1, L3, L5.
b Dorsal view, dermatomes L1, L3, S2.
c Ventral view, dermatomes T12, L2, L4, S1.
d Dorsal view, dermatomes T12, L2, L4, S1.
Distinct areas of the skin are provided with sensory innervation by a single spinal cord segment. These cutaneous areas are referred to as

dermatomes. Since the cutaneous nerves of the lower limb convey sensory fibres from several spinal cord segments, the borders of the dermatomes do not correspond with the areas supplied by the cutaneous nerves (→ Fig. 4.144). In contrast to the belt-like orientation of the dermatomes of the trunk, dermatomes on the **anterior aspect of the lower limb** are obliquely oriented in a lateral superior to medial inferior direction, and longitudinally on the **posterior aspect** (see Development, → Fig. 3.5).

Clinical remarks

The localisation of the dermatomes are extremely important in the **diagnosis of the very common disc prolapses.** Disc prolapses mainly occur in the lower lumbar spine and can damage the nerve roots of L4–S1. While the nerve fibres from the segment **L4** inner-

vate the **medial side of the foot,** the **big toe** and the **second toe are supplied by the L5** segment. The whole lateral side of the foot, including the **little toe,** is provided with sensory innervation by **S1**.

Plexus lumbalis

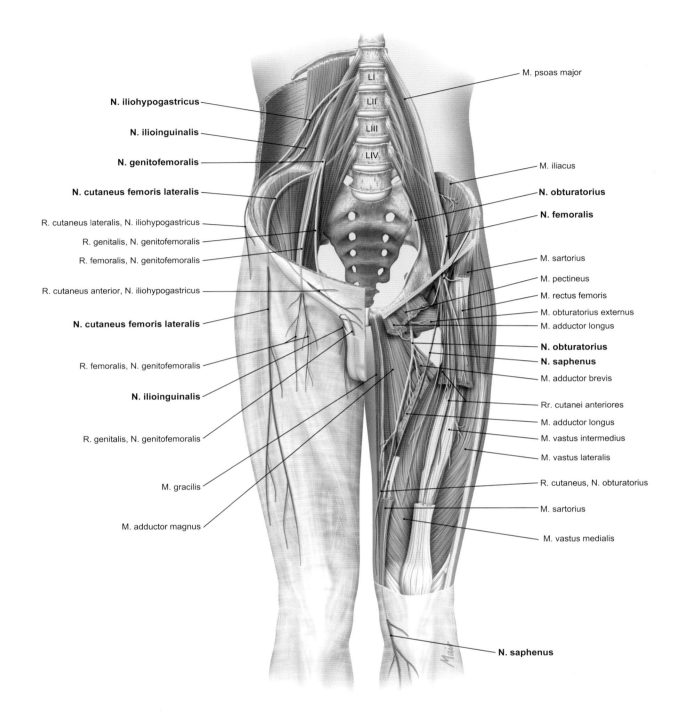

N. iliohypogastricus

N. ilioinguinalis

N. genitofemoralis

N. cutaneus femoris lateralis

R. cutaneus lateralis, N. iliohypogastricus

R. genitalis, N. genitofemoralis

R. femoralis, N. genitofemoralis

R. cutaneus anterior, N. iliohypogastricus

N. cutaneus femoris lateralis

R. femoralis, N. genitofemoralis

N. ilioinguinalis

R. genitalis, N. genitofemoralis

M. gracilis

M. adductor magnus

LI
LII
LIII
LIV

M. psoas major

M. iliacus

N. obturatorius

N. femoralis

M. sartorius

M. pectineus

M. rectus femoris

M. obturatorius externus

M. adductor longus

N. obturatorius

N. saphenus

M. adductor brevis

Rr. cutanei anteriores

M. adductor longus

M. vastus intermedius

M. vastus lateralis

R. cutaneus, N. obturatorius

M. sartorius

M. vastus medialis

N. saphenus

Fig. 4.146 Pathway and innervation areas of the nerves of the Plexus lumbalis (T12–L4); ventral view. The cutaneous branches are highlighted in purple. [S700-L127]

The **N. iliohypogastricus** and the **N. ilioinguinalis** (somewhat more caudally) run behind the kidney across the M. quadratus lumborum, and then pass anteriorly between the M. transversus abdominis and the M. obliquus internus. Both innervate the lower parts of these abdominal muscles. In addition, the N. iliohypogastricus provides sensory innervation to the skin above the inguinal ligament, while the N. ilioinguinalis supplies the anterior parts of the external genitalia. The **N. genitofemoralis** pierces the M. psoas major, crosses below the ureter and then divides into a lateral **R. femoralis,** which passes through the Lacuna vasorum and provides sensory innervation to the skin below the inguinal ligament, while the medial **R. genitalis** runs through the inguinal canal to the scrotum. The R. genitalis provides sensory innervation to the anterior parts of the external genitalia and to the M. cremaster in men. The **N. cutaneus femoris lateralis** passes laterally through the Lacuna musculorum and provides sensory innervation to the lateral side of the thigh. The **N. femoralis** passes medially through the Lacuna

musculorum, where it subdivides in a fan-like manner. Its Rr. cutanei anteriores innervate the skin on the anterior side of the thigh. The Rr. musculares innervate the ventral group of the hip (M. iliopsoas) and thigh muscles (M. sartorius and M. quadriceps femoris), as well as part of the M. pectineus. Its terminal branch is the **N. saphenus,** which enters the adductor canal (→ Fig. 4.173) and leaves it through the Septum intermusculare vastoadductorium on the medial side of the knee joint to supply sensory innervation to the medial and anterior aspects of the lower leg. The **N. obturatorius** initially runs medially of the M. psoas major and then passes through the Canalis obturatorius (→ Fig. 4.173) to the medial aspect of the thigh. Here it sends a muscle branch to the M. obturatorius externus and divides into two branches, the R. anterior and R. posterior (lying in front of and behind the M. adductor brevis), which innervate the muscles of the adductor group. The R. anterior ends with a cutaneous branch supplying the medial aspect of the thigh, whereas the R. posterior also innervates the joint capsule of the knee.

→ T 42

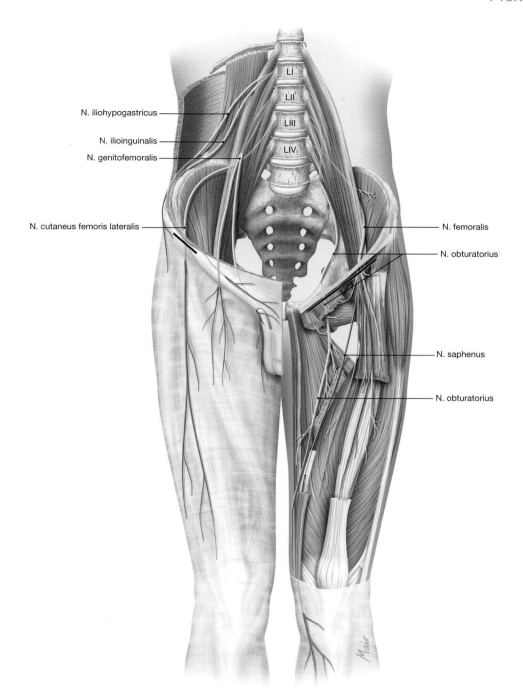

N. iliohypogastricus

N. ilioinguinalis

N. genitofemoralis

N. cutaneus femoris lateralis

LI
LII
LIII
LIV

N. femoralis

N. obturatorius

N. saphenus

N. obturatorius

Fig. 4.147 Lesion sites of nerves of the Plexus lumbalis; ventral view. The cutaneous branches are shown in purple. Common lesion sites are marked with black bars. [S700-L127]

→ T 42

Clinical remarks

Lesions of the **N. iliohypogastricus, N. ilioinguinalis** and **N. genitofemoralis** are rare due to their protected location. Because of their close proximity to the kidney and the ureter, however, certain diseases of the kidney (inflammation of the renal pelvis, pyelonephritis, or kidney stones) may result in **pain radiating** into the inguinal region or the external genitalia.

In the case of anterior surgical access to the hip joint or its constriction under the inguinal ligament by tight trousers, the **N. cutaneus femoris lateralis** can be damaged. This may result in a sensory loss or pain along the lateral aspect of the thigh **(meralgia paraesthetica).**

The **N. femoralis** is most often damaged in the groin due to surgical interventions or diagnostic procedures (heart catheterisation). In ad-

dition to restricted hip flexion, complete loss of knee extension makes it impossible to climb stairs. The patellar tendon reflex (knee-jerk reflex) fails and the sensory function of the anterior thigh and medial lower leg is absent.

The **N. obturatorius** is at risk when passing through the Canalis obturatorius. Besides a pelvic fracture, prolapses of the abdominal viscera (hernias) or advanced ovarian cancer can also be the cause of lesions. As a result of the failure of the adductor muscles, the upright stance becomes unsteady, and closing and crossing the legs becomes impossible. Sensory functions of the medial thigh can be impaired. Dysesthesias may also occur, which mimic diseases of the knee joint **(ROMBERG's knee phenomenon).**

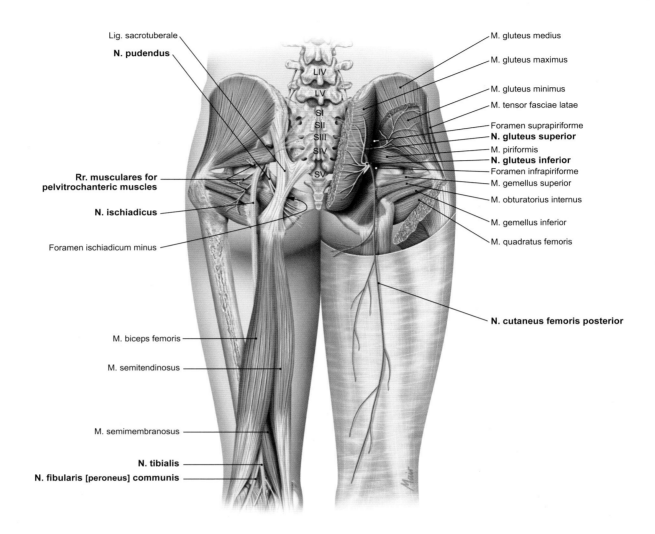

Lig. sacrotuberale

N. pudendus

Rr. musculares for pelvitrochanteric muscles

N. ischiadicus

Foramen ischiadicum minus

M. biceps femoris

M. semitendinosus

M. semimembranosus

N. tibialis

N. fibularis [peroneus] communis

M. gluteus medius

M. gluteus maximus

M. gluteus minimus

M. tensor fasciae latae

Foramen suprapiriforme

N. gluteus superior

M. piriformis

N. gluteus inferior

Foramen infrapiriforme

M. gemellus superior

M. obturatorius internus

M. gemellus inferior

M. quadratus femoris

N. cutaneus femoris posterior

Fig. 4.148   Pathway and innervation areas of nerves of the Plexus sacralis (L4–S5, Co1); dorsal view. The cutaneous branches are shown in purple. [S700-L127]

The **N. gluteus superior** exits the lesser pelvis through the Foramen suprapiriforme and provides motor innervation to the small gluteal muscles (the most important abductors and medial rotators of the hip joint) and the M. tensor fasciae latae. The **N. gluteus inferior** exits through the Foramen infrapiriforme and innervates the M. gluteus maximus, the strongest extensor and external rotator of the hip joint.

The **N. ischiadicus** is the strongest nerve of the human body. It consists of two divisions (N. tibialis and N. fibularis communis) which are joined only by their connective tissue sheath (epineurium) to form one trunk over a variable pathway. The N. ischiadicus exits the pelvis through the Foramen infrapiriforme and runs below the M. biceps femoris to the popliteal fossa of the knee.

In most cases the **N. tibialis** and **N. fibularis communis** separate where they transfer to the distal third of the thigh. Occasionally (in approx. 12 %), both nerves already exit the pelvis separately (high division) in which case the N. fibularis communis often pierces the M. piriformis. In the thigh, the N. tibialis provides motor innervation to the hamstring muscles and to the posterior head of the M. adductor magnus. The N. fibularis only innervates the Caput breve of the M. biceps femoris in the thigh. With both these trunks, the N. ischiadicus provides motor innervation to all muscles of the lower leg and foot as well as sensory innervation to the whole lower leg (except medially, where it is supplied

by the N. saphenus from the N. femoralis) and the foot (with the exception of the medial side).

After exiting the Foramen infrapiriforme, the **N. cutaneus femoris posterior** sends the sensory Nn. clunium inferiores to the skin of the lower buttocks. Then it continues its subfascial pathway to approximately the middle of the thigh and provides sensory innervation to the posterior thigh.

The pathway of the **N. pudendus** is relatively complicated. After exiting the Foramen infrapiriforme it winds around the Spina ischiadica with its eponymous blood vessels and passes medially through the Foramen ischiadicum minus into the Fossa ischioanalis. Here it runs laterally inside a fascial duplication of the M. obturatorius internus (ALCOCK's canal). The N. pudendus innervates the external sphincter of the anal canal (M. sphincter ani externus) as well as all the perineal muscles and provides sensory innervation to the posterior parts of the external genitalia (penis/clitoris).

The muscle branches to the pelvitrochanteric muscles also exit via the Foramen infrapiriforme, while the muscle branches to the pelvic floor and the parasympathetic Nn. splanchnici pelvici do not leave the lesser pelvis. The small cutaneous branches pierce the Lig. sacrotuberale (N. cutaneus perforans) or the M. ischiococcygeus (N. anococcygeus) and are of minor significance.

→ T 42

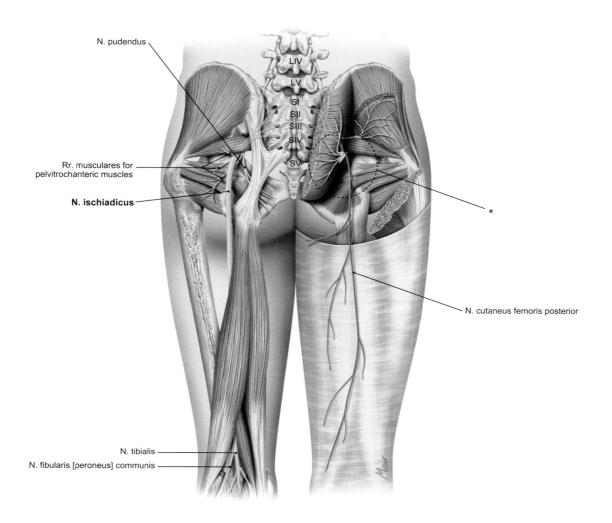

N. pudendus

Rr. musculares for pelvitrochanteric muscles

N. ischiadicus

LIV
LV
SI
SII
SIII
SIV
SV

*

N. cutaneus femoris posterior

N. tibialis

N. fibularis [peroneus] communis

Fig. 4.149 Lesion sites of the most important nerves of the Plexus sacralis; dorsal view. The cutaneous branches are shown in purple. [S700-L127]

Nerve lesions at the exit from the pelvis, e. g. due to incorrect intragluteal injection, are shown here on the right side of the body.
* damage due to incorrect intragluteal injection

Clinical remarks

Lesions of the nerves of the Plexus sacralis – Part 1 (Part 2 → Fig. 4.152)

In the case of a **high division** of the N. ischiadicus, the **N. fibularis communis** can be compressed while passing through the M. piriformis. The resulting pain can mimic a disc hernia. Apart from intragluteal injections, the **N. ischiadicus** can also be damaged by compression during prolonged sitting or, in the case of pelvic fractures, dislocations and hip operations. The resulting paralysis of the hamstring muscles restricts the extension of the hip joint, but more importantly, the flexion and rotation in the knee joint. If both the N. tibialis and the N. fibularis are damaged completely, all the muscles of the leg and the foot are paralysed and **standing or walking is impossible.** When lifting the leg while walking, the foot is dragged

(steppage gait). Standing on tiptoes is no longer possible. In addition, the sensory innervation of the lower leg (except anterior medial) and the foot is almost completely absent (for isolated lesions of the N. tibialis → Fig. 4.153 or N. fibularis → Fig. 4.154). The damage of individual muscle branches to the pelvitrochanteric muscles, as well as lesions of the cutaneous branches, are functionally insignificant. The **muscle branches** to the pelvic floor and especially the parasympathetic **Nn. splanchnici pelvici** may however be injured during surgical procedures in the lesser pelvis, such as the excision of the rectum or the prostate gland. Insufficiency of the pelvic floor can result in **faecal** and **urinary incontinence.** Damage to the parasympathetic nerves can cause **erectile dysfunction** in men and problems with the **Corpus cavernosum of the clitoris** in women.

Intragluteal injection

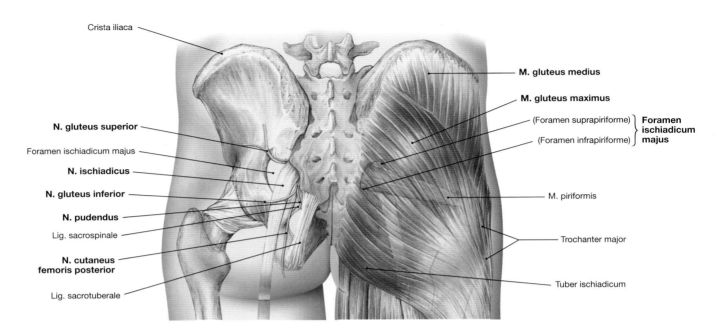

Crista iliaca

N. gluteus superior

Foramen ischiadicum majus

N. ischiadicus

N. gluteus inferior

N. pudendus

Lig. sacrospinale

N. cutaneus
femoris posterior

Lig. sacrotuberale

M. gluteus medius

M. gluteus maximus

(Foramen suprapiriforme) } **Foramen ischiadicum majus**

(Foramen infrapiriforme) }

M. piriformis

Trochanter major

Tuber ischiadicum

Fig. 4.150 Surface projection of the skeletal contours and the N. ischiadicus in the gluteal region. [S700]
In the case of an incorrect intragluteal injection into the M. gluteus maximus, all the neurovascular pathways that exit the Foramen ischiadicum majus are potentially at risk. Only the A. and V. pudenda interna as well as the N. pudendus, which pass through the Foramen ischiadicum minus into the Fossa ischioanalis, are relatively well-protected. Therefore, injections should always be given into the M. gluteus medius (→ Fig. 4.151).

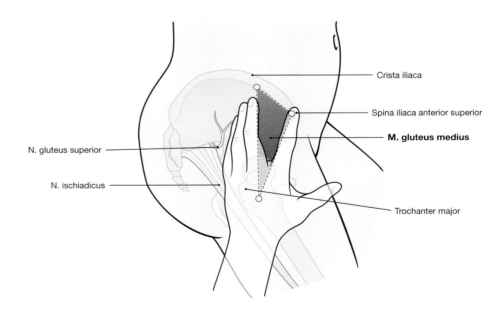

Crista iliaca

Spina iliaca anterior superior

M. gluteus medius

N. gluteus superior

N. ischiadicus

Trochanter major

Fig. 4.151 Intragluteal injection (according to von HOCHSTETTER). [S700-L126]
To be absolutely sure of preventing any lesion of the neurovascular pathways in the gluteal region, the intragluteal injection is given into the triangular field between the two spread-out fingers and the Crista iliaca, as shown here. The index finger is placed on the Spina iliaca anterior superior, and the palm of the hand lies on the Trochanter major. However, the muscle branch of the N. gluteus superior, running to the M. tensor fasciae latae, still remains at risk.

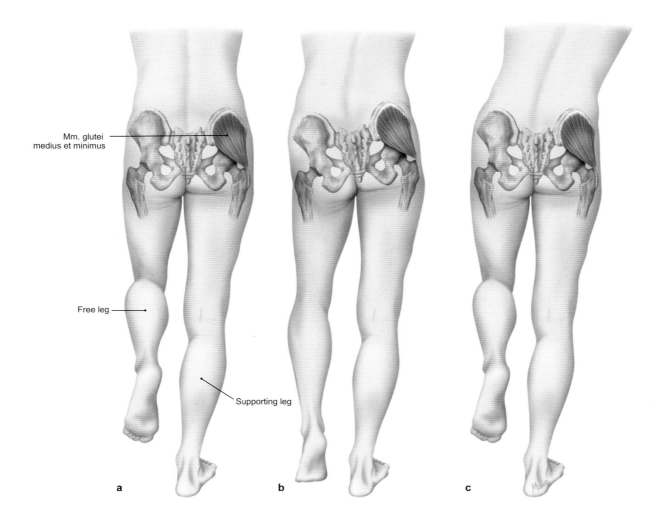

Mm. glutei medius et minimus

Free leg

Supporting leg

a   b   c

Fig. 4.152a–c   TRENDELENBURG sign and DUCHENNE sign (limp) indicating a weakness or paralysis of the small gluteal muscles, on the right side. [S700-L127]/[G1060-001]
a The gluteal muscles abduct the ipsilateral leg if the body weight is shifted to the other leg. In the one-legged stance, the muscles of the same side stabilise the pelvis and prevent it dropping to the opposite side (side of the free or non-supported leg).

b With functional insufficiency of the small gluteal muscles, such as in hip dysplasia or due to lesions of the N. gluteus superior, the pelvis drops to the healthy side when standing on the leg of the affected side **(TRENDELENBURG sign).**
c While walking, the pelvis of the healthy side is elevated by shifting the trunk towards the affected side **(DUCHENNE sign or limp).**

Clinical remarks

Lesions of nerves of the Plexus sacralis – Part 2 (Part 1 → Fig. 4.149) Due to the protected pathway of the **N. pudendus,** nerve lesions are rare, yet can lead to insufficiency of the perineal and sphincter muscles of the bladder and rectum, resulting in **incontinence,** and the sensory deficiency of the external genitalia can cause **disorders of sexual function.** When giving birth, the loss of sensation in the perineal region and the external genitalia may even be a desirable effect and is therefore induced by performing a **pudendal nerve block.** The Spina ischiadica is palpated through the vagina, and the N. pudendus is completely anaesthetised by injection of a local anaesthetic approximately 1 cm lateral and cranial of the Spina ischiadica before it enters the ALCOCK's canal. This procedure has become less important since the introduction of epidural anaesthesia, with the injection of local anaesthetics into the epidural space of the lower spinal cord. In the case of an **incorrect intramuscular injection** in the gluteal region, the neurovascular pathways passing through the Foramina

supra- and infrapirifome can be damaged. In addition to the blood vessels, the Nn. glutei superior and inferior, the N. cutaneus femoris posterior and the N. ischiadicus may be affected. The intragluteal injection according to von HOCHSTETTER is applied into the M. gluteus medius (→ Fig. 4.151). Lesions of the **N. gluteus superior** can lead to paralysis of the small gluteal muscles (the most important abductors and medial rotators of the hip) as well as of the M. tensor fasciae latae. Dysfunctions of the small gluteal muscles make the one-legged stance on the affected side impossible, because the pelvis tilts to the healthy side **(TRENDELENBURG sign).** If the **N. gluteus inferior** is damaged, the M. gluteus maximus, the strongest extensor of the hip joint, becomes impaired or paralysed. With normal gait, this can largely be compensated for by the hamstring muscles. However, climbing stairs, jumping and running are hardly possible anymore. Lesions of the **N. cutaneus femoris posterior** compromise the sensory innervation on the dorsal aspect of the thigh.

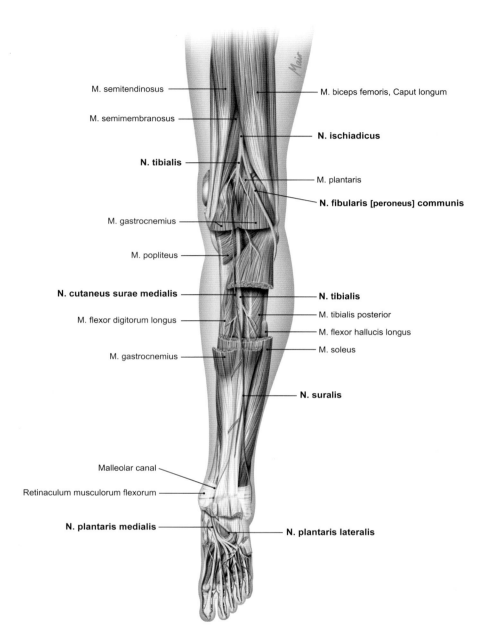

M. semitendinosus

M. semimembranosus

N. tibialis

M. gastrocnemius

M. popliteus

N. cutaneus surae medialis

M. flexor digitorum longus

M. gastrocnemius

Malleolar canal

Retinaculum musculorum flexorum

N. plantaris medialis

M. biceps femoris, Caput longum

N. ischiadicus

M. plantaris

N. fibularis [peroneus] communis

N. tibialis

M. tibialis posterior

M. flexor hallucis longus

M. soleus

N. suralis

N. plantaris lateralis

Fig. 4.153   N. tibialis: sensory innervation by cutaneous nerves (purple), and motor innervation by muscle branches, right side; dorsal view. [S700-L127]

The **N. ischiadicus** often divides at the transition from the middle to the distal third of the thigh into the medial **N. tibialis** and the lateral **N. fibularis communis.** The N. tibialis portion innervates the dorsal muscles of the thigh (hamstring muscles and dorsal part of the M. adductor magnus). The N. tibialis continues the pathway of the N. ischiadicus in the direction of the popliteal fossa of the knee, passes between the heads of the M. gastrocnemius below the tendinous arch of the M. soleus **(Arcus tendineus musculi solei),** and runs together with the A. and V. tibialis posterior between the superficial and deep flexors

to the medial ankle. In the popliteal fossa, the **N. cutaneus surae medialis** branches off to the medial calf, continues in the distal calf as **N. suralis** and along the lateral side of the foot as the **N. cutaneus dorsalis lateralis,** whereby it usually receives a communicating branch from the N. fibularis communis. When passing underneath the Retinaculum musculorum flexorum **(malleolar canal or tarsal tunnel),** the N. tibialis divides into its two terminal branches **(Nn. plantares medialis** and **lateralis** for the innervation of the sole of the foot. Thus, the N. tibialis provides motor innervation to all flexor muscles of the calf and all plantar muscles as well as sensory innervation to the middle calf and, after forming the N. suralis, to the lower calf and the lateral side of the foot.

Clinical remarks

Lesions of the N. tibialis are rare, but may occur with injuries to the knee joint or due to nerve compression in the **malleolar canal/tarsal tunnel** associated with tibial fractures or ankle joint injury **(posterior tarsal tunnel syndrome).** The tarsal tunnel syndrome is associated with burning pain in the sole of the foot and a loss of function of the plantar muscles. Flexion, adduction and spreading the toes are impossible. Paralysis of the Mm. interossei and Mm. lumbricales re-

sults in a **claw foot deformity.** In the case of nerve lesions in the knee region, all the flexor muscles of the lower leg are also paralysed (absent ACHILLES tendon reflex). The plantar flexion is strongly restricted and only supported to a minor degree by the fibular muscle group. This results in a **fixed pronation** of the foot, as well as a **pes calcaneus** in which the foot remains in a dorsiflexed position and it is not possible to stand on tiptoes.

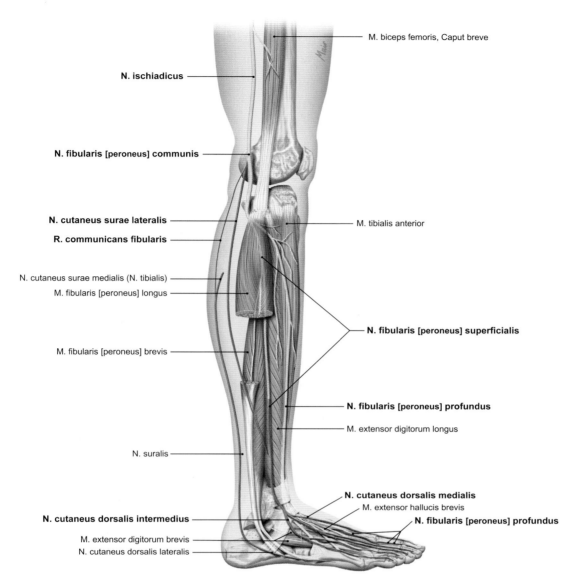

Fig. 4.154   N. fibularis communis: sensory innervation by cutaneous nerves (purple) and motor innervation by muscle branches, right side; lateral view. [S700-L127]

After the division of the **N. ischiadicus** at the transition from the middle to the distal third of the thigh, the **N. fibularis communis** passes through the popliteal fossa and turns around the head of the fibula in the fibularis compartment, where it divides into its two terminal branches (Nn. fibulares superficialis and profundus). The N. fibularis only innervates the short head of the M. biceps femoris at the upper thigh. Prior to the division into its terminal branches, the N. fibularis communis usually sends the **N. cutaneus surae lateralis** to supply the skin of the lateral calf as well as a communicating branch to the N. cutaneus surae medialis.

The **N. fibularis superficialis** continues its pathway inside the lateral compartment of the leg and innervates the fibular muscles before piercing the fascia of the distal lower leg and dividing into the two sensory terminal branches (**Nn. cutanei dorsales medialis** and **intermedius**) for the dorsum of the foot.

The **N. fibularis profundus** passes into the extensor compartment and runs with the A. tibialis anterior to the dorsum of the foot. On its way, it innervates the extensors of the leg and of the dorsum of the foot, and sends a sensory terminal branch to the first interdigital space.

Clinical remarks

Lesions of the N. fibularis communis are the most common nerve lesions of the lower limb. They can be caused by fractures of the proximal fibula, a plaster cast that is too tight, or by crossing the legs. The resulting paralysis of the extensor muscles causes the tips of the toes to point downwards (**weak dorsal flexion of the foot with equinus deformity**). To compensate for this, patients use increased knee flexion to raise their lower leg higher (**steppage gait**) or swing the leg forward in a circular movement. Due to the paralysis of the fibular muscles, the foot remains in a **supinated position**. The sensory perceptions in the lateral calf and the dorsum of the foot are lost.

The **N. fibularis profundus** can be damaged in the case of compartment syndrome, in which a traumatic swelling of the extensor mus-

cles (**tibialis anterior syndrome**) leads to compression of the nerve and its accompanying blood vessels. In this case, the fascia of the lower leg must be split. Lesions of the N. fibularis profundus are also associated with equinus deformity and steppage gait. However, the sensory function is only compromised in the first interdigital space! In the case of an **anterior tarsal tunnel syndrome**, compression of the sensory terminal branches under the Retinaculum musculorum extensorum results in dysaesthesia in the first interdigital space.

Isolated lesions of the **N. fibularis superficialis** are less common (e.g. due to trauma to the fibular muscles), in which case the paralysis of the fibular muscles results in a **supinated position** of the foot. This leads to sensory losses on the dorsum of the foot, with only the sensitivity in the first interdigital space still intact.

Arteries of the pelvis and thigh

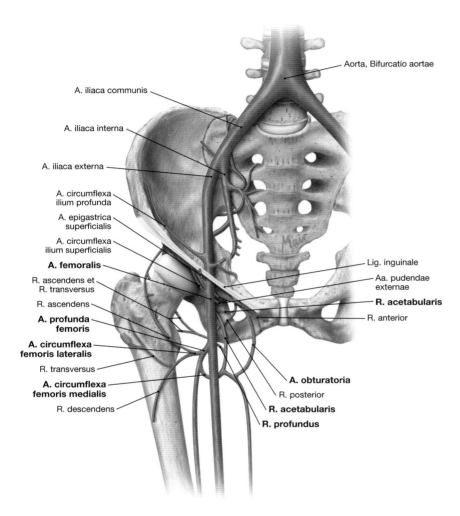

A. iliaca communis

A. iliaca interna

A. iliaca externa

A. circumflexa
ilium profunda

A. epigastrica
superficialis

A. circumflexa
ilium superficialis

A. femoralis

R. ascendens et
R. transversus

R. ascendens

**A. profunda
femoris**

**A. circumflexa
femoris lateralis**

R. transversus

**A. circumflexa
femoris medialis**

R. descendens

Aorta, Bifurcatio aortae

Lig. inguinale

Aa. pudendae
externae

R. acetabularis

R. anterior

A. obturatoria

R. posterior

R. acetabularis

R. profundus

Arteries of the lower limb

Branches of the A. iliaca externa:
- A. epigastrica inferior
  - A. cremasterica/A. ligamenti teretis uteri
  - R. pubicus (anastomosis with A. obturatoria)
- A. circumflexa ilium profunda

Branches of the A. femoralis:
- A. epigastrica superficialis
- A. circumflexa ilium superficialis
- Aa. pudendae externae
- A. profunda femoris
  - A. circumflexa femoris medialis
  - A. circumflexa femoris lateralis
  - Aa. perforantes (usually three)
- A. descendens genus

Branches of the A. poplitea:
- A. superior medialis genus
- A. superior lateralis genus
- A. media genus
- Aa. surales
- A. inferior medialis genus
- A. inferior lateralis genus

Branches of the A. tibialis anterior:
- A. recurrens tibialis posterior
- A. recurrens tibialis anterior
- A. malleolaris anterior medialis
- A. malleolaris anterior lateralis
- A. dorsalis pedis
  - A. tarsalis lateralis
  - Aa. tarsales mediales
  - A. arcuata (Aa. metatarsales dorsales → Aa. digitales dorsales; A. plantaris profunda → Arcus plantaris profundus)

Branches of the A. tibialis posterior:
- A. fibularis
  - R. perforans
  - R. communicans
  - Rr. malleolares laterales
  - Rr. calcanei
  - A. nutricia fibulae and A. nutricia tibiae
- Rr. malleolares mediales
- Rr. calcanei
- A. plantaris medialis
  - R. superficialis
  - R. profundus (→ Arcus plantaris profundus)
- A. plantaris lateralis (→ Arcus plantaris profundus with Aa. metatarsales plantares → Aa. digitales plantares)

Fig. 4.155 Arteries of the pelvis and thigh, right side; ventral view. [S700-L127]
The **A. iliaca communis** divides into the A. iliaca externa and A. iliaca interna in front of the sacroiliac joint. The **A. iliaca externa** provides the A. epigastrica inferior and the A. circumflexa ilium profunda to the ventral abdominal wall and then passes underneath the inguinal ligament. It then continues as **A. femoralis,** the artery supplying the entire leg, whereby the thigh, including the femoral head, is supplied by its strongest branch, the **A. profunda femoris,** of which the proximal branches (Aa. circumflexae femoris medialis and lateralis) wind around the femo-

ral neck. The **A. iliaca interna** also participates in the supply of the thigh and buttock region (→ Fig. 4.158): the **Aa. gluteae superior and inferior** exit dorsally via the segments of the Foramen ischiadicum majus and anastomose there with the branches of the A. profunda femoris. In contrast, the **A. obturatoria** passes ventrally through the Canalis obturatorius onto the medial side of the anterior thigh. With great variability it anastomoses via a R. pubicus with an eponymous branch from the A. epigastrica inferior. If this connection of blood vessels is well-developed, the term **Corona mortis** is used, because interventions in the groin could lead to fatal bleeding in the past.

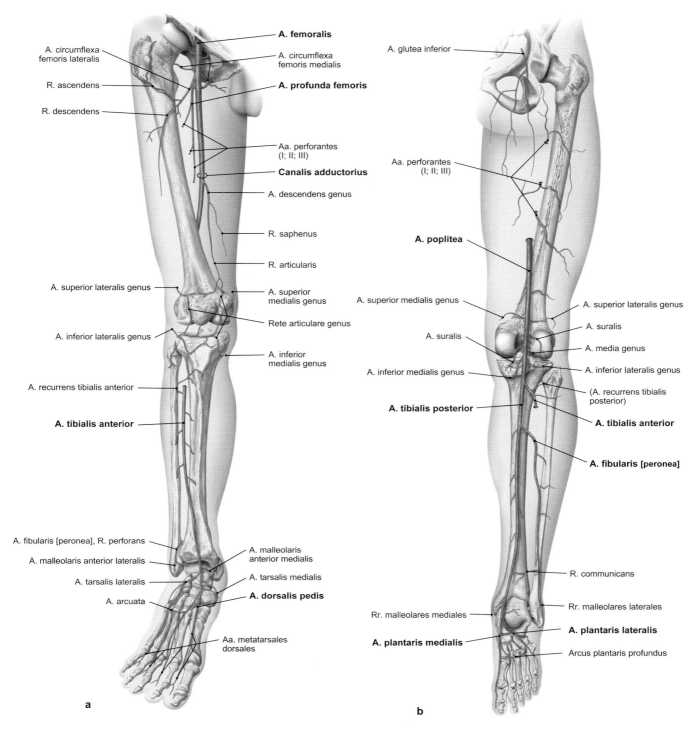

A. circumflexa femoris lateralis
R. ascendens
R. descendens

A. femoralis
A. circumflexa femoris medialis
A. profunda femoris
Aa. perforantes (I; II; III)
Canalis adductorius
A. descendens genus
R. saphenus
R. articularis

A. superior lateralis genus
A. superior medialis genus
Rete articulare genus
A. inferior lateralis genus
A. inferior medialis genus

A. recurrens tibialis anterior
A. tibialis anterior

A. fibularis [peronea], R. perforans
A. malleolaris anterior lateralis
A. tarsalis lateralis
A. arcuata
A. malleolaris anterior medialis
A. tarsalis medialis
A. dorsalis pedis
Aa. metatarsales dorsales

a

A. glutea inferior
Aa. perforantes (I; II; III)
A. poplitea
A. superior medialis genus
A. suralis
A. inferior medialis genus
A. tibialis posterior
A. superior lateralis genus
A. suralis
A. media genus
A. inferior lateralis genus
(A. recurrens tibialis posterior)
A. tibialis anterior
A. fibularis [peronea]
R. communicans
Rr. malleolares laterales
A. plantaris lateralis
Arcus plantaris profundus
Rr. malleolares mediales
A. plantaris medialis

b

Fig. 4.156a and b   Arteries of the leg, right side. [S700-L127]
a Ventral view.
b Dorsal view.
The **A. iliaca externa** runs in front of the sacroiliac joint from the A. iliaca communis. It continues underneath the inguinal ligament in the Lacuna vasorum as the **A. femoralis,** which is labelled as the **A. poplitea** (supplying vessel of the knee joint) after passing through the adductor canal. This artery passes below the tendinous arch of the M. soleus, between the superficial and deep flexors of the lower leg and divides

into the **A. tibialis posterior,** which continues its pathway, and into the **A. tibialis anterior,** which reaches the anterior extensor compartment via the Membrana interossea cruris. On the dorsum of the foot it continues as the **A. dorsalis pedis.** The A. tibialis posterior releases the **A. fibularis** as a large blood vessel supplying the lateral ankle, and continues its pathway towards the medial ankle and the malleolar canal/tarsal tunnel, via which it arrives in the sole of the foot, where it divides into its terminal branches **(Aa. plantares medialis** and **lateralis).**

Clinical remarks

A complete physical examination includes palpation of the arterial **pulses** of the A. femoralis (in the groin), the A. poplitea (in the popliteal fossa), the A. dorsalis pedis (on the dorsum of the foot, lateral

to the tendon of the M. extensor hallucis longus), and the A. tibialis posterior (behind the medial malleolus) to exclude any occlusion of the blood vessels due to **arteriosclerosis** or blood clots **(emboli).**

Arteries of the thigh

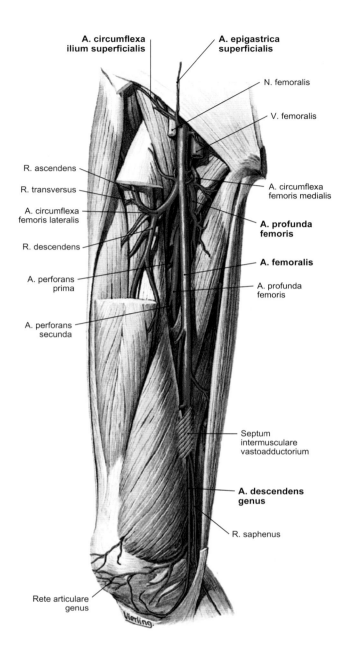

A. circumflexa ilium superficialis

A. epigastrica superficialis

N. femoralis

V. femoralis

R. ascendens

R. transversus

A. circumflexa femoris lateralis

R. descendens

A. perforans prima

A. perforans secunda

A. circumflexa femoris medialis

A. profunda femoris

A. femoralis

A. profunda femoris

Septum intermusculare vastoadductorium

A. descendens genus

R. saphenus

Rete articulare genus

Fig. 4.157   Branches of the A. femoralis, right side; ventral view; after removal of the M. sartorius and splitting of the M. rectus femoris. [G1066-O1109]

The **A. femoralis** runs between the N. femoralis (lateral) and the V. femoralis (medial) and has five branches:

- The **A. epigastrica superficialis** is a thin epifascial vessel and supplies the lower abdominal wall.
- The **A. circumflexa ilium superficialis** is an epifascial vessel, running laterally along the inguinal ligament.
- The **Aa. pudendae externae** supply the external genitalia (Rr. labiales/Rr. scrotales anteriores).

- The **A. profunda femoris** is the strongest branch and runs medially.
- The **A. descendens genus** originates in the adductor canal and supplies the knee joint and the skin in the knee region.

The **A. profunda femoris** is the main vessel supplying the hip joint and thigh. The other branches of the A. femoralis do not contribute to the arterial supply of the thigh. With its branches **(Aa. circumflexae femoris medialis** and **lateralis, Aa. perforantes)** the A. profunda femoris supplies the femur, the femoral neck and head as well as all the ventral and dorsal groups of the thigh muscles and parts of the gluteal region. The branches can also come directly from the A. femoralis.

Clinical remarks

The femoral artery is tapped when performing a **left ventricular catheterisation,** in which the catheter is inserted into the left heart chamber in order to assess the ejection volume of the ventricle and the condition of the coronary arteries.

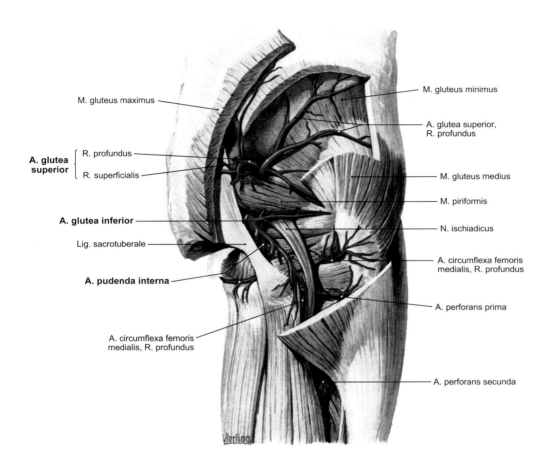

M. gluteus maximus

M. gluteus minimus

A. glutea superior, R. profundus

A. glutea superior
R. profundus
R. superficialis

M. gluteus medius

M. piriformis

A. glutea inferior

N. ischiadicus

Lig. sacrotuberale

A. circumflexa femoris medialis, R. profundus

A. pudenda interna

A. perforans prima

A. circumflexa femoris medialis, R. profundus

A. perforans secunda

Fig. 4.158 Arteries of the gluteal region, right side; dorsal view; after removal of the Mm. glutei maximus and medius. [G1066-O1109] The gluteal region and the dorsal thigh are supplied by parietal branches of the **A. iliaca interna** (→ Fig. 7.15) and the **A. profunda femoris.** Dorsal parietal branches of the **A. iliaca interna:**

* The **A. glutea superior** leaves the pelvis through the Foramen suprapiriforme and supplies the gluteal muscles. It passes laterally between the Mm. glutei medius et minimus.
* After passing through the Foramen infrapiriforme, the **A. glutea inferior** runs to the M. gluteus maximus.

Branches of the **A. profunda femoris:**

* **A. circumflexa femoris medialis:** its R. profundus supplies the posterior parts of the adductor and hamstring muscles, and the femoral head.
* **A. circumflexa femoris lateralis:** its R. ascendens runs to the gluteal muscles and to the femoral neck. It anastomoses with the A. circumflexa femoris medialis and the Aa. gluteae superior and inferior.
* **Aa. perforantes** (typically three): pierce the adductor and hamstring muscles.

The branches of the A. iliaca interna (including the A. obturatoria) anastomose with each other and with the A. profunda femoris, so that collateral circulations can be created.

Clinical remarks

In different sections of the leg, **collateral circulations** are formed by arterial anastomosis. The connections of the A. profunda femoris with branches of the A. iliaca interna show a great variability, but in emergency situations they allow the A. femoralis to be tied off proximally to the A. profunda femoris.

Arteries of the popliteal fossa and the dorsal lower leg

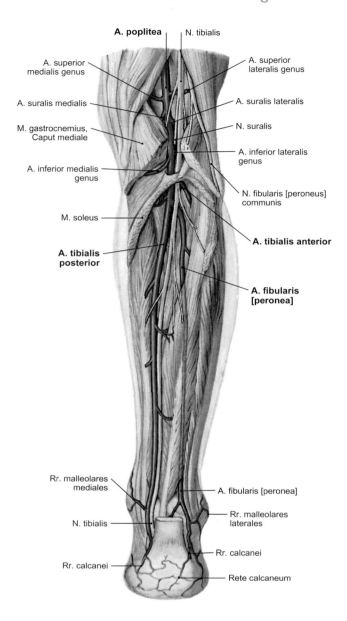

A. poplitea

N. tibialis

A. superior
medialis genus

A. superior
lateralis genus

A. suralis medialis

A. suralis lateralis

M. gastrocnemius,
Caput mediale

N. suralis

A. inferior lateralis
genus

A. inferior medialis
genus

N. fibularis [peroneus]
communis

M. soleus

A. tibialis
posterior

A. tibialis anterior

A. fibularis
[peronea]

Rr. malleolares
mediales

A. fibularis [peronea]

Rr. malleolares
laterales

N. tibialis

Rr. calcanei

Rr. calcanei

Rete calcaneum

Fig. 4.159 Branches of the A. poplitea and A. tibialis posterior, right side; dorsal view after removal of the superficial calf muscles. [B500]

After passing through the adductor hiatus, the A. femoralis continues its pathway in the popliteal fossa as the **A. poplitea.** It releases various branches, which form a vascular plexus in front of the knee joint (Rete articulare genus):

- **Aa. superior medialis and lateralis genus** around the medial/lateral femoral condyle
- **A. media genus** to the knee joint
- **Aa. inferiores medialis and lateralis genus** to the proximal tibia/head of the fibula
- **Aa. surales** to the calf muscles.

Terminal branches:

- **A. tibialis anterior:** passes through the Membrana interossea cruris (→ Fig. 4.160).
- **A. tibialis posterior:** continues the pathway of the A. poplitea and releases the following branches before passing through the malleolar canal/tarsal tunnel to the sole of the foot:
  - **A. fibularis:** the strongest branch descending along the dorsal side of the fibula; together with the **Rr. malleolares laterales** it supplies the lateral ankle and with the **Rr. calcanei** the lateral side of the heel.
  - **Rr. malleolares mediales** and **Rr. calcanei** supply the medial ankle and the medial side of the heel.

Clinical remarks

In contrast to the **collateral circulations** in the gluteal region, the connections of the **Rete articulare genus** in the knee region (which is fed by the recurrent arteries of the leg and the third perforating artery of the A. profunda femoris), are not sufficient to supply the leg in the case of an occlusion of the A. poplitea. In contrast, the **arterial arch around the ankle** is generally well-developed, so that the supply to the foot is not acutely at risk if either of the two Aa. tibiales or the A. fibularis is occluded.

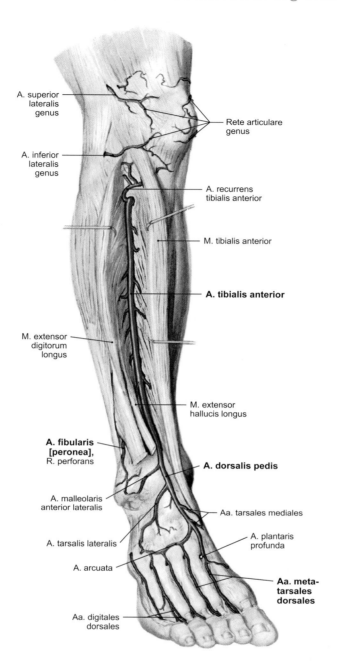

A. superior
lateralis
genus

Rete articulare
genus

A. inferior
lateralis
genus

A. recurrens
tibialis anterior

M. tibialis anterior

A. tibialis anterior

M. extensor
digitorum
longus

M. extensor
hallucis longus

**A. fibularis
[peronea],**
R. perforans

A. dorsalis pedis

A. malleolaris
anterior lateralis

Aa. tarsales mediales

A. tarsalis lateralis

A. plantaris
profunda

A. arcuata

**Aa. meta-
tarsales
dorsales**

Aa. digitales
dorsales

Fig. 4.160 Branches of the A. tibialis anterior and of the A. dorsalis pedis, right side; ventral view after spreading of the extensor muscles of the leg and removal of the tendons of the Mm. extensores digitorum longus and hallucis longus. [B500]

The **A. tibialis anterior** pierces the Membrana interossea cruris and descends in the extensor compartment before it continues on the dorsum of the foot as the A. dorsalis pedis. It has four branches:

- **A. recurrens tibialis anterior** and **A. recurrens tibialis posterior:** these vessels run before and after their passage through the Membrana interossea back to the knee joint.
- **A. malleolaris anterior medialis** and **A. malleolaris anterior lateralis:** with the branches of the A. tibialis posterior and of the A. fibu-

laris, these arteries complete the vascular plexus of the medial and lateral ankles (malleoli).

The **A. dorsalis pedis** also has four branches:

- **A. tarsalis medialis** and **A. tarsalis lateralis** to the medial and lateral sides of the foot
- **A. arcuata:** forming an arch, it runs laterally and releases the Aa. metatarsales dorsales which continue as Aa. digitales dorsales to the toes.
- **A. plantaris profunda:** connects with the Arcus plantaris profundus of the sole of the foot.

Clinical remarks

Due to the rich blood supply of the **tibia** (by the Vasa nutricia), it is possible to administer large volumes of fluid via an **intraosseous access** if in emergency situations no peripheral access can be found.

The cannula is inserted medially to the Tuberositas tibiae in the Condylus medialis tibiae.

Lower limb

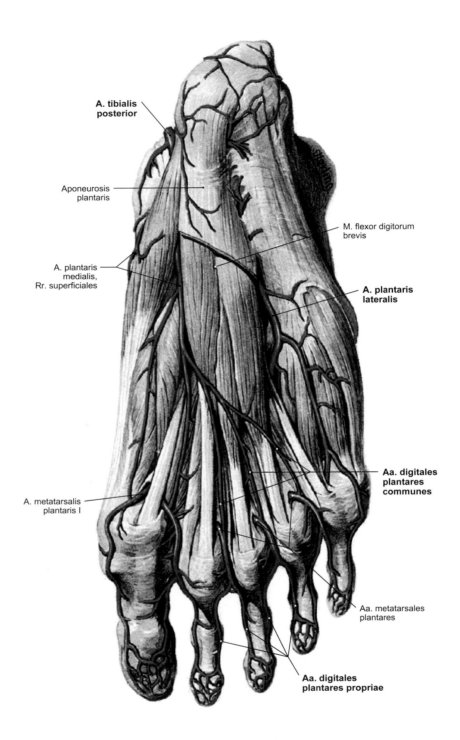

A. tibialis
posterior

Aponeurosis
plantaris

M. flexor digitorum
brevis

A. plantaris
medialis,
Rr. superficiales

A. plantaris
lateralis

Aa. digitales
plantares
communes

A. metatarsalis
plantaris I

Aa. metatarsales
plantares

Aa. digitales
plantares propriae

Fig. 4.161 Superficial arteries of the sole of the foot, right side; plantar view after removal of the plantar aponeurosis. [G1066-O1109]
After passing through the malleolar canal/tarsal tunnel, the **A. tibialis posterior** divides into its two terminal branches in the sole of the foot:

- **A. plantaris medialis:** runs medially of the M. flexor digitorum brevis.
- **A. plantaris lateralis:** runs laterally underneath the M. flexor digitorum brevis. Both vessels together form the Arcus plantaris profundus (→ Fig. 4.162).

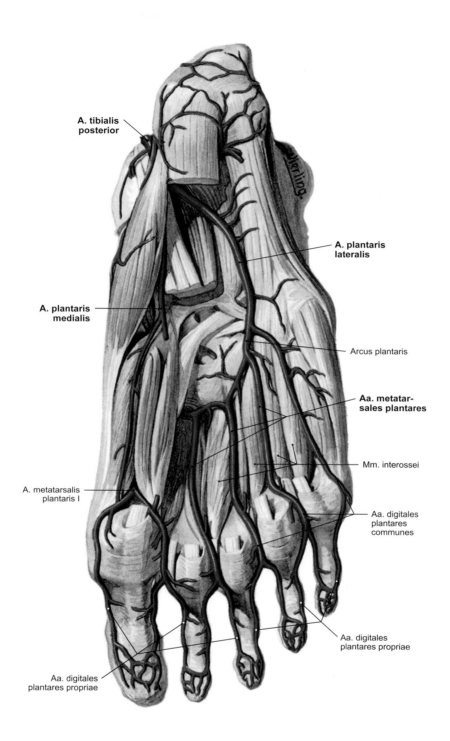

A. tibialis posterior

A. plantaris lateralis

A. plantaris medialis

Arcus plantaris

Aa. metatarsales plantares

Mm. interossei

A. metatarsalis plantaris I

Aa. digitales plantares communes

Aa. digitales plantares propriae

Aa. digitales plantares propriae

Fig. 4.162 Deep arteries of the sole of the foot, right side; plantar view after removal of the plantar aponeurosis, the M. flexor digitorum brevis and the tendons of the Mm. flexores digitorum longus and hallucis longus. [G1066-O1109]

The A. plantaris lateralis forms the arterial arch of the sole of the foot **(Arcus plantaris profundus),** which is completed by a deep branch of the A. plantaris medialis. The Aa. metatarsales plantares of the deep arterial arch supply the plantar side of the toes, together with the Aa. digitales plantares communes and the Aa. digitales plantares propriae.

Veins of the leg

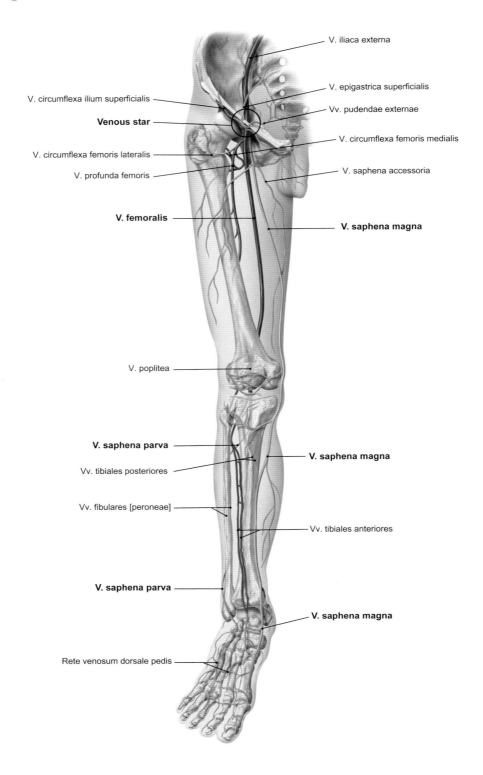

V. iliaca externa

V. epigastrica superficialis

Vv. pudendae externae

V. circumflexa femoris medialis

V. saphena accessoria

V. circumflexa ilium superficialis

Venous star

V. circumflexa femoris lateralis

V. profunda femoris

V. femoralis

V. saphena magna

V. poplitea

V. saphena parva

V. saphena magna

Vv. tibiales posteriores

Vv. fibulares [peroneae]

Vv. tibiales anteriores

V. saphena parva

V. saphena magna

Rete venosum dorsale pedis

Fig. 4.163 Veins of the leg, right side; ventral view. [S700-L127]
The veins of the **deep venous system** (dark blue) **accompany** the corresponding **arteries.** In the lower leg, two veins usually accompany the respective arteries, whereas in the thigh and the popliteal fossa only one concomitant vein is found. The **superficial venous system** of the lower limb (light blue) consists of **two main vascular trunks** which collect the blood from the dorsum and the sole at the sides of the foot. The **V. saphena magna** originates at the medial sides of the foot, anterior to the medial ankle and runs along the medial side of the lower leg and thigh to the Hiatus saphenus (→ Fig. 4.176). In the area of the so-called **venous star** it collects several tributaries (see below) from the inguinal region and drains deep inside into the V. femoralis.

On the dorsal aspect, the **V. saphena parva** starts at the lateral side of the foot **behind** the lateral ankle and runs via the middle of the calf into the popliteal fossa, where it drains into the V. poplitea. The V. saphena magna and the V. saphena parva are connected via variable branches.
Tributaries of the V. saphena magna in the area of the venous star:
*   V. epigastrica superficialis
*   V. circumflexa ilium superficialis
*   V. saphena accessoria (inconstant and variable)
*   Vv. pudendae externae.

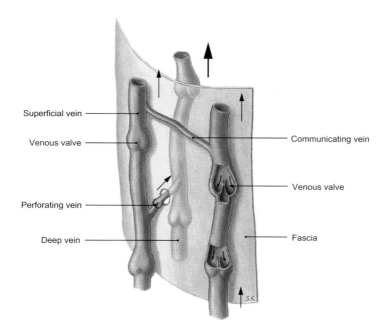

Fig. 4.164 Superficial and deep veins of the leg with venous valves: structural principle. [S700-L238]
There is a **superficial** epifascial **venous system** in the limbs, as well as a **deep subfascial venous system** which accompanies the respective arteries. Both systems are connected by perforating veins **(Vv. perforantes).** As **venous valves** direct the blood flow from the superficial towards the deep veins, the majority of the blood (85 %) is transported

back to the heart by the deep veins of the leg. Of the many perforating veins, three groups are of particular clinical significance:
- DODD's perforating veins: medial aspect of the thigh, in the middle third
- BOYD's perforating veins: medial aspect of the proximal lower leg (below the knee)
- COCKETT's perforating veins: medial aspect of the distal lower leg.

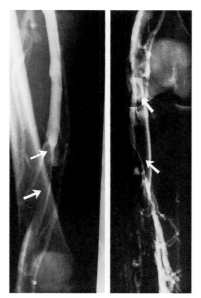

Fig. 4.165 Acute venous thrombosis in the leg with a large thrombus plug (arrows) in the V. femoralis. [R236]

Clinical remarks

As the blood mainly flows via the deep veins of the legs to the heart, there is the risk that in the case of **deep vein thrombosis,** blood clots can be transported to the lung, resulting in a potentially fatal **pulmonary embolism.** An inflammation of the superficial veins **(thrombophlebitis),** e.g. due to prolonged confinement in bed is, however, in most cases a harmless condition.
In the clinic, the V. femoralis is often used as access route for a **right cardiac catheterisation** because the catheter can be inserted into this vein and pushed forward into the right ventricle. In contrast, the superficial veins can be used in **bypass surgery** to bridge occluded sections of the coronary arteries.
Dilation of the superficial veins **(varicosis)** with the formation of swollen varicose veins **(varices)** is a common condition. These are usually the result of a connective tissue weakness with insufficiency

of the venous valves, but can also be secondary to a thrombosis with occlusion of the deep veins in the leg. This distinction is important, because the surgical removal of varicose veins **(varicose vein stripping)** should only be carried out in deep veins that are open. [E288]

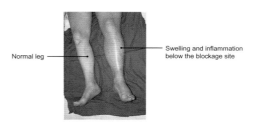

Neurovascular pathways

Lymphatic vessels of the leg

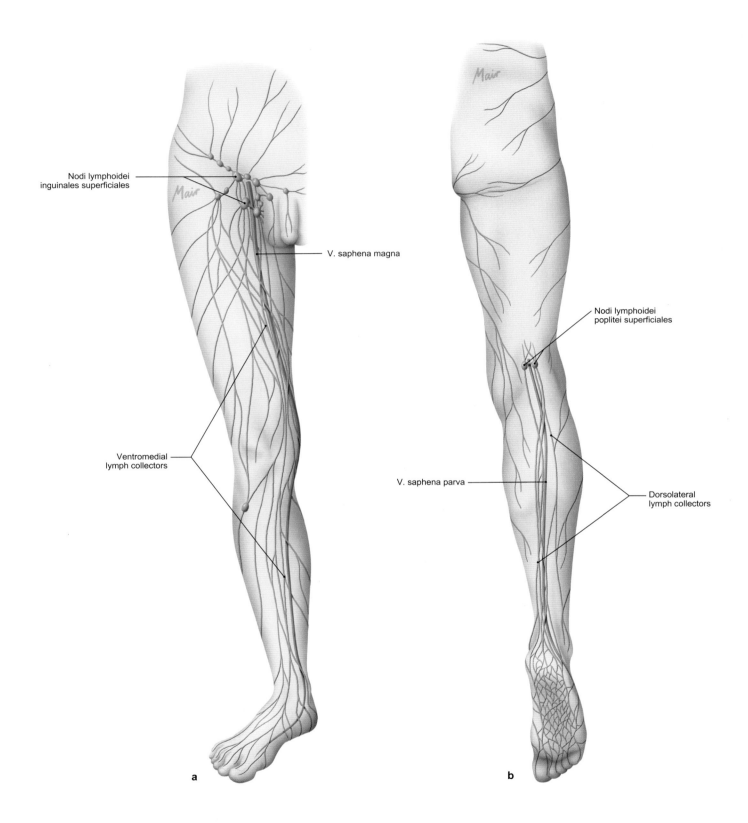

Nodi lymphoidei
inguinales superficiales

V. saphena magna

Ventromedial
lymph collectors

Nodi lymphoidei
poplitei superficiales

V. saphena parva

Dorsolateral
lymph collectors

a

b

Fig. 4.166a and b Superficial lymphatic vessels of the leg, right side. [S700-L127]
a Ventral view.
b Dorsal view.
Along the veins of the leg there is a **superficial** and a **deep** network of lymphatic vessels with interposed lymph nodes in certain places which act as **lymph collectors.** The superficial **ventromedial system** alongside the V. saphena magna is the main lymphatic drainage system of the lower limb and drains into the superficial inguinal lymph nodes **(Nodi lymphoidei inguinales superficiales)** (→ Fig. 4.172). The smaller **dor-**

solateral system drains only the lateral side of the foot. It runs adjacent to the V. saphena parva and flows to the lymph nodes of the popliteal fossa **(Nodi lymphoidei poplitei superficiales** and **profundi),** and from there it drains into the deep inguinal lymph nodes **(Nodi lymphoidei inguinales profundi).** The deep collecting systems drain directly into the deep popliteal and inguinal lymph nodes.
While the venous drainage of the leg mainly occurs via the deep veins, the major part of the lymph is drained via the superficial collecting system.

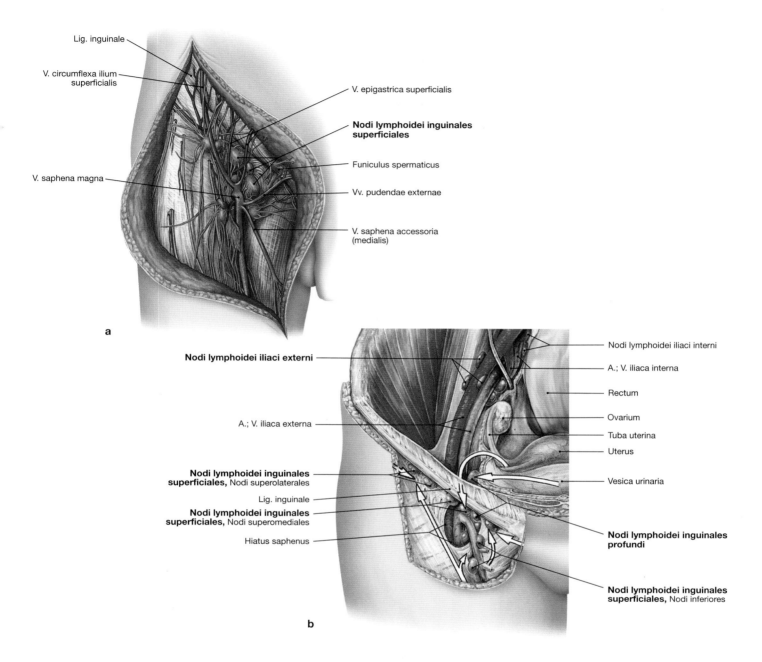

Lig. inguinale

V. circumflexa ilium superficialis

V. saphena magna

V. epigastrica superficialis

Nodi lymphoidei inguinales superficiales

Funiculus spermaticus

Vv. pudendae externae

V. saphena accessoria (medialis)

a

Nodi lymphoidei iliaci externi

A.; V. iliaca externa

Nodi lymphoidei inguinales superficiales, Nodi superolaterales

Lig. inguinale

Nodi lymphoidei inguinales superficiales, Nodi superomediales

Hiatus saphenus

Nodi lymphoidei iliaci interni

A.; V. iliaca interna

Rectum

Ovarium

Tuba uterina

Uterus

Vesica urinaria

Nodi lymphoidei inguinales profundi

Nodi lymphoidei inguinales superficiales, Nodi inferiores

b

Fig. 4.167a and b Superficial lymph nodes of the inguinal region, Regio inguinalis, right side; ventral view. [S700]

a Lymph nodes of the Regio inguinalis.

b Catchment area of the Regio inguinalis.

The groin harbours 4–25 superficial inguinal lymph nodes **(Nodi lymphoidei inguinales superficiales),** from which the lymph is drained into one to three deep inguinal lymph nodes, located medially of the V. femoralis **(Nodi lymphoidei inguinales profundi),** and then further into the Nodi lymphoidei iliaci externi in the pelvis. The superficial inguinal lymph nodes form a **vertical strand** along the V. saphena magna and a **horizontal strand** underneath the inguinal ligament.

The inguinal lymph nodes are not only the regional lymph nodes for most of the **leg** but also collect the lymph from the lower quadrants of the **abdominal wall** and the **back,** as well as the **perineal region** and the **external genitalia.** The lymph from the **lower parts of the anal canal** and the **vagina,** as well as from the **uterus** and the adjacent uterine tubes (via lymphatic vessels along the Lig. teres uteri) also drains into the inguinal lymph nodes.

Clinical remarks

Palpation of the lymph nodes is part of a complete physical examination. The inguinal lymph nodes represent the regional lymph nodes for nearly the entire leg. For the lateral side of the foot and the calf, the first lymph node station is located in the popliteal fossa but these are frequently non-palpable lymph nodes. Metastatic tumour cells can reach the inguinal region from all the above-mentioned lymph node areas and from the anal canal and the internal female sex organs. In men, however, only the lymph flow from the external genitalia (penis, scrotum) is directed to the inguinal lymph nodes, while the lymph from the testes is drained into the lumbar lymph nodes via the spermatic cord.

Superficial vessels and nerves of the inguinal region and thigh

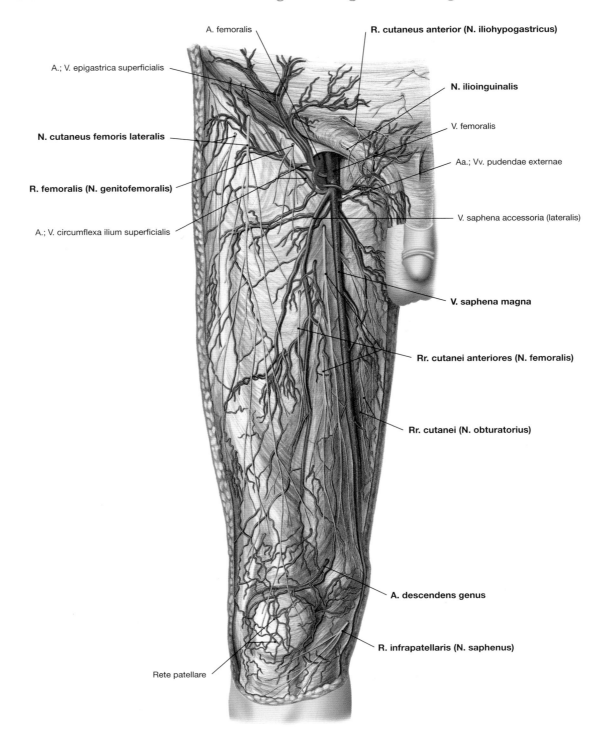

A. femoralis

A.; V. epigastrica superficialis

N. cutaneus femoris lateralis

R. femoralis (N. genitofemoralis)

A.; V. circumflexa ilium superficialis

R. cutaneus anterior (N. iliohypogastricus)

N. ilioinguinalis

V. femoralis

Aa.; Vv. pudendae externae

V. saphena accessoria (lateralis)

V. saphena magna

Rr. cutanei anteriores (N. femoralis)

Rr. cutanei (N. obturatorius)

A. descendens genus

R. infrapatellaris (N. saphenus)

Rete patellare

Fig. 4.168   Epifascial vessels and nerves of the inguinal region, Regio inguinalis, the anterior thigh, Regio femoris anterior, and knee, Regio genus anterior, right side; ventral view. [S700]
With dissections in this area, the pathways of the cutaneous nerves and of the epifascial veins should especially be considered. The **N. ilioinguinalis** emerges from the inguinal canal above the inguinal ligament. The **R. cutaneus anterior** of the **N. iliohypogastricus** can be found just cranially. The **V. saphena magna** ascends along the medial side of the thigh and flows into the V. femoralis at the Hiatus saphenus. Here the vein collects several tributaries from the inguinal region, forming the so-called **venous star** (→ Fig. 4.161). These veins usually accompany thin arterial branches from the A. femoralis. Laterally of the A.

femoralis, the **R. femoralis** of the **N. genitofemoralis** passes through the Lacuna vasorum. Medially of the Spina iliaca anterior superior, the **N. cutaneus femoris lateralis** passes through the Lacuna musculorum and innervates the lateral side of the thigh with its branches. The **Rr. cutanei anteriores** of the **N. femoralis** penetrate the fascia at different points and innervate the anterior side of the thigh. Medially of the V. saphena magna, several small **cutaneous branches of the N. obturatorius** supply a variable area on the medial aspect of the thigh. Medially below the knee, the fascia is pierced by the **R. infrapatellaris** from the **N. saphenus.** Just above the patella, the thin A. descendens genus runs to the Rete patellare.

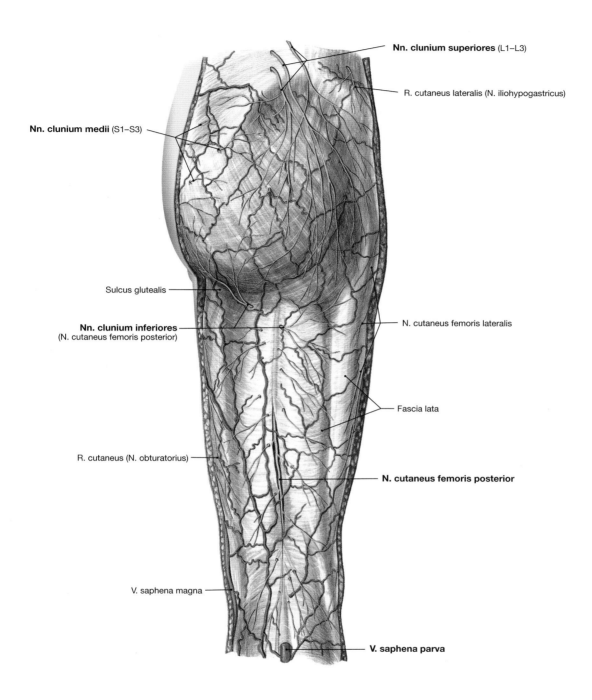

Nn. clunium superiores (L1–L3)

R. cutaneus lateralis (N. iliohypogastricus)

Nn. clunium medii (S1–S3)

Sulcus glutealis

Nn. clunium inferiores
(N. cutaneus femoris posterior)

N. cutaneus femoris lateralis

Fascia lata

R. cutaneus (N. obturatorius)

N. cutaneus femoris posterior

V. saphena magna

V. saphena parva

Fig. 4.169 Epifascial vessels and nerves of the gluteal region, Regio glutealis, thigh, Regio femoris posterior, and popliteal fossa, Fossa poplitea, right side; dorsal view. [S700]
There are no significant epifascial veins on the posterior side of the thigh. The V. saphena parva of the lower leg flows into the subfascial V. poplitea in the popliteal fossa. The skin of the gluteal region is innervated by three groups of cutaneous nerves. The **Nn. clunium superiores** (Rr. posteriores from L1– L3) pass laterally of the autochthonous muscles of the back across the iliac crest. The **Nn. clunium medii** (Rr. posteriores from S1–S3) penetrate the M. gluteus maximus at its origin on the posterior side of the sacrum. In contrast, the **Nn. clunium inferiores** are branches of the N. cutaneus femoris posterior and ascend around the caudal side of the M. gluteus maximus. The **N. cutaneus femoris posterior** itself descends in the middle of the thigh, mostly piercing the fascia half way down, in order to provide sensory innervation to the posterior thigh.

Vessels and nerves of the lower leg

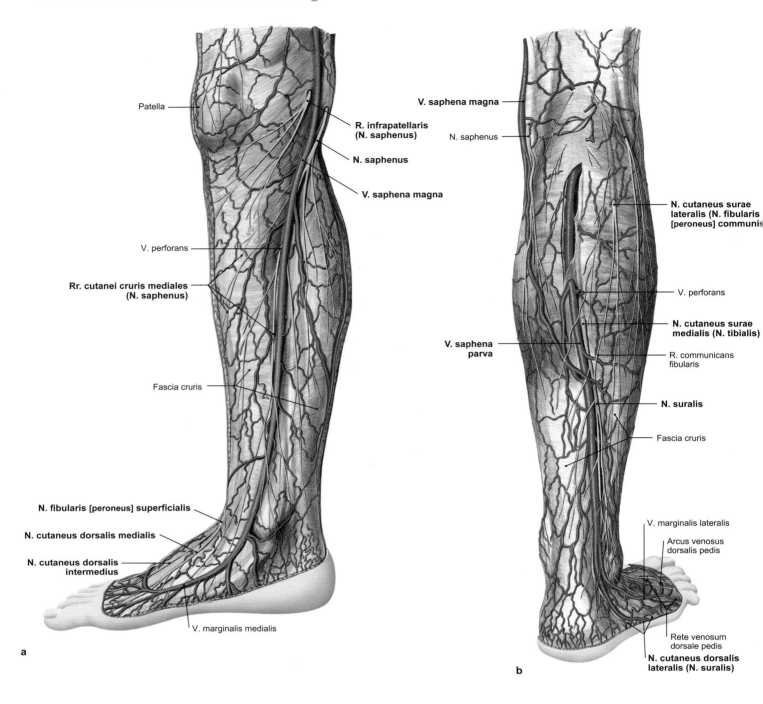

Patella

R. infrapatellaris (N. saphenus)

N. saphenus

V. saphena magna

V. perforans

Rr. cutanei cruris mediales (N. saphenus)

Fascia cruris

N. fibularis [peroneus] superficialis

N. cutaneus dorsalis medialis

N. cutaneus dorsalis intermedius

V. marginalis medialis

a

V. saphena magna

N. saphenus

N. cutaneus surae lateralis (N. fibularis [peroneus] communis)

V. perforans

N. cutaneus surae medialis (N. tibialis)

R. communicans fibularis

V. saphena parva

N. suralis

Fascia cruris

V. marginalis lateralis

Arcus venosus dorsalis pedis

Rete venosum dorsale pedis

N. cutaneus dorsalis lateralis (N. suralis)

b

Fig. 4.170a and b   Epifascial veins and nerves of the lower leg, Regio cruris, and the foot, Regio pedis, right side. [S700]

a Medial view. The **V. saphena magna** originates from the medial side of the foot anterior to the medial ankle and ascends along the medial side of the lower leg and thigh. On the medial side of the knee, the **N. saphenus** pierces the fascia. Its main trunk joins the V. saphena magna dorsally and runs distally along the vein, where it divides into its sensory **Rr. cutanei cruris mediales,** which provide sensory innervation to the anterior and medial aspects of the lower leg and down to the medial side of the foot. The **R. infrapatellaris** of the N. saphenus passes ventrally of the V. saphena magna through the fascia and innervates the skin below the patella. In the distal third of the lateral aspect of the lower leg, the **N. fibularis superficialis** penetrates the fascia and di-

vides into its two terminal branches (**Nn. cutanei dorsales medialis** and **intermedius**), which continue on the dorsum of the foot.

b Dorsolateral view. On the posterior side of the lower leg, the **V. saphena parva** emerges from the epifascial veins of the lateral side of the foot, and ascends behind the lateral ankle on the posterior side of the lower leg, penetrating the fascia in the popliteal fossa to flow into the V. poplitea. It runs alongside the **N. cutaneus surae medialis,** a branch of the N. tibialis, which in the distal third of the lower leg continues in a distal direction as **N. suralis.** This nerve usually receives a communicating branch from the **N. cutaneus surae lateralis** or directly from the N. fibularis communis. The terminal branch of the N. suralis is the **N. cutaneus dorsalis lateralis,** which innervates the lateral side of the dorsum of the foot.

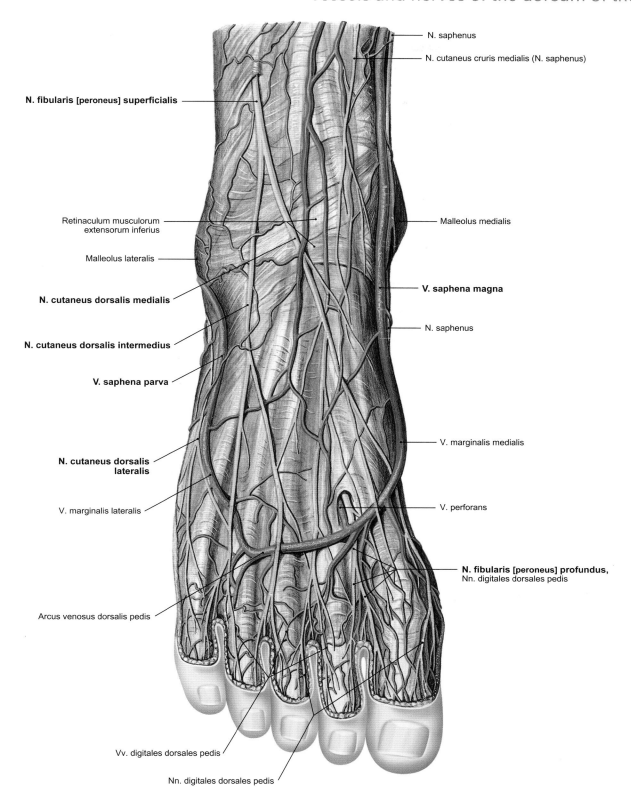

N. saphenus

N. cutaneus cruris medialis (N. saphenus)

N. fibularis [peroneus] superficialis

Retinaculum musculorum
extensorum inferius

Malleolus medialis

Malleolus lateralis

N. cutaneus dorsalis medialis

V. saphena magna

N. cutaneus dorsalis intermedius

N. saphenus

V. saphena parva

V. marginalis medialis

**N. cutaneus dorsalis
lateralis**

V. marginalis lateralis

V. perforans

N. fibularis [peroneus] profundus,
Nn. digitales dorsales pedis

Arcus venosus dorsalis pedis

Vv. digitales dorsales pedis

Nn. digitales dorsales pedis

Fig. 4.171 Epifascial veins and nerves of the dorsum of the foot, Dorsum pedis, right side; dorsal view in relation to the Dorsum pedis. [S700]
The **V. saphena magna** originates from the epifascial veins of the dorsum of the foot at the medial side, and thus is a continuation of the Arcus venosus dorsalis. The smaller **V. saphena parva** emerges on the lateral side of the foot. At the distal end of the leg, the **N. fibularis su-** **perficialis** passes laterally through the fascia, and generally only thereafter divides into the **Nn. cutanei dorsales medialis** and **intermedius,** which provide sensory innervation to the dorsum of the foot and the toes. The lateral side of the foot is innervated by the **N. cutaneus dorsalis lateralis** from the N. suralis. Only the first interdigital space receives its sensory innervation from the terminal branches of the **N. fibularis profundus** that penetrate the fascia here.

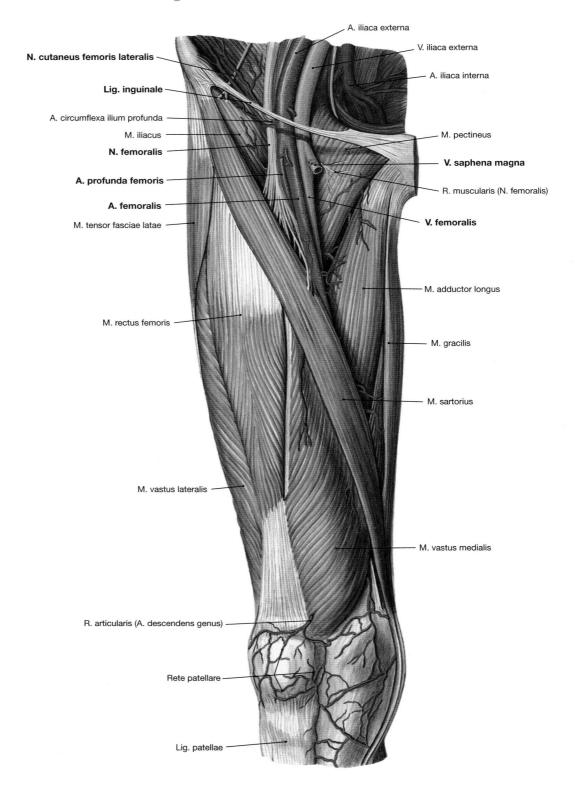

N. cutaneus femoris lateralis

Lig. inguinale

A. circumflexa ilium profunda

M. iliacus

N. femoralis

A. profunda femoris

A. femoralis

M. tensor fasciae latae

M. rectus femoris

M. vastus lateralis

R. articularis (A. descendens genus)

Rete patellare

Lig. patellae

A. iliaca externa

V. iliaca externa

A. iliaca interna

M. pectineus

V. saphena magna

R. muscularis (N. femoralis)

V. femoralis

M. adductor longus

M. gracilis

M. sartorius

M. vastus medialis

Fig. 4.172 Vessels and nerves of the thigh, Regio femoris anterior, right side; ventral view. [S700]
After removal of the Fascia lata, the individual muscles and the subfascial vessels and nerves are displayed in the femoral triangle **(Trigonum femorale).** The femoral triangle is limited proximally by the inguinal ligament **(Lig. inguinale),** medially by the M. adductor longus and laterally by the M. sartorius.
From medially to laterally, the V. femoralis, the A. femoralis and the N. femoralis pass below the inguinal ligament. The **V. femoralis** flows into the **V. saphena magna.** The **A. femoralis** provides the **A. profun-** da femoris as well as sending various small arteries into the inguinal area, 3–6 cm below the inguinal ligament. In the Fossa iliopectinea, the **N. femoralis** branches out in a fan-like pattern, where it provides, besides the **N. saphenus,** which continues the pathway of the N. femoralis below the M. sartorius, various **Rr. musculares** for the ventral muscle group of the thigh and the M. pectineus, as well as the sensory **Rr. utanei anteriores,** supplying the skin on the anterior aspect of the thigh. Medially of the Spina iliaca anterior superior, the **N. cutaneus femoris lateralis** enters the Lacuna musculorum below the inguinal ligament.

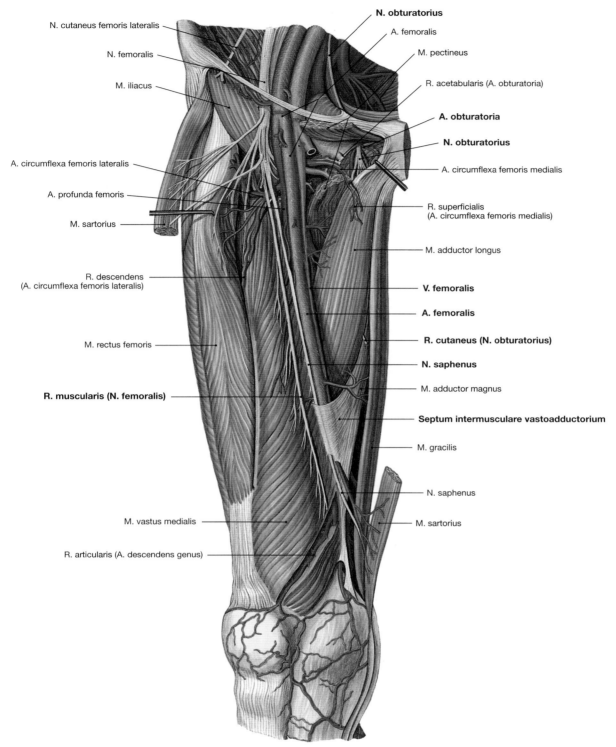

N. cutaneus femoris lateralis

N. femoralis

M. iliacus

A. circumflexa femoris lateralis

A. profunda femoris

M. sartorius

R. descendens
(A. circumflexa femoris lateralis)

M. rectus femoris

R. muscularis (N. femoralis)

M. vastus medialis

R. articularis (A. descendens genus)

N. obturatorius

A. femoralis

M. pectineus

R. acetabularis (A. obturatoria)

A. obturatoria

N. obturatorius

A. circumflexa femoris medialis

R. superficialis
(A. circumflexa femoris medialis)

M. adductor longus

V. femoralis

A. femoralis

R. cutaneus (N. obturatorius)

N. saphenus

M. adductor magnus

Septum intermusculare vastoadductorium

M. gracilis

N. saphenus

M. sartorius

Fig. 4.173 Vessels and nerves of the anterior thigh, Regio femoris anterior, right side, ventral view; after partial removal of the M. sartorius and severing of the M. pectineus. [S700]
The **A.** and **V. femoralis** and the **N. saphenus** can be followed until they enter the adductor canal **(Canalis adductorius).** The entrance of the adductor canal is formed by the M. vastus medialis, the M. adductor longus as well as by the **Septum intermusculare vastoadductorium** which spans these muscles and the M. adductor magnus. By splitting the M. pectineus, the outlet of the **Canalis obturatorius** through which the **N. obturatorius** and the **A. and V. obturatoria** leave the pelvis, becomes visible.

Clinical remarks

Lesions of the CNS or cerebral strokes may result in **spasticity.** The muscle tone of the adductors innervated by the N. obturatorius may be raised to such an extent that the legs cannot be spread and walking and standing become impossible. To relieve their spasticity, the individual muscles can be relaxed by botulinum injections. These injections inhibit the signal transmission at the motor endplates.

However, sometimes it is more effective to irreversibly damage the **N. obturatorius with phenol injections.** The needle is hereby inserted a few centimetres lateral to the pubic symphysis and below the inguinal ligament, to inject the N. obturatorius where it exits from the Canalis obturatorius.

Vessels and nerves of the thigh

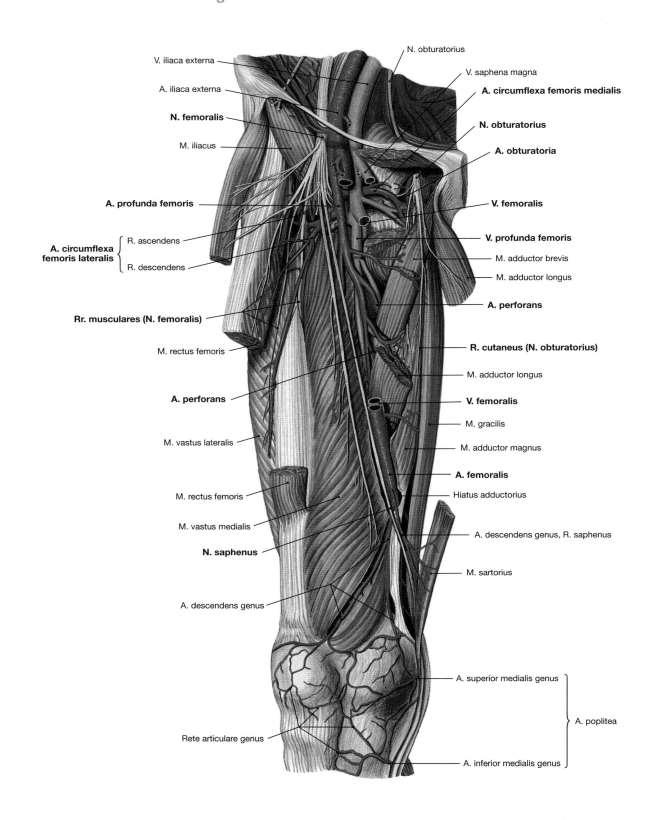

V. iliaca externa

A. iliaca externa

N. femoralis

M. iliacus

A. profunda femoris

A. circumflexa femoris lateralis { R. ascendens / R. descendens }

Rr. musculares (N. femoralis)

M. rectus femoris

A. perforans

M. vastus lateralis

M. rectus femoris

M. vastus medialis

N. saphenus

A. descendens genus

Rete articulare genus

N. obturatorius

V. saphena magna

A. circumflexa femoris medialis

N. obturatorius

A. obturatoria

V. femoralis

V. profunda femoris

M. adductor brevis

M. adductor longus

A. perforans

R. cutaneus (N. obturatorius)

M. adductor longus

V. femoralis

M. gracilis

M. adductor magnus

A. femoralis

Hiatus adductorius

A. descendens genus, R. saphenus

M. sartorius

A. superior medialis genus

} A. poplitea

A. inferior medialis genus

Fig. 4.174 Vessels and nerves of the anterior thigh, Regio femoris anterior, right side; ventral view; after partial removal of the M. sartorius and the M. rectus femoris as well as after severing the M. pectineus and M. adductor longus. The adductor canal is largely opened. [S700]

The **A. profunda femoris** with its branches can be seen here. This artery originates 3–6 cm below the inguinal ligament and is the main supplying vessel of the thigh and femoral head (→ Fig. 4.52, → Fig. 4.157). Its branches are the **Aa. circumflexae femoris medialis** and **lateralis,** which sometimes also originate independently from the A. femoralis.

The A. circumflexa femoris medialis supplies the femoral neck and head with a deep branch, as well as the adductor muscles and the proximal parts of the hamstring muscles. It anastomoses with the **A. obturatoria,** which also contributes to the blood supply of the adductor muscles and the hip socket (acetabulum). The ascending R. ascendens of the A. circumflexa femoris lateralis supplies the lateral muscles of the hip, and its R. descendens supplies the anterior muscles of the thigh. The main trunk of the A. profunda femoris is descending and usually releases three **Aa. perforantes** that pass onto the posterior side of the thigh to supply the deep adductor and hamstring muscles.

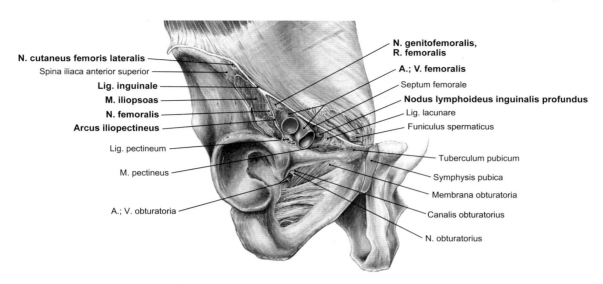

N. cutaneus femoris lateralis
Spina iliaca anterior superior
Lig. inguinale
M. iliopsoas
N. femoralis
Arcus iliopectineus
Lig. pectineum
M. pectineus
A.; V. obturatoria

N. genitofemoralis, R. femoralis
A.; V. femoralis
Septum femorale
Nodus lymphoideus inguinalis profundus
Lig. lacunare
Funiculus spermaticus
Tuberculum pubicum
Symphysis pubica
Membrana obturatoria
Canalis obturatorius
N. obturatorius

Fig. 4.175 Lacunae musculorum and vasorum, right side; oblique section at the level of the inguinal ligament; ventral view. [S700]
The space between the Os coxae and the **Lig. inguinale** (Fossa iliopectinea) is divided by the **Arcus iliopectineus,** which connects the inguinal ligament to the pelvic bones, into the lateral **Lacuna musculorum** and the **medial Lacuna vasorum.** The Lacuna musculorum is almost completely occupied by the **M. iliopsoas.** On this muscle lie two

nerves, the **N. cutaneus femoris lateralis,** which is closely lateral to the Spina iliaca anterior superior, and medially, the **N. femoralis.** In the Lacuna vasorum lie (from lateral to medial) the **R. femoralis** of the **N. genitofemoralis,** the **A. femoralis,** the **V. femoralis,** and the deep inguinal lymph nodes **(Nodi lymphoidei inguinales profundi),** which are located most medially.

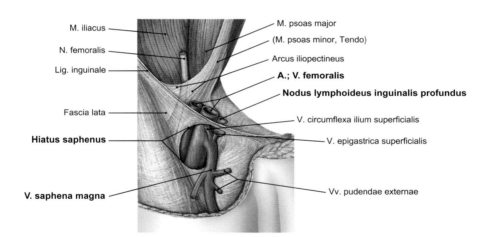

M. iliacus
N. femoralis
Lig. inguinale
Fascia lata
Hiatus saphenus
V. saphena magna

M. psoas major
(M. psoas minor, Tendo)
Arcus iliopectineus
A.; V. femoralis
Nodus lymphoideus inguinalis profundus
V. circumflexa ilium superficialis
V. epigastrica superficialis
Vv. pudendae externae

Fig. 4.176 Hiatus saphenus and Lacuna vasorum, right side; ventral view; after removal of the anterior abdominal wall, the Fascia iliaca and the abdominal viscera. [S700]

The Hiatus saphenus is an opening in the Fascia lata for the passage of the V. saphena magna before it flows into the V. femoralis. The deep inguinal lymph nodes **(Nodi lymphoidei inguinales profundi)** are located most medially in the Lacuna vasorum.

Clinical remarks

The **topography of the Fossa iliopectinea** is of great importance for diagnostic and therapeutic interventions. From medially (**i**nner side) to laterally, the large vessels are arranged in the following sequence: **V.** femoralis, **A.** femoralis and **N.** femoralis (**iVAN**). As the pulse of the A. femoralis is easily palpable, access to the V. femoralis is gained by piercing the skin about 1 cm medial of the artery, when a cardiac catheter is inserted into the right ventricle via the V. femoralis. The N. femoralis runs laterally to this artery, which is punctured, for example, to test the arterial blood gases as well as for a left heart catheterisation, and these procedures can damage the nerve.
The deeply located inguinal lymph nodes lie far to the medial side. It is here where an Anulus femoralis would present a penetration site in the case of a **femoral hernia.** Compared to inguinal hernias, this type of hernia is rare and occurs more frequently in women.

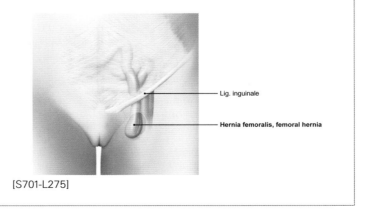

Lig. inguinale
Hernia femoralis, femoral hernia

[S701-L275]

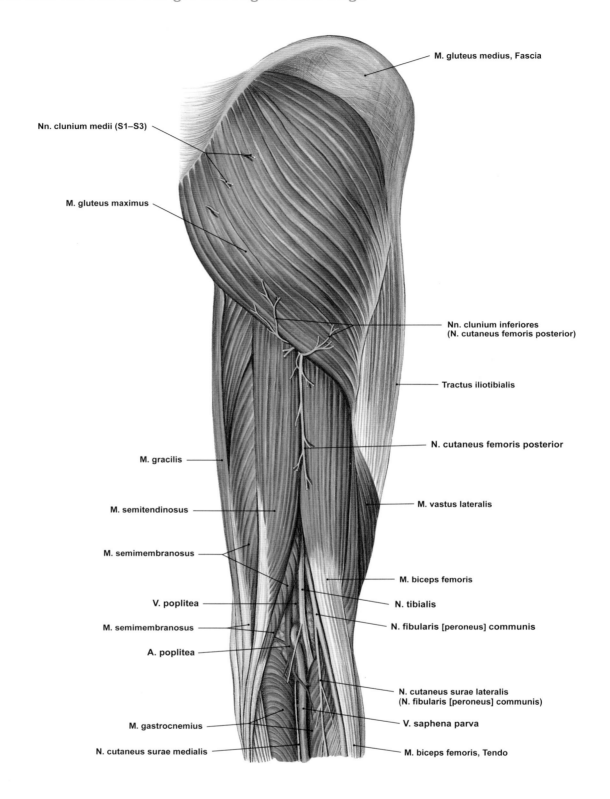

M. gluteus medius, Fascia

Nn. clunium medii (S1–S3)

M. gluteus maximus

Nn. clunium inferiores
(N. cutaneus femoris posterior)

Tractus iliotibialis

N. cutaneus femoris posterior

M. gracilis

M. vastus lateralis

M. semitendinosus

M. semimembranosus

M. biceps femoris

V. poplitea

N. tibialis

M. semimembranosus

N. fibularis [peroneus] communis

A. poplitea

N. cutaneus surae lateralis
(N. fibularis [peroneus] communis)

V. saphena parva

M. gastrocnemius

N. cutaneus surae medialis

M. biceps femoris, Tendo

Fig. 4.177 Vessels and nerves of the gluteal region, Regio glutealis, the posterior thigh, Regio femoris posterior, and popliteal fossa, Fossa poplitea, right side; dorsal view; after removal of the Fascia lata. [S700]

The **N. cutaneus femoris posterior** provides sensory innervation to the posterior aspect of the thigh. At the lower edge of the M. gluteus maximus, the nerve enters the groove between the M. biceps femoris and the M. semitendinosus, and runs below the fascia (subfascial) to the middle of the thigh; this has to be considered in dissections. On the

distal thigh, the two muscles diverge and confine the popliteal fossa **(Fossa poplitea).** As a continuation of the A. and V. femoralis, the A. and V. poplitea enter the popliteal fossa after exiting the adductor canal, and they join the terminal branches of the N. ischiadicus (N. tibialis and N. fibularis communis). In the popliteal fossa, the **N. fibularis communis** runs furthest laterally and superficially, and the **N. tibialis,** the **V. poplitea** and the **A. poplitea (NVA)** follow medially into the depths. The V. saphena parva ascends along the median line of the lower leg to the popliteal fossa and drains into the V. poplitea.

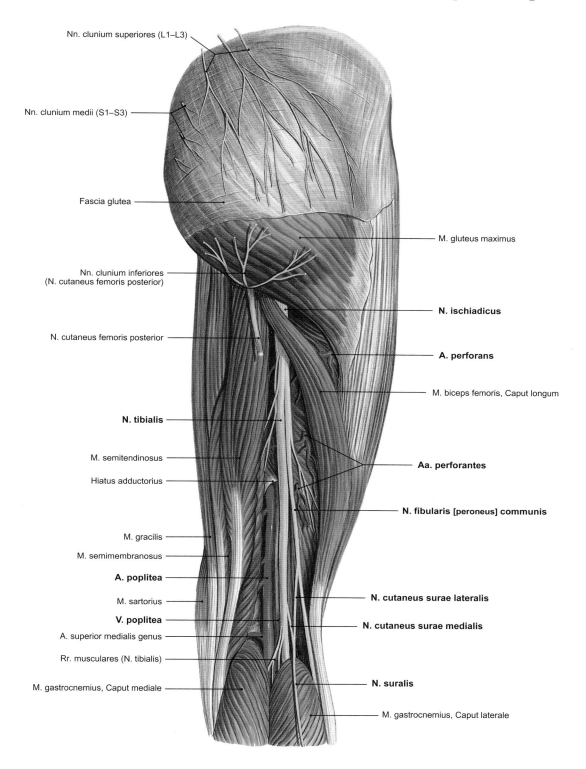

Nn. clunium superiores (L1–L3)

Nn. clunium medii (S1–S3)

Fascia glutea

Nn. clunium inferiores
(N. cutaneus femoris posterior)

N. cutaneus femoris posterior

N. tibialis

M. semitendinosus

Hiatus adductorius

M. gracilis

M. semimembranosus

A. poplitea

M. sartorius

V. poplitea

A. superior medialis genus

Rr. musculares (N. tibialis)

M. gastrocnemius, Caput mediale

M. gluteus maximus

N. ischiadicus

A. perforans

M. biceps femoris, Caput longum

Aa. perforantes

N. fibularis [peroneus] communis

N. cutaneus surae lateralis

N. cutaneus surae medialis

N. suralis

M. gastrocnemius, Caput laterale

**Fig. 4.178 Vessels and nerves of the gluteal region, Regio glutea-
lis, the thigh, Regio femoris posterior, and popliteal fossa, Fossa
poplitea, right side;** dorsal view; after removal of the Fascia lata and
lateral deflection of the Caput longum of the M. biceps femoris. [S700]
Guided by the M. biceps femoris, the **N. ischiadicus** descends along
the thigh. Usually at the level of the distal third (or significantly higher,
as shown here), the N. ischiadicus divides into two terminal branches,
of which the **N. tibialis** continues the pathway, while the **N. fibularis
communis** turns laterally and winds around the fibular head below the
popliteal fossa, before entering the fibular compartment. Mostly in the
popliteal fossa, the N. tibialis releases the **N. cutaneus surae medialis,**
and the N. fibularis communis releases the **N. cutaneus surae lateralis,** both providing sensory innervation to the calf. The **N. suralis** is
formed by the N. cutaneus surae medialis, which usually receives a
communicating branch from the N. cutaneus surae lateralis. At the
thigh, the **Aa. perforantes** of the A. profunda femoris penetrate the M.
adductor magnus laterally of the N. ischiadicus, in order to supply the
hamstring muscles.

Vessels and nerves of the gluteal region and thigh

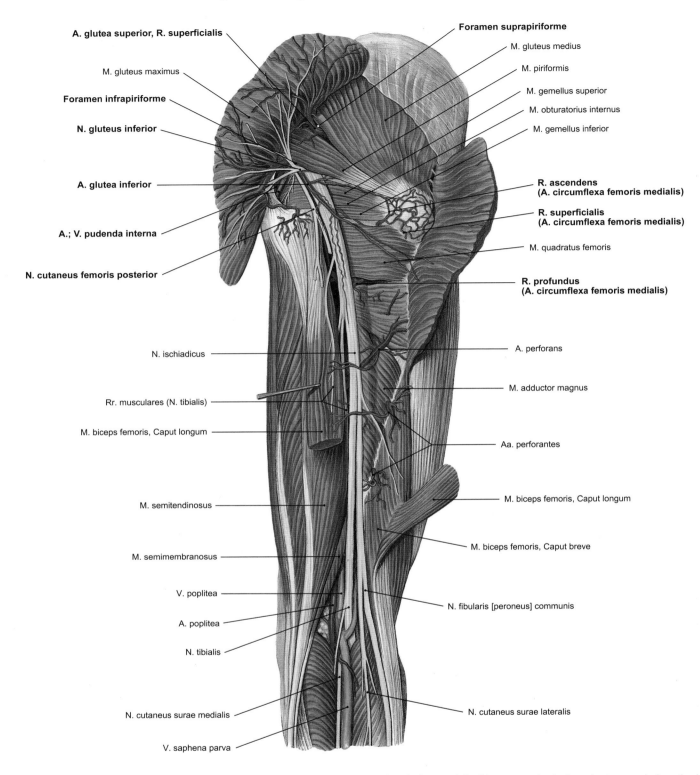

A. glutea superior, R. superficialis

M. gluteus maximus

Foramen infrapiriforme

N. gluteus inferior

A. glutea inferior

A.; V. pudenda interna

N. cutaneus femoris posterior

N. ischiadicus

Rr. musculares (N. tibialis)

M. biceps femoris, Caput longum

M. semitendinosus

M. semimembranosus

V. poplitea

A. poplitea

N. tibialis

N. cutaneus surae medialis

V. saphena parva

Foramen suprapiriforme

M. gluteus medius

M. piriformis

M. gemellus superior

M. obturatorius internus

M. gemellus inferior

R. ascendens
(A. circumflexa femoris medialis)

R. superficialis
(A. circumflexa femoris medialis)

M. quadratus femoris

R. profundus
(A. circumflexa femoris medialis)

A. perforans

M. adductor magnus

Aa. perforantes

M. biceps femoris, Caput longum

M. biceps femoris, Caput breve

N. fibularis [peroneus] communis

N. cutaneus surae lateralis

Fig. 4.179 Vessels and nerves of the gluteal region, Regio glutealis, the thigh, Regio femoris posterior, and popliteal fossa, Fossa poplitea, right side; dorsal view; after severing the M. gluteus maximus and the Caput longum of the M. biceps femoris. [S700]
Together with the **N. cutaneus femoris posterior** and the **N. gluteus inferior,** as well as with the **A.** and **V. glutea inferior,** the **N. ischiadicus** passes through the Foramen infrapiriforme. They are accompanied by the **N. pudendus** and the **A.** and **V. pudenda interna,** but immedi-

ately wind around the Lig. sacrospinale, in order to pass below the Lig. sacrotuberale and enter the Fossa ischioanalis via the Foramen ischiadicum minus. The N. gluteus inferior innervates the M. gluteus maximus. The **N. gluteus superior** passes together with the **A.** and **V. glutea superior** via the Foramen suprapiriforme but remains in the layer below the M. gluteus medius, which it innervates, along with the deep vascular branches.

Clinical remarks

The topography of the gluteal region explains why **intramuscular injections** should be administered in the **M. gluteus medius** and not in the M. gluteus maximus – the injection may otherwise cause

bleeding or lesions of the nerves that are important for movements of the hip (Nn. glutei superior and inferior) and the leg (N. ischiadicus).

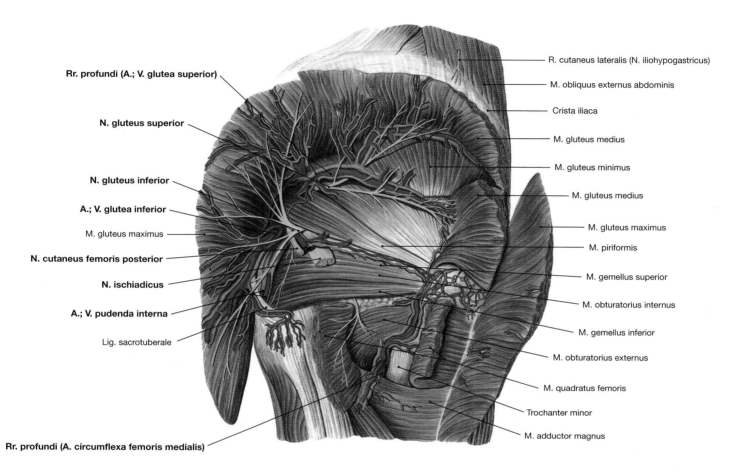

Rr. profundi (A.; V. glutea superior)

N. gluteus superior

N. gluteus inferior

A.; V. glutea inferior

M. gluteus maximus

N. cutaneus femoris posterior

N. ischiadicus

A.; V. pudenda interna

Lig. sacrotuberale

Rr. profundi (A. circumflexa femoris medialis)

R. cutaneus lateralis (N. iliohypogastricus)

M. obliquus externus abdominis

Crista iliaca

M. gluteus medius

M. gluteus minimus

M. gluteus medius

M. gluteus maximus

M. piriformis

M. gemellus superior

M. obturatorius internus

M. gemellus inferior

M. obturatorius externus

M. quadratus femoris

Trochanter minor

M. adductor magnus

Fig. 4.180 Vessels and nerves of the gluteal region, Regio glutealis, and the thigh, Regio femoris posterior, right side; dorsal view; after severing and partial removal of the Mm. glutei maximus and medius, and removal of the N. ischiadicus after its passage through the Foramen infrapiriforme. [S700]
Severing the M. gluteus medius exposes the **N. gluteus superior** which passes through the Foramen suprapiriforme together with the **A.** and **V. glutea superior** and then runs laterally between the M. gluteus medius and the deeper M. gluteus minimus to the M. tensor fasciae latae, thereby innervating all these muscles. At different points, several branches of the **A. circumflexa femoris medialis** emerge between the pelvitrochanteric hip muscles. The deep branches of this artery cross the muscles and anastomose with the gluteal arteries.

Clinical remarks

The topography of the gluteal region is particularly important for **hip joint surgery** needing dorsal access. If at all possible, the pelvitrochanteric muscles (in particular the M. quadratus femoris and M. obturatorius externus) should not be severed to prevent any damage to the A. circumflexa femoris medialis as the most important blood vessel supplying the femoral head.

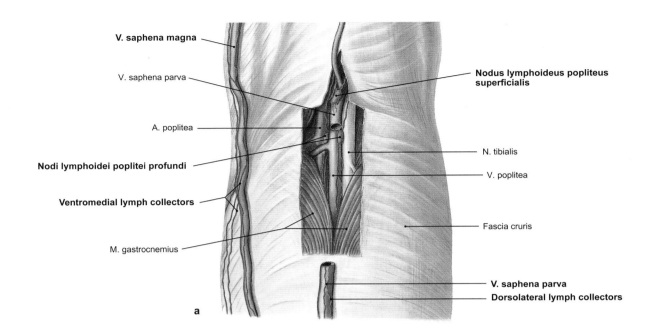

V. saphena magna

V. saphena parva

A. poplitea

Nodi lymphoidei poplitei profundi

Ventromedial lymph collectors

M. gastrocnemius

Nodus lymphoideus popliteus superficialis

N. tibialis

V. poplitea

Fascia cruris

V. saphena parva
Dorsolateral lymph collectors

a

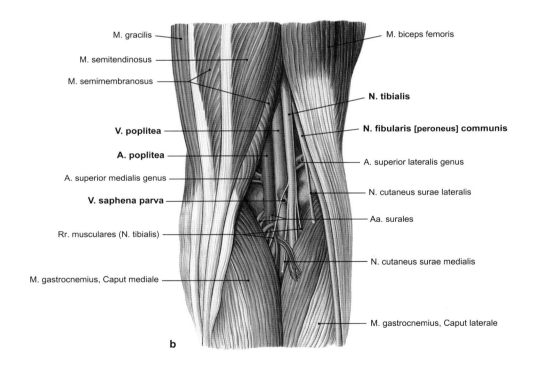

M. gracilis

M. semitendinosus

M. semimembranosus

V. poplitea

A. poplitea

A. superior medialis genus

V. saphena parva

Rr. musculares (N. tibialis)

M. gastrocnemius, Caput mediale

M. biceps femoris

N. tibialis

N. fibularis [peroneus] communis

A. superior lateralis genus

N. cutaneus surae lateralis

Aa. surales

N. cutaneus surae medialis

M. gastrocnemius, Caput laterale

b

Fig. 4.181a and b Vessels and nerves of the popliteal fossa, Fossa poplitea, right side; dorsal view. [S700]
a View after partial ablation of the fascia.
b View after complete ablation of the fascia.
In the popliteal fossa, the **N. fibularis communis** runs laterally and superficially, whereas the **N. tibialis,** the **V. poplitea** and the **A. poplitea (NVA)** run medially and in greater depth. The **V. saphena parva** ascends along the median line of the lower leg to the popliteal fossa and drains into the V. poplitea. The **dorsolateral lymphatic bundle** follows the pathway of the V. saphena parva, while the **V. saphena magna** ascends along with the stronger **ventromedial lymphatic bundle.** The first lymph node station for the dorsolateral lymphatic bundle consists of the **Nodi lymphoidei poplitei superficiales** and **profundi** (→ Fig. 4.166).

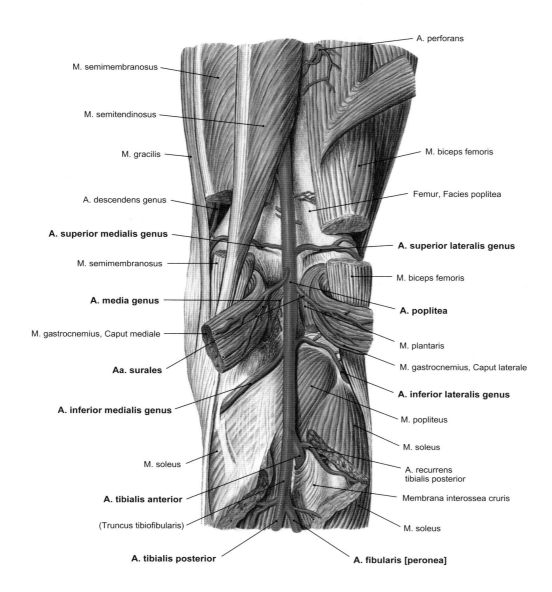

M. semimembranosus

M. semitendinosus

M. gracilis

A. descendens genus

A. superior medialis genus

M. semimembranosus

A. media genus

M. gastrocnemius, Caput mediale

Aa. surales

A. inferior medialis genus

M. soleus

A. tibialis anterior

(Truncus tibiofibularis)

A. tibialis posterior

A. perforans

M. biceps femoris

Femur, Facies poplitea

A. superior lateralis genus

M. biceps femoris

A. poplitea

M. plantaris

M. gastrocnemius, Caput laterale

A. inferior lateralis genus

M. popliteus

M. soleus

A. recurrens tibialis posterior

Membrana interossea cruris

M. soleus

A. fibularis [peronea]

Fig. 4.182 Arteries of the popliteal fossa, Fossa poplitea, right side; dorsal view; after partial removal of the muscles covering them. [S700]

The **A. poplitea** supplies the knee joint. Its branches above (Aa. superiores medialis and lateralis genus) and below (Aa. inferiores medialis and lateralis genus) the joint space form 'crown-like' vascular plexuses which supply the Rete articulare genus at the front of the knee. At the level of the knee joint, the A. media genus branches off to the knee joint. The Aa. surales supply the calf muscles. Below the popliteal fossa, the A. poplitea passes between the two heads of the M. gastrocnemius and divides into its terminal branches below the tendinous arch of the M. soleus. The **A. tibialis posterior** continues in this direction, while the **A. tibialis anterior** passes through the Membrana interossea cruris into the anterior extensor compartment.

Clinical remarks

The section of the A. poplitea between the outlet of the A. tibialis anterior and the origin of the A. fibularis, running from the A. tibialis posterior, is also known by its clinical term as the **Truncus tibiofibularis**.

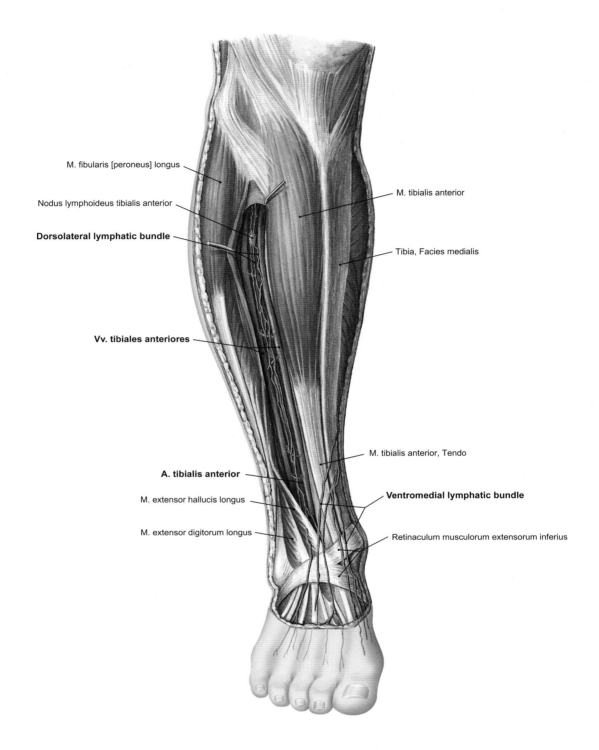

M. fibularis [peroneus] longus

Nodus lymphoideus tibialis anterior

Dorsolateral lymphatic bundle

Vv. tibiales anteriores

A. tibialis anterior

M. extensor hallucis longus

M. extensor digitorum longus

M. tibialis anterior

Tibia, Facies medialis

M. tibialis anterior, Tendo

Ventromedial lymphatic bundle

Retinaculum musculorum extensorum inferius

Fig. 4.183 Vessels and lymphatic vessels of the lower leg, Regio cruris anterior, right side; ventral view; after spreading apart the extensor muscles. [S700]
This figure shows sections of the superficial and deep lymphatic systems: the **superficial lymphatic vessels** form the ventromedial lymphatic bundle and join the V. saphena magna at the medial side of the foot, while the dorsolateral lymphatic bundle runs with the V. saphena parva along the lateral side of the foot. The **deep lymphatic vessels** accompany the deep veins and arteries in the three muscle compartments as shown here for the extensor compartment.

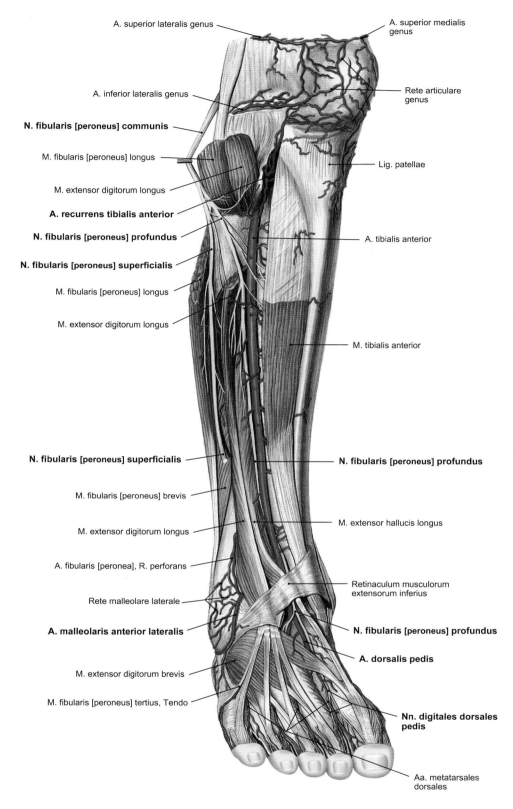

A. superior lateralis genus

A. inferior lateralis genus

N. fibularis [peroneus] communis

M. fibularis [peroneus] longus

M. extensor digitorum longus

A. recurrens tibialis anterior

N. fibularis [peroneus] profundus

N. fibularis [peroneus] superficialis

M. fibularis [peroneus] longus

M. extensor digitorum longus

N. fibularis [peroneus] superficialis

M. fibularis [peroneus] brevis

M. extensor digitorum longus

A. fibularis [peronea], R. perforans

Rete malleolare laterale

A. malleolaris anterior lateralis

M. extensor digitorum brevis

M. fibularis [peroneus] tertius, Tendo

A. superior medialis genus

Rete articulare genus

Lig. patellae

A. tibialis anterior

M. tibialis anterior

N. fibularis [peroneus] profundus

M. extensor hallucis longus

Retinaculum musculorum extensorum inferius

N. fibularis [peroneus] profundus

A. dorsalis pedis

Nn. digitales dorsales pedis

Aa. metatarsales dorsales

Fig. 4.184 Vessels and nerves of the lower leg, Regio cruris anterior, right side; ventral view; after removal of the Fascia cruris and severing the Mm. extensor digitorum longus and fibularis longus. [S700]

The **A. tibialis anterior** descends in the extensor compartment between the M. extensor digitorum longus and the M. tibialis anterior, and then continues as **A. dorsalis pedis** on the dorsum of the foot. After releasing the **A. recurrens tibialis posterior** on the posterior aspect of the lower leg, it releases the **A. recurrens tibialis anterior** after crossing through the Membrana interossea cruris. At the level of the ankles, it sends out the **Aa. malleolares anteriores medialis** and **lateralis** to supply the malleolar vascular networks, which may represent a sufficient collateral circulation if one of the arteries of the lower leg is occluded.

The **N. fibularis communis** winds laterally around the head of the fibula and enters the fibular muscle compartment. Here it divides into two branches, of which the **N. fibularis superficialis** descends into the fibular compartment, innervating the two fibular muscles and piercing the Fascia cruris in the distal third of the leg. In contrast, the **N. fibularis profundus** enters the extensor compartment where it accompanies the A. tibialis anterior. It provides motor innervation to all the extensors of the leg and the dorsum of the foot, and innervates the first interdigital space with its sensory terminal branches.

Clinical remarks

The **N. fibularis communis** can be **damaged near the fibular head** (by proximal fibular fractures, plaster casts or crossed legs). The resulting paralysis of the extensor muscles causes the tips of the toes to drop (**equinus or foot-drop deformity,** Clinical remarks → Fig. 4.154. This is the most common nerve lesion of the lower limb!

Vessels and nerves of the popliteal fossa and the lower leg

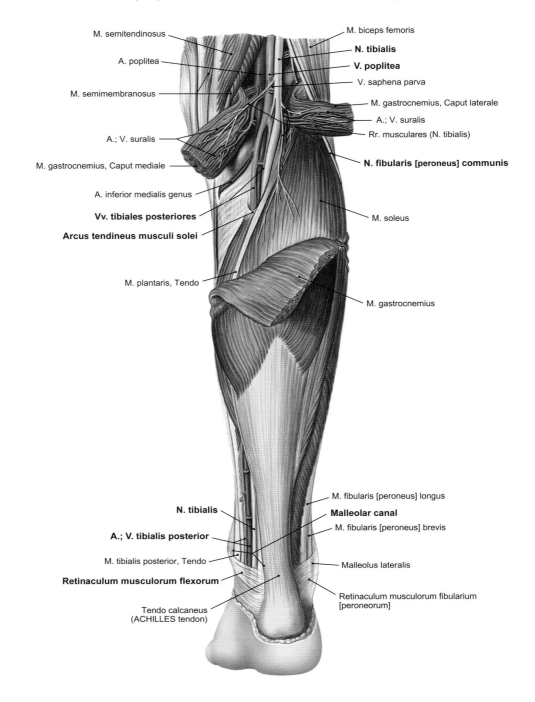

M. semitendinosus

A. poplitea

M. semimembranosus

A.; V. suralis

M. gastrocnemius, Caput mediale

A. inferior medialis genus

Vv. tibiales posteriores

Arcus tendineus musculi solei

M. plantaris, Tendo

N. tibialis

A.; V. tibialis posterior

M. tibialis posterior, Tendo

Retinaculum musculorum flexorum

Tendo calcaneus
(ACHILLES tendon)

M. biceps femoris

N. tibialis

V. poplitea

V. saphena parva

M. gastrocnemius, Caput laterale

A.; V. suralis

Rr. musculares (N. tibialis)

N. fibularis [peroneus] communis

M. soleus

M. gastrocnemius

M. fibularis [peroneus] longus

Malleolar canal

M. fibularis [peroneus] brevis

Malleolus lateralis

Retinaculum musculorum fibularium
[peroneorum]

Fig. 4.185 Vessels and nerves of the popliteal fossa, Fossa poplitea, and posterior aspect of lower leg, Regio cruris posterior, right side; dorsal view; after removal of the Fascia cruris and severing the M. gastrocnemius. [S700]

The **A. tibialis posterior** passes below the tendinous arch of the M. soleus (Arcus tendineus musculi solei) together with its two accompanying veins and the **N. tibialis** and descends into the layer between the superficial and deep flexors of the lower leg to the medial malleolus, and continues through the **malleolar canal/tarsal tunnel** below the Retinaculum musculorum flexorum to the sole of the foot.

Clinical remarks

The **N. tibialis** can be compressed in the malleolar canal (**tarsal tunnel syndrome,** Clinical remarks → Fig. 4.154). This causes a burning pain in the sole of the foot and a loss of function of the plantar muscles of the foot. Flexion, adduction and spreading the toes apart are no longer possible. Paralysis of the Mm. interossei and Mm. lumbricales results in a **claw foot deformity.**

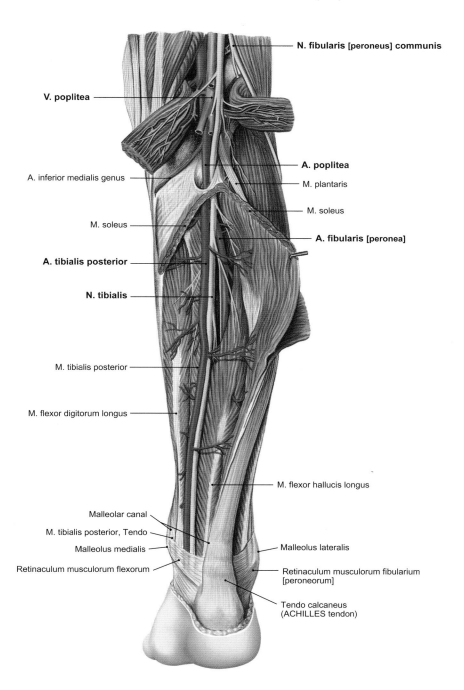

- N. fibularis [peroneus] communis
- V. poplitea
- A. inferior medialis genus
- M. soleus
- A. tibialis posterior
- N. tibialis
- M. tibialis posterior
- M. flexor digitorum longus
- Malleolar canal
- M. tibialis posterior, Tendo
- Malleolus medialis
- Retinaculum musculorum flexorum
- A. poplitea
- M. plantaris
- M. soleus
- A. fibularis [peronea]
- M. flexor hallucis longus
- Malleolus lateralis
- Retinaculum musculorum fibularium [peroneorum]
- Tendo calcaneus (ACHILLES tendon)

Fig. 4.186   Vessels and nerves of the popliteal fossa, Fossa pop-litea, and the lower leg, Regio cruris posterior, right side; dorsal view; after severing the Mm. gastrocnemius and soleus. [S700]

Shortly after passing underneath the tendinous arch of the M. soleus, the **A. tibialis posterior** releases the A. fibularis, its most important branch, directed to the lateral malleolus.

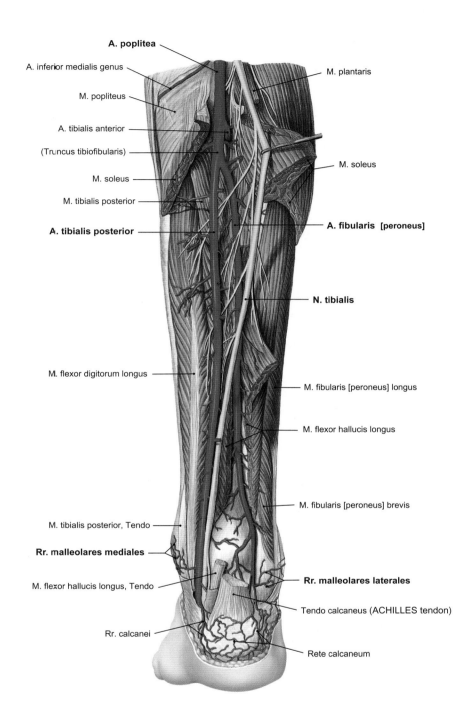

A. poplitea

A. inferior medialis genus

M. popliteus

A. tibialis anterior

(Truncus tibiofibularis)

M. soleus

M. tibialis posterior

A. tibialis posterior

M. flexor digitorum longus

M. tibialis posterior, Tendo

Rr. malleolares mediales

M. flexor hallucis longus, Tendo

Rr. calcanei

M. plantaris

M. soleus

A. fibularis [peroneus]

N. tibialis

M. fibularis [peroneus] longus

M. flexor hallucis longus

M. fibularis [peroneus] brevis

Rr. malleolares laterales

Tendo calcaneus (ACHILLES tendon)

Rete calcaneum

Fig. 4.187 Vessels and nerves of the lower leg, Regio cruris posterior, right side; dorsal view; after removal of the Fascia cruris and severing the Mm. gastrocnemius, soleus and flexor hallucis longus. [S700]

The **A. tibialis posterior** descends along with the **N. tibialis** between the superficial and deep flexors of the leg to the medial malleolus, and then continues by passing through the **malleolar canal/tarsal tunnel** underneath the Retinaculum musculorum flexorum to the sole of the foot. The **Rr. malleolares mediales** branch off to the medial malleolus. On its way to the lateral malleolus, the **A. fibularis** pierces the M. flexor hallucis longus and runs in the deepest layer directly on the Membrana interossea cruris. Together with the branches of the Aa. tibiales anterior and posterior, the **Rr. malleolares laterales** complete the vascular circle around the ankle, which provides a sufficient collateral circulation in the case of a vascular occlusion.

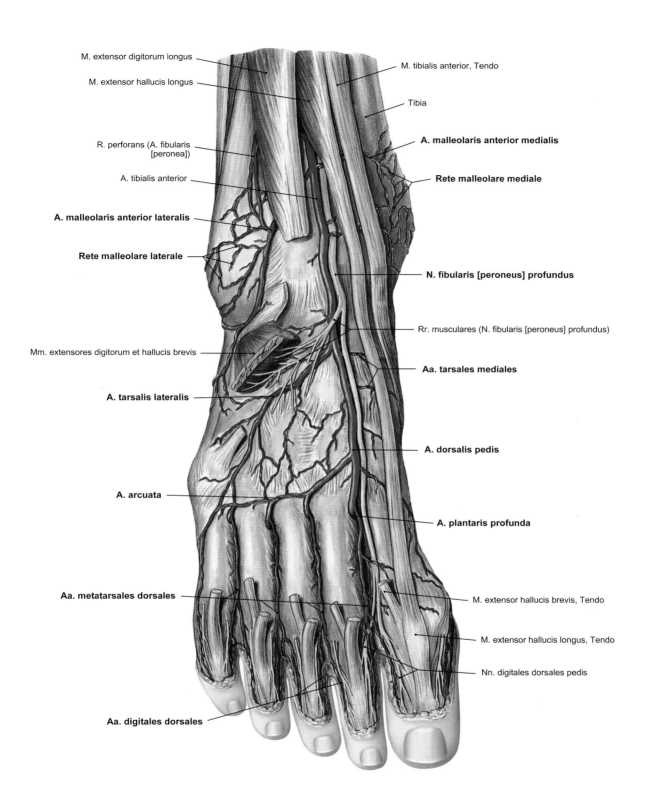

M. extensor digitorum longus

M. extensor hallucis longus

R. perforans (A. fibularis [peronea])

A. tibialis anterior

A. malleolaris anterior lateralis

Rete malleolare laterale

Mm. extensores digitorum et hallucis brevis

A. tarsalis lateralis

A. arcuata

Aa. metatarsales dorsales

Aa. digitales dorsales

M. tibialis anterior, Tendo

Tibia

A. malleolaris anterior medialis

Rete malleolare mediale

N. fibularis [peroneus] profundus

Rr. musculares (N. fibularis [peroneus] profundus)

Aa. tarsales mediales

A. dorsalis pedis

A. plantaris profunda

M. extensor hallucis brevis, Tendo

M. extensor hallucis longus, Tendo

Nn. digitales dorsales pedis

Fig. 4.188 Vessels and nerves of the dorsum of the foot, Dorsum pedis, right side; dorsal view in relation to the dorsum of the foot af-ter removal of the tendons of the M. extensor digitorum longus as well as the short extensors of the toes. [S700]

The **A. tibialis anterior** continues on the dorsum of the foot as the **A. dorsalis pedis.** It is accompanied by the **N. fibularis profundus,** which innervates the extensors of the leg and of the dorsum of the foot, and then divides into its sensory terminal branches to supply the first interdigital space. In the ankle region, the A. tibialis anterior supplies the vascular networks around the malleoli (Rete malleolare mediale and Rete malleolare laterale) with the **Aa. malleolares anteriores medialis** and **lateralis.** The **A. dorsalis pedis** sends several smaller Aa. tarsales mediales and a single A. tarsalis lateralis to the tarsal bones, and contin-ues as A. arcuata which forms an arch on its way to the lateral side of the foot and releases the Aa. metatarsales dorsales. These arteries re-lease the Aa. digitales dorsales which supply the toes. The A. plantaris profunda participates in the blood circulation of the sole of the foot by supplying the Arcus plantaris profundus.

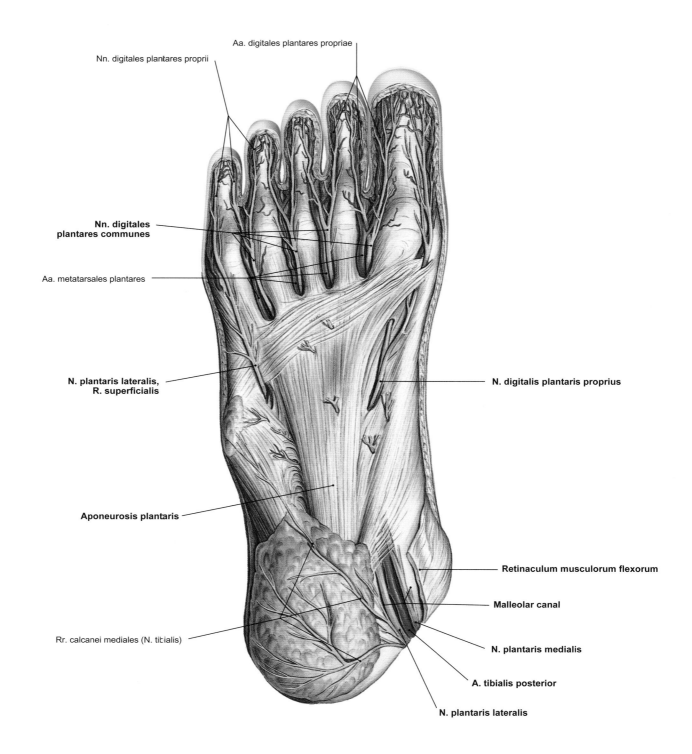

Nn. digitales plantares proprii

Aa. digitales plantares propriae

Nn. digitales plantares communes

Aa. metatarsales plantares

N. plantaris lateralis, R. superficialis

N. digitalis plantaris proprius

Aponeurosis plantaris

Retinaculum musculorum flexorum

Malleolar canal

Rr. calcanei mediales (N. tibialis)

N. plantaris medialis

A. tibialis posterior

N. plantaris lateralis

Fig. 4.189 Superficial layer of the arteries and nerves of the sole of the foot, Planta pedis, right side; plantar view. [S700]
Early on at the medial malleolus, the **N. tibialis** divides into its two terminal branches **(Nn. plantares medialis** and **lateralis)** on its pathway through the **malleolar canal/tarsal tunnel** underneath the Retinaculum musculorum flexorum. These terminal branches branch out into several Nn. digitales plantares. The N. plantaris lateralis divides in a sim-

ilar way to the N. ulnaris in the hand, into a R. superficialis and a R. profundus. The N. plantaris medialis has an additional branch, the **N. digitalis plantaris proprius,** at the medial side of the foot. These sensory branches pass between the longitudinal fibres of the plantar aponeurosis (Aponeurosis plantaris). The A. tibialis posterior only divides once it reaches the sole of foot.

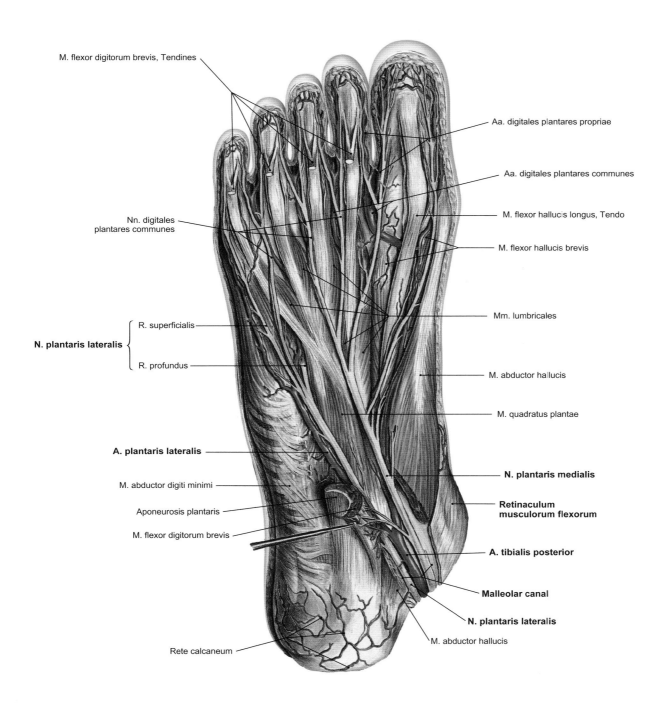

M. flexor digitorum brevis, Tendines

Aa. digitales plantares propriae

Aa. digitales plantares communes

Nn. digitales plantares communes

M. flexor hallucis longus, Tendo

M. flexor hallucis brevis

R. superficialis

Mm. lumbricales

N. plantaris lateralis

R. profundus

M. abductor hallucis

M. quadratus plantae

A. plantaris lateralis

N. plantaris medialis

M. abductor digiti minimi

Retinaculum musculorum flexorum

Aponeurosis plantaris

M. flexor digitorum brevis

A. tibialis posterior

Malleolar canal

N. plantaris lateralis

M. abductor hallucis

Rete calcaneum

Fig. 4.190 Medial layer of the arteries and nerves of the sole of the foot, Planta pedis, right side; plantar view. [S700]
The M. flexor digitorum brevis and the M. abductor hallucis have been split to expose the neurovascular structures of the malleolar canal/tarsal tunnel.

The **Nn. plantares medialis** and **lateralis** are accompanied by eponymous vessels from the A. tibialis posterior. The blood vessels run below the M. flexor digitorum brevis in the intermediate layer of the neurovascular pathways to the toes. Along the way, the nerves provide muscle branches to the short plantar muscles.

497

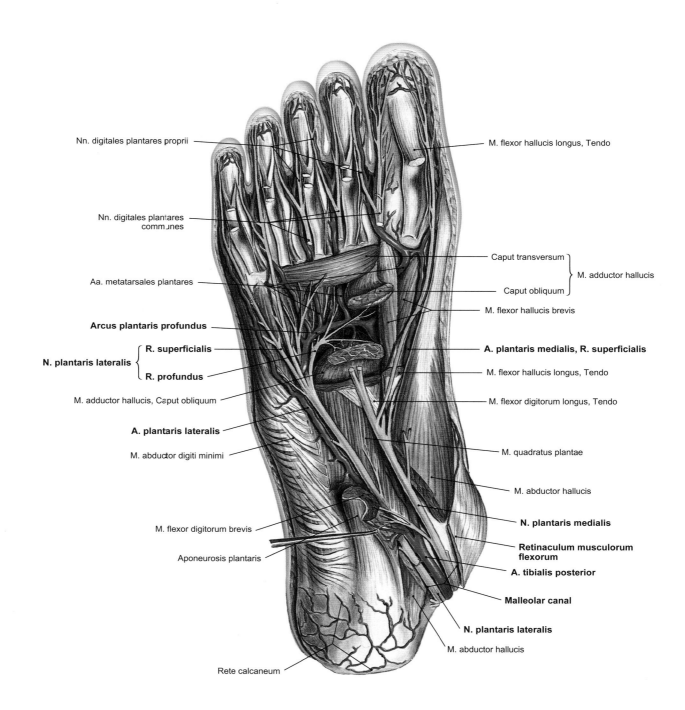

Nn. digitales plantares proprii

M. flexor hallucis longus, Tendo

Nn. digitales plantares communes

Aa. metatarsales plantares

Caput transversum
Caput obliquum
} M. adductor hallucis

M. flexor hallucis brevis

Arcus plantaris profundus

N. plantaris lateralis { **R. superficialis**
R. profundus

A. plantaris medialis, R. superficialis

M. flexor hallucis longus, Tendo

M. adductor hallucis, Caput obliquum

M. flexor digitorum longus, Tendo

A. plantaris lateralis

M. abductor digiti minimi

M. quadratus plantae

M. abductor hallucis

N. plantaris medialis

M. flexor digitorum brevis

Retinaculum musculorum flexorum

Aponeurosis plantaris

A. tibialis posterior

Malleolar canal

N. plantaris lateralis

M. abductor hallucis

Rete calcaneum

Fig. 4.191 Deep layer of the arteries and nerves of the sole of the foot, Planta pedis, right side; plantar view. [S700]
The M. flexor digitorum brevis and the M. abductor hallucis have been split to expose the neurovascular structures in the **malleolar canal/ tarsal tunnel.** In addition, the Caput obliquum of the M. adductor hallucis has been cut, so that the deep plantar arch **(Arcus plantaris profundus)** and the **R. profundus of the N. plantaris lateralis** become visible.

The Arcus plantaris profundus is a continuation of the A. plantaris lateralis and receives further blood supply from the R. profundus of the A. plantaris medialis and of the A. plantaris profunda, which in turn originates from the A. dorsalis pedis. Together with the R. profundus of the N. plantaris lateralis, it forms an arch and runs on the Mm. interossei of the sole of the foot in the deep layer of the neurovascular pathways.

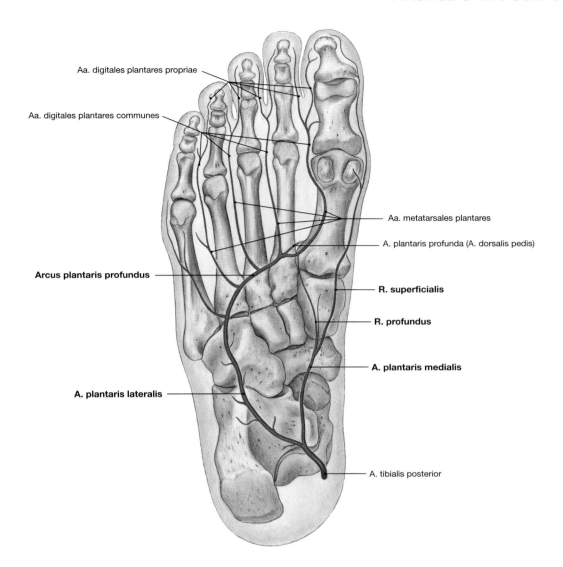

Aa. digitales plantares propriae

Aa. digitales plantares communes

Arcus plantaris profundus

A. plantaris lateralis

Aa. metatarsales plantares

A. plantaris profunda (A. dorsalis pedis)

R. superficialis

R. profundus

A. plantaris medialis

A. tibialis posterior

Fig. 4.192 Arteries of the sole of the foot, Planta pedis, right side; plantar view. [S700]
The sole of the foot is supplied by the terminal branches of the A. tibialis posterior. The **A. plantaris medialis** provides a **R. superficialis** to the medial side of the foot and a **R. profundus** to connect with the **Arcus plantaris profundus.** This arterial arch is a direct continuation of the **A. plantaris lateralis.**

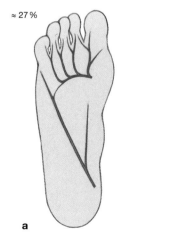

≈ 27 %

a

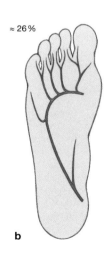

≈ 26 %

b

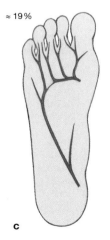

≈ 19 %

c

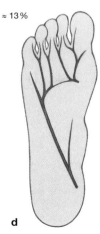

≈ 13 %

d

Fig. 4.193a–d Variations in the arterial supply of the toes, right side; plantar view. [S700]
a The Arcus plantaris profundus can receive most of its blood supply from the A. dorsalis pedis of the dorsum of the foot via the A. plantaris profunda.

b Observed at a similar frequency as above, the A. tibialis posterior can provide the main blood supply to the Arcus plantaris profundus.
c, d Alternatively, both arterial systems can contribute to the blood supply of the toes.

Hip joint, oblique section

Lower limb

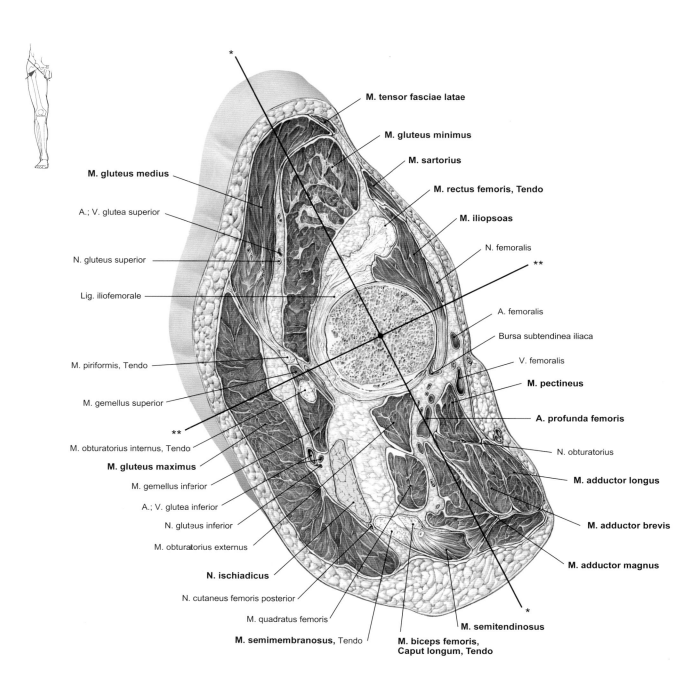

M. tensor fasciae latae

M. gluteus minimus

M. sartorius

M. rectus femoris, Tendo

M. iliopsoas

N. femoralis

A. femoralis

Bursa subtendinea iliaca

V. femoralis

M. pectineus

A. profunda femoris

N. obturatorius

M. adductor longus

M. adductor brevis

M. adductor magnus

M. gluteus medius

A.; V. glutea superior

N. gluteus superior

Lig. iliofemorale

M. piriformis, Tendo

M. gemellus superior

M. obturatorius internus, Tendo

M. gluteus maximus

M. gemellus inferior

A.; V. glutea inferior

N. gluteus inferior

M. obturatorius externus

N. ischiadicus

N. cutaneus femoris posterior

M. quadratus femoris

M. semimembranosus, Tendo

M. biceps femoris, Caput longum, Tendo

M. semitendinosus

Fig. 4.194 Thigh, Femur, oblique section through the hip joint, right side; distal view with illustration of the movement axes of the hip joint. [S700]

The oblique section through the thigh at the level of the femoral head shows the position of the individual muscle groups in relation to the femoral head and the movement axes. The **M. gluteus maximus** is located dorsally of the hip joint, whereas the smaller gluteal muscles **(Mm. glutei medius** and **minimus)** may run in part ventrally of the longitudinal and transverse axes of the hip joint. This position explains why the M. gluteus maximus acts as an external rotator and extensor of the hip, while the smaller gluteal muscles can also flex the hip and are the strongest medial rotators. The **M. iliopsoas** is located anterior to the transverse axis and is the most important flexor of the hip joint. It is functionally supported by the **anterior group of femoral muscles**

(M. sartorius, M. rectus femoris), by the M. tensor fasciae latae as well as by the superficial **adductor muscles** (Mm. adductores longus and brevis, M. pectineus, main part of the M. adductor magnus). As the dorsal part of the M. adductor magnus already lies behind the transverse axis, it acts as an extensor together with the hamstring muscles, to which it belongs functionally and also according to its innervation. Cross-sections of the limbs make it easy to visualise the positional relationships of the neurovascular structures in different compartments or layers. The **N. ischiadicus** initially lies underneath the M. gluteus maximus after leaving the lesser pelvis. Anteriorly, the **A. profunda femoris** is covered by the M. pectineus.

* transverse axis of movement in the hip joint
** sagittal axis of movement in the hip joint

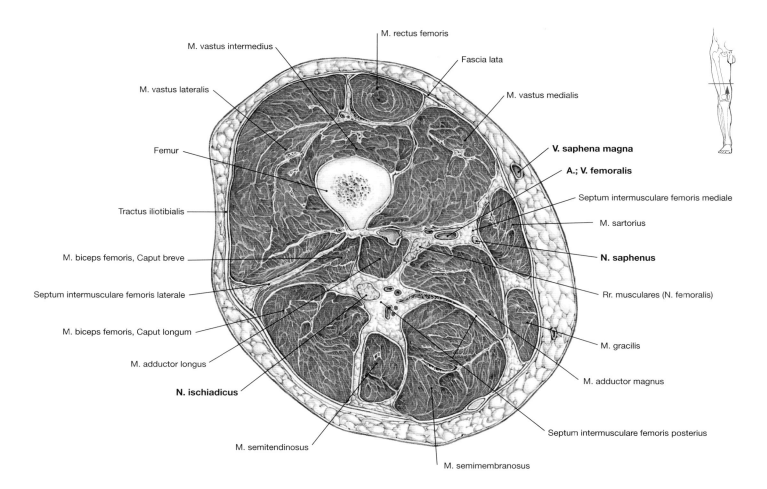

M. rectus femoris

M. vastus intermedius

Fascia lata

M. vastus lateralis

M. vastus medialis

Femur

V. saphena magna

A.; V. femoralis

Tractus iliotibialis

Septum intermusculare femoris mediale

M. sartorius

M. biceps femoris, Caput breve

N. saphenus

Septum intermusculare femoris laterale

Rr. musculares (N. femoralis)

M. biceps femoris, Caput longum

M. gracilis

M. adductor longus

M. adductor magnus

N. ischiadicus

Septum intermusculare femoris posterius

M. semitendinosus

M. semimembranosus

Fig. 4.195 Thigh, femur, right side; cross-section through the middle of the thigh; distal view. [S700]
In this cross-section the **three muscle groups of the thigh** can be identified. The anterior group includes the M. quadriceps femoris and the M. sartorius. The adductor muscles are located medially and the hamstring muscles dorsally.

The **V. saphena magna** is found in the epifascial subcutaneous adipose tissue on the medial side of the thigh. The **A.** and **V. femoralis** pass together with the **N. saphenus** through the adductor canal (Canalis adductorius) of the M. quadriceps. The adductor canal is limited dorsally by the Mm. adductores longus and magnus, and covered medially by the M. vastus medialis, and ventrally by the M. sartorius. The **N. ischiadicus** is dorsally located below its key muscle, the M. biceps femoris.

Lower limb

4

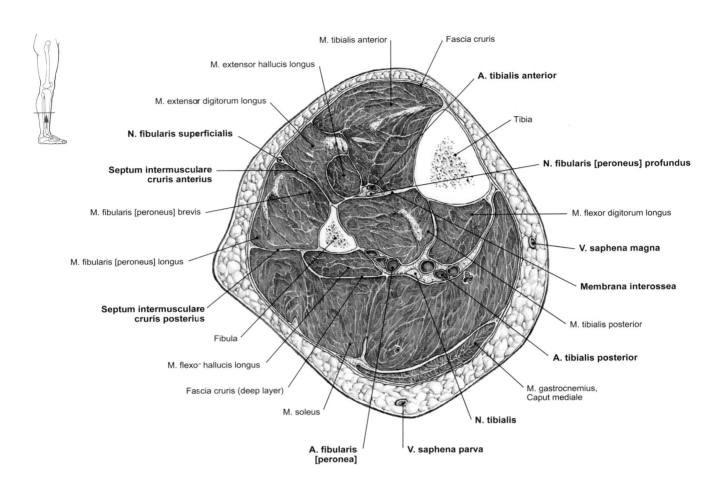

M. tibialis anterior

Fascia cruris

M. extensor hallucis longus

A. tibialis anterior

M. extensor digitorum longus

Tibia

N. fibularis superficialis

N. fibularis [peroneus] profundus

Septum intermusculare cruris anterius

M. fibularis [peroneus] brevis

M. flexor digitorum longus

V. saphena magna

M. fibularis [peroneus] longus

Membrana interossea

Septum intermusculare cruris posterius

M. tibialis posterior

Fibula

A. tibialis posterior

M. flexor hallucis longus

M. gastrocnemius, Caput mediale

Fascia cruris (deep layer)

M. soleus

N. tibialis

A. fibularis [peronea]

V. saphena parva

Fig. 4.196 Lower leg, Crus, right side; cross-section through the middle of the leg; distal view. [S700]
Together with the connective tissue septa attached to the bones of the lower leg, the Fascia cruris forms **osteofibrous tubes or compart-** **ments.** The neurovascular pathways between the muscle bellies of the individual muscle groups run in these compartments.
The anterior (extensor) compartment, which contains the N. fibularis profundus together with the A. tibialis anterior, has the highest clinical relevance.

Clinical remarks

Compression syndrome (compartment syndrome) most often occurs in the anterior (extensor) compartment, less often in the lateral (fibular) compartment.

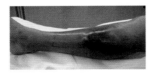

a

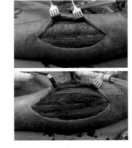

b

a Post-traumatic swelling of the extensor muscles or a long walk can compress and damage the supplying vessels and nerves to the muscles. In addition to pain, there may also be a pulse deficit of the A. dorsalis pedis, originating in the A. tibialis anterior. But most frequently, the compression causes a lesion of the N. fibularis profundis (Clinical remarks → Fig. 4.154) with resulting functional (extension) deficits in the talocrural joint and loss of sensory perception in the first interdigital space. [E993]
b The treatment requires an urgent splitting of the fascia, which, however, requires long-term immobilisation of the open leg. To confirm the diagnosis, the pressure in the compartments should be measured with a pressure sensor. [E475]

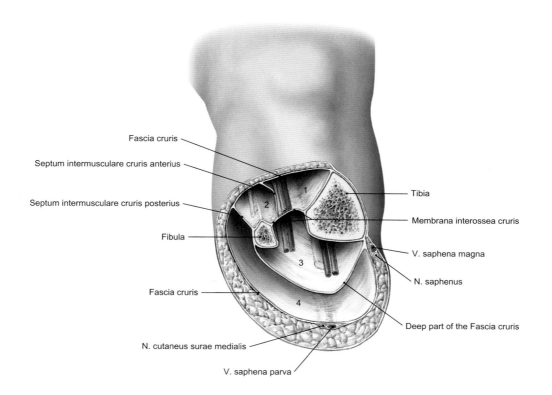

Fascia cruris

Septum intermusculare cruris anterius

Septum intermusculare cruris posterius

Fibula

Fascia cruris

N. cutaneus surae medialis

V. saphena parva

Tibia

Membrana interossea cruris

V. saphena magna

N. saphenus

Deep part of the Fascia cruris

1 Anterior (extensor) compartment:
A.; V. tibialis anterior
N. fibularis profundus
M. tibialis anterior
M. extensor digitorum longus
M. extensor hallucis longus
M. fibularis [peroneus] tertius

2 Lateral (fibular) compartment:
N. fibularis superficialis
M. fibularis [peroneus] longus
M. fibularis [peroneus] brevis

3 Posterior (deep or flexor) compartment:
A.; V. tibialis posterior
A.; V. fibularis
N. tibialis
M. flexor digitorum longus
M. tibialis posterior
M. flexor hallucis longus

4 Posterior (superficial) compartment:
M. triceps surae
M. plantaris

Fig. 4.197 Lower leg, crus, right side; cross-section through the middle of the leg showing the osteofibrous tubular compartments; distal view. [S700]
The Fascia cruris is attached to the bones of the lower leg by fibrous connective tissue septa. These septa confine and keep osteofibrous tubes, which are known as **compartments,** separated from each other. They contain the neurovascular pathways which run between the muscle bellies of the individual muscle groups. The Septum intermusculare anterius divides the anterior extensor compartment from the lateral fibular muscle compartment, which in turn is separated from the superficial flexors by the Septum intermusculare posterius. A deep layer of the

Fascia cruris separates the superficial from the deep flexors, which are anteriorly adjacent to the Membrana interossea cruris. In the **anterior (extensor) compartment,** the N. fibularis profundus is accompanied by the A. tibialis anterior and the Vv. tibiales anteriores. The N. fibularis superficialis is located in the **lateral (fibular) compartment.** In the **deep posterior (flexor) compartment,** the N. tibialis together with the A. tibialis posterior and the Vv. tibiales posteriores can be found, as well as the A. and V. fibularis, which are covered by the M. flexor hallucis longus and which are embedded between the muscles. In the epifascial layer, the V. saphena magna runs on the medial side of the leg, and the V. saphena parva on the dorsal side.

Sample exam questions

To check that you are completely familiar with the content of this chapter, sample questions from an oral anatomy exam are listed here.

Show the sections and most important structures of the femur on the skeleton:

- Which muscles insert at the Trochanter major and Trochanter minor?
- How does the curvature of the femoral condyles influence the flexion movement in the knee joint and its stabilisation by the collateral ligaments?

Explain the structure of the knee joint on an articular model:

- Which skeletal elements articulate with each other?
- Which ligaments stabilise the knee joint and with which clinical tests can they be evaluated?
- Which types of joint are specifically involved?
- Which movements can be carried out and to what extent (range of motion)?
- Which orientation do the movement axes have?
- Which muscles are important for the individual movements?

Show the muscle groups of the lower leg:

- What is the position of the muscles in relation to the axes of the ankle joints and how does this influence their function?
- Explain the course of the M. triceps surae, including its origin and insertion.

How is it innervated and which movements are affected when it fails?

Show the N. fibularis communis and explain its pathway on the dissection.

- Explain its innervation area.
- Where is it damaged most often?
- Which clinical picture can be expected with a nerve lesion in the area of the fibular head, e. g. in the case of a high fracture of the fibula?

What arterial pulses can you palpate in a clinical examination of the lower limb?

- Show the vessels branching off the A. femoralis and explain their supply areas.

How is the venous system of the leg organised?

- Where can you as a physician insert a cardiac catheter?

Explain the lymphatic drainage on the leg:

- How are the lymph nodes in the groin organised?
- Which body regions do they drain?

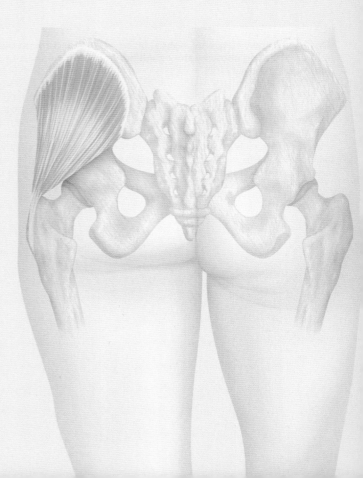

Appendix

Index. 506

Index

Page numbers are in **bold** when the corresponding entries on that page are also in bold.

A

Abdomen 4
- CT angiogram 74
Abdominal muscles **156**
- CT **154**
- deep layer **151**
- middle layer **149**, **150**
- oblique **159**
- superficial layer **149**
Abdominal musculature
- prune belly syndrome 88
Abdominal wall
- anterior **188**
-- inner wall **155**
-- muscles 141, 142
-- newborn 188, 194
- dermatomes 186
- Fascia endothoracica **144**
- hernias 151
- innervation **186**
- posterior
-- muscles **158**
-- Plexus lumbosacralis 195
- structure 193
Abduction 7
- arm 10
- carpometacarpal joint 232
- extremities 8
- finger 10
- hip joint 376
- jaw 8
- knee joint **386**
- leg 10
- shoulder joint 220, 221
- thumb 10, 234
- toe joint 413
Access, operative
- cervical spine 180
- lumbar spine 181
Acetabular rim plane angle **373**
Acetabulum 352, **354**, 355
- acetabular rim plane 373
- retroversion 373
- structure 355
- X-ray image 358
ACHILLES tendon 401, 402, 403, 409, 414, 416,
    436, 439, 440, 441, 442, 443, 445, 492, 493,
    494
- rupture 441
AC joint see Acromioclavicular joint
AC joint separation 217
Acromioclavicular joint 216
- arm elevation 222
- classification of TOSSY 217
- injury 217
- X-ray image 217
Acromion 132, **207**, **218**, **219**, 224, 236, 237,
    238, 239, 246, 247, 315
- shoulder, roof 246
- surface anatomy 84
- X-ray image 217, 223
Acropodium 22
Actin filament 40
Adduction 7
- arm 10
- carpometacarpal joint 232
- extremities 8
- finger 10
- hip joint 376
- jaw 8
- knee joint **386**
- leg 10
- shoulder joint 220, 221
- thumb 10, 234
- toe joint 413

Adductor canal 423, 481, 482, 501
Adductor stress load in knee 418
Adipose tissue 183
Adminiculum lineae albae 188
Adolescent 6
Adolescent kyphosis 124
Adrenal glands
- endocrine system **59**
Afferent **63**
- dermatome 66
- somatic sensory 63
Age-related kyphosis 124
Ala ossis
- ilii 153, 354, 355
-- X-ray image 353
- sacri 108, 110
ALCOCK canal
- pudendal nerve block 461
ALLEN test 303
Amastia 182
Amnion 19
Amniotic cavity 18, 19
Amphiarthrosis 32
- characteristics 32
- sacroiliac joint 352
Ampulla ductus deferentis 188
Anamnesis **5**
Anastomosis
- cavocaval 163
- portocaval 56
- thoracic wall veins 162
- trunk wall veins 162
Anchylosis 31
Angiogram
- abdomen 74
- CT 74
- kidneys **73**
- pelvis 74
Angulus
- acromii scapulae 207
- costae 92
- inferior scapulae 207
-- landmarks 84
- infrasternalis 86
-- surface anatomy 85
- lateralis scapulae 207
- mandibulae
-- X-ray image 124
- sterni (LUDOVICI) 86, **90**, **111**
-- orientation point 90
-- surface anatomy 85
- subpubicus 352, 368
- superior scapulae 207
- venosus 57
Ankle joint
- fracture 400
- range of movement 36
Annular ligament
- finger 275
- radius **225**, **262**
-- head **225**, **229**
Ansa
- cervicalis 314
- subclavia 69
Antebrachium see Forearm
Anterior 9
Anterior drawer test 389
Anteversion
- arm 11
- hip joint 376
- shoulder joint 220, 221
Anulus
- fibrosus 114, 115, 117, 121, 122
-- BECHTEREW disease 117
-- development 89
-- lamellae 121

Anulus
- inguinalis
-- profundus 188, 189, **190**, **191**
--- borders **190**
--- inguinal hernia 189, 193
-- superficialis 149, 150, **189**, **190**, 193, 194
--- borders **190**
--- Crus laterale 151
--- Crus mediale 151
- umbilicalis 86, 141, 142, 149, **153**, 154, 187, 194
Aorta 146, 179
- abdominalis 157
-- CT 129
- Bifurcatio aortae 464
- development 88
- thoracica **165**
-- branches 161
Aortic isthmus stenosis 161
Ape hand **291**
Apertura
- pelvis
-- inferior 350
-- superior **350**, 351, 352
- thoracis
-- inferior **90**
-- superior **90**, **148**
Apex
- capitis fibulae 363
-- X-ray image 380
- dentis 99
- ossis sacri 108, 109
- patellae 361
-- X-ray image 70, 380
Apical 9
Aplasia 182
Aponeurosis
- dorsalis 79
- musculi bicipitis brachii 201, 248, **249**, 250,
    254, 324, 329
- palmaris 201, **266**, 301, **332**, 337
- plantaris **401**, **408**, 409, 448, 449, 451, 470,
    496, 497, 498
Apophysis 24
- blood supply 24
Appendicitis 17
Appendix vermiformis 16, 17
Arachnoidea mater
- cranialis 173
- spinalis 173, 174, **176**, 177, 178
ARANTIUS, duct (Ductus venosus) 55
ARANTIUS, ligament of (Lig. venosum) 55
Arch of the foot
- bones 408
- tension 404, 406, 439, 449
Arcus
- anterior atlantis **98**, 99, 118
- aortae 50, 55, 69
-- X-ray image 70
- costalis 86, 90, 91, 142
-- surface anatomy 85
- ductus thoracici 57
- iliopectineus 188, 369, 422, **483**
- palmaris
-- profundus 294, **301**, **303**, 334
-- superficialis 294, 301, 302, 303, 333, **337**
- plantaris 471
-- profundus 465, **498**, **499**
- posterior atlantis **98**
- pubicus 352, 368
- tendineus musculi
-- levatoris ani 418
-- solei 441, **492**
- venosus
-- dorsalis pedis 478, 479
-- palmaris
--- profundus 305
--- superficialis 304

Arcus
– vertebrae **97**, 113, 116, 177
–– axis 98, 99
–– Pediculus, X-ray image 126
–– vertebrae
––– lumbalis 138
––– thoracicae 104, 175
Area intercondylaris
– anterior **362**
– posterior 362
Areola mammae **182**
ARLT shoulder repositioning 223
Arm
– abduction 222
– anteversion 11
– arteries 294
– bones and joints **204**
– carrying angle 204, 228
– cutaneous innervation **280**
– development 202, 203
– elevation 222
– fascia 201
– lymph vessels 304, 305
– musculature
–– dorsal 237
–– lateral 238
–– ventral 236
– retroversion 11
– surface anatomy 200
– veins 304, 305
Arm buds, flipper-like 202
Arteria(-ae)
– arcuata 465, 469, **495**
– auricularis posterior, R. occipitalis 171
– axillaris 50, 67, 143, 160, 276, **277**, 279, 286,
  294, **296**, 297, **299**, 307, 315, **316**, **318**, 319
–– anastomosis **297**
–– branches 294, **299**
–– pathway 294
–– sections 297, 299
– basilaris 298
– brachialis 50, 279, **294**, 295, 296, 297, **299**,
  300, **301**, 302, 318, 319, **322**, 323, **324**, **325**,
  326, 327, **328**, **329**, **338**
–– branches 294, **300**
–– bypass circulation 295
–– injury 295
–– pathway 294, 300
–– superficialis **311**
–– supply area 300
– carotis
–– communis 50, 69, 160, 164, 180, 277, 296, 298
–– externa 50
–– interna 50
– cervicalis
–– ascendens **296**, 298
–– profunda 164, 172, 298
–– superficialis 187
– circumflexa
–– femoris
––– lateralis 24, 345, 358, **377**, **464**, 465, 466,
  481, **482**
––– medialis 24, 345, 358, **377**, **464**, 465, 466,
  467, 481, **482**, 487
–– humeri
––– anterior 209, 294, **296**, **297**, **299**, 318
––– posterior 170, 209, 294, **296**, **297**, **299**,
  310, 315, **318**, 323
–– ilium
––– profunda **160**, 191, 464, 480
––– superficialis 187, 464, **466**, 476
–– scapulae **170**, **296**, **297**, 299, **315**, **323**
––– anastomosis 297
––– axillary space 170, 299, 323
– collateralis
–– media 294, **300**, **323**
–– radialis 294, 295, **300**, 322, **325**, **328**, 330
––– R. anterior **323**
––– R. posterior **323**

Arteria(-ae) collateralis
–– ulnaris
––– inferior 294, 295, **300**, 301, 302, **319**
––– superior 294, 295, **300**, 301, 302, **319**,
  324, 325, 338
– comitans nervi mediani 294, **302**, 327, 339
– descendens genus 465, **466**, **476**, 482, 489
–– R. saphenus 482
– digitales
–– dorsales
––– manus 301, 335, **337**
––– pedis 469, **495**
–– palmares
––– communes 294, 301, 302, 303, **332**, **333**,
  337, 340
––– propriae 294, 301, 302, 303, **332**, 333,
  337, 340
–– plantares
––– communes **470**, 471, 497, 499
––– propriae **470**, 471, 496, 497, 499
– dorsalis
–– pedis 50, **465**, **469**, **491**, **495**
––– branches 464, 469, 495
––– pulse 465
–– scapulae 298, 321
––– anastomosis 297, 298
––– pathway 298
– ductus deferentis 189
– epigastrica
–– inferior 153, **160**, **166**, **187**, 188, 189, 190,
  191, 193
–– superficialis **187**, 464, **466**, 476
–– superior 153, **160**, 165, 166, **187**, 194
– femoralis 50, 74, 156, 159, 188, 190, 423, **464**,
  465, **466**, 476, **480**, **481**, **482**, **483**, 500, **501**
–– branches **464**, 466
–– location in cross-section 501
–– pulse 465
–– ventricular catheter 466
– fibularis [peronea] 50, **465**, **468**, **489**, **493**,
  494, **502**, 503
–– branches 464
–– pathway 494
–– R. perforans 465, **469**, 491
– glutea
–– inferior 465, **467**, **486**, **487**, 500
––– pathway 467
–– superior **467**, 500
––– pathway 467
––– R. profundus 467
––– R. superficialis **486**
– iliaca
–– communis 50, 69, 464
––– dextra 74
––– pathway 464
––– sinistra 74
–– externa 50, 160, **166**, 188, 190, 464, 475,
  480, 482
––– branches **464**
––– dextra 74
–– interna 50, 464, 475, 480
––– branches 467
––– collateral circulation 467
––– dextra 74
––– sinistra 74
– inferior
–– lateralis genus **391**, 465, 468, 469, **489**, 491
–– medialis genus **391**, 465, 468, 482, **489**,
  492, 493, 494
–– intercostalis 144, 164, 194
–– anterior 146
–– posterior 145, 146, **161**, **165**, 179
–– Rr. collaterales 146
–– Rr. cutanei laterales 146
–– Rr. perforantes anteriores 146
–– suprema 165, 298
– interossea
–– anterior 294, **302**, 330, 335, **337**
–– communis 50, 294, 295, **302**, **326**, **327**
––– branches **302**

Arteria(-ae) interossea
–– posterior 257, 294, **302**, **330**, **331**, **337**
–– recurrens 294, 295, 302, 328, **331**
––– origin 302
– lienalis 74
– lumbalis **179**
– malleolaris anterior
–– lateralis 465, 469, **491**, **495**
–– medialis 465, **495**
– mammaria(-ae)
–– interna 160, **161**, 164, 165, 166, 187
––– bypass 166
–– laterales **184**, 307
– media genus **391**, 465, **489**
–– R. anterior 391
–– R. posterior 391
– mesenterica
–– inferior 50, 69
–– superior 50, 69, 74
– metacarpales
–– dorsales 335, 336
–– palmares **303**, **334**, **337**, 340
– metatarsales
–– dorsales 465, **469**, 491, **495**
–– plantares 470, **471**, 496, 498, 499
– musculophrenica **160**, **165**, 166
– obturatoria 188, **464**, **481**, **482**, 483
–– femoral head supply 345
– occipitalis 170, 171, 172
–– R. mastoideus 171
–– R. occipitales 171
– ovarica 50
– perforans(-tes) **464**, 465, **482**, **485**, 486, 489
–– prima 466, 467
–– secunda 466, 467
– pericardiacophrenica **160**, 166
– phrenica inferior 157
– plantaris
–– lateralis 465, **470**, **471**, **497**, **498**, **499**
–– medialis **465**, **471**, **499**
––– branches 464
––– R. superficialis 470, **498**
–– profunda 469, **495**, 499
– poplitea 50, 75, **391**, 395, **396**, 430, 441, **465**,
  468, **484**, **485**, 486, 488, **489**, 492, **493**, **494**
–– branches **464**, 468, 489
–– pathway 489
–– pulse 465
– princeps pollicis 294, 303, 332, **334**
– profunda
–– brachii 50, **170**, 294, 296, 297, **300**, **318**,
  319, **322**, **323**, **338**
––– R. deltoideus 322
––– triangular interval 170
–– cervicis 298
–– femoris 50, 74, 377, **464**, **465**, **466**, **480**,
  481, **482**, **500**
––– branches 464, **467**
––– collateral circulation 467
––– femoral head supply 345
––– pathway 482
– pudenda
–– externa 187, 464, 476
–– interna **467**, **486**, **487**
– pulmonalis
–– X-ray image 70
– radialis 50, **294**, **295**, **300**, 301, **302**, 303,
  312, **324**, **325**, 326, 327, 328, 329, **333**, **334**,
  335, **336**, **339**
–– branches 294, **301**
–– indicis 294, 303, 332, **334**
–– pathway 294, 301, 325, 336
–– R. carpalis dorsalis **335**, 336
–– R. palmaris superficialis 326, 327, **333**, **336**
– recurrens
–– radialis 294, 295, 300, 301, 302, **325**, 326,
  327, 328
–– tibialis
––– anterior 465, 469, **491**
––– posterior 465, 489

Appendix

Arteria(-ae) recurrens
– – ulnaris 294, 295, 302, 326, 327, 329, 330
– – – pathway **302**
– renalis 50, 69
– – dextra 61, 74
– – sinistra 61, 74
– spinalis anterior **177**
– – R. radicularis anterior 177
– subclavia 50, 69, 164, 165, 277, 279, **296**, 297, 298
– – anastomosis 297
– – branches 294, **298**
– – dextra **160**
– – sinistra 160
– subscapularis **160**, 294, **296**, **297**, **299**, 318
– – pathway **296**
– superior
– – lateralis genus 465, 468, 469, 488, **489**, 491
– – – femur epiphysis 24
– – medialis genus 465, 468, 482, 485, 488, **489**, 491
– – – femur epiphysis 24
– suprascapularis **296**, **297**, 298, 321, **323**
– – anastomosis 297
– – pathway 296, **298**
– suralis(-es) 465, 488, **489**, 492
– – lateralis 468
– – medialis 468
– tarsalis(-es)
– – lateralis 465, 469, **495**
– – mediales 465, 469, **495**
– testicularis 50, 188, 190, **191**, 194
– thoracica
– – interna 146, 160, **161**, 164, **165**, **166**, 184, **187**, **298**
– – – branches 160
– – – bypass 166
– – – Rr. intercostales anteriores 166
– – – supply area **298**
– – lateralis **160**, 184, **187**, **296**, **297**, **299**, 307, **308**, **315**, **316**, 317
– – – pathway 296
– – superior 160, 296, **297**, **299**, 317
– thoracoacromialis **160**, 294, **296**, **297**, **299**, **316**
– – anastomosis 297
– – branches **297**
– – R. pectoralis **184**, **315**
– thoracodorsalis **160**, **296**, 299, **315**, **316**
– thyroidea inferior 298
– – supply area **298**
– tibialis
– – anterior 50, **465**, **468**, **469**, **489**, **490**, 491, 494, 495, **502**, 503
– – – branches **464**, 469, 491
– – – pathway 469, 491
– – posterior 50, **465**, **468**, **470**, **471**, **489**, **492**, **493**, **494**, **496**, **497**, **498**, 499, **502**, 503
– – – branches **464**, 468, 470
– – – pathway 492, 494
– – – pulse 465
– transversa
– – cervicis 298
– – branches 298
– – colli **298**
– – – R. profundus 298
– – – R. superficialis **296**, 298, 317
– ulnaris 50, 291, **293**, 294, **295**, **300**, 301, **302**, **303**, **324**, **325**, 326, 327, 329, **332**, **333**, **334**, 339
– – branches 294, **302**, 326
– – pathway 294, 302, 325
– – R. carpalis dorsalis 326, 327, 333, **335**
– – R. palmaris profundus **334**
– umbilicalis(-es) 55, 188, **194**
– vertebralis 121, 123, 160, 164, 170, **172**, **173**, 180, **298**
– – Pars
– – – atlantica **140**, **173**, 298
– – – intracranialis 298
– – – prevertebralis 298
– – – transversaria **173**, 298

Arteria(-ae) vertebralis
– – supply area **298**
– vesicalis superior **194**
Arteries 49
– ALLEN test 303
– arm 294
– – collateral circulation 295
– axilla 308, 314, 316, 317, 318, 319
– axillary space
– – lateral 170
– – medial 170
– back **170**, 171
– back of the hand 335, 336
– blood flow 52
– blood pressure 53
– cardiopulmonary system 48
– chest wall 316, 317
– circulatory system **50**
– cross-sectional diameter 52
– cubital fossa 328
– diameter 52
– dorsum of the foot 469, 495
– elbow 329
– epigastric 166
– extremity
– – upper 294, 295
– forearm 324, 325, 326, 327, 330, 331
– gluteal region 467, 487
– hand **303**
– high-pressure system 48, 49, 53
– inguinal canal **189**
– inguinal region 476, 483
– intercostal space 146
– intravasal pressure 52
– knee 476
– leg 464, 465
– – collateral circulation 467
– long bones 24
– lower leg 468, 469, 490, 491, 492, 493, 494
– lower limb 464, 465, 467
– neck 171, 172, 173
– number 52
– occipital region 172
– palmar arch 303
– palm of the hand 332, 333, 334
– pelvis 464
– popliteal fossa 468, 484, 485, 486, 488, 489, 492, 493, 494
– pulse 50
– shoulder **296**, 297, **323**
– sole of the foot 470, 471, 496, 497, 498, 499
– thigh 464, 466, 467, 476, 480, 481, 482, 485, 486, 487
– thoracic wall **161**, 164, **165**
– trunk wall
– – anterior 160, 166, 187
– – dorsal **170**
– upper arm 318, 319, **322**
– vertebral canal 174, 178, **179**
– vessel pressure 53
Arterioles
– blood flow 52
– cross-sectional diameter 52
– diameter 52
– intravasal pressure 52
– number 52
Arthritis 31
Arthrodesis **31**
Arthrography 31
Arthroplasty 31
Arthroscopy 31, 398
– knee joint 398
Arthrosis 31, 98
– ankle joint **399**
– Coxa valga/vara 359
– knee joint 361, 379
– scaphoid fracture 230
Arthrotomy 31
Articular effusion 35

Articulatio(-nes)
– acromioclavicularis 204, **205**, 214, 216, **219**, 246
– – arm elevation **222**
– – injury 217
– – X-ray image 217, 223
– atlantoaxialis 99
– – lateralis **99**, **119**, **120**
– – – Capsula articularis 118, **120**
– – mediana **99**
– – – anterior **118**
– – – posterior **118**
– atlantooccipitalis **99**, **119**, **120**
– – Capsula articularis 118
– – range of movement 99
– bicondylaris
– – knee joint 393
– calcaneocuboidea 348
– capitis costae **104**, 106, **114**, 115, 116
– – X-ray image 125
– carpi **230**
– carpometacarpalis(-es) 204, 214, **230**
– – pollicis 214, **230**, **231**
– conoidea 33
– costochondrales 90
– costotransversaria **104**, 106, **114**, 115, 116
– – X-ray image 125
– costovertebrales **114**, **115**, **116**
– – ligaments **116**
– cotylica
– – hip joint 376
– coxae 348, 368, **374**
– – blood supply **377**
– – Capsula articularis **373**
– – LAUENSTEIN projection 375
– – ligaments 373
– – range of movement **376**
– – X-ray image **375**
– cricoarytenoidea 31
– cubiti 204, 214, **225**
– – bony parts **225**
– – range of movement **227**
– – rotational movements **227**
– – X-ray image **226**
– cuneocuboidea 348
– cuneonavicularis 348
– cylindrica 33
– digiti manus **232**
– ellipsoidea **33**
– femoropatellaris 348, 361, **378**, **396**
– femorotibialis 348, **378**
– genus 348, **378**, **396**
– – arthroscopy 398
– – Capsula articularis 388, 433
– – coronary scan 397
– – cross-section 396
– – cruciate ligaments 389
– – ligamentous apparatus 385
– – menisci 390
– – outer ligaments 381, 382
– – range of movement 393
– – sagittal section 395, 397
– – synovial bursae 383, 384
– – X-ray image **380**
– humeri 204, 214, **218**, **219**, **220**, **224**, 247, 320
– – luxation **223**
– – X-ray image **223**
– humeroradialis 204, 214, **225**
– humeroulnaris 204, 214, **225**
– intercarpales 214
– interchondrales 90
– intercuneiformes 348
– intermetacarpales 214
– interphalangea(-ae)
– – manus 214, **232**
– – – distalis 79, 204, 232
– – – proximalis 204, 232
– – pedis 348
– lumbosacralis 90
– mediocarpalis 204, 214, 230
– metacarpophalangeae 204, 214, **231**, 232

Articulatio(-nes)
- metatarsophalangeae 348, **407**
- ovoidea **33**
- pedis 406, 407
- plana **33**
- radiocarpalis 204, 214, 230
- radioulnaris
-- distalis 204, 214, **229**, 230, 231
--- Capsula articularis 229
-- proximalis 204, 214, **225**, **229**
- sacrococcygea **90**, 109
- sacroiliaca **90**, 348, 350, 352, **368**, **369**, **371**, **372**, 418
-- joint structure 32
-- X-ray image 127, 353, 375
- sellaris **33**
- spheroidea **33**
- sternoclavicularis(-es) 86, **112**, **205**, 214
-- Discus articularis **112**
-- X-ray image 215
- sternocostales 90, 112
- subtalaris 348, **401**, **404**
-- MRI **401**
-- X-ray image **405**
- talocalcaneonavicularis 348, **404**
-- ligaments 404
-- X-ray image 405
- talocruralis 348, **401**
-- ligaments 402, 403
-- MRI **401**
-- X-ray image 405
- talonavicularis
-- MRI 401
- tarsi transversa (CHOPART's joint) **364**, **366**
- tarsometatarsales (LISFRANC's joint) 348, **364**, **366**
- tibiofibularis 348, 362, 378, 399
-- proximalis 378
-- X-ray image 380
- trochoidea **33**
- zygapophysialis 101, 102, 106, 372
-- CT 129
-- X-ray image 124, 126, 127
Arytenoid cartilage, ossified 31
Athelie 182
Atlantoaxial joint, intermediate 118
Atlanto-occipital joint(s) 99
Atlas 90, 95, 99, 101, 118, 120
- Arcus
-- anterior, X-ray image 124
-- posterior 118, 119, 139, 172, 173
--- X-ray image 124
- assimilation 94, 98
- KLIPPEL-FEIL syndrome 129
- Massa lateralis 120
- occipital joint 99
- Proc. transversus 136, 140
- Tuberculum posterius 136, 139
-- X-ray image 124
Atlas arch
- fractures 98
- front 98
- rear 98
Atrium
- dextrum 55
-- X-ray image 70
- sinistrum 55
Auricula sinistra, X-ray image 70
Auscultation 16
Autopodium 22
- evolution 23
Avulsion fracture **353**
Axilla **314**, 315
- lateral **247**
- lymph nodes **306**
-- level **307**
- lymph vessels **306**
- nerves 308, 318, 319
- topography 316, 317
- vessels 308, 318, 319

Axillary space
- lateral 170, **247**, **252**, **320**, **321**, 323
-- content **321**
- medial 170, **247**, **252**, **320**, **321**, 323
-- content **321**
Axis 90, 95, 99, 101, 118, 119, 120, 123
- Arcus vertebrae 120
- Corpus vertebrae 119
-- X-ray image 124
- Dens
-- X-ray image 124
- human body 7
-- joints 33
- KLIPPEL-FEIL syndrome 129
- occipital joint 99
- Proc. spinosus 118, 139
-- X-ray image 124
- Proc. transversus 140
Azygos system **163**

B

Back (*see* Dorsum)
- cutaneous nerves 169
- dermatomes 169
- nerves **170**, 171
- vessels **170**, 171
Back muscles
- autochthonous 135, 180, 181
-- development 88
-- schematic 134
- deep 135, 136, 137, 138
-- schematic 134
- superficial **132**
Back of the hand
- arteries 335
- nerves **313**, 335, 336
- tendon compartments 261, 262
- tendon sheaths **265**
- vessels **313**
Back of the knee 6
Backpack palsy 241
BAKER's cyst 384
Ball-and-socket joint
- clavicular joint **205**, 214
- hip joint 374, 376
- humeroradial joint 214, 225, 227
- metacarpophalangeal joint 214, **233**
- metatarsophalangeal joint 413
- shoulder joint 214, 218, 221
- sternoclavicular joint 112
Ball joint **33**
BARTHOLIN's gland 60
Basal 9
Basal ganglia 64
Basipodium 22
Basis
- ossis
-- metatarsi 364
-- sacri 108, 109
--- X-ray image 126, 353
- patellae 361
-- X-ray image 70, 380
- phalangis
-- manus 212
-- pedis 364
BECHTEREW disease 117
Benediction sign 291
BENNINGHOFF arcade scheme 32
Biceps tendon, rupture **249**
Bifid rib 92
Bifurcatio
- aortae 50, 74
- tracheae
-- X-ray image 70
Blastocyst cavity 18
Blistering 77
Block vertebra 89

Blood
- circulation, fetal 55
- clot 54
- pressure 53
-- system **48**
BOCHDALEK triangle (Trigonum lumbocostale) 157, 158
- hernia 158
Body proportion, normal **6**
Body surface, projection of the organs **16**, **17**
Bone lamellae 27
Bone marrow 28
- aspiration 23
- red 28
- tap (puncture) 111
- yellow 28
Bones **20**
- accessory 21
- aerated 21
- basic structure 27
- compact 24
- compression load 25
- desmal 29
- development 29, 203
- flat 21
- irregular 21
- long 21
- membrane 27
- osteoblasts 27
- sesamoid 21
- short 21
- spongy 24
- structure 24
- subchondral 32
- tap (puncture) 111
- tendon insertion site 45
- trabeculae 24
- vector forces 25
BOTALLO's duct 55
BOTALLO's foramen 55
Bottle sign 291
Bow-leg deformity (Genu varum) 348
- mechanical axis 349
- uneven load 349
Boxer fracture **230**
BOYD's perforating veins 473
Brachial plexus 276
Brachial pulse **50**
Brachium *see* Arm
Brain
- hemispheres 64
- magnetic resonance imaging 75
- ventricle 64
Brainstem 64
Breast
- cancer 185
-- localisation 185
- female **182**
-- blood supply **184**
-- development 182
-- lymph drainage 184
-- mammography 185
-- structure **183**
Bronchus principalis dexter/sinister
- X-ray image 70
Bucket handle tear, meniscus 392
Bulbourethral glands 60
Bulge 78
Bursa
- acromialis 34
- anserina **384**, 425
- bicipitoradialis 225, 255
- infrapatellaris profunda 34, 381, **383**, **384**
- intratendinea **210**
- ischiadica musculi obturatorii interni 431
- musculi
-- coracobrachialis 239
-- gastrocnemii **384**
-- semimembranosi **384**, 441, 442, **443**

Appendix

Bursa
- olecrani **210**
- poplitea **384**
- prepatellaris 395
- shoulder joint 224
- subacromialis 218, 224, 239
- subcoracoidea 224
- subcutanea 34
-- calcanea 448
-- coccygea 170
-- infrapatellaris **384**, 414, 422
-- olecrani 201
-- prepatellaris **384**, 396, 414
-- sacralis 170
-- spinae iliacae posterioris superioris 170
- subdeltoidea 224, 247
- subfascialis prepatellaris **383**
- subligamentosa 34
- subpoplitea **383**
- subtendinea 34, **210**
-- iliaca 424, 425, 500
-- musculi
--- gastrocnemii medialis 441, 442, **443**
--- sartorii 425
--- subscapularis 219, 224, 239
--- prepatellaris 422
- suprapatellaris **381**, **383**, **384**, 395
-- arthroscopy 398
- synovialis 34, 219
- trochanterica musculi glutei
-- maximi 429, 430, 431
-- medii 431
Bursitis
- mechanical loading 383
- olecrani **210**
- rheumatoid arthritis 35
Bypass circulation, aortic isthmus stenosis 161
Bypass surgery 473

C

Calcaneus **364**, **365**, **366**, **367**, 401, 403, 404, 408
- arch of the foot 408
- bone core formation 29
- MRI 401
Callus 26
Calx [Regio calcanea] 13
- surface anatomy 347
Calyx renalis 61
Canalis
- adductorius 423, **465**, 481, 482, 501
- carpi 269, **291**, 339
- inguinalis **190**
-- content **189**
-- walls **189**
- nervi hypoglossi 119
- nutricius 24
- obturatorius **368**, 373, 374, **425**, 433
- sacralis **108**, **109**
-- MRI 130
- vertebralis 175
-- arteries **179**
-- content **176**, **178**
-- MRI 130
-- veins **179**
Capillaries 49, 52
- blood flow 52
- cross-sectional diameter 52
- fluid exchange 52
- intravasal pressure 52
- number 52
Capillary network 58
Capitulum humeri **208**, **225**
- X-ray image 226
Capsula articularis 34
- articulationis
-- atlantoaxialis lateralis 119
-- atlantooccipitalis 119, 120

Capsula articularis articulationis
-- capitis costae 114
-- coxae 374
-- cubiti **225**
-- genus 381, 388
-- humeri 219, **220**, 239
-- interphalangeae distalis 79
-- sternoclavicularis 112, 214
- structure 32
Capsule, lymph nodes 58
Caput 4, 5, 42
- breve musculi bicipitis
-- brachii 47, 246, 248, 318
-- femoris 428
- costae 92, 104, 114
-- X-ray image 125
- epididymidis 191
- femoris **356**, 357, 359, 373, 374
-- sinistra 74
-- X-ray image 353, 358, 375
- fibulae 362, **363**, 378, 381, 382, 399, 414, 417, 422, 439
-- MRI 397
-- surface anatomy **346**, **347**
-- X-ray image 70, 380
- humeri **208**, 209, **218**
-- X-ray image 217, 223
- laterale musculi
-- gastrocnemii 39, 436
-- tricipitis brachii 47, 248
- longum musculi
-- bicipitis brachii 47, 246, 248, 318
--- rupture 249
-- bicipitis femoris 39, 428
-- tricipitis brachii 47, 248
- mediale musculi
-- gastrocnemii 39, 436
-- tricipitis brachii 47, 248
- obliquum musculi adductoris hallucis 401, 451, 498
- ossis metatarsi 364
- phalangis
-- manus 212
-- pedis 364
- profundum musculi flexoris pollicis brevis 267
- radii **211**
-- Circumferentia articularis **211**
-- X-ray image 226
- rectum musculi recti femoris 373, 424
- reflexum musculi recti femoris 373, 424
- sonography 72
- superficiale musculi flexoris pollicis brevis 267
- tali 364, 365, 366, **367**, 401
-- X-ray image 405
- transversum
-- musculi adductoris hallucis 267, 449, 450, 451, 498
-- musculi adductoris pollicis 268
- ulnae 210, 229, 262, 264, 272
-- Proc. styloideus ulnae 201
Caput medusae 56
Cardiovascular system 48
- prenatal 55
Carina tracheae, X-ray image 70
Carotid pulse **50**
Carpal tunnel **290**, **291**, 339
- syndrome **291**, 333
Carpometacarpal joint
- movements 230
- of the thumb 234
- range of movement **232**, 234
- type 214
Carpus 204, 212
- cross-section **339**
Carrying angle of the arm 228
Cartilage 34, 385
- tendon insertion site 45
Cartilage bone 29
Cartilaginous **30**

Cartilago(-ines)
- articularis(-es) 24, 75
- costalis(-es) **90**, 91, 112, 147, 150, 151, 194, 214
-- attachment **112**
- cricoidea
-- Lamina
--- X-ray image 124
- thyroidea 180
Cauda equina 62, 138, **174**, **178**
- lumbar puncture 174
- MRI 130
Caudal 9
Cavea thoracis
- anterior wall **147**
- posterior wall **147**
Cavitas
- articularis 32
- glenoidalis **207**, **218**, 239
-- X-ray image 217, 223
- medullaris 24
- serosa scroti **191**, **193**
- symphysialis 372
- synovialis 44
CCD angle (*see* Centrum-collum-diaphyseal angle)
Central 9
Centrum-collum-diaphyseal angle 359, 360
Centrum tendineum diaphragmatis **156**, **157**, 158
Cerebellum 64
Cerebrum, lobes 64
Cervical
- fascia layer 180
- lordosis **95**, 103
- lordotic curve 96
- rib(s) 89, 92
- spine
-- CT 129
-- KLIPPEL-FEIL syndrome 129
-- kyphosis 95
-- lordosis 95, 103
-- mobility 102, **103**
-- normal **101**
-- operative access 180
-- osteophytes 131
-- upper **120**
-- X-ray image 102, **124**
Changes to the sacroiliac joints **352**
Chest (*see* Thorax)
Chest wall
- anterior
-- surface anatomy 85
- lateral
-- lymph vessels 306
-- nerves 308, 316
-- topography 316, 317
-- vessels 308, 316
- movements 91
- skeleton of the trunk 91
Chiasma
- cruris 437, **442**
- plantare 437, **451**
Chickenpox 15
Child body proportions, development phase 6
Chondroblasts 29
Chondrocytes 32
Chondrosis 131
CHOPART's joint (Art. tarsi transversa) **364**, 406
Chorda
- arteriae umbilicalis 153, 187, 188, 193
- dorsalis 19, 88, 89
- obliqua 225, **229**
Chorion 19
- frondosum 19
- laeve 19
Chorionic
- cavity 19
- villus 19
Cingulum
- pectorale 204
- pelvicum 90, 348

Circulation
- terminal 49
Circulatory system 48
- arteries **50**
- functions 52
- low-pressure system 51
Circumduction
- shoulder joint 10
Circumferentia articularis 210, 211, 225, 229
Cisterna
- cerebellomedullaris 173
- chyli 57
Clavicula 21, 34, 47, 89, 112, 142, 201, 204, 205, 214, 218, 236, 238, 246, 249, 250, 251, 283, 297, **315**
- bone core formation 29
- Corpus 86
- projection onto the chest wall 85
- structure of the extremities 22
- surface anatomy 85
- X-ray image 70, 215, 217, 223
Clavicular joint
- lateral 214, 216
-- injury 217
-- X-ray image 217
- medial 214
-- X-ray image 215
Claw foot deformity **462**, 492
Claw hand **293**
Claw toe deformity 407
Clitoris 60
Cloacal membrane 19
Clubfoot, congenital 409
Coalitio 31
Coccyx, injuries 110
COCKETT's perforating veins 473
Cold-light source 398
Collagen fibres
- fibrils 32
- microfibrils 43
- tendon insertion site 45
Collateral bypass, aortic isthmus stenosis 161
Collateral circulation
- elbow area 295
- hip region 467
- knee joint 468
- scapular anastomoses 297
COLLES fracture 211
Collum 4, 5
- anatomicum 208, **209**
- chirurgicum 208, **209**
- costae 92, 104, 114
- femoris **356**, 357, 359, 373
-- X-ray image 353, 358, 375
- fibulae **363**, 378
- radi **211**, **225**, 229
-- X-ray image 226
- scapulae 207
-- X-ray image 223
- tali 366, **367**
-- X-ray image 405
Colon 16, 17, 71
- contrast agent imaging 71
Columna vertebralis
- cervicalis
-- X-ray image 102
- nerves **178**
- thoracica 105
Compact bone(s) **24**
- adjustment 25
- compression load 25
Compartment 502, 503
- anterior 503
- deep posterior 503
- lateral 503
- syndrome 502
Compressive trabeculae 25

Computed tomography **73**
- angiogram 74
- cervical spine **129**
- lumbar spine 129, **130**
Concha nasalis
- inferior
-- CT 73
- media, CT 73
Condyloid joint
- hand joint 214
- wrist joint 230
Condylus
- humeri **208**
- lateralis **356**, 357, 361, **362**, 381, 389
-- femoris **378**
--- X-ray image 70
-- tibiae **378**
--- X-ray image 70
- medialis **356**, 357, 361, **362**, 381, 389
-- femoris **378**
--- X-ray image 70
-- tibiae **378**
--- X-ray image 70
- occipitalis **98**
Congenital clubfoot **202**
Conjugata
- diagonalis 351
- vera 351
Connecting stalk 19
Connective tissue
- bone 29
- subsynovial 32
Connexus intertendinei **264**, 265, **272**
Contrast agent imaging, renal angiogram 73
COOPER ligaments **183**
Cor 16, 17, 48, 50, 51, 68
- dermatomes 186
Cornu
- coccygeum 109, 110
- sacrale 108, 109
Coronal plane 7
Corpus callosum 64
Corpus(-ora)
- adiposum infrapatellare 75, 381, 388, 395, 432
- callosum **64**
-- genu 75
-- splenium 75
- claviculae 206
- costae 92
- femoris **356**, 357
-- X-ray image 70, 380
- fibulae 363, 399
-- X-ray image 70, 380
- humeri **208**, 250
- mammae 142
- ossis
-- ilii **354**, 355
--- X-ray image 375
-- ischii 354, 355
-- metatarsi 364, 444
-- pubis **354**, 355
- phalangis
-- manus 212, 340
-- pedis 364
- radii **211**, 262
- sterni 91, **111**, 112, 147
-- fissure formation 89
-- projection onto the chest wall 85
-- surface anatomy 85
- tali 366, **367**
- tibiae 399
-- X-ray image 70, 380
- ulnae **210**, **262**
- unguis 79
- vertebrae **97**, 98, **99**, 100, 104, 107, 116, 121, 175, 177
-- CT 129
-- Epiphysis anularis **100**
-- Facies intervertebralis 104, 107

Corpus(-ora) vertebrae
-- vertebrae
--- cervicalis 91, 131
--- lumbalis 91, 130
-- X-ray image 125
Cortex
- cerebri 64
- renalis 61
Cortex (hair) 78
Cortical bone 24
- tendon insertion site 45
Costa(-ae) 21, 89, 91, 92, 93, 104, 113, 115, 116, 133, 136, 137, 138, 140, 143, 144, 145, 148, 151, 157, 153, 159, 166, 175, 277, 283
- fluctuantes 89, 90, 93
- prima 91, 93
- projection onto the chest wall 85
- spuriae 89, 90, 93
- verae 89, 90, 93
- X-ray image 70, 125, 126, 127
Costovertebra joint **114**, **115**
- inspiration 91
- ligament(s) **116**
Coupling, arteriovenous **54**
COWPER's glands 60
Coxa 348
- valga **359**, 360
-- load 359
-- spongy bone structure 359
-- X-ray image **360**
- vara 359, **360**
-- arthrosis 359
-- femoral neck fracture 359
-- load 359
-- spongy bone structure 359
-- X-ray image **360**
Coxa profunda 373
Coxarthrosis 359
- development 373, 376
Cranial 9
Cranial suture 30
Cranium 64
Cremasteric reflex 189
Crena ani 13
Cricoid cartilage, ossified 31
Crista
- capitis costae 92
- colli costae 92
- iliaca 13, 132, 133, 156, 159, 170, 352, **354**, **355**, 414, 418, **429**, 430, 460, 487
-- bone marrow aspiration 28
-- intragluteal injection 460
-- Labium externum 417
-- landmarks 84
-- surface anatomy 84
-- X-ray image 353
- intertrochanterica 356, 359
-- X-ray image 353
- medialis fibulae 363
- musculi supinatoris 210
- obturatoria 354, 355
- occipitalis externa 98
- pubica 354
- sacralis
-- lateralis **108**
-- medialis [intermedia] **108**
-- mediana **108**, 109
--- X-ray image 126
- supraepicondylaris
-- lateralis 208
--- X-ray image 226
-- medialis 208
--- X-ray image 226
- tuberculi
-- majoris **208**
-- minoris 208
Cruciate ligament(s) 275
- flexor tendons of the finger 275
- injury **389**

Crus 4, 5, 348
– lateral anuli inguinalis superficialis **189**
– medial anuli inguinalis superficialis **141**, **189**
CT angiogram 74
– abdomen 74
– pelvis 74
Cubita 204
Cubital fossa
– nerves 310, 312, 328
– veins 310, 312
–– variations 311
– vessels 328
Cubital pulse **50**
Cubital tunnel 329
– syndrome 292, 293
Cutaneous covering 76
– layers **77**
Cuticle(s) 78, 79
Cuticula 79
Cutis 76, 77, 194
– structure 76
Cytotrophoblast 18

D

Deep vein thrombosis **54**
Dens
– axis **98**, 99, 101, 118, 119, 123
–– dislocation 119
–– subluxation 119
– fracture 100
– hypoplasia 100
Depression
– arm 8
– shoulder girdle 205
Dermatomes 15, 66, **88**, 169
– abdominal wall 186
– arm 281
– development 88, 203
– disc prolapse 455
– extremity
–– dorsal side 203
–– upper 281
–– ventral side 203
– leg 455
– limb
–– lower 455
– thoracic wall 186
– ventral-axial border 203
Dermis **76**, 77, 78, 79, 144
– blistering 77
– functions 76
– hair 78
Descensus testis 188, 192
– disorders 192
Dexter 9
Diameter
– anatomica 350, 351
– conjugate
–– birth 351
– diagonalis 350, 351
–– birth 351
– transversa 350, 351
– vera 350, 351
Diaphragm 16, 17, 144, 155, **156**, **157**, **159**, 166
– Centrum tendineum 147, 159
– Cupula
–– X-ray image 70
– dermatomes 186
– expiration 91
– hernia 158
– inspiration 91
– Pars costalis 159
– passageways **158**
Diaphragmatic hernia 158
Diaphysis 24
– blood supply 24

Diarthrosis
– facet joint 102
– types 32
Digitus(-i) 212
– anularis 200
– manus, Ossa 204
– medius 200
–– cross-section 340
– minimus 200
– pedis, Ossa 348
– surface anatomy 346
DIP *see* Distal interphalangeal joint
Directions of movement 7, 8
Disc 34
– degenerative changes 122
– hernia 122
–– Foramen intervertebrale 175
– prolapse 122, 131
–– dermatome localisation 455
–– Foramen intervertebrale 175
–– MRI **131**
– protrusion 122
Discus 34
– articularis 34, **214**, **229**, **230**
– interpubicus **372**
– intervertebralis 34, 95, 102, 106, 113, 114,
  115, 116, **117**, 118, 120, **121**, **122**, 123
–– Anulus fibrosus **176**, 178
–– cervicalis 121, **123**
–– CT 129
–– lumbalis 121, **122**
–– MRI 130
–– X-ray image 124
Dislocation 208
– CHOPART's joint 364
– LISFRANC's joint 364
– patella **379**
Distal 9
Distal interphalangeal joint
– finger 233
–– muscles 235, 273
DODD's perforating veins 473
Dog-like figure
– lumbar vertebra 127
Dorsal 9
Dorsal aponeurosis 273
– finger 264, 272, 274
–– extension 232, 273
–– flexion 273
– hand **272**
–– structure **272**
– palm of the hand 270
Dorsal extension 232
– ankle joint 411, 412
– distal interphalangeal joint 233
– hand 10
– metacarpophalangeal joint 233
– proximal interphalangeal joint 233
– toe joint 413
– wrist joint 232, 235
Dorsalis-pedis pulse **50**
Dorsiflexion 8
Dorsum
– manus 13, 200
–– nerves **313**, 335, 336
–– tendons **264**
–– vessels **313**, 335, 336
– pedis 12, 13
–– nerves 479, 495
–– surface anatomy 346, 347
–– vessels 479, 495
Dorsum of the foot
– fasciae 414
– musculature 446, 447
– nerves 479, 495
– vessels 479, 495
Drawer test 394
DUCHENNE sign 461

Ductus
– arteriosus (BOTALLI) 55
– deferens 60, 188, 189, 190, 191, **193**, 194
– lactiferi **183**
– lymphaticus dexter 57
– thoracicus 57, 157
–– confluence (opening) **317**
– venosus (ARANTII) 55
Duodenum 16
Dura mater 118
– cranialis 118
– spinalis 122, 173, 174, **176**, 177, 178
DVT **54**
Dysregulation, autonomic 68
Dystonia **423**

E

Ectoderm 19, 203
Efferent 63
Effusion 394
Elbow
– arteries 329
– nerves 309, 329
– veins 309
Elbow joint 214, **225**
– bony parts **225**
– dislocation 228
– evolution 23
– extension 11
– flexion 11
– HUETER triangle **228**
– range of movement **227**
– rotational movements **227**
– X-ray image 70, **226**
Elevation 7
– extremities 8
– shoulder girdle 205
– shoulder joint 221, 222
Ellipsoidal joint
– wrist joint 234
Embolus **54**
Embryoblast 18
Embryonic development **18**
– gastrulation **19**
– germ disc 18
Eminentia
– iliopubica 354
– intercondylaris 362, 378
–– X-ray image 380
Encephalon 62, 64
Endometrium
– capillaries 18
– glands 18
Endomysium 40
Endosteum 27
Entoderm 19
Epiblast 18
Epicondylus
– lateralis
–– femoris **356**, 361, 378, 396
––– X-ray image 70, 380
–– humeri **208**, 225, 238, 251, 259, 260, 261,
  262, 310, 322, 330, **356**
––– HUETER triangle 228
––– X-ray image 226
– medialis
–– femoris **356**, 357, 361, 378, 386, 396
––– X-ray image 70, 380
–– humeri **200**, **208**, 225, 249, 250, 254, 255,
  256, 257, 292, 319, 324, 329
––– HUETER triangle 228
––– X-ray image 226
Epidermis **76**, 77, 78, 79
Epididymis 60, 193
Epiglottis, X-ray image 124
Epimer **88**
Epimysium 40
Epineurium 176

Epiorchium 193
Epiphyseal plate injuries 29
Epiphysis 24, 30
– anularis 97, 104, **107**, 117
– blood supply 24
– distalis 24
– proximalis 24
Epitendineum 44
Eponychium 79
Equinus deformity 491
ERB's palsy 199, 278
Erector system, deep back muscles 134
Eversion 412
– ankle joint 411
– extremities 8
– foot 11
Extension 7
– ankle joint 412
– carpometacarpal joint 232
– cervical spine 103
– elbow joint 11, 227
– finger 233
–– muscles 235, 273
– knee joint 10, 393
– occipital joint 99
– pelvis 8
– spine 8, 102, 152
– thumb 234
–– muscles 235, 273
– trunk 152
Extensor compartment 503
Extensors, development 88
External ligament
– ankle joint 402, 403
–– injury 402
– knee joint **385**, 386
–– injury 386
External rotation
– extremities 8
– knee joint 393
– shoulder joint 10, 220, 221
Externus 9
Extremitas
– acromialis claviculae 206
– sternalis claviculae 206
Extremity
– clubfoot 202
– development 202
– directions of movement 8
– limb girdle 22
– longitudinal growth 203
– lower
–– bone core formation 29
–– dermatomes
––– development 203
–– evolution 23
–– main lines 9
–– ossification 203
–– structure 22
– structure **22**
– upper
–– arteries 294
–– bone core formation 29
–– bones and joints **204**
–– cutaneous innervation **280**
–– dermatomes 281
––– development 203
–– evolution 23
–– main lines 9
–– ossification 203
–– structure 22

F

Facet joint 102
– cervical spine 102
– lumbosacral joint 102
– positioning 102
– thoracic spine 102

Facial pulse **50**
Facies
– anterior
–– patellae 361
–– radii 211
–– ulnae 210
– anterolateralis humeri 208
– anteromedialis humeri 208
– articularis
–– acromialis 206
–– anterior axis **98**, **99**
–– calcanea
––– anterior 367
––– media 367
––– posterior 367
–– capitis
––– costae 92
––– fibulae 363
–– carpalis 211, 229
–– clavicularis 207, 218
–– cuboidea 367
–– fibularis 362
–– inferior
––– atlantis 98
––– tibiae 362, 363, 399, 403
––– vertebrae **107**, 114
–– malleoli
––– lateralis 363, 399, 403
––– medialis 362, 363, 399, 403
–– navicularis 367
–– patellae 361
–– posterior axis **99**
–– sternalis claviculae 206
–– superior
––– atlantis 98
––– vertebrae 100, 102, 115
–– talaris
––– anterior calcanei 367, **404**
––– media calcanei 367, **404**
––– posterior calcanei 367, **404**
–– tuberculi costae 92
– auricularis ossis sacri **108**, **109**, **354**
– costalis scapulae 207
– glutea **355**
– intervertebralis 114, 117
–– inferior **107**
–– superior **107**
–– X-ray image 124, 125, 126, 127
– lateralis
–– fibulae 363
–– radii 211
–– tibiae 362
– lunata 354, 355, 374
– malleolaris
–– lateralis 366, 367
–– medialis 366, 367
– medialis
–– fibulae 363
–– ulnae 210
– patellaris femoris 356, 361, 381
– pelvica 109
– poplitea femoris 356, 357, 378
–– X-ray image 380
– posterior
–– fibulae 363
–– humeri 209
–– radii 211
–– scapulae 207
–– tibiae 362
–– ulnae 210
– sacropelvica 354
– symphysialis **354**, 371
Faecal incontinence 459
Fallen arches 409
FALLOPIAN ligament 156
False joint (pseudoarthrosis) 31
Falx inguinalis 188
Fascia(-ae) 42
– antebrachii **201**, 249, 250, 332
– axillaris 141, 306

Fascia(-ae)
– brachii 141, **201**, 308, 338
– clavipectoralis 141, **315**
– cremasterica **193**
– cruris **414**, 440, 478, 488, 502, 503
–– deep layer 502
– deltoidea 132, 133
– dorsalis pedis **414**
– endothoracica **144**, **145**
– glutea 142, 414, 429, 485
– infraspinata 132, 133, 135, 238, 251
– lata **414**, 422, 423, 424, 429, 477, 483, 501
– nuchae 172
– pectoralis **183**, 239
–– Hiatus venae cephalicae 239
– phrenicopleuralis 144
– spermatica
–– externa 189, **191**, **192**, **193**, 194
–– interna 191, **192**, **193**, **194**
– superficialis 193
– thoracica
–– externa 144, **145**
–– interna **145**
– thoracolumbalis **117**, **132**, 133, 134, 135, 136, **138**, 142, **429**
–– CT 129
–– Lamina profunda **137**, 138, 153
–– Lamina superficialis **137**, 138, 153
–– MRI 130
– transversalis 136, 151, **153**, 156, 159, 166, 181, 188, **189**, **190**, 191, **192**, 193
–– sectioned edge 188
Fasciculus(-i)
– lateralis plexus brachialis 67, 276, **277**, 278, 279, 284, **236**, 287, 290, 315, **318**
–– arm nerves 286
–– plexus lesion 199
– longitudinalis
–– aponeurosis plantaris **448**
–– inferior ligamenti cruciformis atlantis 119
–– superior ligamenti cruciformis atlantis 119
– medialis plexus brachialis 67, 276, 277, 278, 279, 284, **286**, 290, 292, 315, **318**
–– arm nerves 286
–– plexus lesion 199
– posterior plexus brachialis 67, 276, **277**, 278, 279, 284, 285, **286**, 288, 315, **318**
–– arm nerves 286
–– plexus lesion 199
– transversi
–– aponeurosis plantaris **448**
Fatty bone marrow **28**
Female reproductive organs **60**
Femoral
– gliding surface 396
– hernia 189, **483**
– neck
–– angle **359**
–– anteversion 357
–– fracture 358
––– arterial damage **377**
–– retroversion 357
–– torsion angle 357
– pulse **50**
– triangle 480
Femur 4, 5, 21, 75, 348, **356**, **357**, 378, 381, 382, 385, 386, 387, 395, 396, 425, 501
– adjustment **25**
– bone core formation 29
– centrum-collum-diaphyseal angle **359**
– Condylus
–– articular surfaces 361
–– lateralis 382
––– arthroscopy 398
––– MRI 397
––– X-ray image 380
–– medialis 382
––– arthroscopy 398
––– MRI 397
––– X-ray image 380

Femur
– Corpus
–– X-ray image 375
– cross-section 500, 501
– distal **361**
– evolution 23
– Facies
–– patellaris
––– arthroscopy 398
–– poplitea 442, 489
– Fossa poplitea 433
– fracture 345
– hip fracture 358
– Linea aspera 433
– proximal **359**
–– centrum-collum diaphyseal angle 360
– shaft axis 348
– spongy bone structure 359
– structure 22, 24
– Substantia
–– compacta
––– X-ray image 358
–– medullaris
––– X-ray image 358
– torsion angle 357
– X-ray image 353, **358**
Fertilisation 18
Fetus
– sonography **72**
– spine 96
Fibrae intercrurales **141**, 149, **189**
Fibrous joints **30**
Fibula 21, 42, 348, **362**, **363**, 378, 381, 382, 384, 385, 386, 387, **399**, 400, 402, 403, 445, 502, 503
– articular surface **363**
– bone core formation 29
– distal
–– X-ray image 400
– evolution 23
– Margo interosseus 442, 443
– structure of the extremities 22
– WEBER fracture 400
– X-ray image 405
Fibular 9
Fibular compartment 503
Filtration pressure, effective **52**
Filum terminale **178**
Finger 212
– development 202
– extension
–– muscles 235, 273
– flexion
–– muscles 235, 273
– flexor mechanism 274
– flexor tendons apparatus 275
Finger joints **232**
– distal joints 214, 232
– extensor muscles **273**
– flexor muscles **273**
– ligaments **232**
– metacarpophalangeal joints 214, 232
– middle joints 214
– proximal joints 232
– range of movement **233**
Fissura sterni congenita 111
Fixed pronation 462
Flat arches, foot deformity 409
Flatfoot deformity, acquired 409
Flexion 7
– ankle joint 412
– carpometacarpal joint 232
– cervical spine 103
– elbow joint 11, 227
– extremities 8
– finger 233
–– muscles 235, 273
– knee joint 10, 393
– occipital joint 99

Flexion
– pelvis 8
– spine 8, 102, 152
– thumbs 234
–– muscles 235, 273
– trunk 152
Flexor compartment 503
Flexors, development 88
Fontanelle
– large 30
– small 30
Fonticulus
– anterior 30
– posterior 30
Foot
– clubfoot 202
– deformity 409
– development 202
– eversion 11
– inversion 11
– joints 406, 407
– longitudinal arch 408, 409
– main lines 9
– musculature 438, 439
– nerves 478, 479
– plantar aponeurosis 448
– sagittal section 401
– tendon sheaths 444, 445
– transverse arch 408, 409
– vessels 478, 479
Foot *see* Pes
Foot drop deformity **491**
Foramen(-ina)
– costotransversarium 104, 116
– infrapiriforme 418, **429**, 430, 431, 458, 460, **486**
– intervertebrale 95, **106**, 114, 117, 118, 121, 124, 175
–– CT 129
–– disc prolapse 175
–– narrowing 106, 175
–– spinal nerve 176
–– X-ray image 126
– ischiadicum
–– majus **369**, 370, **371**, **429**, **460**
–– minus **369**, 370, **371**, 418, **429**, 431, 458
– magnum 98, 173
– nutricium 24, 206, 210, 211, 362, 363
– obturatum **354**, **369**, 371
–– sinistrum 74
–– X-ray image 353, 375
– ovale 55
– sacralia
–– anteriora **108**
––– X-ray image 127
–– posteriora **108**, 109
– suprapiriforme 418, **429**, 430, 458, 460, **486**
– transversarium **98**, **99**, **100**
–– CT 129
– venae basivertebralis 117
– venae cavae 147, **156**, 157
– vertebrale 98, 100, 104, **107**, 115
–– axis 99
–– CT 129, 130
Forearm 200, 204
– arteries 324, 325, 326, 327, 330, 331
– bone
–– shaft axis 204
– compartments 42
– cross-section **339**
– cutaneous innervation 280
– diagonal axis 204
– fascia 201
– musculature
–– dorsal **258**, **259**, 260, 261, 262
–– radial **258**
–– ventral **253**, **254**, **255**, **256**, **257**
– nerves 312, 324, 325, 326, 327, 330, 331
– surface anatomy 4, 5
– veins 312

Forefoot 364
Fossa
– acetabuli 354, **355**, 374
–– X-ray image 353, 375
– axillaris **314**, 315
–– blood vessels 308, 318, 319
–– lymph nodes **306**
––– level **307**
–– lymph vessels **306**
–– nerves 308, 318, 319
–– topography 316, 317
– coronoidea 208
–– X-ray image 226
– epigastrica
–– surface anatomy 85
– iliaca 354
– iliopectinea 483
– infraclavicularis 201
– infraspinata **207**
– inguinalis
–– lateralis **155**, 188, 193
––– inguinal hernia 193
–– medialis **155**, 188, 193
––– inguinal hernia 189
– intercondylaris 356, 357, 361, 378
–– X-ray image 380
– malleoli lateralis 363
– olecrani 209
–– X-ray image 226
– ovalis 55
– poplitea 414, 431
–– nerves 477, 484, 485, 486, 488, 492, 493, 494
–– vessels 477, 484, 485, 486, 488, 489, 492, 493, 494
– radialis 208
– subscapularis **207**
– supraspinata **207**
– supravesicalis **155**, 188, 193
– trochanterica 356, 357, 359
Fovea
– articularis 211
– capitis femoris 356, 357, 359
–– X-ray image 353, 358, 375
– costalis 104
–– inferior **104**, 113, 114
–– processus transversi **104**, 106, 114, 115, 116, 177
–– superior 104, 106, 113, 114, 116
– dentis 98
– radialis **264**, **272**, 336
Fracture **26**
– diagnostics 208
– healing
–– primary 26
–– secondary 26
– hip 358
– humerus 208, 209
– intertrochanteric 358
– radius 211
– ribs
–– resuscitation 91
FROHSE, arcade of 288, 325
FROMENT sign 293
Frontal 9
– lobes 64
– plane 7, 205
Fundus gastricus
– herniated 159
– X-ray image 70
Funiculus
– spermaticus **141**, 149, 150, 151, 188, 189, **190**, 195, 414, 475, 483
–– content **191**
–– coverings **193**
– umbilicalis 55, 194
Funny bone 209, 292, 329

G

Galea aponeurotica 78
Ganglion(-ia)
– cervicale
–– medium 69
–– superius 69
– cervicothoracicum [stellatum] 68, 69, 278
–– plexus lesion 199
– ciliare 68
– coeliacum 68, 69
– impar 69
– mesentericum
–– inferius 68
–– superius 68
– oticum 68
– pelvica 69
– pterygopalatinum 68
– sensorium nervi spinalis 65, 174, 175, 176, 177, 178
– spinale 67, 122
– stellatum [cervicothoracicum] 68, 69, 278
–– plexus lesion 199
– submandibulare 68
– trunci sympathici 65, 175, 177, 178
Gaster 16, 17
– contrast agent imaging 71
– dermatomes 186
– Pars cardiaca 158
Gastrulation 19
General lamellae 27
Genitalia, accessory 60
Genu 348
– valgum (knock-knee deformity) 348
–– mechanical axis 349
–– osteoarthritis 349
–– uneven load 349
– varum (bow-leg deformity) 348
–– mechanical axis 349
–– uneven load 349
Germ disc 18, 19
Gibbus 124
– deformity 96
GIMBERNAT ligament (Lig. lacunare) 190
Ginglymus 33
Glandula(-ae)
– areolares 182
– bulbourethralis 60
– mammaria 183
– oris 68
– parathyroidea, endocrine system 59
– suprarenalis 68, 181
–– endocrine system 59
– thyroidea 16
–– endocrine system 59
–– Lobus sinister 180
–– scintigraphy 72
– urethralis 60
– vesiculosa 60
– vestibularis
–– major 60
–– minor 60
Gluteal region
– hip joint surgery 487
– intragluteal injection 460
– nerves 477, 484, 485, 486, 487
– projection of the skeletal contours 460
– vessels 477, 484, 485, 486, 487
Gluteus muscles
– small 427, 430
–– course 500
–– DUCHENNE sign 461
–– innervation 458
–– TRENDELENBURG sign 427, 461
Gomphoses 30
Gonarthrosis 349, 359, 361, 379, 392
Goose bumps 78
GRYNFELT-LESSHAFT-LUSCHKA triangle 133
GRYNFELT lumbar hernia 133
Guard nodes 185

Gubernaculum testis 192, 194
GUYON's canal 292, 293, 332
– syndrome 293, 333
Gynaecomastia 182

H

Hair
– bulbus 78
–– root sheath 78
– colour 78
– cuticles 78
– follicle 76, 78
–– structure 78
– funnel 78
– papilla 78
– root 76, 78
– shaft 76, 78
Hairless skin 76
Hairy skin 76, 77
Hallux
– surface anatomy 346
– valgus 407
Hammer toe deformity 407
Hamulus ossis hamati 212, 231, 291, 293
Hand
– arteries 303, 337
– cutaneous innervation 280
– development 202
– dorsal aponeurosis 272
– joints 231
– main lines 9
– musculature 266, 267, 269, 270, 271
– pronation 11
– skeleton 212
– supination 11
– tendon sheaths 268
–– variants 268
Hand, back of the
– arteries 336
– tendons 264
Hangman's fracture 100
HAVERSIAN canal 27
Head joint(s) 120
– ligaments 118, 119, 120
Head of rib joint 114
HEAD's zone 186
– herpes zoster 186
Heart
– musculature 41
– valves 48
Heart see Cor 48
Hemiarthrosis uncovertebralis 123
Hemispheres 64
Hemivertebra 89, 129
HENLE's layer 78
Hepar 16, 17, 55, 144, 145
– dermatomes 186
Hernia 193
– axial 159
– diaphragm 158
– lateral, indirect 193
– lumbar 133
– medial, direct 193
Hernia diaphragmatia vera 158
Hernia diaphragmatica spuria 158
Herniated discs
– diagnosis 281
Herpes zoster 186
HESSELBACH
– ligament (Lig. interfoveolare) 188
– triangle (Trigonum inguinale) 188
–– inguinal hernia 189
Hiatal hernia 158
– paraoesophageal 159
Hiatus
– adductorius 424, 425, 433, 482, 485
– aorticus 156, 157, 158
– basilicus 304

Hiatus
– oesophageus 156, 157
– sacralis 108, 109
– saphenus 475, 483
–– Fascia cribrosa 414
High-pressure system 49, 53
Hilus 58
Hindfoot 364
Hinge joint 33
– ankle joint 410
– distal finger joint 214
– humeroulnar joint 214, 225
– metacarpophalangeal joint of the thumb 214
– middle finger joint 214
– talocrural joint 401
Hip
– dislocation, central 355
– dysplasia 373
– joint 374
–– axes of movement 500
–– blood supply 377
–– cross section 500
–– instability 418
–– ligamentous apparatus 373
–– movements 376
–– musculature 376, 415, 416, 417, 418
––– dorsal 426, 427, 429, 430, 431
––– medial 421
––– pelvitrochanteric group 427
––– ventral 419, 420, 422, 423, 424, 425
–– range of movement 376
–– surgery 487
–– X-ray image 375
Hip bone see Os coxae
Hips see Hip joint
HOFFA's fat pad (Corpus adiposum infrapatellare) 75, 381
Horizontal plane 7
HORNER's syndrome
– plexus lesion 278
HUETER triangle 228
Humeral head, fracture 208
Humeral shaft
– axis 204
– fracture 208, 322
– lateral axillary space 170
Humeroradial joint 214, 227
Humeroulnar joint 214, 227
Humerus 21, 47, 204, 208, 209, 218, 225, 246, 247, 252, 263, 320, 324, 338
– bone core formation 29
– Corpus 239
– development 203
– evolution 23
– fracture 208, 209
– MRI 338
– rotational axis 204
– structure of the extremities 22
– X-ray image 70, 208, 226
Humerus head, repositioning with shoulder dislocation 223
Hunchback 96, 124
HUXLEY's layer 78
Hydrocele 191
Hydrostatic indifference point 53
Hyperkyphosis 96
Hyperlordosis 96, 124
– shortening of the psoas muscle 418
Hypoblast 18
Hypomer 88
Hypomochlion 44
– patella 361
Hyponychum 79
Hypophysis, endocrine system 59
Hypothalamus, endocrine system 59
Hypothenar 200, 236, 266, 339
– atrophy 333
– eminence 266
– musculature 37
H-zone 40

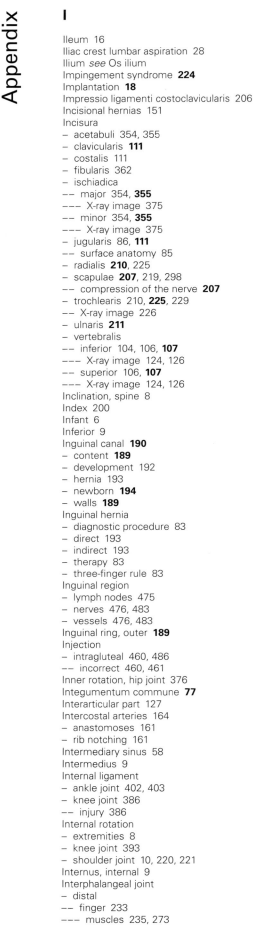

I

Ileum 16
Iliac crest lumbar aspiration 28
Ilium *see* Os ilium
Impingement syndrome **224**
Implantation **18**
Impressio ligamenti costoclavicularis 206
Incisional hernias 151
Incisura
– acetabuli 354, 355
– clavicularis **111**
– costalis 111
– fibularis 362
– ischiadica
–– major 354, **355**
––– X-ray image 375
–– minor 354, **355**
––– X-ray image 375
– jugularis 86, **111**
–– surface anatomy 85
– radialis **210**, 225
– scapulae **207**, 219, 298
–– compression of the nerve **207**
– trochlearis 210, **225**, 229
–– X-ray image 226
– ulnaris **211**
– vertebralis
–– inferior 104, 106, **107**
––– X-ray image 124, 126
–– superior 106, **107**
––– X-ray image 124, 126
Inclination, spine 8
Index 200
Infant 6
Inferior 9
Inguinal canal **190**
– content **189**
– development 192
– hernia 193
– newborn **194**
– walls **189**
Inguinal hernia
– diagnostic procedure 83
– direct 193
– indirect 193
– therapy 83
– three-finger rule 83
Inguinal region
– lymph nodes 475
– nerves 476, 483
– vessels 476, 483
Inguinal ring, outer **189**
Injection
– intragluteal 460, 486
–– incorrect 460, 461
Inner rotation, hip joint 376
Integumentum commune **77**
Interarticular part 127
Intercostal arteries 164
– anastomoses 161
– rib notching 161
Intermediary sinus 58
Intermedius 9
Internal ligament
– ankle joint 402, 403
– knee joint 386
–– injury 386
Internal rotation
– extremities 8
– knee joint 393
– shoulder joint 10, 220, 221
Internus, internal 9
Interphalangeal joint
– distal
–– finger 233
––– muscles 235, 273
– proximal
–– fingers II–V 233
––– dislocation 234
––– muscles 235, 273

Interphalangeal joint proximal
–– thumbs 234
––– muscles 235, 273
Intersectiones tendineae 150, 151
Intersegmental blood vessel(s), development 89
Interstitial lamellae 27
Intervertebral disc **121**
– cervical 121, **123**
– lumbar 121, **122**
Intestinal tube 88
Intestine
– embryonic gut 19
– fetal gut 19
Intestinum
– crassum
–– dermatomes 186
–– tenue 17, 68
–– dermatomes 186
Intra-articular, ligament(s), anterior 34
Intra-articular disc 34
Inversion 412
– ankle joint 411
– extremities 8
– foot 11
Ischialgia 454
Ischium *see* Os ischii
Isthmus glandulae thyroideae 72

J

Jejunum 16
Joint **20**
– aspiration 31
– auxiliary structures 34
– capsule 32
–– functions 43
–– structure **32**
– cartilage
–– hyaline 32
––– structure **32**
– cavity 32
– ligaments
–– acromioclavicular joint 217
––– injury 217
–– elbow joint 225, 228
–– sternoclavicular joint 214
– lips 34
– neutral-zero-method **36**
– plane **33**
– prosthesis 31
– range of movement 36
– reaction force vector 25
– structure **32**
– synovial **32**
– types 33
Junctura
– cartilaginea [synchondrosis] **30**
– fibrosa [syndesmosis] **30**
– ossea [synostosis] **30**
– synovialis [Articulatio, diarthrosis] 32
Juvenile kyphosis 96

K

Kidneys 61
– angiogram **73**
– functions 61
KLIPPEL-FEIL syndrome 129
KLUMPKE's palsy **199**, 278
Knee joint **378**
– arthroscopy 398
– capsule 388
– collateral ligament
–– lateral 387
–– medial 386
– coronary scan 397
– cross-section 396
– cruciate ligaments 389

Knee joint
– development 202
– effusion 394
– evolution 23
– extension 10, 393
– external ligaments **385**
– external rotation 393
– flexion 10, 393
– internal rotation 393
– lateral ligaments 386, 387
– ligamentous apparatus 385
– magnetic resonance imaging **75**
– menisci 390
– movements 393
– musculature 393, 432, 433
– outer ligaments 381, 382
– range of movement 36, 393
– sagittal section 395, 397
– stiffening 36
– synovial bursae 383, 384
– X-ray image 70, **380**
Knock-knee deformity (Genu valgum) 348
– mechanical axis 349
– osteoarthritis 349
– uneven load 349
Kyphosis 96, 124
– cervical spine 95
– sacral vertebra 95

L

Labia minora/majora vulvae 60
Labium
– externum cristae iliacae 354, 355
– internum cristae iliacae 354, 355
– laterale lineae asperae 356
– mediale lineae asperae 356
– superius 72
Labrum 34
– acetabuli **374**
– glenoidale 34, **218**, 239
Lacuna
– musculorum **188**, 369, 483
–– content 483
– vasorum 156, **188**, 195, 369, 483
–– content 483
Lamellar bone 27
Lamina
– anterior vaginae musculi recti abdominis 149, 150, 153
– arcus vertebrae **97**, 100, **104**, **107**, 115, 116, 117, 138, 174
–– CT 129, 130
–– disc prolapse surgery 181
– cribrosa 195
– parietalis tunicae vaginalis testis 191, 193
– posterior vaginae musculi recti abdominis 150, 151, 153
– prevertebralis fasciarum cervicalium 180
– profunda fasciae thoracolumbalis 138
– superficialis
–– fasciae thoracolumbalis 138
–– fasciarum cervicalium 180
– visceralis tunicae vaginalis testis 191, 193
LANDSMEER ligament 274
LANGER's lines, of skin tension 14
Lateral 9
– flexion
–– cervical spine 103
–– spine 8, 102, 152
–– trunk 10, 152
Laterotrusion
– jaw 8
LAUENSTEIN projection 375
Left ventricular catheterisation **466**
Leg
– arteries 464, 465
– bones 348
– cutaneous nerves 454
– dermatomes 455

Leg
– development 202
– fasciae 414
– joints 348
– lymphatic vessels 474
– mechanical axis 349
– musculature 415, 416
– skin innervation
–– segmental 455
– surface anatomy 346, 347
Leg veins 472, 473
– BOYD's perforating veins 473
– COCKETT's perforating veins 473
– deep
–– X-ray image 473
– DODD's perforating veins 473
– thrombosis 473
Lever arm 47
Ligamentous apparatus
– ankle joint 402, 403
– head joints 118, 119, 120
– hip joint 376
– knee joint 379
– sacroiliac joint 352
– spine 117
– talocrural joint 401
– uncovertebral joint 123
Ligaments
– BECHTEREW disease 117
– functions 43
– hip joint 373, 376
– knee joint 381
– structure 43
Ligamentum(-a)
– acromioclaviculare **216**, 218, **219**, 239
–– AC joint separation 217
– alaria **119**
– anterolaterale **387**
– anulare radii **225**, 229, **262**
– apicis dentis **118**, **119**
– arcuatum
–– lateral (lateral arcuate ligament) 156, **157**, **158**, 195
–– medial (medial arcuate ligament) **157**, **158**
–– medial (psoas arcade) 156
–– medianum 157
– arteriosum (BOTALLI) 55
– atlantooccipitale lateral 120
– bifurcatum **402**, **404**
– calcaneocuboideum 402, **404**
–– plantare **406**, **407**
– calcaneofibulare 402, 403, 404
– calcaneonaviculare 402, **404**
–– plantare 401, 402, **404**, **406**, **407**, **408**, 409
– capitis **113**, **114**, **115**, **116**
–– femoris 371, **373**, **374**
–– fibulae
––– anterius 389, 399
––– posterius 382
– capitis costae radiatum
–– BECHTEREW disease 117
– carpi
–– palmare 291, 292, 293
–– radiatum **231**
– carpometacarpalia
–– dorsalia **231**
–– palmaria **231**, 291, 293
– collaterale **232**
–– carpi
––– radiale **230**, **231**
––– ulnare **230**, **231**
–– fibulare **381**, **382**, 383, 384, **387**, 388, 389, 391, 394, 396
––– MRI 397
–– genus lateralis 34, **385**
–– manus 231
–– mediale **385**
–– mediale [deltoideum] **402**, 404
––– Pars tibiocalcanea **403**
––– Pars tibiotalaris posterior **403**

Ligamentum(-a) collaterale
–– pedis **406**
–– radiale **225**, **262**
–– tibiale **381**, **382**, 383, **386**, 388, 389, 391, 394, 396
––– meniscofemoral fibres 386
––– meniscotibial fibres 386
––– MRI 397
–– ulnare **225**
– conoideum **216**, 218, **219**, 239
–– AC joint separation 217
– coracoacromiale 34, **218**, **219**, 224, 239, 246
–– shoulder, roof 246
– coracoclaviculare **216**, 218, 249
–– AC joint separation 217
– coracohumerale 34, 218, **219**, **220**, 224, 239
– costoclaviculare **112**, **214**
– costotransversarium **113**, **115**, 137
–– BECHTEREW disease 117
–– lateral **115**, **116**
–– superius 115, **116**, 136
– costoxiphoidea 141, 149
– cruciatum
–– anterius 34, 75, **382**, **385**, **388**, **389**, 390, 391, 394, 395
––– arthroscopy 398
––– injury **389**
––– MRI 397
–– posterius **382**, 383, **385**, **388**, **389**, 390, 391, 394
––– injury **389**
––– MRI 397
– cruciforme atlantis **119**
–– rupture 119
– cuboideonaviculare
–– dorsale 402, 404
–– plantare 406, 407
– cuneocuboideum dorsale 404
– cuneonavicularia
–– dorsalia 402, 404
–– plantaria 406
– denticulatum 173, 176, 177
– falciforme hepatis 153, **155**, 188
– flavum 34, **115**, **116**, **117**, 137, 174, **176**, 178
–– CT 129
– fundiforme penis **141**, 189
– glenohumeralia 219
– iliofemorale 368, **373**, **374**, 424, 500
–– functions 373
– iliolumbale 136, 174, **368**, **369**, **370**, **372**
– inguinale 150, 156, 188, 189, **190**, 368, **369**, 370, 414, 418, 422, 464, 475, **480**, **483**
–– surface anatomy 346
– intercarpalia
–– dorsalia **231**
–– interossea **230**
– interclaviculare **112**, **214**
– intercuneiformia dorsalia 404
– interfoveolare (HESSELBACH's ligament) 188
– interspinale 34, **115**, **117**, 118, 136, 174
–– BECHTEREW disease 117
–– CT 129
– intertransversaria **116**, 136, 137, 174
– ischiofemorale **373**, **374**
–– functions 373
– lacunare (GIMBERNAT ligament) 188, 190, 483
– longitudinale
–– anterius **113**, 115, **116**, **117**, 118, **120**, 121, 122, 138, 147, 153, 177, 178, 368
––– BECHTEREW disease 117
–– posterius **113**, 115, **117**, 118, 122, 177, 178, 179
– lumbocostale 158
– meniscofemorale
–– anterius **390**
–– posterius **382**, 383, **390**
– meniscotibiale
–– anterius 390
–– posterius 390

Ligamentum(-a)
– metacarpale(-ia)
–– dorsalia **231**
–– interossea **230**
–– palmaria 231
–– transversum
––– profundum 231
––– superficiale 266, 332
– metatarsale(-ia)
–– dorsalia 402
–– plantaria **407**
–– transversum
––– profundum 402, **406**, **407**
––– superficiale **448**
– nuchae 118, 135, **140**
– palmaria 231, **232**
– patellae 75, 361, **381**, 383, 386, 387, 388, 390, **395**, 414, 417, 420, 422, 423, 424, 432, 438, 439, 480, 491
–– MRI 397
– pectineum 483
– pisohamatum 231
– pisometacarpale **231**
– plantare longum **401**, **402**, **406**, **408**, 409, 451
–– MRI **401**
– plantaria **406**
– popliteum
–– arcuatum **382**, 383, 441
–– obliquum **382**, 383, 441, 442
– pubicum
–– inferius **368**, 370, 371, **372**
–– superius **368**, 369, **372**
– pubofemorale **373**, **374**
–– functions 373
– radiocarpale
–– dorsale **231**
–– palmare **231**
– reflexum **141**, 149, **189**
– retinaculare
–– obliquum 275
–– transversum 275
– sacrococcygeum posterius
–– profundum 370
–– superficiale 370
– sacroiliacum
–– anterius **368**, 369, **371**, **372**
–– interosseum **370**, **371**, **372**
–– posterius **370**, **371**, **372**
– sacrospinale 351, **369**, **370**, **371**, 373, 460
– sacrotuberale 136, 351, **369**, **370**, **371**, 373, 418, **429**, 430, 431, 458, 460, 467, 487
– sternoclaviculare anterius 34, **112**, **214**
– sternocostale
–– intraarticulare 112
–– radiatum **112**
– supraspinale **115**, **116**, **117**, 136, 139, 370
– suspensorium(-ia)
–– mammaria (COOPER ligaments) **183**
–– penis **141**
– talocalcaneum
–– interosseum **401**, 402, **404**
––– MRI **401**
–– laterale 402
–– mediale **403**
–– posterius 403
– talofibulare
–– anterius **402**, 404
–– posterius **403**
– tarsi plantaria **407**
– tarsometatarsalia
–– dorsalia 402, 404
–– plantaria 406, **407**
– teres
–– hepatis 55, 153, **155**, 188
–– uteri **168**
– tibiofibulare
–– anterius 399, 402, **403**, 444
–– posterius 402, 403

Ligamentum(-a)
– transversum
–– acetabuli **374**
–– atlantis **99**, **118**, 119
–– genus 389, **390**
–– scapulae
––– inferius 321, 323
––– superius 207, 216, 219, 220, 246, 249, 321, 323
– transversum atlantis
–– rupture 119
– trapezoideum **216**, 218, **219**, 239
–– AC joint separation 217
– ulnocarpale palmare **231**
– umbilicale
–– medial 191
–– medianum (Chorda urachi) 153, 191, 193
– venosum (ARANTII) 55
Limb
– free 22
– girdle
–– evolution 23
– lower
–– arteries 464, 465
–– bones 348
–– cutaneous nerves 454
–– dermatomes 455
–– joints 348
–– lymphatic vessels 474
–– mechanical axis 349
–– skin innervation 455
–– surface anatomy 346, 347
Limbus acetabuli 354, **355**
Linea(-ae)
– alba **141**, **149**, **153**, 154, 188, 189
– arcuata 151, 155, 188, 194, 350, **354**, 371
–– X-ray image 353
– aspera **356**, 357
–– compression load 25
–– Labium mediale 359
– axillaris
–– anterior 9, 87
–– posterior 9, 85
– epiphysialis 24
–– MRI 401
–– X-ray image 380, 405
– glutea
–– anterior 355
–– inferior 355
–– posterior 355
– intercondylaris 356
– intermedia 354
–– cristae iliacae 354, 355
– intertrochanterica 356
–– X-ray image 358
– mediana
–– anterior 9, 87
–– posterior 9, 85
– medioclavicularis 9, 87
–– surface anatomy 85
– musculi solei 362, 399
– parasternalis 9, 87
– paravertebralis 9, 85
– pectinea 356, 359
– scapularis 9, 85
– semilunaris 151
– sternalis 9, 87
– supracondylaris
–– lateralis 356
–– medialis 356
– terminalis **350**, **351**, 352, 371
–– Diameter transversa 351
–– X-ray image 375
– transversae **108**
– trapezoidea **206**
Lingua
– X-ray image 124
Lingual tonsil *see* Tonsilla lingualis
LISFRANC's joint **364**, 406

LITTRÉ glands 60
Lobuli glandulae mammariae **183**
Lobus(-i)
– frontalis **64**
–– sinister 75
– glandulae
–– mammariae **183**
–– thyroideae 72
– occipitalis **64**, 75
– parietalis 64
– temporalis **64**, 75
Long hair 78
Longitudinal
– arch
–– foot 408, 409
––– tension 408
– axis 7
– ligament (spine)
–– front 113
–– rear 113
– rupture
–– meniscus 392
Lordosis
– cervical spine 95, 103
– lumbar spine 95
– spine 96
Lower leg
– compartments 42
– cross-section 502, 503
– fasciae 414
– musculature 434, 435, 436, 437, 438, 439, 440, 441, 442, 443
– nerves 478, 490, 491, 492, 493, 494
– vessels 478, 490, 491, 492, 493, 494
Lower thigh bones
– connections 399
Low-pressure system **48**, 49, 51, **53**
Lumbalisation 94
Lumbar
– hernia 133
– lordosis **95**
– lordotic curve 96
– puncture 174
– rhombus (MICHAELIS rhomboid) 90
– ribs 89, 93, 106
– spine
–– CT 129, **130**
–– ligaments **113**
–– lordosis 95
–– MRI **130**, **131**
–– operative access 181
–– SCHOBER, method of 152
–– vertebral canal **174**
–– X-ray image 126, 127
– vertebra **106**, **107**
–– X-ray image 127
Lumbosacral joint
– mobility 102
Lunula 79
LUSCHKA's joint 123
Luxatio
– subcoracoidea 223
Luxation 208
Lymph
– capillaries 57
– collecting nodes 57
– collectors
–– arm
––– deep 305
––– superficial 304, 306
–– leg 474, **488**
– duct 57
– node artery 58
– node(s) 57, 58
–– axilla **307**
–– axillary 167
–– B-region 58
–– carcinoma 185
–– examination 58

Lymph node(s)
–– genital region of the woman 168
–– inguinal 167
––– inflammations 168
––– tumours 168
–– inguinal region 475
–– Mamma 184
––– level 184
–– palpation 307, 475
–– regional 57
–– station
––– dorsolateral **488**
––– ventromedial **488**
–– structure **58**
–– T-region 58
–– trunk wall 167
–– veins 58
–– vessels
––– arm 304, 305
––– axilla **306**
–– genital region of the woman 168
–– Mamma 184
–– ovary 168
–– trunk wall 167
–– uterine FALLOPIAN tube 168
–– uterus 168
–– vagina 168
Lymphadenectomy 307
Lymphatic
– bundle
–– deep anterior **490**
–– leg 490
–– ventromedial **490**
– valves **57**
– vessels
–– inguinal region 475
–– leg 474
–– lymph system 57
–– system **57**
Lymphocyte 58
Lymphoedema 52

M

Macrocirculation 48
Macrophage 58
Magnetic resonance imaging 75
– brain 75
– knee joint **75**
– lumbar spine **130**, **131**
– thoracic spine **130**
MAISONNEUVE fracture **399**
Malleolar
– canal 462, **492**, **493**, **496**, **497**, **498**
–– tibial compression 492
– fork 399
Malleolus
– lateralis **363**, **399**, 400, 402, 403, 438, 439, 440, 444, 446, 447, 448, 479, 492, 493
–– surface anatomy 346, **347**
–– X-ray image 405
– medialis **363**, **399**, 400, 403, 438, 440, 441, 442, 444, 446, 448, 479, 493
–– surface anatomy 346, **347**
–– X-ray image 405
MALT (mucosa associated lymphatic tissue) 58
Mamma **182**
– blood supply **184**, 187
– carcinoma 185
– lymph nodes 185
– development 182
– lymph drainage 184
– mammography 185
– structure **183**
Mammary
– gland 183
–– aplasia 182
–– blood supply **184**
–– lymph drainage 184
– hypertrophy 182

Mammography 185
– breast cancer 185
Mandibula 21
Manubrium sterni 91, **111**, 112, 147, 148, 166, 214
– projection onto the chest wall 85
– surface anatomy 85
– X-ray image 215
Manus 4, 5, 204
– arteries **303**, **337**
– cutaneous innervation 280
– development 202
– dorsal aponeurosis **272**
– joints **231**
– main lines 9
– musculature 266, 267, 269, 270, 271
– pronation 11
– skeleton 212
– supination 11
– tendon sheaths **268**
–– variants 268
Marginal ridge 203
Margo
– anterior 362
–– fibulae 363
–– radii 211
–– tibiae **346**
– falciformis 414
– interosseus
–– fibulae 363
–– radii **211**, 229
–– tibiae 362
–– ulnae **210**, 229
– lateralis
–– humeri 208
–– scapulae 207
––– X-ray image 223
– liber unguis 79
– medialis
–– humeri 208
–– scapulae 207
–– tibiae 362
– posterior
–– fibulae 363
–– radii 211
–– ulnae 210
– superior scapulae 207
Massa lateralis atlantis 98
Matrix
– pili 78
– unguis 79
Maxilla 21
MCP see Metacarpophalangeal joint
– finger 233
–– muscles 235, 273
– thumbs
–– muscles 235, 273
Mechanical axis, leg 349
Medial 9
– meniscus
–– injury 392
Median 9
– plane 7, 205
Mediotrusion
– jaw 8
Medulla
– oblongata 69
– ossium
–– flava 28
–– rubra 28
– spinalis 62, 64, 122, 173, 175, **177**, 199, 278
–– dorsal root **66**
Medullary sinus 58
MEISSNER corpuscles 76
Melanin (hair) 78
Melanocytes 78
Membrana
– atlantooccipitalis
–– anterior **118**, **120**
–– posterior **118**, **120**, 140
– fibrosa capsulae articularis 32, **225**, **388**, 391
– intercostalis interna 136, 147

Membrana
– interossea
–– antebrachii **229**, **262**, 331, 335, 337, 339
–– cruris 30, 42, 382, **399**, 400, 403, 489, **502**, 503
– obturatoria **368**, 371, 373, 374, 483
– subpleuralis [SIBSON fascia] 144
– synovialis capsulae articularis **32**, **388**
– tectoria **118**
Membrum
– inferius 4, 5
–– bones and joints 348
– superius 4, 5
–– bones and joints **204**
Meniscus(-ci) 34, 385, 391
– injury 392
– lateralis 34, 382, 383, 385, 389, **390**, 392
–– arthroscopy 398
–– attachment **388**
–– MRI 397
– medialis 34, 383, 385, **386**, 389, **390**, 392
–– attachment **388**
–– injury 392
–– MRI 397
– movability 390
– ruptures 392
– supply 391
Meralgia
– paraesthetica 457
Mesoderm 19, 88
Mesorchium
– testicular torsion 191
Mesotendineum 44, 340
Metacarpal
– joints **230**
– ligaments 231
Metacarpophalangeal joint
– finger 233
–– muscles 235, 273
– movements **233**
– thumb 234
–– muscles 235, 273
Metacarpus 212
– cross-section **340**
Metaphysis
– blood supply 24
– distalis 24
– proximalis 24
Metapodium 22
Metatarsophalangeal joint, range of movement 413
Metatarsus 348
MICHAELIS
– rhombus of 13, 90
Microcirculation 48, 49
Microfibril, collagen 43
Middle finger, cross-section **340**
MIKULICZ line 349
Milk line **182**
Mineralisation zone 32
MOHRENHEIM's fossa (Trigonum clavipectorale) 315
MORGAGNI hernia 158
Morula 18
Motion segment
– spine 89, 102
Movement
– musculature 37
– scapulohumeral 222
Muscle(s) **20**
– fascia 42
– fibre
–– red 41
–– types 41
–– white 41
– insertion 42
– lever 47
– line of force 42
– origin 42
– phasic 37
– shoulder girdle 132

Muscle(s)
– skeletal musculature 41
– smooth 41
– stiffness and ache 46
– strain 46
– tendon insertion site 45
– tonic 37
– trunk 132
– types 41
– virtual lever 42
Muscular pump **54**
Musculature
– arm 236, 237, 238
– back
–– deep 135
––– schematic 134
–– superficial **132**
– chest **238**
– dorsal
–– hips 426, 427, 429, 430, 431
–– thigh 428, 429, 430, 431
– dorsum of the foot 446, 447
– dystonia **256**
– foot 438, 439
– forearm
–– dorsal **258**, **259**, 260, 261, 262
–– radial **258**
–– ventral **253**, **254**, **255**, **256**, **257**
– hand 266, 267, 269, 270, 271
– heart muscles 41
– hips 415, 416, 417, 418
– ischiocrural 430
–– thigh 428
– knee joint 432, 433
– leg 415, 416
– lower leg 434, 435, 436, 437, 438, 439, 440, 441, 442, 443
– medial
–– hips 421
–– thigh 421, 422, 423, 424, 425
– mimic 37
– palm of the hand 266, 267, 269, 270, 271
– pelvitrochanteric
–– hips 427
– rotator cuff 239
– shoulder 236, 237, **242**, 243, **244**, 245, 246, **247**
–– dorsal **251**, **252**
– shoulder girdle 132, 240, 246, 247
– skeletal musculature 41
– smooth 41
– sole of the foot 449, 450, 451
– spasticity 256
– spinoscapular 240
– thigh 417, 418
– trunk 132
– types **41**
– upper arm (Brachium)
–– dorsal **248**, **252**, **259**, 260
–– ventral **248**, **249**, **250**, **251**
– ventral
–– hips 419, 420, 422, 423, 424, 425
–– thigh 422, 423, 424, 425
Musculoskeletal system **20**
Musculus(-i)
– abdominis 141, 142, **149**, **150**, **151**, **156**, **159**
–– CT **154**
–– functions 152
– abductor
–– digiti minimi
––– manus 39, 266, 267, 268, 269, 334, 340
––– pedis 444, 446, 447, **449**, 450, 451, 497, 498
–– hallucis 445, 448, **449**, 450, 451, 497, 498
––– Tendo 445
–– pollicis
––– brevis 266, 267, 268, 269, 290, 333, 334, 336
––– longus 39, 201, 235, 237, 238, 254, 255, 256, 258, 259, 260, **261**, **262**, 269, 288, 303, 330, 331, 335, **336**, 337, 339, 340

Musculus(-i)
- adductor
-- brevis 421, **424**, 425, 456, 482, **500**
-- hallucis 451, 498
--- Caput 401, 449, 450, 498
-- longus 37, 38, 415, 418, 421, **422**, 423, 424, 425, 456, 480, 481, 482, **500**, 501
-- magnus 39, 395, 418, 421, **424**, **425**, 429, 430, **431**, 433, 456, 481, 482, 486, 487, **500**, 501
--- hip joint 376
--- Tendo 382, 383, 425, 433
-- minimus 39, **425**, 429, 430, **431**
-- pollicis 238, 269, 292, 333, 334, 335, 336, 340
--- brevis 38
--- Caput transversum 267, 268
--- thenar 267
- anconeus 39, 201, 237, 238, 248, 252, 259, 260, 261, 262, 331
- arrector pili 68, 76, 78
- articularis genus 381
- biceps 46
-- brachii 37, 38, 142, 200, 201, 236, 238, 246, 250, **251**, 252, 254, 255, **263**, 287, 318, **319**, 322, 324, 328, 329, 338
--- aponeurosis 300, 301
--- Caput 143, 201, 218, 219, 224, 239, 246, 248, **249**, 250, 252
--- elbow joint 227
--- functions 248
--- lever arm 47
--- MRI 338
--- supination 263
--- Tendo 225, 229, **249**, 254, 255, 256, 257, **263**, 324, 325
-- femoris 39, 396, 416, 428, 439, 440, 441, 442, 458, 484, 488, 489, 492
--- Caput 417, 418, 429, **430**, **431**, 433, 462, 463, 485, 486, 500, 501
--- knee joint 393
--- Tendo 382, 383, 433, 443, 484
- biventer 46
- brachialis 38, 47, 142, 201, 236, 238, 248, **249**, 250, **251**, 252, 254, 255, 256, 257, 259, 260, 287, 288, 300, **319**, 322, 324, 325, 326, 327, 329, 338
-- functions 248
-- lever arm 47
-- MRI 338
-- Tendo 255
- brachioradialis 37, 38, 200, 201, 236, 237, 238, 249, 250, **251**, 252, 254, 255, 256, 257, 258, **259**, 260, 261, **263**, 288, 301, 324, 325, 328, 329, 339
-- functions 258
-- lever arm 47
-- pronation 263
-- supination 263
-- Tendo 201, 254, 255, 256, 257, 267
- buccinator 38
- colli **140**
- coracobrachialis 143, 239, 246, 248, **249**, **250**, 277, 279, 287, 296, 314, **318**, **319**, 338
-- functions **248**
- corrugator supercilii 38
- cremaster 141, 149, 150, **189**, 190, **191**, **192**, **193**, 194
-- reflex 189
- dartos 194
- deltoideus 37, 38, 39, 141, 142, 143, 170, 200, 201, 236, 237, 238, 239, 245, **246**, 247, 249, 250, **251**, 252, 285, 316, 322
-- arm abduction 222
-- atrophy of plexus lesion 199
-- fascia 308
-- functions 245
-- paralysis **285**

Musculus(-i) deltoideus
-- Pars
--- acromialis 245
--- clavicularis 245, **315**
--- spinal s 245
-- plexus lesion 278
-- shoulder dislocation 223
-- shoulder joint 220
-- surface anatomy 84
- depressor
-- labii inferioris 38
-- supercilii 38
- digastricus
-- Venter posterior 136, 139, 140
- dorsi 175
-- CT 129
-- deep layer 136, 137
-- schematic 134
-- superficial layer 135
- epicranius 172
- erector spinae 133, 135, **137**, 138, 154
-- functions 135
-- schematic 134
-- surface anatomy 84
- extensor
-- carpi
--- radialis 39, 201, 235, 236, 237, 238, **251**, 252, 254, 255, 256, 257, 258, **259**, 260, **261**, 262, 264, 272, 288, 324, 328, 330, 331, 336, 339
--- ulnaris 37, 39, 201, 235, 237, 258, **259**, **260**, 261, 262, 264, 272, 330, 331, 335, 339
-- digiti minimi 37, 39, 201, 258, **260**, **261**, 264, 288, 339, 340
--- dorsal extension 235
--- finger extension 273
--- functions 258
--- Tendo **259**, 272, 330, 339
-- digitorum
--- brevis pedis 38, 438, 439, 444, 445, **446**, **447**, 463, 491
--- digiti minimi 261
--- longus pedis 401, 412, 414, 415, 434, **438**, **439**, 444, 445, 446, 447, 463, 469, 490, 491, 495, 502
--- manus 37, 39, 201, 235, 237, 238, 258, **259**, **260**, 261, **264**, 265, 270, **272**, 273, 274, 275, 288, 328, 330, 331, 336, 337, 339, 340
--- pedis 495
-- hallucis
--- brevis 38, 438, 439, 444, 445, **446**, **447**, 463, 495
--- longus 38, 412, 414, 415, 434, **438**, **439**, 444, 445, 446, 447, 469, 490, 491, 495, 502
-- indicis 39, 258, **261**, **262**, 288
--- dorsal extension 235
--- finger extension 273
--- functions 258
--- Tendo 339
-- pollicis
--- brevis 39, 201, 235, 237, 238, 255, 258, 259, 260, **261**, **262**, **264**, **272**, 273, 288, 330, 331, 335, **336**, 339, 340
--- longus 39, 201, 235, 237, 238, 258, 259, **261**, **262**, **264**, **272**, 273, 288, 331, 335, **336**, 337, 339, 340
- fibularis [peroneus]
-- brevis 412, 435, **438**, **439**, 443, 445, 463, 491, 492, 494, 502
--- functions **435**
--- Tendo 4C2, 404, 407, **439**, **444**, 445, 446, 447
-- longus 37, 38, 39, 412, 415, 435, **438**, **439**, 441, 442, 445, 463, 490, 491, 492, 494, 502
--- ankle joint 435
--- functions 435
--- Tendo 401, **407**, 409, **439**, 450, **451**
-- tertius 447
--- Tendo **438**, 439, **444**, 445, 446, 447, 491

Musculus(-i)
- flexor
-- carpi
--- radialis 37, 38, 201, 235, 236, 238, 253, **254**, **255**, 256, 257, 263, 269, 290, 291, 293, 303, 324, 326, 327, 333, 334, 339
--- ulnaris 37, 38, 39, 201, 235, 236, 253, **254**, **255**, **256**, 257, 259, 260, 261, 262, 267, 268, 292, 301, 302, 303, 324, 326, 327, 333, 334, 339
-- digiti minimi 267
--- brevis 268, 269, 449, 450, 451
--- hypothenar 266
-- digitorum
--- brevis 401, 408, 445, **449**, 450, 451, 470, 497, 498
--- longus 39, 401, 412, 437, **441**, **442**, 443, **450**, 451, 462, 493, 494, 498, 502
--- profundus 79, 235, 236, **253**, 257, 267, **269**, 271, 273, 274, 275, 290, **291**, 292, 293, 302, 329, 337, 339, 340
--- superficialis 235, 236, 253, **254**, 255, **256**, 257, 267, **269**, 271, 273, 274, 275, 290, **291**, 293, 324, 325, 326, 327, 337, 339, 340
-- hallucis
--- brevis 449, 450, **451**, 497, 498
--- longus 39, 401, 409, 412, 437, **441**, **442**, 443, 449, **450**, 451, 462, 493, 494, 497, 498, 502
-- pollicis
--- brevis 266, 267, 268, 269, 290, 292, 333, 334, 340
--- longus 235, 253, 254, 255, 256, **257**, 267, 269, 273, 290, **291**, 293, 324, 339, 340
- fusiformis 46
- gastrocnemius 38, 39, 395, 414, 416, 436, 438, **439**, **441**, 462, 484, 488, 492
-- Caput
--- laterale 382, 383, 384, 396, 417, 430, 431, 433, **440**, 441, 442, 485, 488, 489, 492
--- mediale 382, 384, 396, 415, 430, 431, 432, 433, **440**, 441, 442, 443, 468, 485, 488, 489, 492, 502
-- surface anatomy 347
-- Tendo 414
-- walking 413
- gemellus
-- inferior 39, 427, **429**, 430, 431, 458, 486, 487, 500
-- superior 39, 427, **429**, 430, 431, 458, 486, 487, 500
- gluteus
-- maximus 39, 142, 416, 417, 418, 426, **429**, 430, 431, 458, **460**, 467, 484, 485, 486, 487, **500**
--- functions 426
--- hip joint 376
--- incorrect injection 460
--- location on hip joint 500
--- surface anatomy 84, 347
--- Tractus iliotibialis 345
-- medius 39, 153, 416, 423, 424, 425, 427, **429**, **430**, 431, 458, **460**, 467, 486, 487, **500**
--- DUCHENNE sign 461
--- fascia **429**, 484
--- functions 427
--- hip joint 376
--- injection 460, 486
--- intragluteal injection **460**
--- location on hip joint 500
--- TRENDELENBURG sign 461
-- minimus 39, 427, **430**, 431, 458, 467, 487, **500**
--- DUCHENNE sign 461
--- functions 427
--- hip joint 376
--- location on hip joint 500
--- TRENDELENBURG sign 461

Appendix

Musculus(-i)
– gracilis 37, 38, 39, 415, 416, 418, 421, **422**, 423, 424, 425, 429, 430, 431, **432**, 433, 440, 456, 480, 481, 482, 484, 485, 488, 489, 501
–– Tendo **396**, 425, 432, 433
– iliacus 153, **156**, 188, 415, 418, 419, 422, 423, 456, 480, 481, 482, 483
–– functions 156
– iliocostalis
–– cervicis 134, **135**, 139, **140**
–– functions 152
–– lumborum 134, **135**, 153
–– thoracis 134, **135**, 170
– iliopsoas 38, 159, 188, 415, 419, **422**, 423, 424, 425, **483**, **500**
–– functions 419
–– hip joint 376
–– location on hip joint 500
–– spasticity (muscle spasms) 419
–– Tendo 431
–– walking 413
– infraspinatus 39, 132, 133, 135, 142, 170, 237, **239**, 243, 246, 247, 252, 282
–– functions 243
–– insertion site 209
–– paralysis 207
–– rotator cuff 224, 239
–– shoulder joint 220
–– Tendo **224**
– intercartilaginei 150, 151
– intercostalis(-es) 153
–– externus(-i) 144, 145, **147**, 148, 150, 151, 246
––– course 147
––– fascia 136
––– functions 147
–– internus(-i) 143, 144, 145, **147**, 148, 149, 246
–– intimus 144
– interfoveolaris
–– fascia 188
– interossei 292, 471
–– dorsales 39, 237, 238, 264, 265, 267, **269**, 270, 272, 273, 274, 275, 334, 335, **336**, **337**, 340, 446, 447
––– abduction 271
––– finger extension 273
––– finger flexion 273
––– finger movement 235
––– functions 270, 272, 451
––– pedis 401, 444, 450, **451**
–– palmares 267, **269**, 270, 272, 273, 274, 275, 334, 337, 340
––– adduction 271
––– finger extension 273
––– finger flexion 273
––– finger movement 235
––– functions 270, 272
–– plantares I–III 449, 450, 451
––– functions 451
– intersectus 46
– interspinales
–– cervicis 134, **136**, 139, 173
–– lumborum 134, **136**
–– thoracis 134
– intertransversarii
–– laterales lumborum 136, 137, 174
–– mediales lumborum 136, 137, 174
–– posteriores 134
––– cervicis 136, 140
––– laterales cervicis 139
–– thoracis 136
– ischiococcygeus [coccygeus] 418
– latissimus dorsi 37, 39, **132**, 133, 135, 138, **141**, 142, 143, 150, 151, 153, 158, 170, 171, 200, 237, 238, 242, **246**, 247, 251, 279, 284, 296, 314, 315, **316**, 318
–– covering defects 132
–– functions 132, **242**
–– surface anatomy 84

Musculus(-i)
– levator(-es)
–– anguli oris 38
–– costarum
––– breves 136, 137
––– functions 152
––– longi 136, 137
–– labii superiores alaeque nasi 38
–– scapulae 39, **47**, **133**, 135, 140, 170, 171, **246**, 247, 282
––– functions 133
––– lifting the shoulders 240
––– shoulder girdle muscles 240
– longissimus
–– capitis 134, **135**, 136, 139, 140, 170, 171, 172
–– cervicis 134, **135**, 139, 140
–– functions 152
–– thoracis 134, **135**, 153, 170
– longus colli 147
– lumbricales
–– manus 266, 267, 268, **269**, 271, 275, 334, 336, 337, 340
––– finger extension 235, 273
––– finger flexion 273, 274
––– functions 271, 272
––– Tendines 270, 272
–– pedis 449, **450**, 451, 497
– masseter 37, 38
– mentalis 38
– multifidus(-i) **136**, **137**, 139, 140, 170, 172
–– cervicis 134
–– functions 152
–– lumborum 134
–– thoracis 134
– nasalis 38
– obliquus
–– capitis
––– inferior 136, 139, **140**, **172**, 173
––– superior 136, 139, **140**, **172**, 173
–– externus abdominis 37, 38, 39, 132, 133, 135, 136, 138, **141**, 142, 143, **149**, 150, 151, 153, 154, 159, 170, 181, 187, 189, 190, 191, 192, 193, 194, 195, 238, 246, 417, 487
––– aponeurosis 141, 142, 149, 153, 154, **189**, 190, 191, 193, 194
––– functions 149, 152
––– rectus sheath 153
–– internus abdominis 38, 39, 133, 135, 136, 138, **149**, **150**, 151, 153, 154, 159, 181, **189**, 190, 191, 192, 193, 194, 195
––– aponeurosis 149, 151, 154
––– course **150**
––– functions **150**, 152
––– rectus sheath 153
– obturatorius
–– externus **425**, 427, **431**, 456, 487, 500
––– hip surgery 487
–– internus 39, 418, 427, **429**, 430, 431, 458, 486, 487
––– Tendo 431, 500
– occipitofrontalis 38
–– Venter occipitalis 172
– omohyoideus
–– Venter
––– inferior 246, 247, 249
––– superior 317
– opponens
–– digiti minimi
––– manus 267, 268, 269, 340
––– pedis 444, 451
–– pollicis 267, 268, 269, 290, 334, 336, 340
––– thenar 266
– orbicularis
–– oculi 38
–– oris 38
– palmaris
–– brevis 38, 266, 301, 332
––– hypothenar 266

Musculus(-i), palmaris
–– longus 38, 201, 236, 253, **254**, **255**, **256**, 263, 290, 324
––– palmar flexion 235
––– Tendo **254**, **255**, 256, 257, 266, 326, 327, 339
– pectineus 38, 415, 421, **422**, 423, 424, 425, 456, 480, 481, 483, **500**
– pectoralis
–– major 37, 38, **141**, **143**, 150, 151, 182, 183, 236, 238, 246, 251, 279, 284, 296, 314, 315, 316, 317, 318, 319
––– covering defects 132
––– fascia 308
––– functions 141, **244**
––– Pars 141, 142, 143, 149, 201, 244, **315**
––– shoulder joint 220
––– Tendo 249, 252
–– minor 38, **143**, 241, **246**, 249, 250, 279, 284, 296, 314, **316**, 317
––– axillary sections 297, 299
––– functions 143, 241
––– lymph nodes level of the Mamma 184, **307**
– pennatus 46
– piriformis 39, 418, 423, 424, 425, 427, **429**, 430, 431, 458, 460, 467, 486, 487
–– Tendo **500**
– plantaris 39, 382, 433, 436, **440**, **441**, 442, 443, 462, 489, 493, 494
–– Tendo **440**, **441**, 492
– planus 46
– popliteus **382**, 384, 395, 436, **442**, **443**, 462, 489, 494
–– aponeurosis 382
–– functions 437
–– Tendo **382**, 383, 388, 391
– procerus 38
– pronator
–– quadratus 253, 254, 255, 256, **257**, 263, 267, 290, 334, 337
––– functions 253
––– pronation 263
–– teres 38, 236, 238, 253, **254**, **255**, **256**, 257, 263, 290, 324, 325, 326, 327, 329, 339
––– Caput 257, **263**, 326, 327
––– elbow joint 227
––– functions 253
––– pronation **263**
––– Tendo 261, 262
– psoas
–– major 138, 153, **156**, 157, 158, 181, 195, 415, 418, 419, 422, 423, 456, 483
––– CT 129
––– functions 152, 156
––– shortening 418
–– minor 153, 156, 158, 422
––– Tendo 156, 418, 483
– pyramidalis **149**, 150, 151, 153, 191, 194
–– functions **149**
–– rectus sheath 153
– quadratus
–– femoris 39, **425**, 427, **429**, 430, **431**, 458, 486, 487, 500
––– hip surgery 487
–– lumborum 138, 153, 154, **156**, 157, 158, 174, 181, 195
––– fascia 133
––– functions 152, 156
–– plantae 401, **450**, 451, 497, 498
––– functions 450
– quadriceps femoris 37, 381, 415, 420, **423**, 439
–– knee joint 393
–– patella function **361**
–– surface anatomy 346
–– Tendo 75, 381, 383, 386, 387, **395**, 414
–– walking 413
– rectus
–– abdominis **149**, **150**, 151, **153**, 154, 155, 166, 181, 187, 188, 191, 193, 194, 246

Appendix

Musculus(-i) rectus abdominis
––– development 88
––– functions **149**, 152
––– Intersectio tendinea 149
––– rectus sheath 153
–– capitis
––– lateralis 139, 140
––– posterior 118, 136, 139, **140**, **172**, 173
–– femoris 37, 38, 395, 415, 417, 418, 420, **422**, 423, 424, 425, 456, 480, 481, 482, 501
––– location on hip joint 500
––– Tendo 373, 374, 423, 424, **500**
––– walking 413
– rhomboideus
–– major 39, **47**, 132, **133**, 135, 171, 172, 240, 247, 282
––– functions 133
––– shrugging the shoulders 240
–– minor 39, **47**, **133**, 171, 172, 247, 282
––– functions 133
––– shoulder girdle muscles 240
––– shrugging the shoulders 240
– risorius 38
– rotatores
–– breves
––– cervicis 134
––– lumborum 134
––– thoracis 134
–– longi
––– cervicis 134
––– lumborum 134
––– thoracis 134
–– thoracis **137**
––– breves **136**
––– longi **136**
– sartorius 37, 38, 142, 415, 417, 418, 420, **422**, 423, 424, 425, **432**, **433**, 456, 480, 481, 482, 485, **500**, 501
–– location on hip joint 500
–– surface anatomy 346
–– Tendo **396**, 424, 425
– scalenus
–– anterior 147, 246, 279, 296, 314, 317
–– medius **140**, 147, 173, 246, 277, 317
–– posterior 135, **140**, 147, 246
– semimembranosus 39, 384, 395, 416, 417, 418, 428, **430**, 431, **432**, 433, 440, 441, 458, 462, 484, 485, 486, 488, 489, 492, 501
–– knee joint 393
–– Tendo 382, 383, **396**, 430, 431, 432, 433, 440, 442, **500**
– semipennatus 46
– semispinalis
–– capitis 134, **135**, **136**, **139**, 140, 171, 172, 173
––– schematic 139
–– cervicis 134, 135, **136**, 139, 172
––– schematic 139
–– functions 152
–– thoracis **136**, 139, **140**
––– schematic 139
– semitendinosus 37, 39, 395, 416, 418, 428, 429, **430**, 431, **432**, **433**, 440, 458, 462, 484, 485, 486, 488, 489, 492, **500**, 501
–– Tendo **396**, 425, 430, 431, 432, 433, 440
– serratus
–– anterior 37, 39, 133, 135, **141**, 142, 143, 144, 145, 149, 150, 158, 182, 194, 238, 241, **246**, 247, 279, 283, 296, 314, 315
––– arm abduction 222
––– arm elevation 222
––– fascia **145**
––– functions 241
––– lesion 241
––– origin 92
––– Scapula alata 283
–– posterior
––– inferior 39, 133, 135, 138
––– superior 133, 135, 170

Musculus(-i)
– soleus 38, 39, 395, 415, 416, 436, 438, **439**, **440**, **441**, **442**, 443, 462, 468, 489, 492, 493, 494, 502
– spinalis
–– capitis 134, **136**
–– cervicis 134
–– functions 152
–– thoracis 134, **135**
– splenius
–– capitis 39, 132, **133**, 134, **135**, 136, **139**, 140, 171, 172
––– schematic 139
–– cervicis 39, **133**, 134, **135**, 139, 140
––– schematic 139
–– functions 152
– sternalis **143**
– sternocleidomastoideus 37, 38, 39, 132, 133, 135, 141, 171, 180, 238, 246, 279, 296, 314, 317
–– Tendo 143
– sternohyoideus **147**
– sternothyroideus 147
– subclavius 143, 241, **246**, 249, 279, 283, 296, 314, 315, 317
– subcostalis 148
– suboccipitales **136**, **139**, **140**
– subscapularis **224**, **239**, 243, **246**, **247**, 249, 250, 279, 284, 296, 314, 318
–– course 247
–– functions **243**
–– rotator cuff **224**, **239**
–– shoulder joint 220
–– Tendo 219, **224**
– supinator 255, 256, 257, 258, **261**, **262**, **263**, 288, 302, 325, 326, 327, 328, 331
–– elbow joint 227
–– functions **258**
–– supination 263
– supraspinatus 39, 218, **224**, **239**, 245, 246, 247, 249, 251, 282
–– functions 245
–– impingement 224
–– insertion site 209
–– paralysis 207
–– rotator cuff 224, **239**
–– shoulder, roof 246
–– Tendo 219, **224**
–– tendon injury 224
– tensor
–– fasciae
––– latae 345
– tensor fasciae latae 37, 38, 39, 142, 159, 414, 415, 417, 420, **422**, 423, 426, 430, 458, 480, **500**
–– functions 420
–– location on hip joint 500
–– surface anatomy 346
– teres
–– major 37, 39, **132**, 133, 135, 142, **170**, 201, 237, 238, 243, **246**, **247**, 249, **251**, **252**, 284, 315, 318, **320**, 321, 322
––– axillary space 170, 321
––– course 247
––– functions **132**, 243
––– surface anatomy 84
–– minor 39, 142, **170**, 224, 237, 238, **239**, 243, 247, 252, 285, **320**, 321
––– axillary space 170, 320, 321
––– functions 243
––– insertion site 209
––– rotator cuff 224, **239**
– thoracis 141, 142, **143**
– tibialis
–– anterior 37, 38, 412, 415, 434, **438**, **439**, 463, 469, 490, 491, 502
––– ankle joint 412
––– functions 434
––– Tendo 401, 402, 407, 414, 438, 439, **444**, 446, 447, 490, 495
––– walking 413

Musculus(-i) tibialis
–– posterior 39, 412, 437, **442**, 443, 462, 493, 494, 502
––– functions **437**
––– Tendo 402, 407, 409, **441**, **442**, 443, **451**, 492, 493, 494
– transversospinales 138
– transversus
–– abdominis 38, 136, 138, 151, 153, 154, 155, 156, 158, 159, 181, **189**, 190, 191, 192, 193, 194, 195
––– aponeurosis 151, 153, 154, 188
––– functions 151
–– thoracis **147**, 166
––– functions **147**
– trapezius 37, 38, 39, **132**, 133, 135, 139, 140, 142, 171, 180, 201, 237, 238, **246**, 247, 250, 251
–– AC joint separation 217
–– arm abduction 222
–– arm elevation 222
–– functions 132, 152
–– Pars
––– ascendens 240
––– descendens 240
––– transversa 240
–– shoulder girdle muscles 240
–– shrugging the shoulders 240
–– surface anatomy 84
– triceps
–– brachii 37, 39, 142, 200, 201, 237, 288
––– axillary space 170, 320, 321
––– Caput 142, **170**, 201, **218**, 238, 239, **247**, 249, **250**, **251**, **252**, 254, 255, 256, 259, 260, 261, 318, 319, **320**, 321, 322, 323, 338
––– elbow joint 227
––– insertion site 210
––– lever arm 47
––– MRI 338
––– radial lesion 289
––– shoulder joint 220
––– Tendo 252, 261
––– triangular interval 320, 321
–– surae 37, 412
––– ankle joint 412
––– functions 440
––– Tendo calcaneus, MRI 401
– vastus
–– intermedius 37, 38, 420, **424**, 425, 456, 501
–– lateralis 37, 38, 415, 417, 420, **422**, 423, 424, 425, 430, 431, 433, 439, 456, 480, 482, 484, 501
–– medialis 37, 38, 395, 415, 420, **422**, 423, 424, 425, 432, 433, 456, 480, 481, 482, 501
Myofibril 40
Myofilament 40
Myosin filament 40
Myotome 88, 89

N

Nail(s) **79**
– bed 79
– brittle 79
– crumbling 79
– dystrophy 79
– mycosis 79
– plate 79
–– white spots 79
– wall 79
Nasus 72
Navel hernia 154
Navicular fracture **230**
Neck (Collum)
– fracture 119
– muscles **136**, 139, **140**
–– short 136, **139**
– nerves 171, 172, **173**
– vessels 171, 172, **173**

Necrosis of the femoral head **377**
Nerve(s)
– axilla 308, 314, 316, 317, 318, 319
– axillary space
–– lateral 170
–– medial 170
– back **170**, 171
– back of the hand **313**, 335, 336
– chest wall 316, 317
– cubital fossa 310, 312, 328
– dorsum of the foot 479, 495
– elbow 309, 329
– fibres
–– afferent 63
–– plexus 67
–– somatic motor 63
–– somatic sensory 63
–– visceral motor 63
–– visceral sensory 63
– foot 478
– forearm 312, 324, 325, 326, 327, 330, 331
– gluteal region 487
– inguinal canal **189**
– inguinal region 476, 483
– injury 66
– intercostal space 146
– knee 476
– lower leg 478, 490, 491, 492, 493, 494
– neck 171, 172, 173
– occipital region 172
– palm of the hand 332, 333, 334
– popliteal fossa 477, 484, 485, 486, 488, 492, 493, 494
– shoulder 309, 310, **323**
– sole of the foot 496, 497, 498
– thigh 476, 477, 480, 481, 482, 484, 485, 486, 487
– trunk wall
–– anterior 187
–– dorsal **170**
– upper arm 318, 319, **322**
– vertebral canal 174, 178
Nervous system
– autonomic 62, **68**
–– disorders 68
– central 62
– enteric 68
– functions 62
– information flow **63**
– peripheral 62
– somatic 62
– structure **62**
Nervus(-i)
– accessorius [XI] **171**, **172**, 279, 314
– anococcygeus 452
– auricularis magnus 170, **171**
–– R. posterior 169
– axillaris 67, **170**, 276, **277**, **279**, **280**, **285**, **286**, 314, 315, 319, 322, **323**
–– axillary space 321, 323
––– lateral 170
–– cutaneous innervation 280
–– humerus fracture 209
–– injury 208
–– lesion **285**
–– pathway 319
–– Plexus brachialis 276
–– segmentation **285**
– cardiacus cervicalis
–– inferior 69
–– medius 69
–– superior 69
– cervicales 65, 173
– clunium
–– inferiores 169, **477**, 484, 485
–– medii 169, **454**, **477**, 484, 485
–– superiores 169, 170, **454**, **477**, 485
– coccygeus 65, 452
– craniales 62

Nervus(-i)
– cutaneus
–– antebrachii
––– lateralis 201, 280, 286, **287**, **309**, **312**, **319**, 322, 323, 332
––– medialis 67, 201, 276, 277, **279**, **280**, **286**, **309**, **312**, 314, 318
––– posterior 201, 280, 286, 288, **309**, **310**, **312**, 313, 322, **323**, 336
–– brachii
––– lateralis 169, 170, 280, **285**, 286, **288**, **310**, **322**, **323**
––– medialis 67, 201, 276, 277, **279**, **280**, **286**, 299, **309**, 310, 312, 314, 317, 318
––– posterior 169, 170, 201, 280, 286, **288**, **310**, 312, **322**, **323**
–– cruris medialis 479
–– dorsalis
––– intermedius 453, 454, **463**, **478**, **479**
––– lateralis 453, 454, 463, **478**, **479**
––– medialis 453, 454, **463**, **478**, **479**
–– femoris
––– lateralis 159, 169, 188, **195**, 452, **453**, **454**, 456, 457, **476**, 477, **480**, 481, **483**
––– posterior 169, 452, **453**, **454**, 458, 459, **460**, 461, **477**, 484, 485, 486, **487**, 500
–– surae
––– lateralis 453, 454, **463**, **478**, 484, **485**, 486, 488
––– medialis 453, **462**, 463, 478, 484, **485**, 486, 488, 503
–– digitales
––– dorsales
–––– manus 280, **288**, 313, 336, 340
–––– pedis 453, 454, 479, **491**, 495
––– palmares
–––– communes 280, 286, **290**, **333**
–––– proprii 280, 286, 332, **333**, 340
––– plantares
–––– communes **496**, 497, 498
–––– proprii 496, 498
–– dorsalis scapulae 171, 172, 276, 277, 279, 282, 314, 321
––– pathway 314
––– Plexus brachialis 276
–– facialis [VII] 68, 69
–– femoralis 159, 188, **195**, **453**, **454**, **456**, 466, **480**, 481, **482**, **483**, 500
––– functions 452, 456
––– lesion 457
––– pathway 456, 480
––– plexus **452**
––– Rr. cutanei anteriores 187, **195**, 454
–– fibularis [peroneus]
––– communis **396**, 452, 453, **454**, **458**, 462, 463, 468, **484**, **485**, 486, **488**, **491**, 492, 493
–––– functions 458, 463
–––– lesion 459, 463, 491
–––– pathway 458, 463, 485, 491
––– profundus 453, **454**, **463**, **479**, **491**, 495, **502**, 503
–––– functions 463
–––– lesion 463
–––– pathway 463, 491
––– superficialis 453, **454**, **463**, **478**, **479**, **491**, **502**, 503
–––– functions 463
–––– lesion 463
–––– pathway 463, 478, 491
–– genitofemoralis **195**, **453**, **454**, **456**
––– cremasteric reflex 189
––– functions 456
––– lesion 457
––– pathway 456
––– plexus 452
––– referred pain 457
––– R. femoralis 187, 190, **195**, 483
––– R. genitalis 189, 190, **191**, **195**
–– glossopharyngeus [IX] 68, 69

Nervus(-i)
– gluteus
–– inferior **453**, **458**, **460**, **486**, **487**, 500
––– functions 452, 458
––– lesion 461
––– pathway 458, 486
––– plexus **452**
–– superior **453**, **458**, **460**, **487**, 500
––– functions 452, 458
––– intragluteal injection 460
––– lesion 461
––– pathway 458, 486, 487
––– plexus **452**
– hypogastricus 69
– iliohypogastricus **195**, **453**, **454**, **456**
–– functions 456
–– lesion 457
–– pathway 456
–– plexus 452
–– R. cutaneus
––– anterior 187, 454
––– lateralis 454
–– referred pain 457
– ilioinguinalis 187, 189, 190, **195**, **453**, **454**, **456**, **476**
–– functions 456
–– lesion 457
–– pathway 456
–– plexus 452
–– referred pain 457
– intercostalis 65, 144, 145, 146, 159, **175**, 177, 194, 276, 280
–– R. cutaneus
––– anterior 146, 187
––– lateralis 187, 279, 314
– intercostobrachialis 170, 201, 277, 279, 280, **309**, 314, **315**, 316
– interosseus antebrachii
–– anterior 286, **290**, **339**
–– posterior **288**, **331**, 335, **339**
– ischiadicus **396**, **453**, **458**, **460**, **462**, **463**, 467, **485**, 486, **487**, **500**, **501**
–– functions **452**, 458
–– high division 459
–– intragluteal injection 460
–– lesion 459
–– location in cross-section 501
–– pathway 458, 485, 486
–– plexus **452**
– laryngeus recurrens 180
–– dexter 69
–– sinister 69
– lumbales 65, **454**
– medianus 67, 201, **263**, 276, **277**, **279**, **280**, **286**, 290, **291**, 293, 299, 300, 301, 302, 314, 317, **318**, **319**, **324**, 325, **326**, **327**, **328**, **329**, **333**, **338**, **339**, 340
–– autonomous area 291
–– benediction sign **291**
–– cutaneous innervation 280
–– lesion **287**
–– pathway 290, 319, 327
–– Plexus brachialis 276
–– R. palmaris **290**, 332, 333
–– segmentation **290**
– musculocutaneus 67, 201, **250**, 276, **277**, **279**, **280**, **286**, **287**, 314, 317, **318**, **319**, 322, 338
–– cutaneous innervation 280
–– lesion **287**
–– pathway 287, 319
–– Plexus brachialis 276
–– segmentation **287**
– obturatorius 188, **195**, **453**, **454**, **456**, 481, 482, 483, 500
–– functions 452, 456
–– lesion **457**
–– pathway 456
–– plexus **452**
–– R. anterior 195
–– R. cutaneus 454

Nervus(-i)
- occipitalis
-- major 170, **171, 172, 173**
-- minor 169, 170, **171**, 279, 314
-- tertius 170, **173**
- oculomotorius [III] 68, 69
- pectoralis
-- lateralis 276, 277, **279**, 284, 314
--- Plexus brachialis 276
-- lesion **284**
-- medialis 276, 277, **279**, 284, 314, **315**
--- Plexus brachialis 276
- phrenicus 276, 277, 279, 298, 314
-- dexter, R. phrenicoabdominalis 157
-- sinister, R. phrenicoabdominalis 157
- plantaris
-- lateralis 401, 453, **462, 496, 497, 498**
--- branches 496
--- R. superficialis **496**
-- medialis 453, **462, 496, 497, 498**
--- branches 496
- pudendus **453, 458, 460**
-- functions 452, 458
-- lesion 459, **461**
-- pathway 458
-- plexus **452**
- radialis 67, **170**, 276, **277, 279**, 280, **286, 288,** 299, 300, 302, 310, 312, 314, **318, 319, 322, 323, 325,** 326, 327, **328, 329,** 336, **338**
-- autonomous area 289
-- branches 323
-- cutaneous innervation 280
-- humerus fracture 209
-- humerus shaft fracture 322
-- injury 208
-- lesion **289**
-- park bench position 209
-- pathway 288
-- Plexus brachialis 276
-- R. profundus **263, 325,** 326, 327, 328, **330, 331,** 335
-- R. superficialis 201, 280, 302, **313, 325,** 326, 327, **328, 330,** 331, 336, **339**
-- segmentation 288
-- triangular interval 170, 321
-- wrist drop **289**
- sacrales 65, **454**
- saphenus 453, **454, 456,** 478, 479, **481, 482, 501,** 503
-- functions **456**
-- lesion 457
-- location in cross-section 501
-- pathway **456**, 478
-- R. infrapatellaris 454
-- Rr. cutanei cruris mediales 454
- scalenus anterior 277
- scrotales anteriores 454
- spinalis 65, 122, 123, 174, 175, 176, 277
-- development 89
-- Fila radicularia 177
-- Ganglion sensorium 121, 173
-- Radix
--- anterior 176, 178
--- posterior 176, 178
-- R. anterior 67, 173, 276
-- R. dorsalis
--- development **88**
-- R. posterior 146, 173
-- Rr. collaterales 146
-- Rr. cutanei laterales 146
-- R. ventralis, development **88,** 89
-- structure **177**
- splanchnicus(-i)
-- lumbales 69
-- major 65, 69, 157, 177
-- minor 69, 157
-- sacrales 69
- subclavius 276, 277, **279,** 283, 314
-- Plexus brachialis 276

Nervus(-i)
- subcostalis **195,** 452
- suboccipitalis 170, **172, 173**
- subscapulares 276, **279,** 284, 314, 318
-- lesions 284
-- Plexus brachialis 276
- supraclaviculares 187, 280
-- intermedii 308
-- laterales 169, 170, 308, 309, 310
-- mediales 308
- suprascapularis 246, 276, 277, **279,** 282, 298, 314, 318, 321, 323
-- compression 207
-- Plexus brachialis 276
- suralis 453, 454, **462,** 463, 468, **478, 485**
-- pathway 478
- thoracicus(-i) 65, 187, 194
-- longus 276, 277, **279,** 283, 314, **315,** 316, 317
--- lesion **241**
-- Plexus brachialis 276
-- R. cutanei posteriores 280
-- Rr. posteriores mediales et laterales 170
- thoracodorsalis 276, 277, **279,** 284, 314, **315, 316,** 318
-- lesions **284**
-- Plexus brachialis 276
- tibialis **396,** 452, **453, 458,** 462, 468, **484, 485,** 486, 488, **492, 493, 494, 502,** 503
-- branches 496
-- functions 458, 462
-- lesion 459, 462, 492
-- pathway 458, 462, 492, 494
- ulnaris 67, 276, 277, 279, **280, 286,** 291, **292, 293,** 299, 301, 302, 314, 317, **318, 319,** 322, 323, 324, **325,** 326, 327, **329,** 330, **332, 333, 334, 338, 339**
-- autonomous area 293
-- claw hand **293**
-- cutaneous innervation 280
-- humerus fracture 209
-- lesion 292, **293,** 333
-- pathway 292, 319, 329
-- Plexus brachialis 276
-- R. dorsalis **292, 313**
-- R. palmaris 332
-- R. profundus **333, 334**
-- R. superficialis **333,** 334
-- segmentation **292**
- vagus [X] 68, 69, 314
Neural tube 88, 89
Neuropathy, autonomic 68
Neurovascular pathway
- Canalis obturatorius 425
- forearm **339**
- malleolar canal 497, 498
- tarsal tunnel 497, 498
- upper arm 300, **338**
- wrist **339**
Neutral-zero-method **36**
Newborn 6
- spine 96
Nipple 142, **182,** 183, 306
- dermatome 186
Nodus(-i) lymphoideus(-i)
- abdominis parietales et viscerales 57
- aortici laterales 168
- axillares 57, **304, 305, 306**
-- apicales **184,** 307, **317**
-- centrales **184, 307, 317**
-- humerales [laterales] **184, 307, 317**
-- pectorales **184, 307, 317**
-- subscapulares **184, 307, 317**
-- superficiales **308**
- brachiales 167
- cavales laterales 168
- cervicales 57
-- anteriores 317
--- superficiales et profundi 317
-- laterales 317

Nodus(-i) lymphoideus(-i)
- cubitales **304,** 306
- deltoidopectoralis 304
- iliaci
-- communes **168**
-- externi **168,** 475
-- interni **168,** 475
- inguinales 57
-- inferiores 168
-- profundi **475, 483**
-- superficiales **168,** 474, **475**
--- inferiores 167, **475**
--- superolaterales 167, **475**
--- superomediales 167, 168, 475
- interpectorales **184, 307**
- lumbales **168**
- paramammarii **184, 307**
- parasternales **184**
- pectorales 167
- pelvis parietales and viscerales 57
- poplitei
-- profundi **488**
-- superficiales 474, **488**
- preaortici 168
- retroaortici 168
- subaortici **168**
- supraclaviculares 317
- tibialis anterior 490
Nucleus(-i)
- basalis 64
- lentiformis
-- Putamen 75
- pulposus 114, 115, 117, **121,** 122
-- development **89**
Nutrient arteries 24

O

Oblique system, deep back muscles 134
Occipital bone **98**
Occipital lobes 64
Occlusion, jaw 8
Oculus 68
Oesophageal varices **56**
Oesophagus 16, 157, 180
- dermatomes 186
- Pars
-- abdominalis 156, 158
-- thoracica 158
Olecranon **200,** 201, **210,** 225, 229, 238, 251, 252, 259, 260, 261, 262, 310, 312, 322, 329, 330
- HUETER triangle 228
- X-ray image 70, 226
Omphalocele 154
One-legged stance 461
Opening angle 396
Opposition 8
- SCHAEFFER's test 10
- test 291, 293
- thumb 10, 234
Orbita 21
- CT 73
Organ
- lymphatic 57
-- primary 58
-- secondary 58
Organa genitalia 68
Os(sa)
- accessoria 21
- brevia 21
- capitatum **212, 213,** 230, 231, 291, 293, 337, 339
-- bone core formation 29
-- X-ray image 213
- carpi 21, 204, **212**
-- development 203
-- evolution 23
-- structure of the extremities 22

Os(sa)
- coccygis 13, 21, 90, **94**, **95**, 109, 110, **352**, 371
-- X-ray image 353
- coxae 21, 90, 348, **352**, **354**, **355**
-- bone core formation 29
-- child **355**
-- evolution 23
-- structure of the extremities 22
-- X-ray image 127
- cuboideum **364**, **365**, **366**, 401, 404, 407, 409
-- arch of the foot 408
-- bone core formation 29
- cuneiforme
-- intermedium **364**, **365**, **366**, 401, 409
--- arch of the foot 408
--- bone core formation 29
-- laterale **364**, **365**, **366**, 409
--- arch of the foot 408
--- bone core formation 29
-- mediale **364**, **365**, **366**, 406, 408, 409
--- arch of the foot 408
--- bone core formation 29
- digitorum [Phalanges]
-- manus 21, 204, **212**
--- bone core formation 29
--- evolution 23
--- structure of the extremities 22
-- pedis 21, **365**, 366
--- bone core formation 29
--- evolution 23
--- structure of the extremities 22
- frontale 21
- hamatum **212**, **213**, 230, 231, 291, 293, 339
-- bone core formation 29
-- X-ray image 213
- hyoideum
-- X-ray image 124
- ilium 154, 188, 350, 352, 372
-- bone core formation 29
-- Crista iliaca, X-ray image 126
-- dextrum 74
-- sinistrum 74
-- X-ray image 127, 375
- irregularia 21
- ischii 21, 350, 352
-- bone core formation 29
- longa 21, **24**
- lunatum **212**, **213**, 230, 231, 337
-- bone core formation 29
-- X-ray image 213
- manus 212
- metacarpi 21, 204, 212, 232, 275
-- cross-section **340**
-- development 203
-- evolution 23
-- I 230, 340
-- II 340
-- III 340
--- Basis 337
-- I–V **212**
-- IV 340
-- IV 340
-- structure of the extremities 22
-- X-ray image 213
- metatarsi 21, 348, **366**
-- evolution 23
-- I 404, 408
-- II 401, 404
-- I–V **365**
-- IV 404
-- V 404
-- structure of the extremities 22
- naviculare **364**, **365**, **366**, 401, 404, 406, 408
-- arch of the foot 408
-- bone core formation 29
-- Facies articularis talaris 404
-- MRI 401
-- X-ray image 405
- occipitale **98**, 99, 118, 119, 120

Os(sa) occipitale
-- Clivus 118
-- Pars
--- basilaris 119, 120
--- lateralis 120
-- X-ray image 124
-- odontoideum 100
- pedis **364**, **366**
- pisiforme **212**, **213**, 231, 267, 269, 333
-- bone core formation 29
-- X-ray image 213
- plana 21
- pneumatica 21
- pubis 188, 350, 352
-- bone core formation 29
-- sinistrum 74
- sacrum 13, 21, 90, **94**, **95**, **109**, 348, 350, **352**, 371, 372, 418
-- Facies dorsalis 132
-- gender differences **109**
-- MRI 130
-- Pars lateralis 174
--- X-ray image 353
-- Proc. articularis superior 174
-- surface anatomy **347**
-- X-ray image 126, 127, 353
- scaphoideum **212**, **213**, 230, 231
-- bone core formation 29
-- tabatière 265
-- X-ray image 213
- sesamoidea 21
-- manus 212, 231
--- X-ray image 213
-- pedis 365, 407
- tarsi 21, 348, **366**
-- evolution 23
-- structure of the extremities 22
- temporale, Proc. mastoideus 173
- trapezium **212**, **213**, 230, 291, 293, 339
-- bone core formation 29
-- X-ray image 213
- trapezoideum **212**, **213**, 230, 231, 291, 293, 339
-- bone core formation 29
-- tabatière 265
-- X-ray image 213
- triquetrum **212**, **213**, 230, 231, 339
-- bone core formation 29
-- X-ray image 213
- zygomaticum 21
Ossification 29
- apophyseal 29
- centre 29
- desmal 203
- diaphyseal 29
- enchondral 29
- endochondral 203
- epiphyseal 29
- perichondral 29
Osteoarthritis 35
- ankle joint 399
- hip joint 373
- knee joint 349, 392
- sacroiliac joint 372
Osteoblasts 27
- bone development 29
Osteochondrosis 131
Osteochondrosis intervertebralis 98
Osteoclasts 27
Osteogenesis 29
- chondral 29
- desmal 29
Osteons 27
Osteophytes
- cervical spine 131
- Foramen
-- intervertebrale 98, 106
-- transversarium 98
- hip joint 376
- Osteochondrosis intervertebralis 98

Osteoporosis 126
- hip fracture 358
Osteosynthesis 26
- external fixator 26
- plate 26
- tension band wiring 26
OTT sign 152
Outer ligaments, knee joint 381, 382
Outer rotation, hip joint 376
Ovar 60, 475
- endocrine system 59
Oviducts 60
Ovoid joint **33**

P

Pain, referred 186
Palatine tonsil *see* Tonsilla palatina
Palmar 9
Palmar aponeurosis 266, 332
Palmar arch
- deep **303**, 334
-- tributary 294, 301, 303
- superficial 333
-- branches 337
-- tributary 301, 302, 303
Palmar flexion 8, 232
- distal interphalangeal joint 233
- hand 10
- metacarpophalangeal joint 233
- proximal interphalangeal joint 233
- wrist joint 232, 235
Palma [Vola] manus 12, 87, 200
- arteries
-- deep 334
-- middle 333
-- superficial 332
- musculature
-- deep 269, 270, 271
-- middle 267
-- superficial **266**
- nerves
-- deep layer 334
-- middle layer 333
-- superficial layer 332
- phlegmon 268
- tendon sheath **268**
-- variants 268
- vessels
-- deep layer 334
-- middle layer 333
-- superficial layer 332
Palm of the hand *see* Palma 12
Pancreas 16
- endocrine system **59**
Papilla mammaria 142, **182**, 183, 306
Paracortical zone [T-cell zone] 58
Parasympathicus 68
- head 68
- pelvis 68
Parathyroid glands, endocrine system **59**
Parietal lobes 64
Park bench position 209, 289
Pars
- abdominalis
-- aortae [Aorta abdominalis] 50, 55, 69, 74, 156
-- ductus thoracici 57
- anularis vaginae tendinis musculi flexoris hallucis longi 449
- ascendens
-- aortae [Aorta ascendens] 50, 69
-- musculi trapezii 39, 132
- cervicalis ductus thoracici 57
- costalis diaphragmatis 145, **156**, **157**
- cranialis 69
- cruciformis vaginae tendinis musculi flexoris hallucis longi 449

Appendix

Pars
– descendens
–– aortae [Aorta descendens] 50, 74
–– ligamenti iliofemoralis 373
–– musculi trapezii 39, 132
– infraclavicularis plexus brachialis **276**, 279, 284
– lateralis ossis sacri 108, 109
– libera membri
–– inferioris 348
–– superioris 204
– lumbalis diaphragmatis
–– Crus dextrum 156, 157, 195
–– Crus intermedium 157
–– Crus laterale 157, 158
–– Crus mediale 157, 158
–– Crus sinistrum 157, 158
– pelvica parasympathici 69
– sternalis diaphragmatis **156**, **157**, 158
– supraclavicularis plexus brachialis **276**, 279, 282
– thoracica
–– aortae [Aorta thoracica] 50, 69, 158, **161**, **165**
––– branches 161
–– ductus thoracici 57
– tibiocalcanea ligamenti collaterale mediale **402**
– tibionavicularis ligamenti collaterale mediale **402**
– tibiotalaris anterior/posterior ligamenti collaterale mediale **402**
– transversa
–– ligamenti iliofemoralis 373
–– musculi trapezii 39, 132
Patella 21, 75, 348, **361**, **378**, 385, 386, 387, 395, 396, 414, 417, 423, 424, 432, 438, 439, 478
– bone core formation 29
– bone types 21
– dislocation **379**
– Facies
–– anterior 381
–– articularis 381
––– arthroscopy 398
––– X-ray image 380
– floating 394
– functions **361**
– MRI 397
– opening angle 396
– surface anatomy **346**
– X-ray image 396
Pecten ossis pubis 156, 350, **354**, 355, 371, 418, 423, 424
Pediculus arcus vertebrae **97**, 115
– cervicalis 100, 121, 124
– lumbalis **107**, 117, 138
–– CT 129, 130
–– X-ray image 126, 127
– thoracicae **104**, 113
–– X-ray image 125
Pelvic
– fracture 353
– girdle (Cingulum pelvicum) 348, 350, 368
– inlet 352
– inner diameter 351
Pelvis 4, **350**, **351**, **352**
– arteries 464
– CT angiogram 74
– deformed
–– rickets 90
– directions of movement 8
– female 350, **351**
–– joints 370
–– ligaments 370
– joints 368, 369
– ligaments 368, 369
– lordotic curve 96
– male 350, **352**
–– X-ray image **353**
– renalis 61
– X-ray image **353**
Pemphigoid 77
Pemphigus 77
Penis 60
Percentile curve 6

Percussion 16
Perforating veins 473
Perfusion pressure 52
Pericardium 158
Perimysium 40
Periost(eum) 24, 27, 32, 176, 178, 340
– blood supply 24
– tendon insertion site 45
Peripheral 9
Peritoneum
– parietale 145, 155, 156, 159, 181, **190**, 191, **192**, 193
– viscerale 145, 194
PERTHES' disease 377
Pes 4, 5, 348
– anserinus
–– profundus 433
–– superficialis 424, 425, 432
– cavus 409
– planus 409
– sagittal section 401
Pes *see Foot*
PETIT lumbar hernia 133
PETIT triangle 133
Phalanx
– distalis
–– manus 204, 212, **213**, 232, 275, 337
––– sagittal section 79
––– X-ray image 213
–– pedis **364**, 365, 366, 401
– media
–– manus 44, 204, **213**, 232, 275, 337
––– X-ray image 213
–– pedis **364**, 365, 366, 401
– proximalis
–– manus 204, 212, **213**, 232, 275, 337
––– X-ray image 213
–– pedis **364**, 365, 366, 401
Pharyngeal membrane 19
Pharyngeal tonsil *see* Tonsilla pharyngea
Pharynx 180
Phlegmon, palm of the hand 268
Pia mater spinalis 174, **176**, 178
Piano key sign 217
PIP (proximal interphalangeal joint)
– dislocation 234
– finger 233
–– muscles 235, 273
– thumbs 234
–– muscles 235, 273
Pivot joint **33**
– ankle joint 410
– radioulnar joint 214
Placenta 55
– Chorion frondosum 19
Planes
– human body 7
Planta pedis 13
– arteries 499
– nerves 496, 497, 498
– surface anatomy 346
– vessels 496, 497, 498
Plantar 9
Plantar aponeurosis 408, 448
Plantar flexion 8
– ankle joint 411, 412
– toe joint 413
Planum
– frontale 7
– sagittale 7
– transversale 7
Platysma 141, 180
Pleura
– parietalis 144
–– Pars
––– costalis 144, **145**
––– diaphragmatica 144, **145**, 158
– visceralis 144
–– pulmonis **145**
Pleural effusion 146

Pleural gap 144
Pleural puncture 146
Plexus
– aorticus abdominalis 69
– autonomic 67
– brachialis 62, **67**, **199**, 276
–– arm nerves 286
–– cervical rib 92
–– distribution 67
–– ERB's palsy 278
–– Fasciculus
––– lateralis 276
––– medialis 276
––– posterior 276
–– formation **67**
–– KLUMPKE's palsy 278
–– lesion **199**, 278
–– nerves **279**
–– Pars
––– infraclavicularis 143, **276**, **286**, 315, **316**
––– supraclavicularis **276**, 286
–– parts 277
–– ultrasound 277
– cardiacus 69
– cervicalis 62, 173
–– R. muscularis 279, 314
– coccygeus 452
– coeliacus 67, 69
– diagram 67
– hypogastricus
–– inferior 68, 69
–– superior 68, 69
– lumbalis 138, 195, 452
–– branches 453
–– nerves **456**
––– lesions 457
–– referred pain 454
– lumbosacralis 62, **195**, 452
–– leg nerves 453
–– referred pain 454
– mesentericus
–– inferior 69
–– superior 67, 69
– oesophageus 69
– pampiniformis 189, 194
– renalis 69
– sacralis 195, 452
–– branches 453
–– nerves 458
––– lesions 459, 461
–– referred pain **454**
– solaris 67
– somatic 67
– venosus
–– areolaris 162, 187
–– pampiniformis **191**
–– sacralis, cavocaval anastomoses 163
–– submucosus 56
–– vertebralis
––– externus **179**
––– internus 174, **176**, **177**, 178, **179**
Plica(-ae)
– alares 381
– axillaris
–– anterior 200
––– surface anatomy 85
–– posterior 200
– infrapatellaris 75
– synovialis 32
–– infrapatellaris 381
– umbilicalis
–– lateralis 153, **155**, 188, 191
–– medialis 153, **155**, 188
–– mediana 153, **155**, 188
– vesicalis transversa 188
Pollex 200
Polymastia 182
Polyneuropathy 66
Polythelia 182
Pons 64, 69

Popliteal fossa
- arteries 489
- nerves 477, 484, 485, 486, 488, 492, 493, 494
- vessels 477, 484, 485, 488, 492, 493, 494
Popliteal pulse **50**
Portal vein circulation 56
Posterior 9
Posterior drawer test 389
Posterior spinous line 101
POUPART ligament 156
Prechordal plate 19
Pregnancy, pelvic diameter 351
Pressure
- colloid osmotic 52
- hydrostatic 52
Primitive node 19
Primitive streak 19
Processus
- accessorius vertebrae
-- lumbalis **107**
-- thoracicae **104**, **106**
- articularis [Zygapophysis]
-- inferior **97**
--- axis 99
--- vertebrae 98, 100, 101, 1C2, 104, **106**, **107**, 116, 117, 121, 124, 126, 127, 129
-- superior **97**
--- axis **98**, 99
--- ossis sacri 108, 109
--- vertebrae 100, 101, 102, **104**, **106**, **107**, 114, 116, 117, 121, 124, 126, 127, 129, 174, 177
- axillaris 184
- coracoideus **207**, 216, **218**, **219**, 220, 224, 239, **246**, 249
-- shoulder dislocation 223
-- shoulder, roof 246
-- X-ray image 217, 223
- coronoideus **210**, **225**, 229
-- X-ray image 226
- costalis vertebrae
-- lumbalis **107**, 121, 138, 157
--- CT 129
--- X-ray image 127
-- thoracicae **106**
--- X-ray image 127
- lateralis
-- tali 364, 367
-- tuberis calcanei 365, 367
- mamillaris **104**, **106**, **107**
-- CT 129
- mastoideus 139
-- X-ray image 124
- medialis tuberis calcanei 365, 366, 367
- posterior tali 366, 367
-- Tuberculum
--- laterale 367
--- mediale 367
-- X-ray image 405
- spinosus **97**, 138
-- axis 98, 99
-- vertebrae
--- cervicalis 84, **100**, 101, 124, 129
--- lumbalis 90, 106, 107, 117, 126, 127, 129, 130, 138
--- thoracicae 84, 104, 116, 175
- styloideus 139, 140
-- radii **200**, **211**, 229, 231
-- ulnae **200**, 210, 229, 231
- transversus **97**
-- atlantis 98, 173
-- axis **99**
-- vertebrae
--- cervicalis 98, 100
--- lumbalis, CT 130
--- thoracicae 104, 114, 116, 125, 129
- uncinatus **100**, **121**, 131
- vaginalis peritonei 188, **192**, **193**
-- persistens 193
- xiphoideus **111**, 147, 157, 194
-- projection onto the chest wall 85

Profundus 9
Prolapse
- laterodorsal 122
- mediodorsal 122
Promontorium **90**, **95**, **108**, 109, 156, **350**, 352
- X-ray image 126
Pronation
- ankle joint 411, 412
- elbow joint 227
- extremities 8
- hand 11
Pronator teres syndrome 291
Prostate 60
Proteoglycans 32
Protraction
- jaw 8
- shoulder girdle 205
Protrusion, jaw 8
Protuberantia occipitalis externa 132, 172
- landmarks 84
Proximal 9
Prune belly syndrome 88
Pseudoarthrosis 31
Pubic symphysis 6, 30, **372**
Pubis see Os pubis
Pudendal nerve block **461**
Pulmo 16, 17, 68, 144, 145
- dexter 55
- sinister 55
Pulmonary circulation 48
Pulmonary embolism 54, 473
Pulse 50
Puncture, bone 111

R

Rachischisis 89
Radial 9
Radial abduction
- extremities 8
- metacarpophalangeal joint 233
- wrist joint 232, 235
Radial pulse **50**
Radial sulcus 288
Radial tunnel 325, 328
Radial zone 32
Radicular syndrome 122
Radioulnar joint
- distal 214, **229**
- proximal 214, **229**
Radius 21, 42, 47, 204, 211, 212, 213, 225, **229**, 230, 231, 259, 260, 261, 262, 263, 264, 267, 269, 272, 337, 339
- bone core formation 29
- development 203
- evolution 23
- Facies anterior 257
- fracture 211
-- X-ray image 211
- head 225
- structure of the extremities 22
- X-ray image 70, 213, 226
Radix
- anterior nervi spinalis 65, 122, 174, 175, **176**, 177
- lateralis 286
- medialis 286
- parasympathica [Nn. splanchnici pelvici] 69
- posterior nervi spinalis 65, 122, 174, 175, **176**, 177
Ramus(-i)
- acetabularis
-- arteriae circumflexae femoris medialis 377, **464**
-- arteriae obturatoriae 481
- acromialis
-- arteriae axillaris 299
-- arteriae thoracoacromialis 160, 297, 316

Ramus(-i)
- anterior
-- arteriae
--- circumflexae femoris medialis 464
--- recurrentis ulnaris 294, 295
-- nervi
--- cutaneus antebrachii medialis 280
--- spinalis 174, 175, 178
- articularis arteriae descendentis genus 465, 480, 481
- ascendens
-- arteriae circumflexae femoris lateralis 377, 464, 465, 466, 482
-- arteriae circumflexae femoris medialis **486**
- bronchiales arteriae thoracicae internae 160
- calcanei
-- arteriae tibialis posterioris 468, 494
-- mediales nervi tibialis 496
- carpalis
- dorsalis
--- arteriae radialis 303
--- arteriae ulnaris 294, 303
-- palmaris
--- arteriae radialis 303
--- arteriae ulnaris 294, 303
- clavicularis
-- arteriae axillaris 299
-- arteriae thoracoacromialis 160, **297**
- collateral s
-- aortae thoracicae 161
-- arteriae intercostalis posterior 144, 165
- communicans
-- albus nervi spinalis 175, **178**
-- arteriae tibialis posterioris 465
-- cum nervo ulnari 286, 333
-- fibularis 453, **463**, 478
-- griseus nervi spinalis 175, **178**
-- nervi spinalis **65**, **175**, 177
-- ulnaris nervi radialis 280
- cutaneus(-i)
-- anterior(-es)
--- nervi 65, 177, 456, **476**
--- pectoralis 280, 308
-- cruris mediales nervi sapheni **478**
-- lateralis(-es) 452
--- aortae thoracicae **161**
--- arteriae lumbalis **179**
--- nervi 65, 169, **175**, 177, 456, 477, 487
--- pectoralis 171, 280, **308**
-- medialis(-es)
--- aortae thoracicae 161
--- arteriae lumbalis **179**
--- nervi spinalis 169, **175**
-- nervi obturatorii 456, 476, 477, **481**, **482**
-- posterior
--- nervi cervicalis 171
--- nervi thoracici 171
- deltoideus
-- arteriae axillaris 299
-- arteriae thoracoacromialis 160, 297
- descendens arteriae circumflexae femoris lateralis 377, 464, 465, 466, 481, 482
- dorsalis
-- aortae thoracicae **161**
-- arteriae lumbalis 174, **179**
-- C2 173
-- nervi ulnaris 280, 286, **312**, 324, **326**, 327, 330
-- venae lumbalis 174
- femoralis nervi genitofemoralis **195**, 452, 454, 456, **476**
-- functions **456**
-- pathway **456**
- genitalis nervi genitofemoralis **195**, 452, 454, 456
-- functions 456
-- pathway 456
- inferior ossis pubis 354, 355, 372, 418
-- X-ray image 353
- infrapatellaris nervi sapheni 476, 478

Appendix

Ramus(-i)
– intercostalis anterior arteriae thoracicae internae **160**, **161**, **165**, 166, 298
– interganglionaris 177
– lateralis nervi spinalis **175**, 178
– malleolares
–– laterales arteriae fibularis 465, 468, **494**
–– mediales arteriae tibialis posterioris 465, 468, **494**
– mammarii
–– lateralis aortae thoracicae 161
–– mediales arteriae thoracicae internae 160, 161, **184**, 298, 307
– medialis nervi spinalis **175**, 178
– mediastinales arteriae thoracicae internae 160
– meningei 65
– meningeus nervi spinalis **175**, 177, **178**
– muscularis(-es)
–– nervi
––– femoralis 480, **481**, 482, 501
––– fibularis profundi 495
––– radialis **331**
––– tibialis 485, 486, 488, 492
–– plexus
––– brachialis 276
––– lumbosacralis 452
––– sacralis **458**, 459
– obturatorius arteriae epigastricae inferioris 160
– oesophagealis 56
– ossis ischii 352, 354, 355 418
–– X-ray image 353
– palmaris
–– nervi
––– mediani 312, 326, 327
––– ulnaris 280, 286, 312
–– profundus arteriae ulnaris 302, 303
–– superficialis arteriae radialis 294, 301, 302, 303
– pectorales
–– arteriae axillaris 299
–– arteriae thoracoacromialis 160, **297**, 316
– perforans(-tes)
–– arcus palmaris profundi 303
–– arteriae
––– fibularis 495
––– thoracicae internae 160. 161, 165, 166, 298
–– venae thoracicae internae 162, 165
– posterior(-es)
–– arteriae
––– circumflexae femoris medialis 464
––– recurrentis ulnaris 294, 295
–– C2 172
–– C3 172
–– C6 170
–– C7 170
–– C8 170
–– nervi
––– cutanei antebrachii medialis 280
––– spinalis 65, 174, **175**, 177, **178**
–– T1 170
–– T12 170
– profundus(-i)
–– arteriae
––– circumflexae femoris medialis **464**, **486**, 487
––– gluteae superioris 467, **487**
––– plantaris medialis **499**
––– transversae cervicis 298
––– transversae colli 171, 172
–– nervi
––– plantaris lateralis 497, 498
––– radialis 286, 288, 289, **331**
––– ulnaris 286, **292**
–– venae gluteae superioris **487**
– pubicus arteriae epigastricae inferioris 160
– saphenus arteriae descendentis genus 465, 466
– spinalis(-es)
–– aortae thoracicae 161
–– arteriae
––– intercostalis posterioris **177**
––– lumbalis **179**

Ramus(-i)
– sternales arteriae thoracicae internae 160, 161, 298
– superficialis
–– arteriae
––– circumflexae femoris medialis 481, **486**
––– gluteae superioris 467
––– plantaris medialis **499**
––– transversae cervicis 298
––– transversae colli 172
–– nervi
––– plantaris lateralis 497, 498
––– radialis 280, 286, 288, 289, **312**
––– ulnaris 286, **292**
– superior ossis pubis 354, 355, 372, 418
–– X-ray image 353
– thymici arteriae thoracicae internae 160
– tracheales arteriae thoracicae internae 160
– transversus arteriae circumflexae femoris lateralis 377, 464, 466
– ventralis
–– arteriae lumbalis 179
–– C2 173
–– nervi spinalis 62, 67
Range of movement joints 36
Recessus
– axillaris 34, 218, 219
– costodiaphragmaticus 145
–– X-ray image 70
– subpopliteus **443**
Reclination
– spine 8
Rectum 16, 17, 68, 156, 475
Rectus sheath 37, **153**
Referred pain 454
Regio
– abdominalis lateralis 12, 87
– analis 13
– antebrachii
–– anterior 12, 87
––– arteries 324, 325, 326, 327
––– nerves 312, 324, 325, 326, 327
––– veins 312
–– posterior 13, 87, 200
––– nerves 312, 330, 331
––– veins 312
––– vessels 330, 331
– axillaris 12, 13, 87
–– Fossa axillaris 200
– brachii
–– anterior 12, 87
––– nerves 309, 310, 318, 319
––– veins 309, 310
––– vessels 318, 319
–– dorsalis
––– nerves **323**
––– vessels **323**
–– posterior 13, 200
––– nerves **322**
––– vessels **322**
– cervicalis
–– anterior 12, 87
–– lateralis 12, 87
–– posterior 13, 84, 85
– cruris
–– anterior 12, 346
––– nerves 490, 491
––– vessels 490, 491
–– medialis
––– nerves 478
––– vessels 478
–– posterior 12, 13
––– nerves 478, 492, 493, 494
––– Sura 347
––– vessels 478, 492, 493, 494
– cubitalis
–– anterior
––– Fossa cubitalis 12, 87
––– nerves 309, 312, 328

Regio cubitalis anterior
––– veins 309, 311, 312
––– vessels 328
–– posterior 13
––– nerves 310, 329
––– veins 310
––– vessels 329
– deltoidea 12, 13, 85, 87, 200
–– nerves 309, 310, **323**
–– veins 309, 310
–– vessels **323**
– epigastrica 12, 87
– femoris
–– anterior 12, 346
––– nerves 476, 480, 481, 482
––– vessels 476, 480, 481, 482
–– posterior 13, 347
––– nerves 477, 484, 485, 486, 487
––– vessels 477, 484, 485, 486, 487
– genus
–– anterior 12, 346
––– nerves 476, 480, 481, 482
––– vessels 476, 480, 481, 482
–– posterior [Fossa poplitea] 13, 347
––– nerves 477, 484, 485, 486, 488, 492, 493, 494
––– vessels 477, 484, 485, 486, 488, 489, 492, 493, 494
– glutealis 13, 85, 347
–– nerves 477, 484, 485, 486, 487
–– vessels 477, 484, 485, 486, 487
– hypochondriaca 12, 87
– inframammaria 12, 87
– infrascapularis 13, 85
– inguinalis 12, 87, 346
–– lymph nodes 475
–– nerves 476
–– vessels 476
– lumbalis 13, 85
– mammaria 12, 87
– mentalis 72
–– sonography 72
– occipitalis 13
– parietalis 13
– pectoralis 12, 87
– pedis
–– nerves 478, 479
–– vessels 478, 479
– presternalis 12, 87
– pubica [Hypogastrium] 12, 87
– sacralis 13, 85
– scapularis 13, 85
– sternocleidomastoidea 12, 87
– surae 13
– thoracica lateralis 316, 317
– umbilicalis 12, 87
– urogenitalis 12, 87
– vertebralis 13, 85
Ren [Nephros] 16, 17, 61, 138, 181
– CT 129
– dermatomes 186
– dexter 61, 74
– functions 61
– sinister 61, 74
Replacement bone 29
Reposition
– extremities 8
– thumb 10
Reproductive organs **60**
Respiratory system 48
Rete
– acromiale 160, 297, 315
– articulare
–– cubiti **295**, 330
–– genus 465, 466, 468, 469, 482, 491
– calcaneum 468, 494, 497, 498
– carpale
–– dorsale 335, 336, **337**
–– palmare **337**

Rete
- malleolare
-- laterale 491, **495**
-- mediale **495**
- patellare 476, 480
- venosum dorsale
-- manus 313
-- pedis 472, 478
Retinaculum
- musculorum
-- extensorum
--- manus 201, 238, 254, 259, 260, **261**, 262, **264**, 265, **272**, 335, **336**
--- pedis 414, **438**, 439, 444, 445, 446, 447, 479, 490, 491
-- fibularium [peroneorum] **439**, 441, 442, 443, 444, 445, 446, 492, 493
-- flexorum
--- manus 236, 266, 267, 268, 269, **291**, **293**, 302, 337, 339
--- pedis **441**, 442, 443, 445, 452, **492**, 493, **496**, **497**, **498**
- patellae
-- laterale **381**, 388, 396, 414
-- mediale **381**, 388, 396, 432
Retraction
- jaw 8
- shoulder girdle 205
Retroversion
- arm 11
- hip joint 376
- shoulder joint 220, 221
Retrusion, jaw 8
Rheumatoid arthritis 35
Rib cartilage, attachment **112**
Rib(s) 92, 93
- abnormality 93
- accessory 89
- anomalies 92
- development 89
- erosion 92
- expiration 91
- false **89**, 90, 93
- fracture
-- resuscitation 91
- free 93
- free floating 89, 90
- inspiration 91
- movement 91
- ossification 91
- real **89**, 90, 93
- two-headed 92
Rickets 90
Right cardiac catheterisation 473
ROCKWOOD classification 217
Rod-like bones 24
ROMBERG's knee phenomenon 457
Root sheath
- connective tissue 78
- inner 78
- outer 78
Rostral 9
Rotation 7
- cervical spine 103
- pelvis 8
- spine 8, 102, 152
Rotator cuff 224
- lesion 224
- muscles **239**
ROTTER lymph nodes (Nodi lymphoidei interpectorales) **184**
RUFFINI corpuscles 76
Rupture, ACHILLES tendon 441

S

Sacralisation 94
Sacral kyphosis **95**, 96

Sacral triangle 13, 90
Sacroiliac joint 352, **372**
- changes **352**
- pain 372
Sacrum **109**
- gender differences **109**
- X-ray image 127
Saddle joint **33**
Sagittal axis 7
Sagittal plane 7
Sarcomere 40
Scaphoid fracture **230**
Scapula 21, 47, 204, 205, 218
- alata **241**, 283
- Angulus inferior 132, 133
-- surface anatomy 84
- Angulus superior
-- X-ray image 70
- arm movement 222
- bone core formation 29
- development 203
- evolution 23
- Margo medialis
-- X-ray image 70
- structure of the extremities 22
- X-ray image 217
Scapular plane 205
SCHAEFFER's test 291
SCHEUERMANN disease 124
SCHEUERMANN kyphosis 96
SCHOBER sign 152
Schoolchild 6
Scintigraphy
- thyroid gland 72
Sclerotisation 131
Sclerotome 88
- caudal **89**
- cranial **89**
Scoliosis 96
- MICHAELIS rhomboid 90
Scrotum 60
Sebaceous gland 78
- drainage pathway 78
Secondary follicle [B-cell zone] 58
Sectional planes, radiological 7
Semen 60
Semi-vertebra (hemivertebra) 129
Senile kyphosis 96
Sentinel lymph (guard) nodes 58, 185, 307
Septum
- femorale 483
- intermusculare
-- brachii
--- laterale **42**, 201, 238, **251**, 252, 259, 260, 261, 322, 338
--- mediale **42**, 201, 249, 250, 254, 255, 256, 257, 290, 292, 318, 338
-- cruris
--- anterius **42**, 438, 439, **502**, 503
--- posterius **42**, 441, **502**, 503
-- femoris
--- laterale 501
--- mediale 501
--- posterius 501
-- vastoadductorium **423**, 466, **481**
- nasi
-- CT 73
- scroti 193
Sesamoid 21
SHARPEY's fibres 27
Shingles (Varizella zoster) 15
Shoulder
- arteries **296**, 297, **323**
- cutaneous innervation 280
- musculature
-- dorsal 237, 240, **242**, 243, 245, **247**, **251**, **252**
-- rotator cuff 239
-- ventral 236, 241, **244**, 246
- nerves 309, 310, **323**

Shoulder
- roof 246
- veins 309, 310
Shoulder corner joint 216
- X-ray image 217
Shoulder girdle 205
- muscles
-- deep 133
-- superficial 132
- musculature
-- dorsal 240, 247
-- ventral 241, 246, 247
- range of movement 205
- structure 22
Shoulder joint 214, **218**, **219**, **220**, **224**
- arm elevation 222
- circumduction 10
- dislocation **223**
- findings **223**
-- repositioning **223**
- external rotation 10
- internal rotation 10
- movements 220
- muscles 220
- range of movement 221
- X-ray image **223**
SIBSON fascia 144
Sinister 9
Sintigraphy
- thyroid gland 72
Sinus(es)
- CT **73**
- frontalis 75
- lactiferi 183
- maxillaris
-- CT **73**
- sagittalis superior **173**
- tarsi **366**
-- X-ray image 405
- transversus **173**
- wall cells 53
Skeletal
- age 29
- musculature 41
-- muscle fibre types **41**
-- structural principle 42
-- structure **40**
Skin 77
- blistering 77
- hairless 76
- hairy 76
- innervation 15
-- back 139
-- lower limb 455
-- upper extremity 280
- segments 15
- structure **76**
- tension lines 14
Sliding hernia 158, 159
Slipping of the vertebrae 106
Snuffbox (Fovea radialis) 265, **336**
- content 265
- tenderness 265
Solar plexus 67
Sole of the foot
- arteries 499
-- deep 471, 498
-- medial 497
-- superficial 470, 496
- musculature
-- deep layer 451
-- middle layer 450
-- superficial layer 449
- nerves
-- deep 498
-- medial 497
-- superficial 496
Somites 38
Sonography, fetus **72**

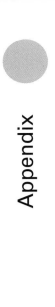

Index

Spasticity 423, **481**
Spatium
- axillare
-- laterale **247**, 320
-- mediale **247**, 320
- epidurale 122, 174, **176**, 178
-- MRI 130
- intercostale 90
- retropubicum 194
- subarachnoideum 174, 176, 177, 178
- subdurale 174, 176, 178
Special lamellae 27
Spermatic cord **190**
- content **191**
- coverings **193**
Spermatocele 191
SPIEGHEL's hernia (SPIEGHELIAN hernia) 151
Spina
- bifida 89
-- occulta 89
- iliaca
-- anterior
--- inferior 352, **354**, **355**
--- superior 74, 86, 141, 142, 149, 150, **346**, 352, **354**, **355**, 369, 414, 417, 418, 424, 460, 483
-- posterior
--- inferior 353, **354**, **355**
--- superior 13, 84, 136, 142, 352, 353, **354**, **355**, 370
- ischiadica 352, **354**, **355**, 429
-- X-ray image 353, 375
- scapulae 132, 142, 201, **207**, 220, **222**, 238, 247, 320
-- landmarks 84
-- surface anatomy 84
Spinal canal stenosis 131
Spinal cord see Medulla spinalis
Spinal nerve 65, 175, 176
- autonomous area 15
- damage 15
- structure **177**
Spine
- development 88, **89**, 96
- directions of movement 8
- flexion 152
- kyphosis 96, 124
- lateral flexion 152
- ligaments 113, 116
- lordosis 96
- metastasis site 125
- mobility 102
- motion segment 102
- nerves **178**
- primitive 88
- range of movement 152
- rotation 152
- Spina bifida 89
Spinous process see Processus spinosus
Splen [Lien] 16, 17
Spondylitis ankylosans 117
Spondylolisthesis 106, 128
Spondylolysis 106, 128
Spondylophytes 131
Spongiosa **24**
- adjustment 25
- trabeculae 27
Spraining the ankle 402
Spring ligament 408
Sprouting 66
Stabilising musculature 37
Stenosing tendonitis 45
Stenosis of the vertebral canal, dermatomes 281
Steppage gait 459, 463
Sternal bars **89**
Sternal tap 111
Sternoclavicular joint **112**
- X-ray image 215
Sternocostal joint, inspiration 91

Sternum 21, **90**, **111**, **112**, 162, 205
- age-related changes 91
- development **89**
- merger disorder 89
- movement 91
- projection onto the chest wall 85
Stratum
- basale 76
- corneum 76
- fibrosum 27
-- vaginae tendinis 44
- granulosum 76
- lucidum 76
- osteogenicum 27
- papillare dermis 76
- reticulare dermis 76
- spinosum 76
- synoviale vaginae tendinis
-- Pars
--- parietalis 44
--- tendinea 44
Stylopodium 22
- evolution 23
Subcapsular sinus [cortical sinus] 58
Subcutis **76**, 77, 78, 79, 144
Subluxation, atlantoaxial 119
Substantia
- compacta 24
-- compression load 25
- spongiosa 24, 361
Subtalar joint 404
- axis 410
- eversion 411
- functions 401
- inversion 411
- joint body 404
- ligament 404
- movement 412
- MRI 401
- muscle action 412
- range of movement 411
- X-ray image 405
Sulcus
- analis 347
- arteriae
-- subclaviae 92
-- vertebralis **98**, 120
- calcanei 367
- costae 92, 114, 146
- glutealis 347, 414, 477
- intermammarius
-- surface anatomy 85
- intertubercularis **208**, 209
-- X-ray image 223
- malleolaris 362, 363, 399
- musculi subclavii 206
- nervi
-- radialis **209**, **252**, **320**
-- spinalis **100**
-- ulnaris **209**
- obturatorius 354
- sinus sigmoidei 118, 119
- tali 367
- tendinis musculi
-- fibularis longi 365, 367
-- flexoris hallucis longi 366, 367
- venae subclaviae 92
Superficialis 9
Superior 9
Supination
- ankle joint 411, 412
- elbow joint 227
- extremities 8
- hand 11
Supination trauma 402
Supinator canal 288, 325, 328
Supinator syndrome 289
Sustentaculum tali 365, 366, **367**, 406
- X-ray image 405

Sutura
- coronalis 7
- sagittalis 7
Sweat glands 78
- apocrine 76
- eccrine 76, 77
Sympathetic trunk 177
- abdomen 68
- neck 68
- pelvis 68
- thorax 68
Sympathicus 68
Symphysis 352
- cartilaginous 30
- intervertebralis **100**
- manubriosternalis **111**, **112**
-- surface anatomy 85
- pubica 30, 90, 159, 188, **350**, 352, **372**, 418, 483
-- Discus interpubicus 368, 371
-- X-ray image 353
- xiphosternalis **111**
-- surface anatomy 85
Synarthrosis 30, 32
- characteristics 32
Synchondrosis
- cartilaginous 30
- costae 112
Syncytiotrophoblast 18
Syndesmosis
- fibrous 30
- tibiofibularis 348, **399**, 400
-- WEBER fracture 400
-- X-ray image 405
Synostosis 30
Synovectomy 31
Synovia 32
Synovial bursa 34
System
- arterial 49
- cardiopulmonary 48
- cardiovascular 48
- endocrine **59**
- intertransverse
-- back muscles 134
- musculoskeletal **20**
- sacrospinal
-- back muscles 134
- spinal
-- back muscles 134
- spinal transverse
-- back muscles 134
- transverse spinal
-- back muscles 134
- venous 49
Systema
- musculosceletale **20**
- sceletale **21**
Systemic circulation 48
- portal vein circulation 56
- veins 51

T

Tabatière (Fovea radialis) 264, 265
- tenderness 265
Talocrural joint 401
- axis 410
- dorsal extension 411
- functions 401
- injuries 402
- ligament(s) 402, 403
- movement 412
- MRI 401
- muscle action 412
- plantar flexion 411
- range of movement 411
- X-ray image 405

Talus **364**, **365**, **366**, **367**, 403, 404, 408
- arch of the foot 408
- bone core formation 29
- MRI 401
- X-ray image 405
Tangential fibre zone 32
Taps, bone 111
Tarsal tunnel 462
- syndrome 462, **463**
- tibial compression **492**
T-arthrodesis 31
Technetium-99 m 72
Tela subcutanea 76
- Panniculus adiposus 153
Temporal lobes 64
Temporal pulse **50**
Tendo 42, 44
- calcaneus (ACHILLES tendon) 401, 402, 403,
  409, 414, 416, 436, 439, 440, 441, 442, 443,
  445, 492, 493, 494
-- rupture 441
- conjunctivus [transverse tendon arcade] 188,
  190
Tendon **20**
- compartment
-- back of the hand 261
-- hand, back of the 262
- functions 43
- insertion site 45
-- chondral-apophyseal 45
-- periostal-diaphyseal 45
-- structure **45**
- structure 43
Tendonitis **45**
Tendon sheath(s) 44
- flexor tendons of the fingers 44
- foot 444, 445
- hand **268**
-- back of the hand **265**
-- palm of the hand **268**
-- variants 268
- structure 44
Tendovaginitis **45**
- stenosans **45**
Tennis elbow 258
Tensile trabeculae 25
Tension lines 14
TEP (total endoprosthesis)
- hip joint 376
Terminal hair 78
Testes 60
- endocrine system 59
- wall structure **193**
Testicular ectopy 192
Testicular torsion 191
Testis 60, 192, 193
- endocrine system 59
- wall structure **193**
Thalamus 64, 75
Thenar 200, 236, 266, 339
- atrophy 333
Thenar eminence 266
Thigh see Femur
- arteries 464, 466, 467
- cross-section 501
- fasciae 414
- musculature 417, 418
-- dorsal 428, 429, 430, 431
-- ischiocrural 428
-- medial 421, 422, 423, 424, 425
-- ventral 422, 423, 424, 425
- nerves 476, 477, 480, 481, 482, 484, 485,
  486, 487
- vessels 476, 477, 480, 481, 482, 484, 485,
  486, 487
Thigh bone, fracture 345
Thoracic aperture
- upper **148**
Thoracic kyphosis **95**, 96

Thoracic spine 105
- ligaments **113**
- mobility 102
- MRI 130
- OTT sign 152
- X-ray image **125**
Thoracic vertebra **104**, **106**
- structural features **104**
Thoracic wall
- anterior
-- arteries **160**
-- dermatomes 186
-- innervation 186
- arteries **161**, 164, **165**
- frontal section 145
- muscles **144**, **145**, **148**
-- deep 143
-- superficial 141, 142
- structure **144**
- veins **162**, **165**
Thorax 4
- anterior wall **147**
- lower edge 6
- musculature **238**
- overview image **70**
- posterior wall **147**
- upper edge 6
Thrombophlebitis 473
Thrombus **54**
Thumb(s)
- abduction 234
- carpometacarpal joint 234
- extension
-- muscles 234, 235, 273
- flexion
-- muscles 235, 273
- opposition 234
- range of movement **234**
Thymus
- endocrine system **59**
Thyroid gland (Glandula thyroidea)
- endocrine system **59**
- scintigraphy 72
Tibia 21, 42, 75, 348, **362**, 363, 378, 381, 382,
  384, 385, 386, 387, 395, **399**, 400, 401, 402,
  403, 414, 442, 443, 495, 502, 503
- articular surface **362**, **363**
- bone core formation 29
- Condylus lateralis 382
-- arthroscopy 398
-- MRI 397
-- X-ray image 380
- Condylus medialis 441, 443
-- MRI 397
-- X-ray image 380
- evolution 23
- Facies medialis 438, 490
- MRI 397, 401
- shaft axis 348
- structure of the extremities 22
- X-ray image 400, 405
Tibial 9
Tibialis anterior syndrome 463
Tibialis-posterior pulse **50**
Tide mark, joint cartilage 32
TKR (total knee replacement)
- knee joint 361
Tonsilla
- lingualis 58
- palatina 58
- pharyngea 58
Torn muscle 46
- fibre 46
Torsion
- angle
-- femoral neck 357
- trunk 152
TOSSY
- classification of 217

Total hip endoprosthesis
- hip joint 345
Trabeculae 24, 58
- compressive 25
- Spongiosa 27
- tensile 25
Trachea 16, 180
- X-ray image 70
Tractus iliotibialis 38, 39, 414, **417**, 420, 422,
  426, **429**, 438, 439, 484, 501
- functions 417
- traction force 345
Transition zone 32
Transverse arch, foot 408, 409
Transverse axis 7
Transverse plane 7
Transverse process see Processus transversus
Transverse rupture
- meniscus 392
Transverse tendon arch 190
TRENDELENBURG sign 427, 461
Triangular interval **252**, **288**, **320**, **321**, 322, 323
- content 321
- nervi radialis 288
Trigger finger 45
Trigonum
- arteriae vertebralis 139, **140**, 172
- clavipectorale 12, 87, 141, 315
- femorale 480
- femoris 12
- inguinale (HESSELBACH's triangle) 188
-- inguinal hernia 193
- lumbale 132, 142
-- inferius (PETIT triangle) **133**
-- superius (GRYNFELT-LESSHAFT-LUSCHKA
   triangle) **133**
- lumbocostale (BOCHDALEK triangle) **157**, **158**
-- hernia 158
- sternocostale **157**, 162
-- hernia 158
Trochanter
- major **356**, 357, 359, 373, 429, 430, 431, 460
-- intragluteal injection 460
-- surface anatomy **346**, **347**
-- X-ray image 353, 358, 375
- minor **356**, 357, 359, 373, 374, **425**, 431, 487
-- X-ray image 353, 358, 375
Trochlea
- fibularis 366, 367
- humeri **208**, 209, **225**
-- X-ray image 226
- tali 364, 366
-- Facies superior 367
-- X-ray image 405
Trophoblast 18
Truncus(-i) 4, 5
- brachiocephalicus 50, 160, 164, 277
- bronchomediastinalis 57, 317
- cerebri 64
- coeliacus 50, 69, 74, 156
- costocervicalis 164, 165, **298**
-- branches **298**
- encephali 64
- inferior plexus brachialis 67, 276, **277**, 278
-- plexus lesion 199
- intestinales 57
- jugularis 57
-- sinister 37
- lumbales 57
- lumbosacralis 195, 452
- medius plexus brachialis 67, 276, **277**, 278
-- plexus lesion 199
- nervi spinalis 65, **175**, 177, 178
-- R. anterior 176, 177, 178
-- R. communicans 176, 178
-- R. meningeus 176, 178
-- R. posterior 176, 177, 178
- pulmonalis 55
-- X-ray image 70

Index

Truncus(-i)
- subclavius 57, 317
- superior plexus brachialis 67, 276, **277**, 278
-- plexus lesion 199
- sympathicus 157, **177**, 195, 278
-- Ganglia
--- lumbalia 69
--- sacralia 69
--- thoracica 69
-- plexus lesion 199
- thyrocervicalis 164, **296**, **298**
- tibiofibularis 489, 494
- vagalis
-- anterior 69, 157
-- posterior 69, 157
Trunk
- extension 152
- flexion 152
- lateral flexion 10, 152
- torsion 152
Trunk/arm muscles
- deep **133**
- superficial 132
Trunk/shoulder girdle muscles
- deep **133**
- superficial **132**
Trunk wall
- anterior
-- arteries **160**, **161**
-- lymph vessels **167**
-- nerves 187
-- veins **162**
-- vessels **166**, 187
- posterior
-- lymph vessels **167**
-- nerves **170**
-- vessels **170**
Tuba uterina 60, 475
Tuber
- calcanei 366, **367**, 406, 407, 439, 440, 441, 442, 449, 450
-- X-ray image 405
- ischiadicum **354**, **355**, 370, 418, 429, 430, 460
-- X-ray image 353, 375
Tuberculum
- adductorium 356, 357, 378
- anterius 98, 99, **100**, 147
-- CT 129
- conoideum **206**
- costae 92, 104, 114
- dorsale 211
- iliacum 355
- infraglenoidale 207
-- X-ray image 223
- intercondylare
-- laterale 362
--- X-ray image 70, 380
-- mediale 362
--- X-ray image 70, 380
- majus **208**, **209**, 219, 220, 224, 239
-- X-ray image 223
- minus **208**, **209**
-- X-ray image 223
- musculi scaleni anterioris 92
- posterius 98, 99, **100**, 120
-- CT 129
- pubicum 352, 354, 355, 483
- supraglenoidale 207
Tuberositas
- deltoidea **208**
- glutea 356, 359, **429**
- iliaca 354
- musculi serrati anterioris 92
- ossis
-- cuboidei 365, 366
-- metatarsi
--- primi 365
--- quinti 364, 365, 366, 404, 444
-- navicularis 365
-- sacri 108, 109

Tuberositas
- phalangis distalis 212, 213, 365
- radii **211**, **225**, 229
-- X-ray image 226
- tibiae 75, **362**, 378, 381, 386, 399, 438, 439
-- surface anatomy **346**
-- X-ray image 380
- ulnae **210**, **225**
Tunica
- dartos 194
- vaginalis testis
-- Lamina
--- parietalis **191**, 194
--- visceralis **191**
Twisting the ankle 402
Twitch muscle fibres
- fast 41
- slow 41
Type-A-synoviocytes 32
Type-B-synoviocytes 32
Type I fibres 41
Type II fibres 41

U

Ulna 21, 42, 47, 204, 210, 212, 213, 225, **229**, 230, 231, 259, 260, 261, 263, 267, 339
- bone core formation 29
- development 203
- evolution 23
- structure of the extremities 22
- X-ray image 70, 213, 226
Ulnar 9
Ulnar abduction
- extremities 8
- metacarpophalangeal joint 233
- wrist joint 232, 235
Ulnar pulse **50**
Ultrasound, Plexus brachialis 277
Umbilical cord 19
Umbilical hernia 154
Umbilicus **153**, **155**
Uncovertebral joint 123
Uncus corporis **100**, **121**
Underlying tissue
- auscultation 16
- percussion 16
Unguis 79
Upper arm
- bones and joints 204
- cross-section 338
- cutaneous innervation 280
- fascia 201
- MRI **338**
- musculature
-- dorsal 248, **252**, **259**, 260
-- ventral **248**, **249**, **250**, **251**
- nerves 309, 310, 318, 319, **322**, **323**
- rotational axis 204
- surface anatomy 4, 5
- veins 309, 310
- vessels 318, 319, **322**, **323**
Upside-down stomach 158
Urachus **194**
Ureter 61, 74, 188
- Pars pelvica 188
Urethra 61
Urinary bladder 61
Urinary incontinence **459**
Urinary tract organs **61**
Uterus 60, 475
- development 18

V

Vagina(-ae) 60
- carotica 180
- communis tendinum musculorum
-- fibularium [peroneorum] **444**, **445**
-- flexorum **268**, **291**, 293
- musculi recti abdominis **153**
-- Lamina
--- anterior **141**, 142, 149, **150**, 151, **153**, 194
--- posterior 151, 166, 194
- synovialis 44
-- digitorum manus **268**
-- vaginae tendinis 44
- tendinis/tendinum 44, 236, 337
-- back of the hand **265**
-- carpalis palmaris 44
-- digiti 340
-- digitorum pedis **445**, 449, 450
-- foot 444, 445
-- intertubercularis 218, 224, 250
-- musculi
--- abductoris **265**, **268**
--- extensoris **265**, 268, **444**, **445**
--- flexoris 44, **268**, 291, 293, 336, **445**, **449**
--- tibialis **444**, **445**
-- palm of the hand **268**
-- structure 44
Vallum unguis 79
Varices 473
Varicocele 191
Varicose veins **56**
- stripping 473
Varicosis 473
Vascular system
- structure 49
Vas/Vasa
- cremasterica 190
- lymphaticum 57
-- afferens 58
-- efferens 58
-- superficialis 306
- testicularia 188
VATER-PACINI corpuscles 76
Veins
- arm 304, 305
- axilla 308, 314, 316, 317, 318, 319
- axillary space
-- lateral 170
-- medial 170
- back **170**, 171
- back of the hand **313**
- blood
-- flow 52
-- pressure 53
- cardiopulmonary system 48
- chest wall 316, 317
- cross-sectional diameter 52
- cubital fossa 310, 312, 328
- diameter 52
- dorsum of the foot 479
- elbow 309
- epigastric 166
- foot 478
- forearm 312, 324, 325
- gluteal region 487
- inguinal
-- canal **189**
-- region 476, 483
- intercostal space 146
- intravasal pressure 52
- knee 476
- leg 472, 473
- lower leg 478, 490, 491, 492, 493, 494
- neck 171, 172, 173
- occipital region 172
- popliteal fossa 484, 485, 486, 488, 492, 493, 494
- shoulder 309, 310

Veins
- systemic circulation 51
- thigh 476, 477, 480, 481, 482, 485, 486, 487
- thoracic wall **165**
- trunk wall
-- anterior 166, 187
-- dorsal **170**
- upper arm 318, 319, **322**
- vertebral canal 174, 178, **179**
- vessel pressure 53
Vellus hair 78
Vena(-ae)
- auricularis posterior 171, 172
- axillaris 51, 143, **162**, **305**, 306, 307, 315, **316**, 317
-- cavocaval anastomoses 163
- azygos 51, 56, 146, 157, 162, **163**, **165**
- basilica 51, 201, **304**, 306, **309**, **311**, 312, **338**, 339
-- antebrachii **304**, 311, **312**, **313**
--- pathway 304
-- MRI 338
-- pathway 309
- basivertebralis 179
- brachialis 51, **305**, 315, **338**
- MRI 338
- brachiocephalica
-- cavocaval anastomoses 163
-- dextra 51, 163, 165
-- sinistra 51, **162**, 163, 165
- cava
-- inferior 51, 55, 56, 61, 157, 158, **162**, 163
--- cavocaval anastomoses 163
--- CT 129
--- venous congestion 163
--- X-ray image 70
-- superior 51, 55, 70, **162**, 163
--- azygos system 163
--- cavocaval anastomoses 163
--- venous congestion 163
- cephalica 51, **141**, **162**, 187, 201, **304**, 305, 306, 308, **309**, 310, **311**, 312, **315**, 316, 317, 338, 339
-- accessibility 309
-- antebrachii **304**, 311, **312**, **313**
--- pathway 304
-- MRI 338
-- pathway 309
- cervicalis
-- profunda 172
-- superficialis 187
- circumflexa
-- femoris
--- lateralis 472
--- medialis 472
-- humeri posterior **170**, 310, 315
--- axillary space 321
--- lateral axillary space 170
-- ilium
--- profunda 163, 191
--- superficialis **162**, 163, **187**, 472, 475, 476, 483
-- scapulae **170**, **315**
--- axillary space 321
--- lateral axillary space 170
- colica sinistra 56
- digitales
-- dorsales pedis 479
-- palmares 305
- epigastrica(-ae)
-- inferior 56, 153, **162**, 163, 166, **187**, 188, 189
--- cavocaval anastomoses 163
--- dextra 190
--- sinistra 191
-- superficialis 56, **162**, 163, **187**, 472, 475, 476, 483
--- cavocaval anastomoses 163
-- superior 153, 162, **166**, **187**, 194
--- cavocaval anastomoses 163

Vena(-ae)
- femoralis 51, 156, 159, 162, 188, 190, 423, 466, **472**, 476, **480**, **481**, **482**, **483**, 500, **501**
-- catheterisation 473
-- cavocaval anastomoses 163
-- dextra 163
-- location in cross-section 501
-- sinistra 163
- fibulares 472, 503
- gastrica 56
- glutea
-- inferior **487**, 500
-- superior 500
- hemiazygos 56, 157, 162, **163**, 165
-- accessoria 162, **163**, 165
- hepatica(-ae) 51, 56, 158
- iliaca
-- communis 51, 56, **162**, 163
--- venous congestion 163
-- externa 51, 162, 163, 188, 190, 472, 475, 480, 482
--- cavocaval anastomoses 163
-- interna 51, 56, 162, 163, 475
--- azygos system 163
--- cavocaval anastomoses 163
-- iliolumbalis 163
- intercostalis(-es) 144, 159, 163, 194
-- anterior 146, 162, **165**
-- posterior 145, 146, 162, **165**
-- Rr. collaterales 146
-- Rr. cutanei laterales 146
-- Rr. perforantes anteriores 146
-- superior
--- dextra 163, **165**
--- sinistra **165**
-- suprema 163
- interossea(-ae) **305**
-- posterior 257
- intervertebralis **179**
- jugularis 317
-- anterior 51
-- externa 51, 171, 317
-- interna 51, 57, 163, 180
- lumbalis(-es) 163
-- ascendens 56, **163**, **179**
- mammaria(-ae)
-- interna **162**, 165, 166
-- laterales **184**, 307
- marginalis
-- lateralis 478, 479
-- medialis 478, 479
- mediana
-- antebrachii 304, 309, **311**, 312, 339
-- basilica 311, 312
-- cephalica 311
-- cubiti 51, 201, **304**, **309**, **311**, **312**
--- taking blood 311
- mesenterica
-- inferior 51, 56
-- superior 51, 56
- metacarpales palmares 305
- musculophrenica 166
- obturatoria 188, 483
- occipitalis 170, 171, 172
- ovarica 51
- paraumbilicales 56, 153, **162**, **187**
- pectorales 162
- perforans 478, 479
- phrenicae inferiores 56, 157
- poplitea 51, 75, 395, **396**, 441, 472, **484**, **485**, 486, 488, **492**, **493**
- portae hepatis 51, 55, **56**
- profunda
-- brachii **170**, 305
--- triangular interval 170, 321
-- femoris 51, 472, **482**
- pudenda(-ae)
-- externae **162**, 163, 187, 472, 475, 476, 483
-- interna **486**, **487**

Vena(-ae)
- pulmonalis(-es)
-- X-ray image 70
- radiales **305**
- rectalis(-es)
-- inferiores 56
-- superior 56
- renalis(-es) 51
-- sinistra 56
- sacralis
-- lateralis 163
-- mediana 163
- saphena
-- accessoria 162, 472
--- lateralis 476
--- medialis 475
-- magna 51, 162, 187, 195, **396**, 414, **472**, 474, 475, **476**, 477, **478**, **479**, 430, 482, **483**, **488**, **501**, **502**, 503
--- location in cross-section 501
--- lymphatic vessels 474
--- pathway 472, 478
--- tributaries 472
-- parva 51, 75, **396**, **472**, 474, **477**, **478**, **479**, **484**, 486, **488**, 492, **502**, 503
--- lymphatic vessels 474
--- pathway 472, 478
- scapularis dorsalis 162, 321
- sigmoidea 56
- spinalis posterior 174
- splenica [lienalis] 51, 56
- subclavia 51, 57, **162**, 163, 279, 296, 299, **305**, 314
- subcostalis 163
- subcutaneae abdominis 137
- subscapularis **315**
- suprascapularis 321
- suralis 492
- testicularis 188, 190
-- dextra 51
-- sinistra 51
- thoracica
-- interna 51, 146, 157, **162**, **165**, 166, 184, **187**
--- cavocaval anastomoses 163
-- lateralis **162**, 184, **187**, 307, **315**, **316**, 317
- thoracoacromialis 162
- thoracodorsalis **162**, **315**, **316**
- thoracoepigastrica **162**, **187**, 305, 306, **308**, **315**, **316**
-- cavocaval anastomoses 163
- tibiales
-- anteriores 51, 472, **490**, 503
-- posteriores 51, 472, **492**, 503
- transversa colli 171
-- R. superficialis 317
- ulnares **305**, **339**
- umbilicalis 55, 188, **194**
- vertebralis 172
- vesicales 194
Venous star **472**
Venous system, superficial 472
Venous valves 54, 473
Venter 42
Ventral 9
Ventriculus
- cerebri 64
-- lateralis 75
- cordis
-- dexter 55
-- sinister 55
--- X-ray image 70
Venule(s)
- blood flow 52
- cross-sectional diameter 52
- diameter 52
- high endothelial 58
- intravasal pressure 52
- number 52
Venus diamond 90

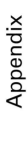

Appendix

Vertebra(-ae)
- cervicalis(-es) **95**
-- I–VII **94**, 101
-- II–VII 100
-- III **94**, 101, 118, 120, 123
--- Corpus vertebrae 120, 124
--- X-ray image **124**
-- V **100**, 180
--- Proc. transversus 173
-- VII 21, 123, 180
--- Corpus vertebrae 124
--- Proc. spinosus 90
- coccygea(-ae)
-- I 110
-- II 110
-- II–V 110
-- III–V 110
- development 89
- lumbalis(-es) **95**
-- Corpus vertebrae 153
--- MRI 130
-- I
--- Arcus vertebrae 137
--- Corpus vertebrae 126, 127, 130
-- I–II 106
-- I–V **94**
--- X-ray image 126, **127**
-- II 71, 181
--- Proc. costalis 174
-- III **107**, 156
--- Proc. spinosus 174
-- IV 74, **107**, 156, 368
--- Proc. spinosus 13
-- V 74
--- Proc. costalis 372
--- Proc. spinosus 84
-- Proc. costalis 137
-- Proc. spinosus 137
-- X-ray image 127
- prominens **95**, **101**
-- landmarks 84
-- Proc. spinosus 123, 132, 140
-- surface anatomy 84
- structural features 104
- structure **97**
- thoracica(-ae) **95**
-- I–XII **94**
-- VI **104**
-- X **104**
-- XII **104**
--- Corpus vertebrae 113
--- Proc. spinosus 132
-- X–XII 106
-- structural features **104**
-- X-ray image **125**
Vertebral arch(es)
- cleft formation 98
- columns
-- lateral 106
- compounds **115**

Vertebral arch(es)
- ligaments 116
Vertebral canal
- arteries **179**
- content **176**, **178**
- nerves 174
- stenosis
-- dermatomes 281
- veins **179**
- vessels 174
Vertebralis triangle 139, 140, 172
Vertebral line 101
Vertebral slippage 128
Vertical axis 7
Vesica
- biliaris [fellea] 17, 55
-- dermatomes 186
- urinaria 61, 68, 156, 188, 190, **194**, 475
-- dermatomes 186
Vessels, terminal **52**
Vestigium processus vaginalis 193
Vincula tendinum **269**
Volar 9
- flexion 8
VOLKMANN's canal 27
von HOCHSTETTER injection 460
V-phlegmon 268
Vulva 60

W

WALDEYER tonsillar ring 58
Walking 413
WALLER's degeneration 66
Walls of the trunk, development **89**
WARD's triangle (neutral fibres) 25
WEBER fracture **399**, 400
- X-ray image 400
Wedge vertebra 89
Wheel joint **33**
Womb 475
Wrist 212
- cross-section **339**
- drop 289
- joint
-- distal 214, 230, 234
-- muscles 235
-- proximal 214, 230, 234
-- range of movement **232**
- joints 230
- ligaments 231

X

X-ray image
- acromioclavicular joint 217
- ankle joint 405
- cervical spine **124**

X-ray image
- contrast agent imaging **71**
- Coxa
-- valga **360**
-- vara **360**
- elbow joint **70**
- femur **358**
- hand 213
- knee joint **70**, **380**
- lumbar spine 126, 127
- Mamma 185
- pelvis 352, **353**
- radius fracture 211
- sacrum 127
- shoulder joint, dislocation 223
- sternoclavicular joint 215
- thoracic spine **125**
- thorax **70**
- WEBER fracture 400

Y

Yolk sac, remnant 19

Z

Zeugopodium 22
- evolution 23
Z-lines 40
Zona
- arcuata 151, **153**
- orbicularis **373**
Zygapophyseal joint **102**
- cervical spine 102
- facet positioning 102
- lumbosacral joint 102
- positioning 102
- thoracic spine 102
Zygapophysis [Proc. articularis]
- inferior **97**
-- axis 99
-- vertebrae
--- cervicalis 98, 100, 101, 102, 124, 129
--- lumbalis **107**, 117, 121, 126, 127, 129
--- thoracicae 104, **106**, 116
- superior **97**
-- axis **98**, 99
-- ossis sacri 108, 109
-- vertebrae
--- cervicalis 100, 101, 102, 124
--- lumbalis **107**, 117, 121, 126, 127, 129, 174
--- thoracicae 104, **106**, 114, 116, 177

All you need for anatomy: compatible with the 17ᵗʰ edition of Sobotta Atlas

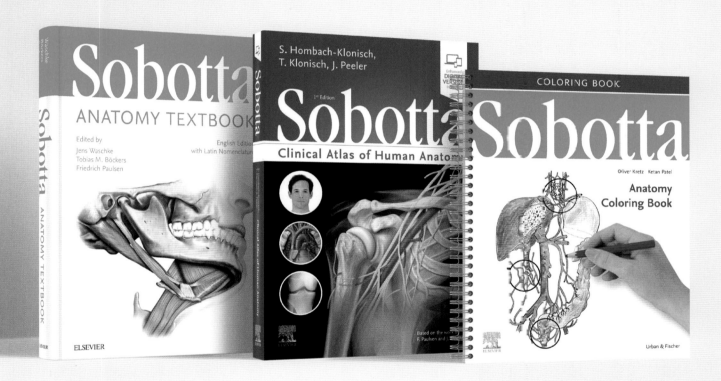

Waschke / Böckers / Paulsen
Sobotta Anatomy Textbook
2018
ISBN 978-0-7020-6760-0

Hombach-Klonisch / Klonisch / Peeler
Sobotta Clinical Atlas of Human Anatomy
2019
ISBN 978-0-7020-5273-6

Kretz / Patel
Sobotta Anatomy Coloring Book
2019
ISBN 978-0-7020-5278-1

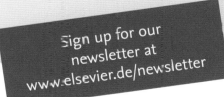
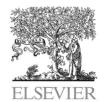

ELSEVIER

These and many other titles as well as the current prices available at your local bookstore and at **shop.elsevier.de**